CASE FILES® Obstetrics and Gynecology

Eugene C. Toy, MD
Assistant Dean for Educational Programs
Director of Doctoring Courses Program
Director of the Scholarly Concentrations
  in Women's Health
Professor and Vice Chair of Medical Education
Department of Obstetrics and Gynecology
McGovern Medical School at The University
  of Texas Health Science Center at Houston
  (UTHealth)
Houston, Texas

Benton Baker III, MD
Fellow, American College of Obstetricians and
  Gynecologists
Retired, Professor of Obstetrics and Gynecology
McGovern Medical School at The University
  of Texas Health Science Center at Houston
  (UTHealth)
Houston, Texas

Patti Jayne Ross, MD
Professor
University of Texas Health Science Center
Department of Obstetrics and Gynecology
McGovern Medical School at The University
  of Texas Health Science Center at Houston
  (UTHealth)
Houston, Texas

John C. Jennings, MD
Professor of Obstetrics and Gynecology
Texas Tech University Health Sciences Center
Odessa, Texas

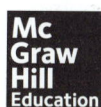

New York   Chicago   San Francisco   Athens   London   Madrid   Mexico City
Milan   New Delhi   Singapore   Sydney   Toronto

Case Files®: Obstetrics and Gynecology, Fifth Edition

Copyright © 2016 by McGraw-Hill Education. All rights reserved. Printed in the United States of America. Except as permitted under the United States Copyright Act of 1976, no part of this publication may be reproduced or distributed in any form or by any means, or stored in a database or retrieval system, without the prior written permission of the publisher.

Previous editions' copyright © 2013, 2009, 2007, 2003 by The McGraw-Hill Companies, Inc. All rights reserved.

Case Files® is a registered trademark of McGraw-Hill Education. All rights reserved.

1 2 3 4 5 6 7 8 9 0   DOC   20 19 18 17 16

ISBN 978-0-07-184872-5
MHID 0-07-184872-X

Notice

Medicine is an ever-changing science. As new research and clinical experience broaden our knowledge, changes in treatment and drug therapy are required. The authors and the publisher of this work have checked with sources believed to be reliable in their efforts to provide information that is complete and generally in accord with the standards accepted at the time of publication. However, in view of the possibility of human error or changes in medical sciences, neither the authors nor the publisher nor any other party who has been involved in the preparation or publication of this work warrants that the information contained herein is in every respect accurate or complete, and they disclaim all responsibility for any errors or omissions or for the results obtained from use of the information contained in this work. Readers are encouraged to confirm the information contained herein with other sources. For example and in particular, readers are advised to check the product information sheet included in the package of each drug they plan to administer to be certain that the information contained in this work is accurate and that changes have not been made in the recommended dose or in the contraindications for administration. This recommendation is of particular importance in connection with new or infrequently used drugs.

This book was set in Adobe Jenson Pro by Cenveo® Publisher Services.
The editors were Catherine A. Johnson and Cindy Yoo.
The production supervisor was Catherine H. Saggese.
Project management was provided by Hardik Popli.
RR Donnelley was printer and binder.
This book is printed on acid-free paper.

Library of Congress Cataloging-in-Publication Data

Names: Toy, Eugene C., author. | Baker, Benton, III, author. | Ross, Patti Jayne, author. | Jennings, John C., author.
Title: Case files. Obstetrics and gynecology / Eugene C. Toy, Benton Baker III, Patti Jayne Ross, John C. Jennings.
Other titles: Obstetrics and gynecology
Description: Fifth edition. | New York : McGraw-Hill Education, [2016] |
   Preceded by Case files. Obstetrics and gynecology / Eugene C. Toy ... [et al.]. 4th ed. c2013. |
   Includes bibliographical references and index.
Identifiers: LCCN 2015042316| ISBN 9780071848725 (pbk. : alk. paper) | ISBN 007184872X (pbk. : alk. paper)
Subjects: | MESH: Gynecology—Case Reports. | Gynecology—Examination
   Questions. | Obstetrics—Case Reports. | Obstetrics—Examination Questions.
Classification: LCC RG111 | NLM WQ 18.2 | DDC 618.0076—dc23 LC record available at
   http://lccn.loc.gov/2015042316

McGraw-Hill Education books are available at special quantity discounts to use as premiums and sales promotions or for use in corporate training programs. To contact a representative, please visit the Contact Us pages at www.mhprofessional.com.

DEDICATION

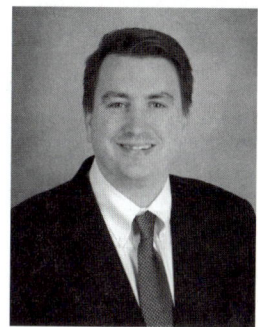

This fifth edition of *Case Files®: Obstetrics and Gynecology* is dedicated to Dr. Sean C. Blackwell, who is my chairman, and whose leadership and friendship I cherish. I have watched him work tirelessly from before dawn to well after dusk, and be available for telephone calls and consultation regardless of the hour. He is the reason I am able to continue to grow as an educator, writer, and teacher. Most precious to me, he strongly supported me (shortly after joining the department full time) to keep my commitment to lead our medical mission team to Cambodia to serve hundreds in the rural province of Kratie. He is probably the biggest reason this edition of *Case Files®: Obstetrics and Gynecology* could see print.

Sean C. Blackwell, MD is a Professor and Chair (appointed 2011) of the Department of Obstetrics, Gynecology and Reproductive Sciences at McGovern Medical School at The University of Texas Health Science Center at Houston (UTHealth). Dr. Blackwell completed his undergraduate degree as a double major in the classics and biology at Wabash College in Crawfordsville, Indiana. He matriculated medical school at the University of Illinois College of Medicine in 1993 and completed both his obstetrics and gynecology residency and maternal fetal medicine fellowship at Wayne State University in Detroit, Michigan. He joined UT Health in 2007, and also serves as the Director of the *Larry C. Gilstrap MD* Center for Perinatal and Women's Health Research and as an Assistant Dean for Healthcare Quality in Perinatal Medicine and Women's Health. Dr. Blackwell is the Chief of Service for Obstetrics and Gynecology for Children's Memorial Hermann Hospital–Texas Medical Center. In 2014, Dr. Blackwell earned his *Six Sigma-Lean* Black Belt at the University of Houston.

Eugene C. Toy, MD

To my Chairman of Obstetrics of Gynecology, Dr. Sean Blackwell, whose work ethic, leadership, and vision inspire everyone around him to excellence and whose heart of generosity touches thousands of pregnant women and their babies.

—ECT

With love and gratitude, to Mom, Joy, Ben, Anne, Jessica, Jim, John, and Col. Alvin Sholk.

—BB III

To Dr. James Knight, and Tulane Medical School, for giving me the opportunity to fulfill my dreams. To my parents, Mary and Jimmy Ross, for their love, inspiration, and devotion.

—PJR

To my wife, Sue Ellen, my three daughters, Beth, Allison, and Amy, their husbands, and my five grandchildren.

—JCJ

Finally, to the wonderful medical students from the McGovern Medical School at The University of Texas Health Science Center at Houston (UTHealth), who graciously gave constructive feedback and enthusiastically received this curriculum.

—THE AUTHORS

CONTENTS

Contributors / vii
Preface / xiii
Acknowledgments / xv
Introduction / xvii
Listing of Cases / xix

Section I
How to Approach Clinical Problems 1
Part 1. Approach to the Patient 3
Part 2. Approach to Clinical Problem Solving 11
Part 3. Approach to Reading 13
Part 4. Approach to Surgery 18

Section II
Cases 19
Obstetric Topics (Cases 1-28) 19
Gynecologic Topics (Cases 29-60) 289

Section III
Review Questions 565

Index / 577

CONTRIBUTORS

Mazen Elias Abdallah, MD
Assistant Professor of Obstetrics and Gynecology
McGovern Medical School at The University of Texas Health Science Center at Houston (UTHealth)
Houston, Texas
Delayed Puberty

Michael T. Adler, MD
Assistant Professor of Obstetrics and Gynecology
McGovern Medical School at The University of Texas Health Science Center at Houston (UTHealth)
Houston, Texas
Amenorrhea, Intrauterine Adhesions

Elizabeth E. Brackett
Medical Student
McGovern Medical School at The University of Texas Health Science Center at Houston (UTHealth)
Houston, Texas
Herpes Simplex Virus Infection in Pregnancy

Shao-Chun R. Chang-Jackson, MD
Assistant Professor of Obstetrics and Gynecology
McGovern Medical School at The University of Texas Health Science Center at Houston (UTHealth)
Houston, Texas
Ectopic Pregnancy

Tamika K. Cross, MD
Resident in Obstetrics and Gynecology
McGovern Medical School at The University of Texas Health Science Center at Houston (UTHealth)
Houston, Texas
Domestic Abuse and Sexual Abuse

Cynthia Donna, MD
Resident in Obstetrics and Gynecology
McGovern Medical School at The University of Texas Health Science Center at Houston (UTHealth)
Houston, Texas
Contraception

Erin G. Dressel
Medical Student
McGovern Medical School at The University of Texas Health Science Center at Houston (UTHealth)
Houston, Texas
Hypertensive Disease in Pregnancy

Amy E. Dudley
Medical Student
McGovern Medical School at The University of Texas
  Health Science Center at Houston (UTHealth)
Houston, Texas
Bacterial Vaginosis

Jenny Duret-Uzodinma, MD
Assistant Professor of Obstetrics and Gynecology
McGovern Medical School at The University of Texas
  Health Science Center at Houston (UTHealth)
Houston, Texas
Pyelonephritis in Pregnancy

Russell Edwards, MD, FACOG
Faculty, Obstetrics and Gynecology Residency Program
The Methodist Hospital—Houston
Houston, Texas
Galactorrhea and Hypothyroidism

Konrad Harms, MD, FACOG
Assistant Clinical Professor of Obstetrics and Gynecology
Weill Cornell Medical College
Program Director,
Obstetrics and Gynecology Residency
The Methodist Hospital—Houston
Houston, Texas
Shoulder Dystocia

Sara B. Holcombe, DO
Assistant Professor of Obstetrics and Gynecology
McGovern Medical School at The University of Texas
  Health Science Center at Houston (UTHealth)
Houston, Texas
Domestic Abuse and Sexual Assault

Steven Blaine Holloway
Medical Student
McGovern Medical School at The University of Texas
  Health Science Center at Houston (UTHealth)
Houston, Texas
Cystitis

Katlyn Hoover
Medical Student
McGovern Medical School at The University of Texas
  Health Science Center at Houston (UTHealth)
Houston, Texas
Placental Abruption

Lina Wael Irshaid
Medical Student
Weill Cornell Medical - Qatar
Dohn, Qatar
Intrauterine Growth Restriction

Randa J. Jalloul, MD, FACOG
Assistant Professor of Obstetrics and Gynecology
McGovern Medical School at The University of Texas
 Health Science Center at Houston (UTHealth)
Houston, Texas
Breast Cancer

Erin Josserand
Medical Student
McGovern Medical School at The University of Texas
 Health Science Center at Houston (UTHealth)
Houston, Texas
Pulmonary Embolism in Pregnancy

Joy Y. Kim, MD
Assistant Professor of Obstetrics and Gynecology
McGovern Medical School at The University of Texas
 Health Science Center at Houston (UTHealth)
Houston, Texas
Contraception

Patricia C. Lenihan
Medical Student
McGovern Medical School at The University of Texas
 Health Science Center at Houston (UTHealth)
Houston, Texas
Approach to Labor
Hypertension in Pregnancy
Pelvic Organ Prolapse
Principal manuscript reviewer

Chunhua Lu, MD, PhD
Resident in Obstetrics and Gynecology
McGovern Medical School at The University of Texas
 Health Science Center at Houston (UTHealth)
Houston, Texas
Breast Cancer

Fangxian Lu, MD, PhD
Assistant Professor of Obstetrics and Gynecology
McGovern Medical School at The University of Texas
 Health Science Center at Houston (UTHealth)
Houston, Texas
Postpartum Hemorrhage

Michael S. MacKelvie, DO
Resident in Obstetrics and Gynecology
McGovern Medical School at The University of Texas
  Health Science Center at Houston (UTHealth)
Houston, Texas
Placenta Accreta

Violet Maldonado
Medical Student
McGovern Medical School at The University of Texas
  Health Science Center at Houston (UTHealth)
Houston, Texas
Preterm Labor

Dalia M. Moghazy, MD
Resident in Obstetrics and Gynecology
The Methodist Hospital—Houston
Houston, Texas
Intrahepatic Cholestasis of Pregnancy

Alyxandra O'Brien, MD
Resident in Obstetrics and Gynecology
McGovern Medical School at The University of Texas
  Health Science Center at Houston (UTHealth)
Houston, Texas
Ectopic Pregnancy

Christine Pan, MD
Resident in Obstetrics and Gynecology
McGovern Medical School at The University of Texas
  Health Science Center at Houston (UTHealth)
Houston, Texas
Postpartum Hemorrhage
Urinary Incontinence

Virginia A. Rauth, MD, MBA
Professor of Obstetrics and Gynecology
Chief of Women's HealthCare at Galveston
University of Texas Medical Branch
Galveston, Texas
Approach to Perimenopause

John W. Riggs, MD, MS, FACOG
Professor of Obstetrics and Gynecology
McGovern Medical School at The University of Texas
  Health Science Center at Houston (UTHealth)
Houston, Texas
Postpartum Endometritis

Reem Sabouni, MD
Resident in Obstetrics and Gynecology
McGovern Medical School at The University of Texas
   Health Science Center at Houston (UTHealth)
Houston, Texas
Amenorrhea, Intrauterine Adhesions
Placenta Previa

Mary Alice Sallman
Medical Student
McGovern Medical School at The University of Texas
   Health Science Center at Houston (UTHealth)
Manuscript reviewer

Viviana C. Salom-Ellis
Medical Student
McGovern Medical School at The University of Texas
   Health Science Center at Houston (UTHealth)
Houston, Texas
Placenta Previa

Priti P. Schachel, MD, FACOG
Associate Program Director
Obstetrics and Gynecology Residency Program
The Methodist Hospital—Houston
Houston, Texas
Intrahepatic Cholestasis of Pregnancy

Nicholas R. Spencer
Medical Student
McGovern Medical School at The University of Texas
   Health Science Center at Houston (UTHealth)
Houston, Texas
Parvovirus Infection in Pregnancy

Lauren Jane Tharp, MD
Administrative Chief Resident in Obstetrics and Gynecology
McGovern Medical School at The University of Texas
   Health Science Center at Houston (UTHealth)
Houston, Texas
Postpartum Endometritis

Aida L. Vigil, MD, MPH
Resident in Obstetrics and Gynecology
McGovern Medical School at The University of Texas
   Health Science Center at Houston (UTHealth)
Houston, Texas
Pyelonephritis in Pregnancy

Joaquin Andres Villegas Inurrigarro
Medical Student
McGovern Medical School at The University of Texas
   Health Science Center at Houston (UTHealth)
Houston, Texas
Septic Abortion

Cristina M. Wallace, MD
Assistant Professor of Obstetrics and Gynecology
McGovern Medical School at The University of Texas
   Health Science Center at Houston (UTHealth)
Houston, Texas
Polycystic Ovarian Syndrome

Amberly Nesbitt Winley, MD
Resident in Obstetrics and Gynecology
McGovern Medical School at The University of Texas
   Health Science Center at Houston (UTHealth)
Houston, Texas
Polycystic Ovarian Syndrome

Nikolaos Zacharias, MD, FACOG
Assistant Professor of Obstetrics and Gynecology
McGovern Medical School at The University of Texas
   Health Science Center at Houston (UTHealth)
Houston, Texas
Placenta Accreta

PREFACE

I have been deeply amazed and grateful to see how the *Case Files*® books have been so well received, and have helped students to learn more effectively. In the 13 short years since *Case Files*®: *Obstetrics and Gynecology* first made it in print, the series has now multiplied to span most of the clinical and basic science disciplines, and been translated into nearly 20 foreign languages. Numerous students have sent encouraging remarks about the changes in the fourth edition, which divided up into Obstetrics in the first half, and Gynecology in the second half to be more "user-friendly" during the clerkship since most students have their rotation divided in those two categories. In this fifth edition, we have retained the grouping of related cases closer together to allow students to use information from one case to reinforce principles to another case, and cross-referenced-related cases. Although space is always a premium, we have also retained and expanded Section III which is a collection of strategic questions that can be used for review, but also to tie in the principles from the cases. Questions have been improved to better reflect the USMLE format, and explanations have been expanded to help the student understand the mechanisms and the reason that the other choices are incorrect. Two completely new cases (Sexual Abuse/Intimate Partner Violence, and Chronic Pelvic Pain) have been written. Updated or new sections include cervical cytology screening, contraception, labor management, hypertension in pregnancy, fetal assessment, and ovarian cancer. This fifth edition has been a collaborative work with my wonderful coauthors and contributors, and with the suggestions from five generations of students. Truly, the enthusiastic encouragement from students throughout not just the United States but worldwide provides me with the inspiration and energy to continue to write. It is thus with humility that I offer my sincere thanks to students everywhere ... for without students, how can a teacher teach?

Eugene C. Toy

ACKNOWLEDGMENTS

The curriculum that evolved into the ideas for this series was inspired by two talented and forthright students, Philbert Yao and Chuck Rosipal, who have since graduated from medical school. It has been a tremendous joy to work with my friend, colleague, and my ob/gyn program director, Dr. Bentor Baker III. It is also a privilege to work with Dr. Ross, who has been a steady hand in administrating the medical student clerkship for so many years. It is a personal honor and with extreme gratitude that I am able to work with Dr. John Jennings, a visionary, brilliant obstetrician gynecologist, leader, and friend. Also, I am awed by the many excellent contributors who continue to work under the deadlines and pleas of perfectionists. I am greatly indebted to my editor, Catherine Johnson, whose exuberance, experience, and vision helped to shape this series. I appreciate McGraw-Hill's believing in the concept of teaching through clinical cases. I am also grateful to Catherine Saggese for her excellent production expertise, and Cindy Yoo for her wonderful editing. At the University of Texas Medical School at Houston, I appreciate the support from my chairman Dr. Sean Blackwell, who is an amazing leader with a brilliant intellect, an unparalleled work ethic, and a generous heart that inspires beyond our department; and Dr. Patricia Butler who as Vice Chair for Educational Programs of our school exemplifies all that is excellent in medical education, and has served as a role model and mentor for me. I appreciate Yaki Bryant, who has faithfully and energetically served as the extraordinary student coordinator for literally thousands and thousands of students at the University of Texas Medical School at Houston. I want to acknowledge the many medical students who have helped to sharpen the focus of this book, especially Patricia Lenihan, who served as principle manuscript reviewer. Most of all, I appreciate my loving wife, Terri, and my four wonderful children, Andy and his wife Anna, Michael, Allison, and Christina, for their patience and understanding.

Eugene C. Toy

INTRODUCTION

Mastering the cognitive knowledge within a field such as obstetrics and gynecology is a formidable task. It is even more difficult to draw on that knowledge, to procure and filter through the clinical and laboratory data, to develop a differential diagnosis, and finally to make a rational treatment plan. To gain these skills, the student often learns best at the bedside, guided and instructed by experienced teachers, and inspired toward self-directed, diligent reading. Clearly, there is no replacement for education at the bedside. Unfortunately, clinical situations usually do not encompass the breadth of the specialty. Perhaps the best alternative is a carefully crafted patient case designed to stimulate the clinical approach and decision making. In an attempt to achieve that goal, we have constructed a collection of clinical vignettes to teach diagnostic or therapeutic approaches relevant to obstetrics and gynecology. Most importantly, the explanations for the cases emphasize the mechanisms and underlying principles, rather than merely rote questions and answers.

This book is organized for versatility: It allows the student "in a rush" to go quickly through the scenarios and check the corresponding answers, and it provides more detailed information for the student who wants thought-provoking explanations. The answers are arranged from simple to complex: a summary of the pertinent points, the bare answers, an analysis of the case, an approach to the topic, a comprehension test at the end for reinforcement and emphasis, and a list of resources for further reading. The clinical vignettes have been arranged as Obstetrical in the first half, and Gynecology in the second half, and related cases grouped together. Section III contains Review Questions designed to require higher level integration of information. A listing of cases is included in Section IV to aid the students who desire to test their knowledge of a specific area, or who want to review a topic including basic definitions. Finally, we intentionally did not use a multiple-choice question (MCQ) format in our clinical case scenarios, since clues (or distractions) are not available in the real world. Nevertheless, several MCQs are included at the end of each case discussion (Comprehension Questions) to reinforce concepts or introduce related topics.

HOW TO GET THE MOST OUT OF THIS BOOK

Each case is designed to simulate a patient encounter with open-ended questions. At times, the patient's complaint is different from the most concerning issue, and sometimes extraneous information is given. The answers are organized into four different parts:

CLINICAL CASE FORMAT: PART I

1. **Summary:** The salient aspects of the case are identified, filtering out the extraneous information. Students should formulate their summary from the case before looking at the answers. A comparison to the summation in the answer will help to improve their ability to focus on the important data, while appropriately

discarding the irrelevant information—a fundamental skill in clinical problem solving.
2. **A Straightforward Answer** is given to each open-ended question.
3. The **Analysis of the Case** is comprised of two parts:
   a. **Objectives of the Case:** A listing of the two or three main principles that are crucial for a practitioner to manage the patient. Again, the students are challenged to make educated "guesses" about the objectives of the case upon initial review of the case scenario, which helps to sharpen their clinical and analytical skills.
   b. **Considerations:** A discussion of the relevant points and brief approach to the specific patient.

PART II

Approach to the Disease Process: It consists of two distinct parts:
   a. **Definitions:** Terminology pertinent to the disease process.
   b. **Clinical Approach:** A discussion of the approach to the clinical problem in general, including tables, figures, and algorithms.

PART III

Comprehension Questions: Each case contains several multiple-choice questions, which reinforce the material, or which introduce new and related concepts. Questions about material not found in the text will have explanations in the answers.

PART IV

Clinical Pearls: Several clinically important points are reiterated as a summation of the text. This allows for easy review, such as before an examination.

LISTING OF CASES

LISTING BY CASE NUMBER

CASE NO.	DISEASE	CASE PAGE
1	Labor (Latent Phase)	22
2	Anemia in Pregnancy (Thalassemia Trait)	42
3	Uterine Inversion	52
4	Shoulder Dystocia	60
5	Fetal Bradycardia (Cord Prolapse)	68
6	Postpartum Hemorrhage	76
7	Serum Screening in Pregnancy	86
8	Twin Gestation with Vasa Previa	96
9	Herpes Simplex Virus Infection in Labor	104
10	Placenta Previa	112
11	Placental Abruption	120
12	Placenta Accreta	128
13	Abdominal Pain in Pregnancy (Ovarian Torsion)	136
14	Pruritus (Cholestasis) of Pregnancy	146
15	Pulmonary Embolus in Pregnancy	154
16	Preeclampsia with Severe Features	166
17	Preterm Labor	180
18	Preterm Premature Rupture of Membranes (PPROM) and Intra-Amniotic Infection	190
19	Parvovirus Infection in Pregnancy	198
20	Chlamydial Cervicitis and HIV in Pregnancy	208
21	Thyroid Storm in Pregnancy	218
22	Intrauterine Growth Restriction	226
23	Pyelonephritis, Unresponsive	236
24	Necrotizing Fasciitis	244
25	Postpartum Endomyometritis	250
26	Breast Abscess and Mastitis	256
27	Diabetes in Pregnancy	264
28	Prenatal Care	278
29	Health Maintenance, Age 66 Years	290
30	Perimenopause	298
31	Sexual Assault	306
32	Ureteral Injury after Hysterectomy	318
33	Pelvic Organ Prolapse	326
34	Fascial Disruption	334

35	Urinary Incontinence	340
36	Salpingitis, Acute	350
37	Chronic Pelvic Pain	362
38	Bacterial Vaginosis	370
39	Syphilitic Chancre	378
40	Urinary Tract Infection (Cystitis)	388
41	Uterine Leiomyomata	394
42	Threatened Abortion and Spontaneous Abortion	404
43	Ectopic Pregnancy	416
44	Contraception	424
45	Abortion, Septic	438
46	Fibroadenoma of the Breast	444
47	Dominant Breast Mass	452
48	Breast, Abnormal Mammogram	460
49	Amenorrhea (Intrauterine Adhesions)	466
50	Galactorrhea Due to Hypothyroidism	474
51	Amenorrhea (Sheehan Syndrome)	482
52	Polycystic Ovarian Syndrome	490
53	Hirsutism, Sertoli–Leydig Cell Tumor	496
54	Pubertal Delay, Gonadal Dysgenesis	504
55	Amenorrhea (Primary), Müllerian Agenesis	512
56	Infertility, Peritoneal Factor	520
57	Postmenopausal Bleeding	530
58	Cervical Cancer	540
59	Ovarian Cancer (Epithelial)	550
60	Lichen Sclerosis of Vulva	560

LISTING BY DISORDER (ALPHABETICAL)

CASE NO.	DISEASE	CASE PAGE
13	Abdominal Pain in Pregnancy (Ovarian Torsion)	136
45	Abortion, Septic	438
49	Amenorrhea (Intrauterine Adhesions)	466
55	Amenorrhea (Primary), Müllerian Agenesis	512
51	Amenorrhea (Sheehan Syndrome)	482
2	Anemia in Pregnancy (Thalassemia Trait)	42
38	Bacterial Vaginosis	370
26	Breast Abscess and Mastitis	256
48	Breast, Abnormal Mammogram	460
58	Cervical Cancer	540
20	Chlamydial Cervicitis and HIV in Pregnancy	208

37	Chronic Pelvic Pain	362
44	Contraception	424
27	Diabetes in Pregnancy	264
47	Dominant Breast Mass	452
43	Ectopic Pregnancy	416
34	Fascial Disruption	334
5	Fetal Bradycardia (Cord Prolapse)	68
46	Fibroadenoma of the Breast	444
50	Galactorrhea Due to Hypothyroidism	474
29	Health Maintenance, Age 66 Years	290
9	Herpes Simplex Virus Infection in Labor	104
53	Hirsutism, Sertoli–Leydig Cell Tumor	496
56	Infertility, Peritoneal Factor	520
22	Intrauterine Growth Restriction	226
1	Labor (Latent Phase)	22
60	Lichen Sclerosis of Vulva	560
24	Necrotizing Fasciitis	244
59	Ovarian Cancer (Epithelial)	550
19	Parvovirus Infection in Pregnancy	198
33	Pelvic Organ Prolapse	326
30	Perimenopause	298
12	Placenta Accreta	128
10	Placenta Previa	112
11	Placental Abruption	120
52	Polycystic Ovarian Syndrome	490
57	Postmenopausal Bleeding	530
25	Postpartum Endomyometritis	250
6	Postpartum Hemorrhage	76
16	Preeclampsia with Severe Features	166
28	Prenatal Care	278
17	Preterm Labor	180
18	Preterm Premature Rupture of Membranes (PPROM) and Intra-Amniotic Infection	190
14	Pruritus (Cholestasis) of Pregnancy	146
54	Pubertal Delay, Gonadal Dysgenesis	504
15	Pulmonary Embolus in Pregnancy	154
23	Pyelonephritis, Unresponsive	236
36	Salpingitis, Acute	350
7	Serum Screening in Pregnancy	86
31	Sexual Assault	306
4	Shoulder Dystocia	60
39	Syphilitic Chancre	378
42	Threatened Abortion and Spontaneous Abortion	404

21	Thyroid Storm in Pregnancy	218
8	Twin Gestation with Vasa Previa	96
32	Ureteral Injury after Hysterectomy	318
35	Urinary Incontinence	340
40	Urinary Tract Infection (Cystitis)	388
3	Uterine Inversion	52
41	Uterine Leiomyomata	394

SECTION I

How to Approach Clinical Problems

Part 1 Approach to the Patient

Part 2 Approach to Clinical Problem Solving

Part 3 Approach to Reading

Part 4 Approach to Surgery

Part 1. Approach to the Patient

The transition from textbook and/or journal article learning to the application of the information in a specific clinical situation is one of the most challenging tasks in medicine. It requires retention of information, organization of the facts, and recall of a myriad of data in precise application to the patient. The purpose of this book is to facilitate this process. The first step is gathering information, also known as establishing the database. This includes taking the history, performing the physical examination, and obtaining selective laboratory examinations or special evaluations such as urodynamic testing and/or imaging tests. Of these, the historical examination is the most important and useful. Sensitivity and respect should always be exercised during the interview of patients.

> **CLINICAL PEARL**
>
> ▶ The history is usually the single most important tool in obtaining a diagnosis. The art of seeking the information in a nonjudgmental, sensitive, and thorough manner cannot be overemphasized.

HISTORY

1. **Basic information:**
    a. **Age:** Age must be recorded because some conditions are more common at certain ages; for instance, pregnant women younger than 17 years or older than 35 years are at greater risk for preterm labor, preeclampsia, or miscarriage.
    b. **Gravidity:** Number of pregnancies including current pregnancy (includes miscarriages, ectopic pregnancies, and stillbirths).
    c. **Parity:** Number of pregnancies that have ended at gestational age(s) greater than 20 weeks.
    d. **Abortuses:** Number of pregnancies that have ended at gestational age(s) less than 20 weeks (includes ectopic pregnancies, induced abortions, and spontaneous abortions).

> **CLINICAL PEARL**
>
> ▶ Some practitioners use a four-digit parity system to designate the number of term deliveries, number of preterm deliveries, number of abortuses, and number of live births (TPAL [Term, Preterm, Abortions, Living] system). For example, G2P1001 indicates gravidity 2 (two pregnancies including the current one), parity 1001; 1 prior term delivery, no preterm deliveries, no abortuses, and 1 living.

2. **Last menstrual period (LMP):** The first day of the last menstrual period. In obstetric patients, the certainty of the LMP is important in determining the gestational age. The estimated gestational age (EGA) is calculated from the LMP or by ultrasound. A simple rule for calculating the expected due date (EDD) is to subtract 3 months from the LMP and add 7 days to the first day of the LMP (eg, an LMP of 1 November would equal an EDD of 8 August). Because of delay in ovulation in some cycles, this is not always accurate.

3. **Chief complaint:** What is it that brought the patient into the hospital or office? Is it a scheduled appointment, or an unexpected symptom such as abdominal pain or vaginal bleeding in pregnancy? The duration and character of the complaint, associated symptoms, and exacerbating and relieving factors should be recorded. The chief complaint engenders a differential diagnosis, and the possible etiologies should be explored by further inquiry. For example, if the chief complaint is postmenopausal bleeding, the concern is endometrial cancer. Thus, some of the questions should be related to the risk factors for endometrial cancer such as hypertension, diabetes, anovulation, early age of menarche, late age of menopause, obesity, infertility, nulliparity, and so forth.

> ### CLINICAL PEARL
>
> ▶ The first line of any obstetric presentation should include age, gravidity, parity, LMP, estimated gestational age, and chief complaint.
>
> Example: A 32-year-old G3P1011 woman, whose LMP was 2 April and who has a pregnancy with an EGA of 32 4/7 weeks' gestation, complains of lower abdominal cramping.

4. **Past gynecologic history:**

    a. **Menstrual history**

        i. Age of menarche (should normally be older than 9 years and younger than 16 years).

        ii. Character of menstrual cycles: Interval from the first day of one menses to the first day of the next menses (normal is 28 ± 7 days, or between 21 and 35 days).

        iii. Quantity of menses: Menstrual flow should last less than 7 days (or be <80 mL in total volume). If menstrual flow is excessive, then it is called heavy menstrual bleeding.

        iv. Irregular *and* heavy menses is called abnormal uterine bleeding (AUB).

    b. **Contraceptive history:** Duration, type, and last use of contraception, and any side effects.

    c. **Sexually transmitted diseases:** A positive or negative history of herpes simplex virus, syphilis, gonorrhea, Chlamydia, human immunodeficiency virus, pelvic inflammatory disease, or human papillomavirus. Number of sexual partners, whether a recent change in partners, and use of barrier contraception.

5. **Obstetric history:** Date and gestational age of each pregnancy at termination, and outcome; if induced abortion, then gestational age and method. If delivered, then whether the delivery was vaginal or cesarean; if applicable, vacuum or forceps delivery, or type of cesarean (low-transverse vs classical). All complications of pregnancies should be listed.

6. **Past medical history:** Any illnesses such as hypertension, hepatitis, diabetes mellitus, cancer, heart disease, pulmonary disease, and thyroid disease should be elicited. Duration, severity, and therapies should be included. Any hospitalizations should be listed with reason for admission, intervention, and location of hospital.

7. **Past surgical history:** Year and type of surgery should be elucidated and any complications documented. Type of incision (laparoscopy vs laparotomy) should be recorded.

8. **Allergies:** Reactions to medications should be recorded, including severity and temporal relationship to medication. Nonmedicine allergies, such as to latex or iodine, are also important to note. Immediate hypersensitivity should be distinguished from an adverse reaction.

9. **Medications:** A list of medications, dosage, route of administration and frequency, and duration of use should be obtained. Prescription, over-the-counter, and herbal remedies are all relevant. Use or abuse of illicit drugs, tobacco, or alcohol should also be recorded.

10. **Review of systems:** A systematic review should be performed but focused on the more common diseases. For example, in pregnant women, the presence of symptoms referable to preeclampsia, such as headache, visual disturbances, epigastric pain, or facial swelling, should be queried. In an elderly woman, symptoms suggestive of cardiac disease, such as chest pain, shortness of breath, fatigue, weakness, or palpitations, should be elicited.

> **CLINICAL PEARL**
>
> ▶ In every pregnancy greater than 20 weeks' gestation, the patient should be questioned about symptoms of preeclampsia (headaches, visual disturbances, dyspnea, epigastric pain, and face/hand swelling).

PHYSICAL EXAMINATION

1. **General appearance:** Cachectic versus well-nourished, anxious versus calm, alert versus obtunded.

2. **Vital signs:** Temperature, blood pressure, heart rate, and respiratory rate. Height and weight are often placed here.

3. **Head and neck examination:** Evidence of trauma, tumors, facial edema, goiter, and carotid bruits should be sought. Cervical and supraclavicular nodes should be palpated.

4. **Breast examination:** Inspection for symmetry, skin or nipple retraction with the patient's hands on her hips (to accentuate the pectoral muscles), and with arms raised. With the patient supine, the breasts should then be palpated systematically to assess for masses. The nipple should be assessed for discharge, and the axillary and supraclavicular regions should be examined for adenopathy.

5. **Cardiac examination:** The point of maximal impulse should be ascertained, and the heart auscultated at the apex of the heart as well as base. Heart sounds, murmurs, and clicks should be characterized. Systolic flow murmurs are fairly common in pregnant women due to the increased cardiac output, but significant diastolic murmurs are unusual.

6. **Pulmonary examination:** The lung fields should be examined systematically and thoroughly. Wheezes, rales, rhonchi, and bronchial breath sounds should be recorded.

7. **Abdominal examination:** The abdomen should be inspected for scars, distension, masses or organomegaly (ie, spleen or liver), and discoloration. For instance, the Grey Turner sign of discoloration at the flank areas may indicate intra abdominal or retroperitoneal hemorrhage. Auscultation of bowel sounds should be accomplished to identify normal versus high-pitched, and hyperactive versus hypoactive sounds. The abdomen should be percussed for the presence of shifting dullness (indicating ascites). Careful palpation should begin initially away from the area of pain, involving one hand on top of the other, to assess for masses, tenderness, and peritoneal signs. Tenderness should be recorded on a scale (eg, 1-4, where 4 is the most severe pain). Guarding, whether it is voluntary or involuntary, should be noted.

8. **Back and spine examination:** The back should be assessed for symmetry, tenderness, or masses. In particular, the flank regions are important to assess for pain on percussion because that may indicate renal disease.

9. **Pelvic examination** (adequate preparation of the patient is crucial, including counseling about what to expect, adequate lubrication, and sensitivity to pain and discomfort):

    a. The external genitalia should be observed for masses or lesions, discoloration, redness, or tenderness. Ulcers in this area may indicate herpes simplex virus, vulvar carcinoma, or syphilis; a vulvar mass at the 5:00 or 7:00 o'clock positions can suggest a Bartholin gland cyst or abscess. Pigmented lesions may require biopsy because malignant melanoma is not uncommon in the vulvar region.

    b. **Speculum examination:** The vagina should be inspected for lesions, discharge, estrogen effect (well-ruggated vs atrophic), and presence of a cystocele or a rectocele. The appearance of the cervix should be described, and masses, vesicles, or other lesions should be noted.

    c. **Bimanual examination:** Initially, the index and middle fingers of the one gloved hand should be inserted into the patient's vagina underneath the cervix, while the clinician's other hand is placed on the abdomen at the uterine

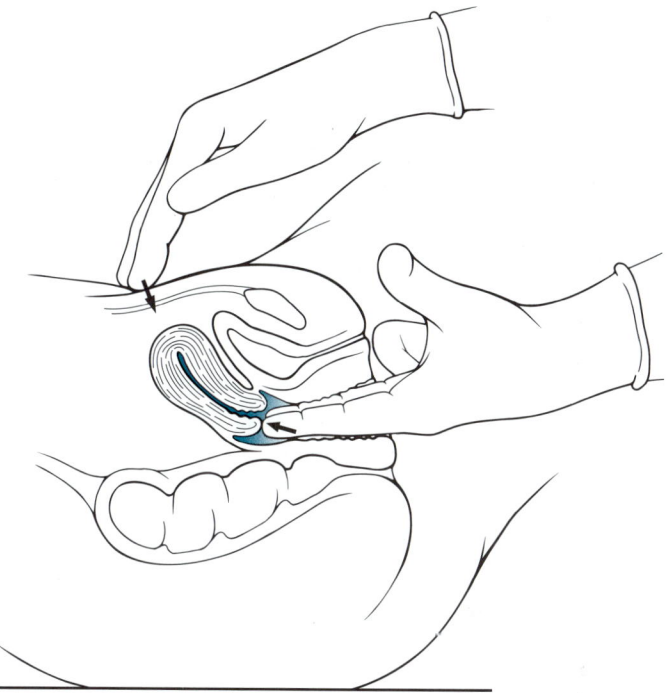

Figure I–1. Bimanual pelvic examination. The examiner evaluates the patient's uterus by palpating her cervix vaginally while simultaneously assessing her uterine fundus abdominally.

fundus. With the uterus trapped between the two hands, the examiner should identify whether there is cervical motion tenderness, and evaluate the size, shape, and directional axis of the uterus. The adnexa should then be assessed with the vaginal hand in the lateral vaginal fornices. The normal ovary is approximately the size of a walnut (Figure I–1).

NOTE: At the time of this writing, there is debate about the utility or necessity of the annual internal pelvic examination for low-risk, nonpregnant, asymptomatic women. While the American College of Physicians states that the internal pelvic examination is not helpful, the American College of Obstetricians and Gynecologists states that there is no definitive evidence either way and that the decision should rest with the patient and her physician.

    d. **Rectal examination:** A rectal examination will reveal masses in the posterior pelvis, and may identify occult blood in the stool. Nodularity and tenderness in the uterosacral ligament can be signs of endometriosis. The posterior uterus and palpable masses in the cul-de-sac can be identified by rectal examination.

10. **Extremities and skin:** The presence of joint effusions, tenderness, skin edema, and cyanosis should be recorded.

11. **Neurologic examination:** Patients who present with neurologic complaints usually require a thorough assessment including evaluation of the cranial nerves, strength, sensation, and reflexes.

> **CLINICAL PEARL**
>
> ▶ The vaginal examination assesses the anterior pelvis, whereas the rectal examination is directed at the posterior pelvis.

12. **Laboratory assessment for obstetric patients:**
    a. Prenatal laboratory tests usually include the following:
        i. **CBC,** or complete blood count, to assess for anemia and thrombocytopenia.
        ii. **Blood type, Rh, and antibody screen** is of paramount importance for all pregnant women; for those women who are Rh negative, RhoGAM is administered at 28 weeks' gestation and at delivery (if the baby proves Rh positive) to prevent isoimmunization.
        iii. **Hepatitis B surface antigen (HBsAg):** Indicates that the patient is infectious. At birth, the newborn should be given hepatitis B immune globulin and hepatitis B vaccine in an attempt to prevent neonatal hepatitis.
        iv. **Rubella titer:** If the patient is not immune to rubella, she should be vaccinated immediately postpartum, because it is a live-attenuated vaccine; this immunization is not given during pregnancy.
        v. **Syphilis nontreponemal test (RPR [rapid plasma reagin] or VDRL [venereal disease research laboratory]):** A positive test necessitates confirmation with a treponemal test such as MHATP (microhemagglutination assay for antibodies to treponema pallidum) or FTA-ABS (fluorescent treponema antibody absorbed). Treatment during pregnancy is crucial to prevent congenital syphilis; penicillin is the agent of choice. Pregnant women who are allergic to penicillin usually undergo desensitization and receive penicillin.
        vi. **Human immunodeficiency virus test:** The screening test is usually the ELISA and, when positive, will necessitate the Western blot or other confirmatory test.
        vii. **Urine culture or urinalysis:** To assess for asymptomatic bacteriuria that complicates 6% to 8% of pregnancies.
        viii. **Pap smear:** To assess for cervical dysplasia or cervical cancer; involves both ectocervical component and endocervical sampling (Figure I–2). Many clinicians prefer the liquid-based media because it may provide better cellular sampling and allows for human papillomavirus subtyping.
        ix. **Assays for *Chlamydia trachomatis* and/or gonorrhea:** traditionally this has been endocervical specimens; however newer technology includes nucleic acid testing of liquid-based Pap smears and vaginal collections with equal sensitivity and specificity as cervical collection. Urine assays are also available at slightly lower sensitivity rate.

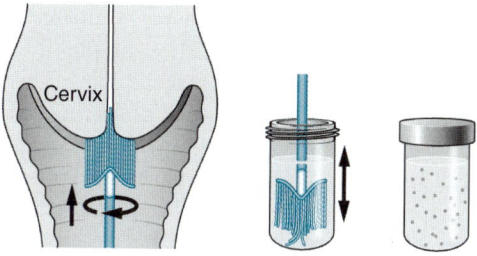

Figure I–2. Pap smear with cytobrush for liquid-based cytology. The brush is used to sample the exocervix and endocervix, and then the brush is rotated and stirred into the fixative, allowing the cervical cells to be dispersed within the fixative solution.

   b. **Timed prenatal tests:**
      i. Serum screening for neural tube defects or Down syndrome offered; usually performed between 16 and 20 weeks' gestation. First-trimester screening for trisomies with serum pregnancy-associated plasma protein-A, beta human chorionic-free gonadotropin (βhCG), and nuchal translucency has gained popularity as well.
      ii. Screening for gestational diabetes at 26 to 28 weeks; generally consists of a 50-g oral glucose load and assessment of the serum glucose level after 1 hour.
      iii. Some practitioners choose to repeat the complete blood count, cervical cultures, or syphilis serology in the third trimester.
      iv. If the culture strategy for group B streptococcus is adopted, then introital cultures are obtained at 35 to 37 weeks' gestation.
13. **Laboratory tests for gynecologic patients:**
    a. Dependent on age, presence of coexisting disease, and chief complaint.
    b. **Common scenarios:**
       i. Threatened abortion: Quantitative hCG and/or progesterone levels may help to establish the viability of a pregnancy and risk of ectopic pregnancy.
       ii. Heavy menstrual bleeding due to uterine fibroids: CBC, endometrial biopsy, and Pap smear. The endometrial biopsy is performed to assess for endometrial cancer and the Pap smear for cervical dysplasia or cancer.
       iii. A woman 55 years or older with an adnexal mass: CA-125 and carcinoembryonic antigen (CEA) tumor markers for epithelial ovarian tumors.
14. **Imaging procedures:**
    a. **Ultrasound examination:**
       i. **Obstetric patients:** Ultrasound is the most commonly used imaging procedure in pregnant women. It can be used to establish the viability of the pregnancy, number of fetuses, location of the placenta, or establish the gestational age of the pregnancy. Targeted examinations can help to examine for structural abnormalities of the fetus.

ii. **Gynecologic patients:** Adnexal masses evaluated by sonography are assessed for size and echogenic texture; simple (fluid filled) versus complex (fluid and solid components) versus solid. The uterus can be characterized for presence of masses, such as uterine fibroids, and the endometrial stripe can be measured. In postmenopausal women, a thickened endometrial stripe may indicate malignancy. Fluid in the cul-de-sac may indicate ascites. The gynecologic ultrasound examination usually also includes investigation of the kidneys, because hydronephrosis may suggest a pelvic process (ureteral obstruction). Saline infusion into the uterine cavity via a transcervical catheter can enhance the ultrasound examination of intrauterine growths such as polyps.

b. **Computed tomography (CT) scan:**
   i. Because of the radiation concerns, this procedure is usually not performed on pregnant women unless sonography is not helpful, and it is deemed necessary.
   ii. The CT scan is useful in women with possible abdominal and/or pelvic masses, and may help to delineate the lymph nodes and retroperitoneal disorders.

c. **Magnetic resonance imaging:**
   i. Identifies soft tissue planes very well and may assist in defining müllerian defects such as vaginal agenesis or uterine didelphys (condition of double uterus and double cervix), and in selected circumstances may also aid in the evaluation of uterine anomalies.
   ii. May be helpful in establishing the location of a pregnancy such as in differentiating a normal pregnancy from a cervical pregnancy.

d. **Intravenous pyelogram:**
   i. Intravenous dye is used to assess the concentrating ability of the kidneys, the patency of the ureters, and the integrity of the bladder.
   ii. It is also useful in detecting hydronephrosis, ureteral stone, or ureteral obstruction.

e. **Hysterosalpingogram:**
   i. A small amount of radiopaque dye is introduced through a transcervical cannula and radiographs are taken.
   ii. It is useful for the detection of intrauterine abnormalities (submucous fibroids or intrauterine adhesions) and patency of the fallopian tubes (tubal obstruction or hydrosalpinx).

CLINICAL PEARL

▶ Sonohysterography is a special ultrasound examination of the uterus that involves injecting a small amount of saline into the endometrial cavity to better define the intrauterine cavity. It can help to identify endometrial polyps or submucous myomata.

Part 2. Approach to Clinical Problem Solving

There are typically four distinct steps that a clinician undertakes to solve most clinical problems systematically:

1. Making the diagnosis.
2. Assessing the severity and/or stage of the disease.
3. Rendering a treatment based on the stage of the disease.
4. Following the patient's response to the treatment.

MAKING THE DIAGNOSIS

The diagnosis is made by careful evaluation of the database, analysis of the information, assessment of the risk factors, and development of the list of possibilities (the differential diagnosis). The process includes knowing which pieces of information are meaningful and which may be thrown out. Experience and knowledge help to guide the physician to "key in" on the most important possibilities. A good clinician also knows how to ask the same question in several different ways, and use different terminology. For example, patients at times may deny having been treated for "pelvic inflammatory disease," but will answer affirmatively to being hospitalized for "a tubal infection." Reaching a diagnosis may be achieved by systematically reading about each possible cause and disease. The patient's presentation is then matched up against each of these possibilities, and each is either placed high up on the list as a potential etiology, or moved lower down because of disease prevalence, the patient's presentation, or other clues. A patient's risk factors may influence the probability of a diagnosis.

Usually, a long list of possible diagnoses can be pared down to two to three most likely ones, based on selective laboratory or imaging tests. For example, a woman who complains of lower abdominal pain *and* has a history of a prior sexually transmitted disease may have salpingitis; another patient who has abdominal pain, amenorrhea, *and* a history of prior tubal surgery may have an ectopic pregnancy. Furthermore, yet another woman with a 1-day history of periumbilical pain localizing to the right lower quadrant may have acute appendicitis.

> **CLINICAL PEARL**
>
> ▶ The first step in clinical problem solving is making the diagnosis.

ASSESSING THE SEVERITY AND/OR STAGE OF THE DISEASE

After ascertaining the diagnosis, the next step is to characterize the severity of the disease process; in other words, describe "how bad" a disease is. With malignancy, this is done formally by staging the cancer. Most cancers are categorized from stage I (least severe) to stage IV (most severe). Some diseases, such as preeclampsia, may be designated as mild or severe. With other ailments, there is a moderate category. With some infections, such as syphilis, the staging depends on the duration and extent of the infection, and follows along the natural history of the infection (ie, primary syphilis, secondary, latent period, and tertiary/neurosyphilis).

> **CLINICAL PEARL**
>
> ▶ The second step in clinical problem solving is to establish the severity or stage of disease. There is usually prognostic or treatment significance based on the stage.

RENDERING A TREATMENT BASED ON THE STAGE OF THE DISEASE

Many illnesses are stratified according to severity because prognosis and treatment often vary based on the severity. If neither the prognosis nor the treatment was influenced by the stage of the disease process, there would not be a reason to subcategorize a disease as mild or severe. As an example, a pregnant woman at 34 weeks' gestation with mild preeclampsia is at less risk from the disease than if she developed severe preeclampsia (particularly if the severe preeclampsia were pulmonary edema or eclampsia). Accordingly, with mild preeclampsia, the management may be expectant, letting the pregnancy continue while watching for any danger signs (severe disease). In contrast, if preeclampsia with severe features complicated this same 34-week pregnancy, the treatment would be magnesium sulfate to prevent seizures (eclampsia) and, most importantly, delivery. It is primarily delivery that "cures" the preeclampsia. In this disease, severe preeclampsia means both maternal and fetal risks are increased. As another example, urinary tract infections may be subdivided into lower tract infections (cystitis) that are treated by oral antibiotics on an outpatient basis, versus upper tract infections (pyelonephritis) that generally require hospitalization and intravenous antibiotics.

Bacterial vaginosis (BV), which has been associated with preterm delivery, endometritis, and vaginal cuff cellulitis (following hysterectomy), does not have a severe or mild substaging. The presence of BV may slightly increase the risk of problems, but neither the prognosis nor the treatment is affected by "more" BV or "less" BV. Hence, the student should approach a new disease by learning the mechanism, clinical presentation, staging, and the treatment based on stage.

> **CLINICAL PEARL**
>
> ▶ The third step in clinical problem solving is that, for most conditions, the treatment is tailored to the extent or "stage" of the disease.

FOLLOWING THE PATIENT'S RESPONSE TO THE TREATMENT

The final step in the approach to disease is to follow the patient's response to the therapy. The "measure" of response should be recorded and monitored. Some responses are clinical such as improvement (or lack of improvement) in a patient's abdominal pain, temperature, or pulmonary examination. Obviously, the student must work on being more skilled in eliciting the data in an unbiased and standardized manner. Other responses may be followed by imaging tests such as a

CT scan to establish retroperitoneal node size in a patient receiving chemotherapy, or a tumor marker such as the CA-125 level in a woman receiving chemotherapy for ovarian cancer. For syphilis, it may be the results of a nonspecific treponemal antibody test RPR titer over time. The student must be prepared to know what to do if the measured marker does not respond according to what is expected. Is the next step to retreat, or to reconsider the diagnosis, or to repeat the metastatic work-up, or to follow up with another more specific test?

> **CLINICAL PEARL**
>
> ▶ The fourth step in clinical problem solving is to monitor treatment response or efficacy, which may be measured in different ways. It may be symptomatic (patient feels better), or based on physical examination (fever), a laboratory test (CA-125 level), or an imaging test (ultrasound for the size of ovarian cyst).

PART 3. Approach to Reading

The clinical problem-oriented approach to reading is different from the classic "systematic" research of a disease. Patients rarely present with a clear diagnosis; hence, the student must become skilled in applying the textbook information to the clinical setting. Furthermore, a reader retains more information when reading with a purpose. In other words, the student should read with the goal of answering specific questions. Likewise, the student should have a plan for the acquisition and use of the information; the process is similar to having a mental "flowchart" and each step sifting through diagnostic possibilities, therapy, complications, and risk factors. There are several fundamental questions that facilitate clinical thinking. These are as follows:

1. What is the most likely diagnosis?
2. What should be your next step?
3. What is the most likely mechanism for this process?
4. What are the risk factors for this condition?
5. What are the complications associated with the disease process?
6. What is the best therapy?
7. How would you confirm the diagnosis?

> **CLINICAL PEARL**
>
> ▶ Reading with the purpose of answering the seven fundamental clinical questions improves retention of information and facilitates the application of "book knowledge" to "clinical knowledge."

WHAT IS THE MOST LIKELY DIAGNOSIS?

The method of establishing the diagnosis has been covered in the previous section. One way of attacking this problem is to develop standard "approaches" to common clinical situations. It is helpful to understand the most common causes of various presentations such as "the most common cause of postpartum hemorrhage is uterine atony." (Clinical Pearls appear at the end of each case.)

The clinical scenario would be something such as:

An 18-year-old G1P0 adolescent female undergoes an uncomplicated vaginal delivery at term. After the placenta is delivered, she has 1500 cc of vaginal bleeding. What is the most likely diagnosis?

With no other information to go on, the student would note that this patient has postpartum hemorrhage (blood loss of >500 mL with a vaginal delivery). Using the "most common cause" information, the student would make an educated guess that the patient has uterine atony.

However, what if the scenario also included the following phrase?

The uterus is noted to be firm.

Now the most likely diagnosis is a genital tract laceration, usually involving the cervix. With a firm well-contracted uterus, atony is not likely.

CLINICAL PEARL

▶ The most common cause of postpartum hemorrhage is uterine atony. Thus, the first step in patient assessment and management is uterine massage to check if the uterus is boggy.

▶ If the uterus is firm, and the woman is still bleeding, then the clinician should consider a genital tract laceration.

▶ Now, the student would use the Clinical Pearl: "The most common cause of postpartum hemorrhage with a firm uterus is a genital tract laceration."

WHAT SHOULD BE YOUR NEXT STEP?

This question is difficult because the next step has many possibilities; the answer may be to obtain more diagnostic information, stage the illness, or introduce therapy. It is often a more challenging question than "What is the most likely diagnosis?" because there may be insufficient information to make a diagnosis and the next step may be to pursue more diagnostic information. Another possibility is that there is enough information for a probable diagnosis, and the next step is to stage the disease. Finally, the most appropriate answer may be to render treatment. Hence, from clinical data, a judgment needs to be rendered regarding how far along one is on the road of:

Make a diagnosis → Stage the disease →
Treat based on stage → Follow response

Frequently, the student is taught to "regurgitate" the information that someone has written about a particular disease, but is not skilled at giving the next step.

This talent is learned optimally at the bedside, in a supportive environment, with freedom to make educated guesses, and with constructive feedback. A sample scenario describes a student's thought process as follows:

1. **Make a diagnosis:** "Based on the information I have, I believe that this patient has a pelvic inflammatory disease because she is not pregnant and has lower abdominal tenderness, cervical motion tenderness, and adnexal tenderness."
2. **Stage the disease:** "I do not believe that this is a severe disease because she does not have high fever, evidence of sepsis, or peritoneal signs. An ultrasound has already been done showing no abscess (tubo-ovarian abscess would put her in a severe category)."
3. **Treat based on stage:** "Therefore, my next step is to treat her with intramuscular ceftriaxone and oral doxycycline."
4. **Follow response:** "I want to follow the treatment by assessing her pain (I will ask her to rate the pain on a scale of 1-10 every day), her temperature, and abdominal examination, and reassess her in 48 hours."

In a similar patient, when the clinical presentation is unclear, perhaps the best "next step" may be diagnostic in nature such as laparoscopy to visualize the tubes. This information is sometimes tested by the dictum, "the gold standard for the diagnosis of acute salpingitis is laparoscopy to visualize the tubes, and particularly seeing purulent material drain from the tubes."

> ### CLINICAL PEARL
> ▶ Usually, the vague query, "What is your next step?" is the most difficult question, because the answer may be diagnostic, staging, or therapeutic.

WHAT IS THE MOST LIKELY MECHANISM FOR THIS PROCESS?

This question goes further than making the diagnosis, but also requires the student to understand the underlying mechanism for the process. For example, a clinical scenario may describe an 18-year-old adolescent female at 24 weeks' gestation, who develops dyspnea 2 days after being treated for pyelonephritis. The student must first diagnose the acute respiratory distress syndrome, which often occurs 1 to 2 days after antibiotics are instituted. Then, the student must understand that the endotoxins that arise from Gram-negative organisms cause pulmonary injury, leading to capillary leakage of fluid into the pulmonary interstitial space. The mechanism is, therefore, endotoxin-induced "capillary leakage." Answers that a student may also entertain, but would be less likely to be causative, include pneumonia, pulmonary embolism, or pleural effusion.

The student is advised to learn the mechanisms for each disease process, and not merely memorize a constellation of symptoms. In other words, rather than solely committing to memorizing the classic presentation of pyelonephritis (fever, flank tenderness, and pyuria), the student should understand that Gram-negative rods, such as *Escherichia coli*, would ascend from the external genitalia to the urethra to the bladder. From the bladder, the bacteria would ascend further to the kidneys and cause an infection in the renal parenchyma. The involvement of the kidney now causes fever (vs an infection of only the bladder, which usually does not induce a fever) and flank tenderness—a systemic response not seen with lower urinary tract infection (ie, bacteriuria or cystitis). Furthermore, the body's reaction to the bacteria brings about leukocytes in the urine (pyuria).

WHAT ARE THE RISK FACTORS FOR THIS CONDITION?

Understanding the risk factors helps the practitioner to establish a diagnosis and to determine how to interpret tests. For example, understanding the risk factor analysis may help to manage a 55-year-old woman with postmenopausal bleeding after an endometrial biopsy shows no pathologic changes. If the woman does not have any risk factors for endometrial cancer, the patient may be observed because the likelihood for uterine malignancy is not so great. On the other hand, if the same 55-year-old woman were diabetic, had a long history of anovulation (irregular menses), was nulliparous, and was hypertensive, a practitioner should pursue the postmenopausal bleeding further, even after a normal endometrial biopsy. The physician may want to perform a hysteroscopy to visualize the endometrial cavity directly and biopsy the abnormal-appearing areas. Thus, the presence of risk factors helps to categorize the likelihood of a disease process.

> ### CLINICAL PEARL
> ▶ When patients are at high risk for a disease, based on risk factors, more testing may be indicated.

WHAT ARE THE COMPLICATIONS ASSOCIATED WITH THE DISEASE PROCESS?

Clinicians must be cognizant of the complications of a disease, so that they will understand how to follow and monitor the patient. Sometimes, the student will have to make the diagnosis from clinical clues, and then apply his or her knowledge of the consequences of the pathologic process. For example, a woman who presents with lower abdominal pain, vaginal discharge, and dyspareunia is first diagnosed as having pelvic inflammatory disease or salpingitis (infection of the fallopian tubes). Long-term complications of this process would include ectopic pregnancy or infertility from tubal damage. Understanding the types of consequences also helps the clinician to be aware of the dangers to a patient. One life-threatening complication of a tubo-ovarian abscess (which is the end-stage of a tubal infection leading to a collection of pus in the region of the tubes and ovary) is rupture of the abscess. The clinical presentation is shock with hypotension, and the appropriate therapy is immediate surgery. In fact, not recognizing the rupture is commonly associated with patient mortality. The student applies this information when she or he sees a woman with a tubo-ovarian abscess on daily rounds, and monitors for hypotension, confusion, apprehension, and tachycardia. The clinician advises the team to be vigilant for any signs of abscess rupture, and to be prepared to undertake immediate surgery should the need arise.

WHAT IS THE BEST THERAPY?

To answer this question, the clinician needs to reach the correct diagnosis, and assess the severity of the condition, and then he or she must weigh the situation to reach the appropriate intervention. For the student, knowing exact dosages is not as important as understanding the best medication, the route of delivery, mechanism of action, and possible complications. It is important for the student to be able to verbalize the diagnosis and the rationale for the therapy. A common error is for the student to "jump to a treatment," like a random guess, and, therefore, he or she is given "right or wrong" feedback. In fact, the student's guess may be correct, but for the wrong reason; conversely, the answer may be a very reasonable one, with only one small error in thinking. Instead, the student should verbalize the steps so that feedback may be given at every reasoning point.

For example, if the question is, "What is the best therapy for a 19-year-old woman with a nontender ulcer of the vulva and painless adenopathy who is pregnant at 12 weeks' gestation?" The incorrect manner of response for the student is to blurt out "azithromycin." Rather, the student should reason it in a way such as the following: "The most common cause of a nontender infectious ulcer of the vulva is syphilis. Painless adenopathy is usually associated. In pregnancy, penicillin is the only effective therapy to prevent congenital syphilis. Therefore, the best treatment for this woman with probable syphilis is intramuscular penicillin (after confirming the diagnosis)."

A related question is, "What would have best prevented this condition?" For instance, if the scenario presented is a 23-year-old woman with tubal factor infertility, then the most likely etiology is *Chlamydia trachomatis* cervicitis which had ascended to the tubes causing damage. The best preventive measure would be a barrier contraception such as condom use.

> ### CLINICAL PEARL
> ▶ Therapy should be logical based on the severity of disease. Antibiotic therapy should be tailored for specific organism(s).

HOW WOULD YOU CONFIRM THE DIAGNOSIS?

In the previous scenario, the woman with a nontender vulvar ulcer is likely to have syphilis. Confirmation can be achieved by serology (RPR or VDRL test) and specific treponemal test; however, there is a significant possibility that patients with primary syphilis may not have developed an antibody response yet, and have negative serology. Thus, confirmation of the diagnosis would be attained with darkfield microscopy. The student should strive to know the limitations of various diagnostic tests, and the manifestations of disease.

PART 4. Approach to Surgery

The student should be generally aware of the various approaches to surgical management of the gynecologic patient. Ways to access the intraabdominal cavity include (a) laparotomy (incision of the abdomen), (b) laparoscopy (using thin, long instruments through small incisions to perform surgery), and (c) robotic surgery (use of the console to direct instruments that have been docked). The latter two are considered minimally invasive approaches.

Some of the relative advantages and disadvantages of laparoscopy versus robotics include:

- Robotics: Better 3D visualization and magnification, better ability to manipulate instruments such as rotating "EndoWrist" stitching, less "fulcrum effect" of long instruments, better ergonomics for surgeon, restoration of eye-target perspective.
- Laparoscopy: Better "feel" of tissue and force used, less expensive, smaller "footprint" of machine, possibly less operative time.

Hysteroscopy is a means to examine or perform surgery on the intrauterine cavity by inserting a distension media in the uterus and using a small, thin scope going through the cervix to visualize the endometrial cavity.

SUMMARY

1. There is no replacement for a meticulous history and physical examination.
2. There are four steps to the clinical approach to the patient: making the diagnosis, assessing severity, treating based on severity, and following response.
3. There are seven questions that help to bridge the gap between the textbook and the clinical arena.

REFERENCES

Cunningham FG, Leveno KJ, Bloom SL, et al. Prenatal care. In: *Williams Obstetrics*. 24th ed. New York, NY: McGraw-Hill; 2014:221-247.

Lentz GM. History, physical examination, and preventive health care. In: Katz VL, Lentz GM, Lobo RA, Gersenson DM, eds. *Comprehensive Gynecology*. 6th ed. St. Louis, MO: Mosby-Year Book; 2012:137-150.

Moore GJ. Obstetric and gynecologic evaluation. In: Hacker NF, Moore JG, eds. *Essentials of Obstetrics and Gynecology*. 6th ed. Philadelphia, PA: Saunders; 2015:12-26.

SECTION II

Cases

CASE 1

A 26-year-old G1P0 woman at 39 weeks' gestation is admitted to the hospital in labor. She is noted to have uterine contractions every 2 to 3 minutes. Her antepartum history is significant for a nonimmune rubella status. On examination, her blood pressure (BP) is 110/70 mm Hg and heart rate (HR) is 80 beats per minute (bpm). The estimated fetal weight is 7 lbs. On pelvic examination, she has been noted to have a change in cervical examinations from 4-cm dilation to 5-cm over the last 2 hours. The pelvis is assessed to be adequate on digital examination.

▸ What is your next step in the management of this patient?

ANSWER TO CASE 1:
Labor (Latent Phase)

Summary: A 26-year-old G1P0 woman at term with an adequate pelvis on clinical pelvimetry, nonimmune rubella status, is in labor. Her cervix has changed from 4- to 5-cm dilation over 2 hours with uterine contractions noted every 2 to 3 minutes.

- **Next step in management:** Continue to observe the labor.

ANALYSIS
Objectives

1. Know the normal labor parameters in the latent and active phase for nulliparous and multiparous patients.
2. Be familiar with the management of common labor abnormalities and know that normal labor does not require intervention.
3. Know that rubella vaccination, as a live-attenuated preparation, should not be administered during pregnancy.

Considerations

This 26-year-old G1P0 woman is at term (defined as between 37 and 42 completed weeks' gestational age). She has not yet reached active phase of labor (generally about 6 cm of dilation) and her cervix has changed from 4 to 5 cm over 2 hours; her contractions are every 2 to 3 minutes. Previously, active phase was defined as beyond 4 cm of cervical dilation; however, recent studies have shown that **active phase cannot be reliably defined until 6 cm of dilation.** In the latent phase of labor, there is no need for intervention; however, if the progress is prolonged or uterine contractions are inadequate, oxytocin is an option. The uterine contraction pattern appears to be every 2 to 3 minutes. Because she has had normal labor, the appropriate management is to observe her course without intervention. The clinical pelvimetry is accomplished by digital palpation of the pelvic bones (passageway). This patient's pelvis was judged on physical examination to be adequate. Unfortunately, this estimation is not very precise, and in clinical practice, the clinician would generally observe the labor of a nulliparous patient. Finally, the nonimmune rubella status should alert the practitioner to immunize for rubella during the postpartum time (since the rubella vaccine is live attenuated and is contraindicated during pregnancy).

APPROACH TO:
Labor Evaluation

DEFINITIONS

LABOR: Cervical change accompanied by regular uterine contractions.

LATENT PHASE: The initial part of labor where the cervix mainly effaces (thins) rather than dilates (usually cervical dilation <6 cm).

ACTIVE PHASE: The portion of labor where dilation occurs more rapidly, usually when the cervix is >6 cm dilation.

ARREST OF ACTIVE PHASE: No progress in the active phase of labor (≥ 6cm) with ruptured membranes for 4 hours with adequate contractions, or 6 hours of inadequate contractions.

STAGES OF LABOR: First stage: onset of labor to complete dilation of cervix. Second stage: complete cervical dilation to delivery of infant. Third stage: delivery of infant to delivery of placenta.

FETAL HEART RATE BASELINE: Normally between 110 and 160 bpm. Fetal bradycardia is a baseline <110 bpm, and fetal tachycardia is exceeding 160 bpm.

DECELERATIONS: Fetal heart rate episodic changes below the baseline. There are three types of decelerations: **early** (mirror image of uterine contractions), variable (abrupt jagged dips below the baseline), and late, which are offset following the uterine contraction.

ACCELERATIONS: Episodes of the fetal heart rate that increase above the baseline for at least 15 bpm and last for at least 15 seconds.

CLINICAL APPROACH TO LABOR

Normal and Abnormal Labor

The **assessment of labor is based on cervical change versus time** (Table 1–1). Normal labor should be expectantly managed. When a labor abnormality is diagnosed, **the three Ps** should be evaluated (powers, passenger, and pelvis). When inadequate

Table 1–1 • NORMAL LABOR PARAMETERS		
	Nullipara (Lower Limits of Normal)	**Multipara (Lower Limits of Normal)**
Latent phase (dilation <6 cm)	≤18-20 h	≤14 h
Active phase	Continued progress	Continued progress
Second stage of labor (complete dilation to expulsion of infant)	≤3 h ≤4 h if epidural	≤2 h ≤3 h if epidural
Third stage of labor	≤30 min	≤30 min

"**powers**" are thought to be the etiology, then **oxytocin** may be initiated to augment the uterine contraction strength and/or frequency. When the latent phase exceeds the upper limits of normal, then it is called a prolonged latent phase. When the cervix has exceeded 6 cm, particularly with near-complete effacement, then the active phase has been reached. Recent studies have shown that as long as there is continued progress of labor in the active phase, in the absence of complications, the labor should be observed. **No cervical dilation for 4 hours in the active phase with rupture of membranes (ROM) and adequate contractions** is called **arrest of active phase.**

When there is **cephalopelvic disproportion**, where the pelvis is thought to be too small for the fetus (either due to an abnormal pelvis or an excessively large baby), **then cesarean delivery must be considered.** When the "powers" are thought to be the factor, then intravenous (IV) oxytocin may be initiated via a dilute titration. Clinically, adequate uterine contractions are defined as contractions every 2 to 3 minutes, firm on palpation, and lasting for at least 40 to 60 seconds (Figure 1–1). Many clinicians choose to use internal uterine catheters to evaluate the adequacy of the powers, a practice that may reduce cesareans. One common assessment tool is to examine a 10-minute window and add each contraction's rise above baseline (each mm Hg rise is called a Montevideo unit). A calculation that meets or exceeds 200 Montevideo units is commonly accepted as an adequate uterine contraction pattern (Figure 1–2).

Fetal Heart Rate Monitoring

Fetal heart rate assessment can help to assess the fetal status. **A normal baseline between 110 and 160 bpm, with accelerations, and variability are indicative of a normal well-oxygenated fetus.** Fetal tachycardia can occur due to a variety of disorders such as maternal fever. Fetal bradycardia, if profound and prolonged, necessitates intervention. The most common decelerations are variable, caused by cord compression. If these are intermittent with abrupt return to baseline, then they can be observed. **Early decelerations**, caused by fetal head compression, are benign. **Late decelerations** are "offset" from the uterine contraction with their onset after the onset of the contraction, the nadir following the contraction peak, and the return to baseline following the contraction resolution. Late decelerations suggest fetal hypoxia, and if recurrent (>50% of uterine contractions), can indicate fetal acidemia. **When late decelerations occur together with decreased variability, then acidosis is strongly suspected** (see Figure 1–3).

An accepted categorization of fetal heart rate patterns is I, II, or III.

- **Category I** is reassuring—normal baseline and variability, no late or variable decelerations.
- **Category II** bears watching—may have some aspect that is concerning but not ominous (eg, fetal tachycardia without decelerations).
- **Category III** is ominous and indicates a high likelihood of severe fetal hypoxia or acidosis—examples include absent baseline variability with recurrent late or variable decelerations or bradycardia, or sinusoidal heart rate pattern (this requires prompt delivery if no improvement).

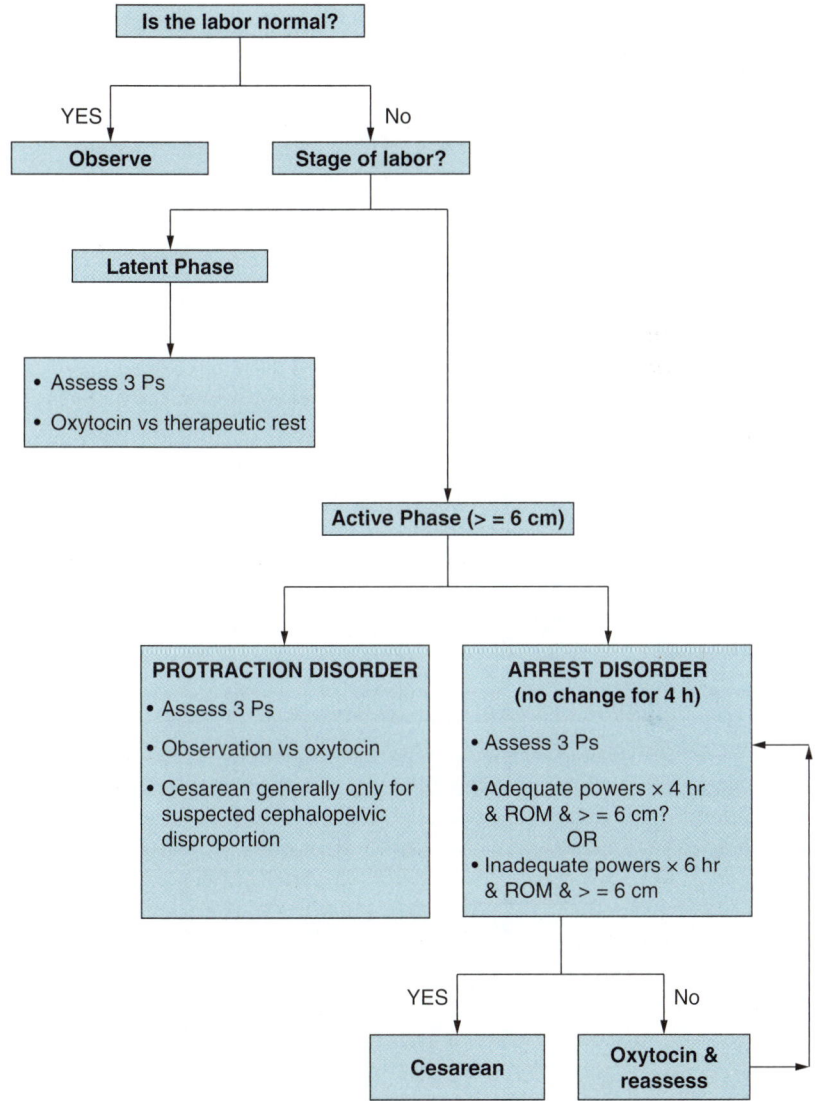

^aAdequate contractions generally >200 Montevideo units or clinically contractions every 2-3 min, firm, lasting 40-60 sec.

Figure 1–1. Algorithm for management of labor.

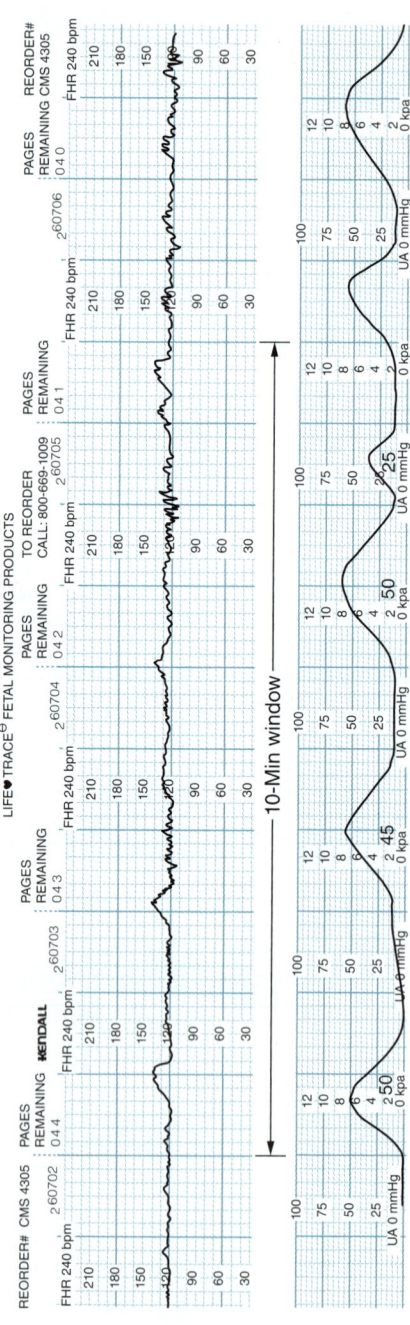

50 + 45 + 50 + 25 = 170 Montevideo units

Figure 1–2. Calculating Montevideo units. Montevideo units are calculated by the sum of the amplitudes (in mm Hg) above baseline of the uterine contractions within a 10-minute window.

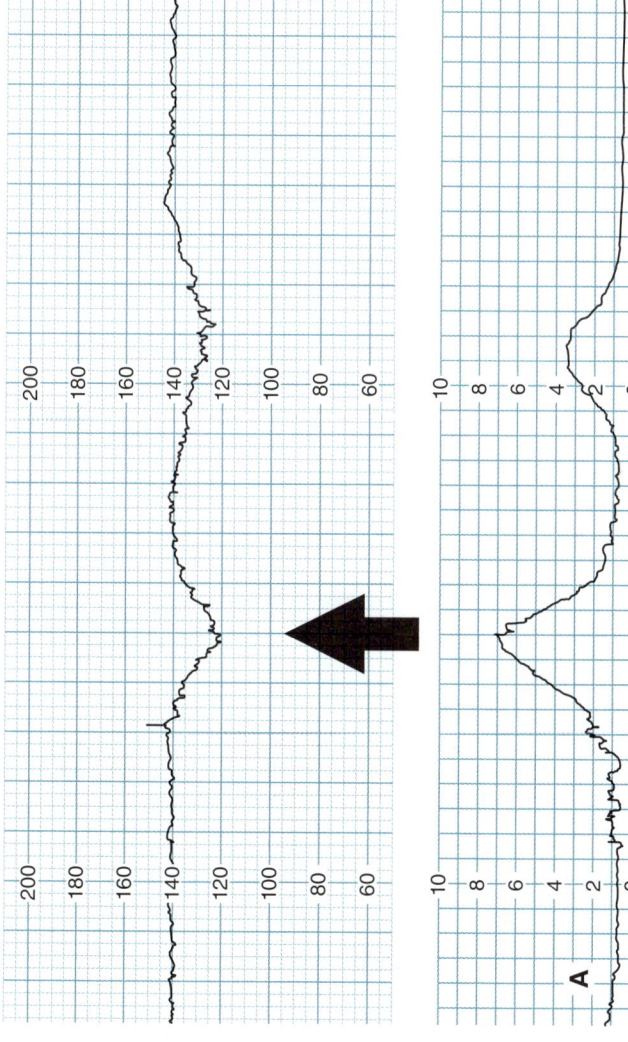

Figure 1–3. Fetal heart rate decelerations. (**A**) Early deceleration—note arrow shows deceleration is gradual and a mirror image to the uterine contraction. (**B**) Late deceleration—note arrow shows deceleration nadir is after the peak of the uterine contraction. (**C**) Variable deceleration—note arrow shows the deceleration is abrupt in its decline and resolution.

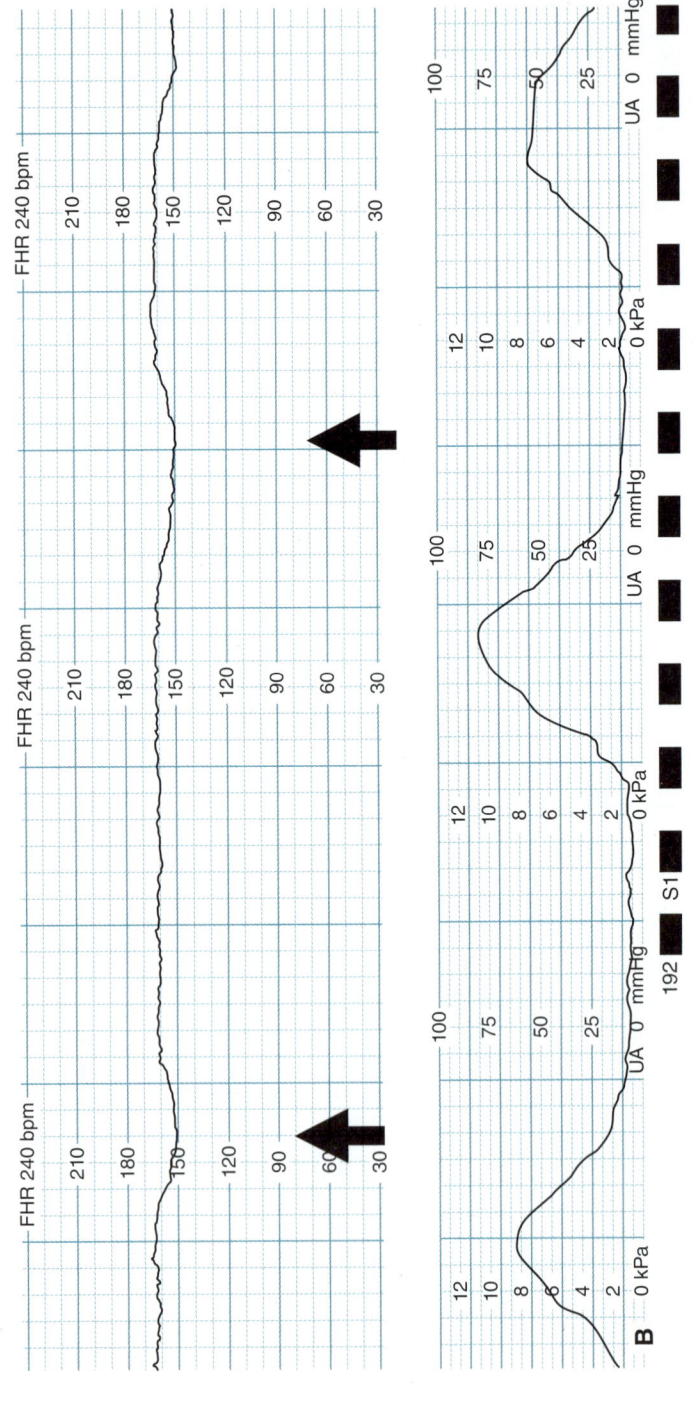

Figure 1–3. (*Continued*)

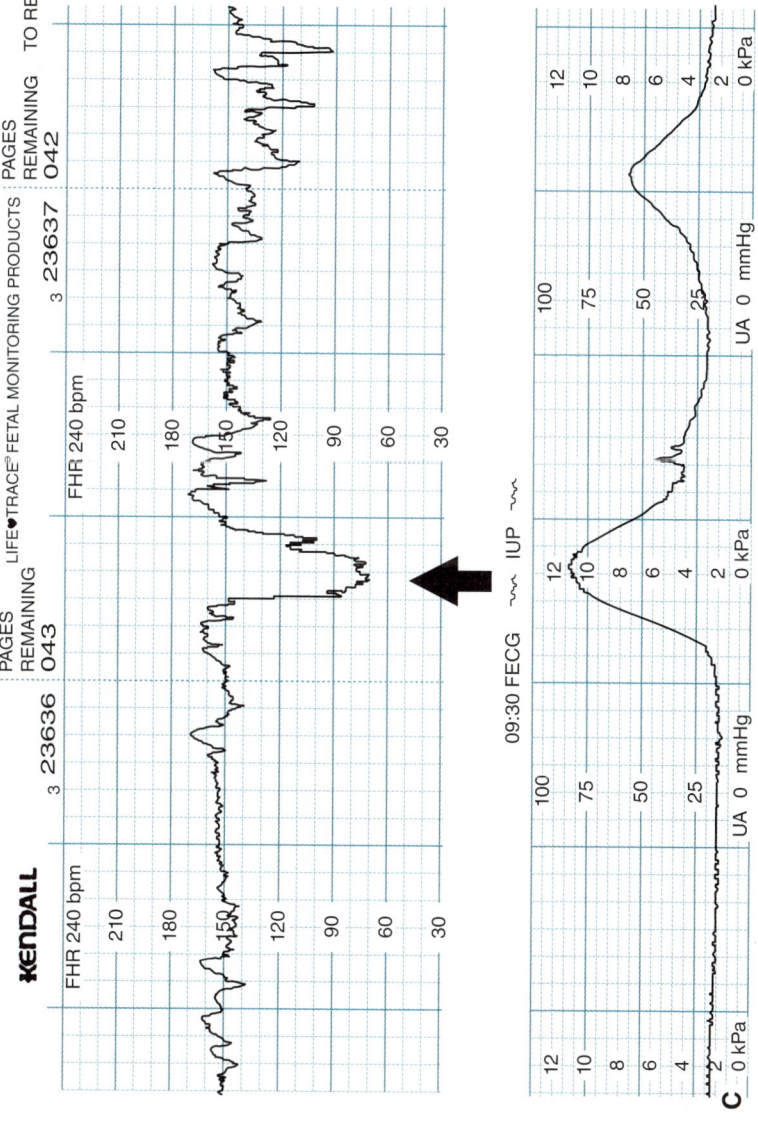

Figure 1–3. (Continued)

Safe Prevention of the Primary Cesarean Delivery

In 2011, one in three deliveries in the US were by cesarean; this rate has steadily increased over the past decades without any significant improvement in maternal or fetal outcome. The reasons in order of frequency **are labor dystocia (34%), abnormal fetal heart rate pattern (23%)**, fetal malpresentation (17%), multiple gestation (7%), and suspected fetal macrosomia (4%). As compared to vaginal delivery, cesarean has a higher overall severe morbidity or mortality rate, and a 3.5-fold increased risk of mortality. To safely reduce the number of primary vertex presenting cesareans, an evidenced based approach should be used for the reasons for abdominal deliveries: **labor arrest and nonreassuring FHR pattern comprise 57% of causes** (See Table 1–2).

Management of FHR Tracing

Category I tracings are reassuring and do not need intervention. **Category III tracings are abnormal and require prompt intervention; if prompt intrauterine resuscitative maneuvers are not curative, imminent delivery is prudent because these tracings are associated with low pH, hypoxia, encephalopathy, and cerebral palsy.**

Most FHR tracings are category II, which can span from a reassuring FHR tracing: normal baseline, moderate variability, accelerations, and mild variable decelerations versus a tracing that is worrisome, such as a tracing showing minimal variability and intermittent deep variable decelerations. **Scalp stimulation inducing an acceleration highly correlates to a normal umbilical cord pH (≥7.20).** Prolonged FHR decelerations (lasting >2 minutes but <10 minutes) often require intervention (see Table 1–3):

Table 1–2 • AFTER REVIEW OF MANY STUDIES, THE CONSORTIUM OF SAFE LABOR MADE THE FOLLOWING RECOMMENDATIONS

1. The traditional definitions of normal latent labor may be kept (20 hours for nulliparous, 14 hours for multiparous), but prolonged latent phase (in the absence of clear cephalopelvic disproportion [CPD]) is not an indication for cesarean.
2. Slow but progressive labor in the first stage of labor (onset to complete dilation) should not be an indication for cesarean.
3. Active phase is defined as cervical dilation ≥**6 cm**.
4. Cesarean for active phase arrest is reserved for women at or beyond 6 cm with ruptured membranes, who fail to progress **despite 4 hours of adequate uterine activity**, or ≥ **6 hours of oxytocin with inadequate uterine activity and no cervical change**.
5. Arrest in the second stage of labor requires at least 2 hours pushing in multiparous and 3 hours pushing in nulliparous (longer duration with epidural or malposition [ie, occiput posterior, OP] as long as progress is documented).
6. **Amnioinfusion** for repetitive variable decelerations may safely reduce the rate of cesarean.
7. Scalp stimulation can help to assess fetal acid–base status when an abnormal or indeterminate (formerly reassuring) FHR pattern (such as minimal variability) is present.
8. External cephalic version should be offered to women after 36 weeks with malpresentation.
9. Cesarean to avoid birth trauma/shoulder dystocia should be limited to estimated fetal weight of ≥5000 g in a nondiabetic woman and 4500 g in a diabetic woman.
10. For persistent occiput posterior or occiput transverse (OT) head positions can be managed by manual rotation of the fetal head, or forceps (but forceps are not as often used now).

Table 1–3 • INTERVENTIONS FOR PROLONGED DECELERATIONS

Etiology	Finding	Intervention
Tachysystole	Uterine contractions >5 /10 min averaged over 30 min	Decrease or stop oxytocin, or administer beta-mimetic agent
Hypotension (such as due to regional anesthesia, ie, epidural)	Low BP following epidural or spinal	IV fluid bolus, or administer vasopressor agent such as ephedrine
Rapid cervical dilation	Labor progression especially descent rapid	Positional changes, observation
Umbilical cord prolapse	Vaginal examination reveals cord through cervix	Elevate presenting part and emergency cesarean
Placental abruption	Uterine tenderness, vaginal bleeding (may be absent with concealed abruption)	Support BP, stabilize patient, consider cesarean if progressive
Uterine rupture	Hx of prior cesarean	Emergency cesarean

COMPREHENSION QUESTIONS

1.1 A 31-year-old G2P1 woman at 39 weeks' gestation complains of painful uterine contractions that are occurring every 3 to 4 minutes. Her cervix has not changed from 6-cm dilation over 3 hours. Which one of the following management plans is most appropriate?

A. Cesarean delivery

B. Intravenous oxytocin

C. Observation

D. Fetal scalp pH monitoring

E. Intranasal gonadotropin therapy

1.2 A 26-year-old G2P1 woman at 41 weeks' gestation has been pushing for 3 hours without progress. Throughout this time, her vaginal examination has remained completely dilated, completely effaced, and 0 station, with the head persistently in the occiput posterior position. Which of the following statements accurately describes the situation?

A. The occiput posterior position is frequently associated with a gynecoid pelvis.

B. The labor progress is normal if the patient does not have an epidural catheter for analgesia, but is abnormal if epidural analgesia is being used.

C. The patient is best described as having an arrest of descent.

D. The bony part of the fetal head is likely to be at the plane of the pelvic inlet.

E. Misoprostol for cervical ripening.

1.3 A 31-year-old G2P1 woman at 40 weeks' gestation has progressed in labor from 5 to 6 cm cervical dilation over 3 hours. Which of the following best describes the labor?

A. Prolonged latent phase
B. Prolonged active phase
C. Arrest of active phase
D. Protracted active phase
E. Normal labor

1.4 A 24-year-old G2P1 woman at 39 weeks' gestation presents with painful uterine contractions. She also complains of dark, vaginal blood mixed with some mucus. Which of the following describes the most likely etiology of her bleeding?

A. Placenta previa
B. Placenta abruption
C. Bloody show
D. Vasa previa
E. Cervical laceration

1.5 A 24-year-old G2P1001 woman at 38 weeks by LMP and supported by a 9-week ultrasound states that her mother is in town for the next 4 days and will be available to assist in taking care of her baby. She requests an induction of labor. Which of the following is the best response to this request?

A. Since the patient is term, there is no increased neonatal complications, but an increased risk of cesarean as compared to spontaneous labor.
B. If the cervix is unfavorable, then prostaglandin ripening would increase the changes for vaginal delivery.
C. Induction at 38 weeks increases neonatal complications as compared to delivery to 39 weeks.
D. The patient's request is reasonable, and induction can be performed with little neonatal or maternal complications.

1.6 A 32-year-old G1P0 woman at 40 weeks' gestational age arrives to the labor floor with frequent and strong contractions. The patient had been seen 24 hours previously and thought to be in latent labor at 2 cm dilated, 70% effaced, fetal vertex at −1 station. She was admitted at 3-cm dilation/80% effacement, −1 station. She undergoes amniotomy, and is started on oxytocin for prolonged latent phase. After 4 hours of oxytocin, she is still at 3-cm dilation, 90% effacement, −1 station. Which of the following is the best management of this patient's labor at this point?

A. Cesarean delivery
B. Continued observation on oxytocin
C. Discharge home with follow-up in 3 days
D. Foley bulb dilation of the cervix

Please match the intervention (A-G) to the clinical situation (1.7-1.10):
  A. Amnioinfusion
  B. Cesarean delivery
  C. Ephedrine
  D. Expectant management
  E. Rupture membranes
  F. Scalp stimulation
  G. Terbutaline

1.7 A 37-year-old G3P2 woman is at 40 weeks' gestation and chronic hypertension. She has been induced with Pitocin and her cervix has been at 3 cm for the past 4 hours. Her fetal heart rate pattern is given below. Which of the following is the best management for this patient? (Figure 1–4)

1.8 A 39-year-old G4P2 Ab1 woman is at 37 weeks' gestation and arrived in active labor. She progressed from 4 to 5 cm over 2 hours. The estimated fetal weight is 7 lb 3 oz, and the pelvis is judged as adequate. The FHR tracing is given below. What is the best next step for this patient? (Figure 1–5)

1.9 An 18-year-old G1P0 woman at 39 weeks' gestation was admitted for labor. She progressed from 4 cm dilation to 6 cm dilation over 2 hours. The FHR tracing is given below. What is your next step in her management? (Figure 1–6)

1.10 A 25-year-old G2P1001 is noted to have a baseline FHR of 150 bpm with moderate variability. She is noted to have repetitive late decelerations shortly after the placement of an epidural catheter for pain control. Her BP is 90/55 mm Hg and HR is 100 bpm. What is the best next step in managing this patient?

ANSWERS

1.1 **C. Observation is best.** This patient has presumably entered into the active phase (6 cm) but not progressed for 3 hours. Also the uterine contraction pattern does not seem adequate since frequency is only every 3 to 4 minutes. We are not told about status of the membranes. Recent studies have indicated that if all other parameters (fetal heart rate tracing) are normal, then cesarean is reserved for active phase arrest with ROM for 4 hours with adequate contractions, or 6 hours with inadequate contractions. Intravenous oxytocin enhances contraction strength and/or frequency, but does not affect cervical dilation. Intranasal gonadotropin therapy is not indicated during any phase of labor.

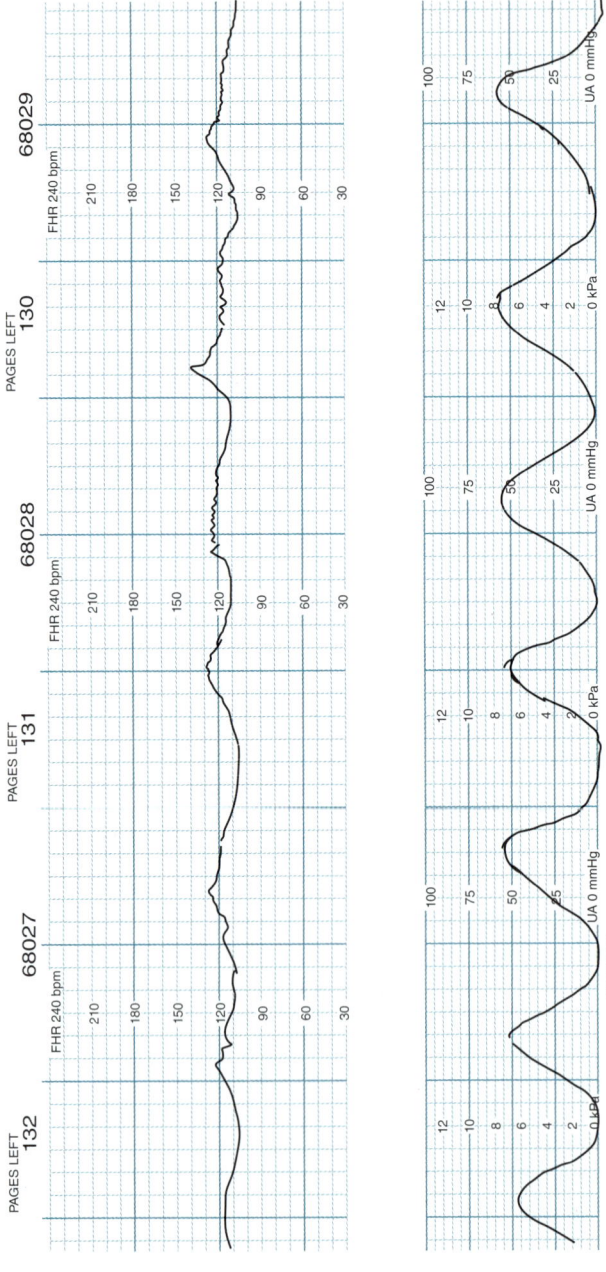

Figure 1–4. FHR tracing (reproduced, with permission, from Eugene C. Toy, MD).

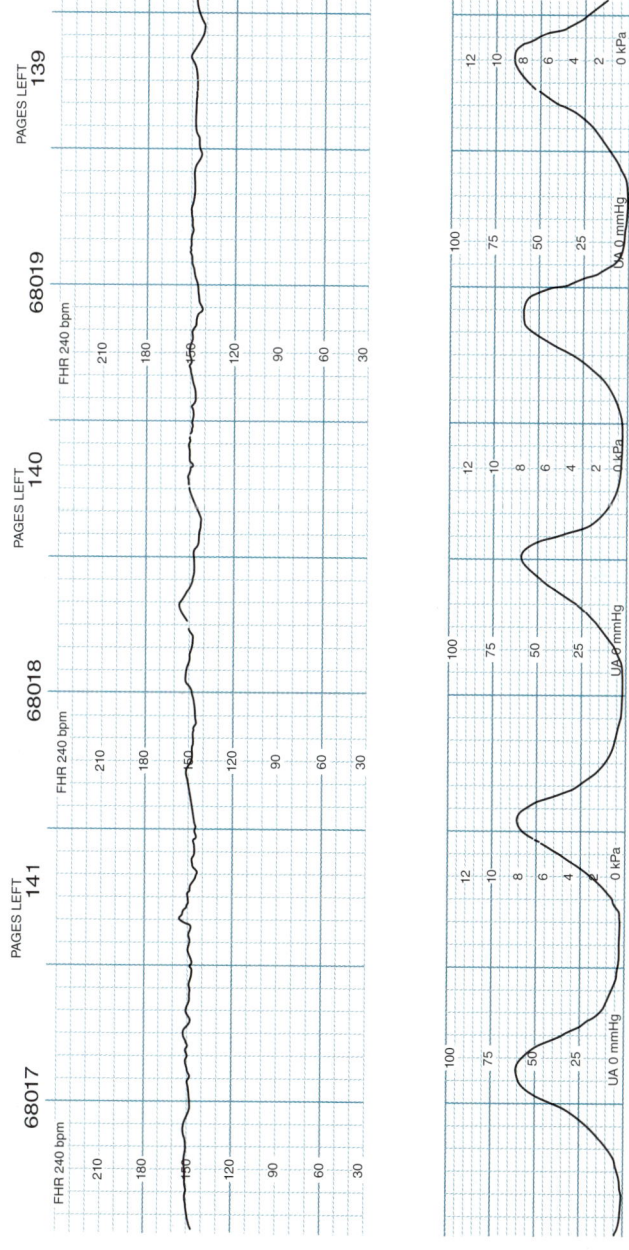

Figure 1–5. FHR tracing (reproduced, with permission, from Eugene C. Toy, MD).

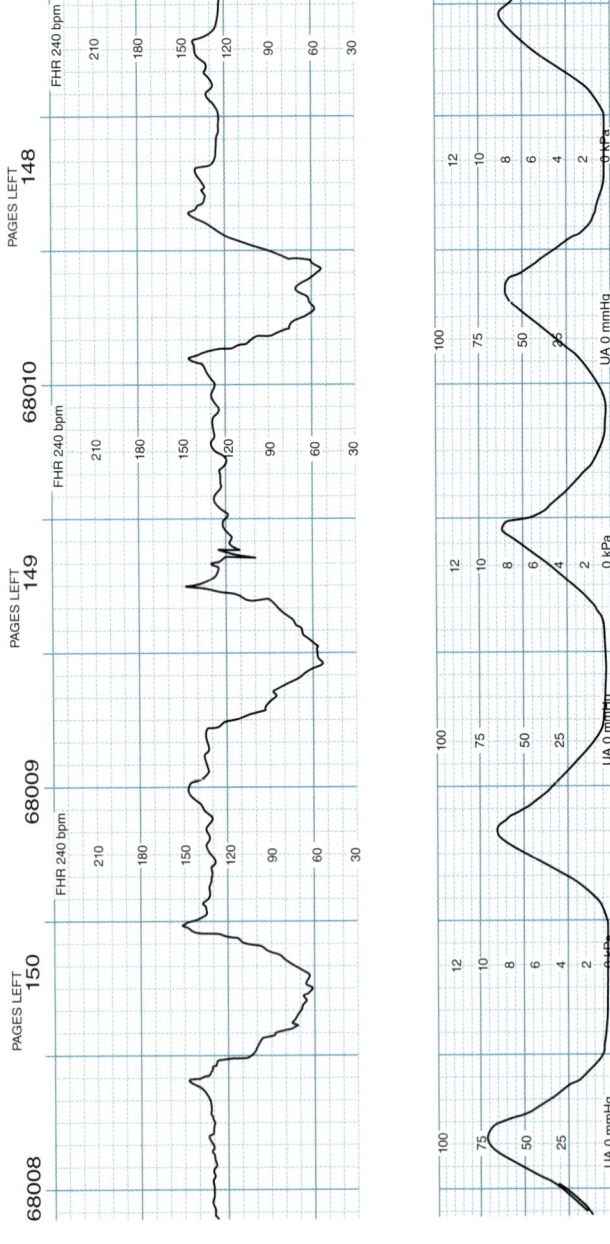

Figure 1–6. FHR tracing (reproduced, with permission, from Eugene C. Toy, MD).

1.2 **C. Arrest of descent.** A 3-hour second stage of labor still is abnormal, even with epidural analgesia. An anthropoid pelvis, which predisposes to the persistent fetal occiput posterior position, is characterized by a pelvis with an anteroposterior diameter greater than the transverse diameter with prominent ischial spines and a narrow anterior segment. The baby is at "0" station, meaning that the presenting part (in most cases, the bony part of the fetal head) is right at the plane of the ischial spines and not at the pelvic inlet. Station refers to the relationship of the presenting bony part of the fetal head in relation to the ischial spines, and not the pelvic inlet. Engagement refers to the relationship of the widest diameter of the presenting part and its location with reference to the pelvic inlet. Manual rotation of the fetal head may be considered in selected circumstances.

1.3 **E. This is normal labor.** This patient is <6 cm dilated, so she is still in the latent phase of labor. The upper limits of normal of latent labor are 20 hours for nullipara and 14 hours for multipara.

1.4 **C. Bloody show** or loss of the cervical mucus plug is often a sign of impending labor. The sticky mucus admixed with blood can differentiate bloody show from antepartum bleeding. Placenta previa, placental abruption, and vasa previa are all associated with antepartum bleeding. A cervical laceration typically occurs during a vaginal delivery. They may be associated with postpartum hemorrhage.

1.5 **C. Increased neonatal complications.** Delivery <39 weeks' gestation, such as by induction of labor or scheduled cesarean, is associated with an increased risk of neonatal complications including increased incidence of neonatal intensive care unit admission, respiratory difficulties, sepsis, hyperbilirubinemia, ventilator use, and hospital stay exceeding 5 days. For this reason, the American College of Obstetricians and Gynecologists (ACOG) and the American Academy of Pediatricians (AAP) recommend against delivery <39 weeks without a medical indication.

1.6 **B. Continued observation on oxytocin** is the best plan for prolonged latent phase, with the same definitions as per Friedman's data (20 hours for nulliparous women and 14 hours for multiparous women). Prolonged latent phase should not be a reason for cesarean delivery, and almost always, a patient will reach the active phase of labor. Once a patient has a favorable cervix (generally beyond 2-3 cm, but also taking into account effacement, softness of the cervix and station), cervical ripening with misoprostol or Foley bulb is not helpful. The patient has ruptured membranes (amniotomy) and therefore is not a candidate to be discharged.

1.7 **G. Terbutaline may be helpful.** This is a uterine contraction pattern of excessive number of contractions or tachysystole. There are seven contractions in the 9-minute window illustrated and late decelerations. The use of a beta-mimetic agent such as terbutaline will bring about uterine relaxation and hopefully resolve the late decelerations. The tachysystole is likely due to excessive oxytocin. Thus, the oxytocin should also be turned off.

1.8 **F. Scalp stimulation may be useful.** This patient is in the latent phase of labor. The FHR strip is category II, indeterminate due to the lack of accelerations and minimal variability; the pattern in and of itself is not necessarily alarming, but when the clinical picture is taken as a whole, it may become worrisome. For instance, if the FHR pattern preceding was category I, this may just be a sleep cycle, and bears reevaluation in 10 minutes; however, if this pattern of minimal variability and lack of accelerations persist, fetal hypoxia may be present. A fetal scalp stimulation inducing an acceleration would be reassuring and allow continued observation of this tracing.

1.9 **A. Amnioinfusion may help with this pattern.** This 18-year-old nulliparous patient is progressing into the active phase of labor. She is having repetitive deep variable decelerations and an amnioinfusion would help to alleviate the cord compression and hopefully, allow for a vaginal delivery. Studies have shown that amnioinfusion for variable decelerations reduces the risk for cesarean.

1.10 **C. The vasopressive sympathomimetic agent ephedrine may help.** This patient is having late decelerations likely due to the hypotension from the epidural analgesia. IV fluid hydration would be the first course of action, and if unsuccessful, then a vasopressor agent such as ephedrine would be useful; theoretically, ephedrine causes vasoconstriction of the peripheral vasculature and spares the uterine arteries. The corrective actions usually lead to resolution of the late decelerations fairly rapidly. The mechanism of the action of epidural-induced hypotension is sympathetic blockade leading to vasodilation. Prior to administration of regional anesthesia, a patient typically will receive an IV fluid bolus as a preventive measure.

CLINICAL PEARLS

▶ The normalcy of labor is determined by assessing the cervical change versus time. Normal labor should be observed.

▶ Cesarean delivery (for labor abnormalities) in the absence of clear cephalopelvic disproportion is generally reserved for arrest of active phase and ROM with adequate uterine contractions for at least 4 hours, or inadequate uterine contractions for at least 6 hours.

▶ Adequate uterine contractions is not a precise definition, but is commonly judged as >200 Montevideo units with an internal uterine pressure catheter, or by uterine contractions every 2 to 3 minutes, firm on palpation, and lasting at least 40 to 60 seconds.

▶ In general, latent labor occurs when the cervix is less than 6 cm dilated and active labor when the cervix is >6 cm dilated.

▶ Early decelerations are mirror images of uterine contractions, caused by fetal head compressions.

- Variable decelerations are abrupt in decline and abrupt in resolution and are caused by cord compression.
- Late decelerations are gradual in shape and are offset from the uterine contractions, caused by uteroplacental insufficiency (hypoxia).
- The normal fetal heart rate baseline is between 110 and 160 bpm.
  - Fetal scalp stimulation inducing an acceleration is reassuring for an umbilical cord pH >7.20.
  - Amnioinfusion can be helpful in the face of repetitive variable decelerations.
  - Category II FHR patterns are the most common and have a wide variety of clinical significance.

REFERENCES

American College of Obstetricians and Gynecologists. Management of intrapartum fetal heart rate tracings. *ACOG Practice Bulletin 116*. Washington, DC; 2010.

American College of Obstetricians and Gynecologists. Safe prevention of the primary cesarean delivery. *Obstetric Care Consensus No. 1*, March 2014.

Cunningham FG, Leveno KJ, Bloom SL, Hauth JC, Gilstrap LC III, Wenstrom KD. Dystocia: abnormal labor and fetopelvic disproportion. In: *Williams Obstetrics*. 23rd ed. New York, NY: McGraw-Hill; 2010:495-520.

Hobel CJ, Zakowski M. Normal labor, delivery, and postpartum care: anatomic considerations, obstetric and analgesia, and resuscitation of the newborn. In: Hacker NF, Gambone JC, Hobel CJ, eds. *Essentials of Obstetrics and Gynecology*. 5th ed. Philadelphia, PA: Saunders; 2009: 91-118.

CASE 2

A 29-year-old G2P1 woman at 20 weeks' gestation is seen for her second prenatal visit. Her antenatal history is unremarkable except for a urinary tract infection treated with an antibiotic 2 weeks ago. The patient was noted to be anemic on her prenatal screen with a hemoglobin level of 9.5 g/dL and a mean corpuscular volume (MCV) of 70 fL. On examination, her blood pressure (BP) is 100/60 mm Hg, heart rate (HR) 80 beats per minute (bpm), and she is afebrile. The thyroid gland appears normal on palpation. The heart and lung examinations are unremarkable. The fundus is at the umbilicus. The fetal heart tones are in the 140- to 150-bpm range. The evaluation of the anemia includes: ferritin level: 90 mcg/L (normal 30-100); serum iron: 140 mcg/dL (normal 50-150); hemoglobin electrophoresis: Hb A1 of 95% and Hb A2 of 5.5% (normal 2.2%-3.5%).

▶ What is the most likely diagnosis?
▶ What is the underlying mechanism?
▶ What is the significance of the anemia to the pregnancy?

ANSWERS TO CASE 2:
Anemia in Pregnancy (Thalassemia Trait)

Summary: A 29-year-old G2P1 woman at 20 weeks' gestation is being seen for prenatal care. On examination, her BP is 100/60, HR 80 bpm, and temperature is normal. Her hemoglobin level is 9.5 g/dL, with an elevated Hb A2 level.

- **Most likely diagnosis:** Anemia due to β-thalassemia minor.
- **Underlying mechanism:** Decreased β-globin chain production.
- **Significance of the anemia to pregnancy:** Although there is a small risk of intrauterine growth restriction, the pregnancy is usually uncomplicated. Because there is risk of the baby developing thalassemia major, genetic testing and evaluation of the father of the baby should be offered.

ANALYSIS
Objectives

1. Know that iron deficiency and thalassemia are common causes of microcytic anemia.
2. Understand that deficiency of folate and vitamin B_{12} are causes of macrocytic anemia.
3. Know the diagnostic approach to anemia in pregnancy.

Considerations

This pregnant patient has a mild anemia, since the hemoglobin level is less than 10.5 g/dL. The red blood cell (RBC) indices give an indication of the etiology. In this case, the MCV is low, microcytic. The most common cause of microcytic anemia is iron deficiency. Typically, with a mild microcytic anemia in the absence of risk factors for thalassemia (such as Southeast Asian ethnicity), a trial of iron supplementation and recheck of the hemoglobin in 3 weeks would be the next step. This is called a therapeutic trial of iron. If the hemoglobin level improves, the evidence supports iron deficiency. If the hemoglobin level does not improve, iron studies and a hemoglobin electrophoresis would be the next step. In this case, iron studies were performed which were normal/high normal, thus eliminating iron deficiency as a cause. The hemoglobin electrophoresis studies strongly suggest β-thalassemia trait (heterozygous for β-thalassemia) with the elevated A2 hemoglobin. If the patient had β-thalassemia homozygous disease, there would have been complications and clinical manifestations since childhood. The patient should now be counseled about her laboratory findings, and referred for genetic counseling, and instructed that her baby has a one in four risk for β-thalassemia disease if the father of the baby also has β-thalassemia trait. Extra iron should not be given, since these patients can be prone to iron overload.

APPROACH TO:
Anemia in Pregnancy Thalassemia

DEFINITIONS

ANEMIA: A hemoglobin level of less than 10.5 g/dL in the pregnant woman.

IRON DEFICIENCY ANEMIA: A fall in hemoglobin level that is due to insufficient iron to meet the increased iron requirements in pregnancy.

THALASSEMIA: A decreased production of one or more of the peptide chains (most common are the α and β chains) that make up the globin molecule. This process may result in ineffective erythropoiesis, hemolysis, and varying degrees of anemia.

HEMOLYTIC ANEMIA: An abnormally low hemoglobin level due to red blood cell destruction, which may be divided into congenital causes and acquired causes.

GLUCOSE-6-PHOSPHATE DEHYDROGENASE DEFICIENCY: An X-linked condition whereby the red blood cells may have a decreased capacity for anaerobic glucose metabolism. Certain oxidizing agents, such as nitrofurantoin, can lead to hemolysis.

CLINICAL APPROACH

Physiology of Pregnancy

Anemia is a common complication in the pregnant woman. It is **most often due to iron deficiency**, partially because of decreased iron stores prior to pregnancy and increased demands for iron (due to fetus need and expanded maternal blood volume). A hemoglobin level below 10.5 g/dL is usually considered a sign of anemia in the pregnant woman, with a mild anemia between 8 and 10 g/dL and severe as less than 7g/dL.

Iron Deficiency

A gravid woman who presents with mild anemia and no risk factors for hemoglobinopathies (African-American, Southeast Asian, or Mediterranean descent) may be treated with supplemental iron and the hemoglobin level reassessed in 3 to 4 weeks. Persistent anemia necessitates an evaluation for iron stores, such as ferritin level (low with iron deficiency) and hemoglobin electrophoresis.

Hemoglobinopathies

The size of the red blood cell may give a clue about the etiology. A microcytic anemia is most commonly due to iron deficiency, although thalassemia may also be causative. Results from a **hemoglobin electrophoresis** can differentiate between the two, and may also indicate the presence of sickle cell trait or sickle cell anemia. The different types of **thalassemias** are classified according to the deficient peptide chain. In β-thalassemia minor, for example, there is a decreased production of the β-globin chain. This particular thalassemia during pregnancy is usually safe for both the mother and fetus, and there is no specific therapy given other than prophylactic folic acid. Patients may be asymptomatic and go their whole life without being aware that they have β-thalassemia minor. Genetic counseling in a patient with a known hemoglobinopathy is important because if the baby inherits a recessive trait from both parents, it will typically be born with a more serious or fatal disease (ie, β-thalassemia major). A neonate born with β-thalassemia major may appear healthy at birth, but as the hemoglobin F level falls (and no β-chains are able to replace the diminishing γ-chains of the fetal hemoglobin), the infant may become severely anemic and fail to thrive if not adequately transfused. The life expectancy with transfusions is somewhere in the third decade.

Whereas the thalassemias are *quantitative* defects in a hemoglobin chain production, sickle cell disease involves a *qualitative* defect that results in a sickle-shaped and rigid hemoglobin molecule. **Sickle cell anemia** is a recessive disorder caused by a point mutation in the β-globin chain in which the amino acid glutamic acid is replaced with valine. This causes improper folding of the hemoglobin molecule, which results in either sickle cell disease (HbSS) or sickle cell trait (HbS), when only the sickle cell trait is inherited. A patient with **sickle cell trait** should not be discouraged to get pregnant as far as risk to her is concerned; however, her baby has a 1:4 chance of inheriting sickle cell disease if the father also has the sickle cell trait. Infants born with sickle cell disease typically do not show signs of being affected until about 4 months. Patients with sickle cell disease usually deal with symptoms related to anemia (ie, fatigue and shortness of breath) and pain. In pregnancy, women with sickle cell disease often have a more intense anemia, more frequent bouts of **sickle cell crisis** (painful vaso-occlusive episodes), and more frequent infections and pulmonary complications. Careful attention must be taken when a pregnant sickle cell patient presents in crisis because some of the symptoms may mimic other common occurrences during pregnancy (ectopic pregnancy, placental abruption, pyelonephritis, appendicitis, or cholecystitis), and they may be missed. All causes of fever, pain, and low Hg laboratory value should be considered before attributing it to a pain crisis. Also, these patients have a higher incidence of fetal growth retardation and perinatal mortality; therefore, serial ultrasonography is recommended.

Macrocytic Anemia

Macrocytic anemias may be due to vitamin B_{12} and folate deficiency. Because vitamin B_{12} stores last for many years, megaloblastic anemias in pregnancy are much more likely to be caused by folate deficiency.

Other Conditions

Less commonly, a woman with glucose-6-phosphate dehydrogenase (G6PD) deficiency may develop hemolytic anemia triggered by various medications such as sulfonamides, nitrofurantoin, and antimalarial agents. Nitrofurantoin is a common medication utilized for uncomplicated urinary tract infections. Affected women usually have dark-colored urine due to bilirubinuria, jaundice, and fatigue due to anemia. G6PD deficiency is more commonly seen in the African-American population.

In the pregnant woman with anemia, jaundice, and thrombocytopenia, the examiner must also consider other hemolytic processes, such as **HELLP (hemolysis, elevated liver enzymes, low platelets) syndrome,** which is a life-threatening condition best treated by delivery. In evaluating anemia, if other hematologic cell lines are also decreased, such as the white blood cell (WBC) count or platelet count, a bone marrow process, such as leukemia or tuberculosis infection of the marrow, should be considered. Bone marrow biopsy may be indicated in these circumstances.

COMPREHENSION QUESTIONS

2.1 A 30-year-old G1P0 woman complains of nausea and vomiting for the first 3 months of her pregnancy. She is noted to have a hemoglobin level of 9.0 g/dL and a mean corpuscular volume of 110 fL (normal 90-105 fL). Which of the following is the most likely etiology of the anemia?

A. Iron deficiency

B. Folate deficiency

C. Vitamin B_{12} deficiency

D. Physiologic anemia of pregnancy

2.2 A 29-year-old G2P1 woman at 28 weeks' gestation, who had normal hemoglobin level 4 weeks ago at her first prenatal visit, complains of 1 week of fatigue and now has a hemoglobin level of 7.0 g/dL. She noted dark-colored urine after taking an antibiotic for a urinary tract infection. Which of the following is the most likely diagnosis?

A. Iron deficiency anemia

B. Thalassemia

C. Hemolysis

D. Folate deficiency

E. Vitamin B_{12} deficiency

2.3 A 33-year-old African-American G1P0 woman at 16 weeks' gestation is diagnosed with sickle cell trait. Her husband also is a carrier for the sickle cell gene. Which of the following best describes the likelihood that their unborn baby will have sickle cell disease?

A. 1/100

B. 1/50

C. 1/10

D. 1/4

2.4 A 36-year-old G2P1 woman at 24 weeks' gestation is noted to have fatigue of 4 weeks' duration. Her hemoglobin level is 8.0 g/dL, leukocyte count is 2.0 cells/µL, and platelet count is 20 000/µL. Which of the following is the most likely diagnosis?
   A. Iron deficiency anemia
   B. HELLP syndrome
   C. Preeclampsia with severe features
   D. Acute leukemia

2.5 A 31-year-old G3P2 woman at 34 weeks' gestation presents to the OB Triage Unit due to nausea and "not feeling well." The BP is 110/82. The fetal heart rate pattern is category 1. The hemoglobin level is 9.0 g/dL leukocyte count of 8000 cells/mL and platelet count is 84 000/fL, ALT of 500 IU/L, AST 550 IU/L, and bilirubin of 2.5 mg/dL. Which of the following is the most likely diagnosis?
   A. Acute leukemia
   B. HELLP syndrome
   C. Hepatitis infection
   D. Preeclampsia with severe features
   E. Viral illness

2.6 A 28-year-old G1P0 woman who is at 32 weeks' gestation with sickle cell anemia is admitted to the hospital for vaso-oclusive pain crisis due to severe pain of the back and hands. She is treated with intravenous fluids and oxygen and pain control. On hospital day 2, she develops acute dyspnea, and has an oxygen saturation level of 85% on room air. Her vital signs are: T 98.2°F, BP 130/80 mm Hg, HR 100 bpm, and RR 36/minute and labored. A chest x-ray shows a new left lower lobe infiltrate. A computed tomography (CT) angiography study is negative. Which of the following is the best treatment for this patient?
   A. Anticoagulation
   B. Antibiotic therapy
   C. Beta-agonist respiratory therapy
   D. Diuretic therapy
   E. Exchange transfusion

ANSWERS

2.1 **B.** This is a macrocytic anemia because the mean corpuscular volume is above normal. Macrocytic anemias include folate deficiency and vitamin B_{12} deficiency; however, folate deficiency is more commonly seen in pregnancy than vitamin B12 deficiency. Iron deficiency is a microcytic anemia (MCV below normal), and it is the most common cause of anemia in pregnancy. Physiologic anemia of pregnancy is a result of the physiologic hemodilution that occurs in the vasculature. There is a disproportionate increase in plasma volume over the increased RBC volume, and this "diluted state" also gives the appearance of a fall in the laboratory values of hemoglobin and hematocrit.

2.2 **C.** This 29-year-old woman at 28 weeks' gestation complains of fatigue. She took an antibiotic for a urinary tract infection and then developed dark-colored urine. She was also probably icteric. Currently, her hemoglobin level is low, reflecting anemia. This constellation of symptoms likely reflects a hemolytic process probably due to G6PD deficiency. The dark urine suggests bilirubinuria. Other causes of hemolysis could include malaria, HELLP syndrome, autoimmune hemolytic anemia, or sickle cell crisis. In this case, the woman ingested an antibiotic, which likely was nitrofurantoin, a commonly prescribed medication for pregnant women. She does not have hypertension, symptoms of systemic lupus erythematosus or other autoimmune diseases, or pain suggestive of sickle cell disease.

2.3 **D.** With autosomal recessive disorders, when both parents are heterozygous for the gene (gene carriers), then there is a 1:4 chance that the offspring will be affected by the disease or will be homozygous for the gene. It is important for expectant mothers, who are at high risk for having sickle cell disease or trait, to get a hemoglobin electrophoresis in addition to other prenatal laboratory tests. They need to know what risks they may have during pregnancy and be counseled on how to have a healthy pregnancy with sickle cell disease. They should also know what kinds of risks they may have in either passing the disease or trait to their children and may seek genetic counseling for this reason. During pregnancy, pain crisis may be more severe, so it is especially important for these women to stay well hydrated and avoid dehydration. There is an increased rate of preterm labor and having a low-birthweight baby in a sickle cell patient, but with proper prenatal care, these women can have perfectly normal pregnancies.

2.4 **D.** Pancytopenia, a reduction in the number of RBCs, WBCs, and platelets circulating throughout the body, suggests a bone marrow process. None of the other answer choices involve low leukocyte counts (leucopenia). Low platelets (thrombocytopenia) may also be a manifestation of severe preeclampsia, and is part of the criteria for HELLP syndrome as well. Iron deficiency anemia involves low hemoglobin levels and is common in pregnancy due to decreased iron stored prior to pregnancy, and increased demands for iron during pregnancy. Since this patient's blood work showed low WBCs, a bone marrow biopsy should be done. A pregnant woman with leukemia may require chemotherapy, which poses a risk of intrauterine growth retardation to the developing fetus. Acute leukemia itself carries a risk for preterm labor, spontaneous abortion, and stillbirth.

2.5 **B.** This patient likely has HELLP syndrome, which is hemolysis, elevated liver enzymes, and low platelets. An elevated serum LDH or evidence of fragmented erythrocytes would "clinch" the diagnosis. It is unlikely to be preeclampsia with normal blood pressure. There is no urine protein given, which would be elevated in preeclampsia. The leukocyte count is normal, speaking against leukemia. A viral illness can lead to mildly low platelets (100 000-120 000/fL), and slightly elevated liver function tests (ALT 100-150 UI/mL), but not to this extent. Acute hepatitis should not affect the platelet count, and usually leads to ALT levels above 1500 IU/mL.

2.6 **E.** This patient likely has acute chest syndrome, which is vaso-occlusive disease of the lungs, leading to a new pulmonary infiltrate, acute dyspnea, and hypoxia. Pneumonia is a possibility but the patient does not have a fever or cough. Pulmonary embolism is less likely due to the negative CT angiography examination, which is treated with anticoagulation. There is no history of asthma or report of wheezing on examination, which would be treated with beta-agonist therapy. Acute chest syndrome that is severe is usually treated with a partial exchange transfusion. Antibiotics are also administered in case pneumonia is present.

CLINICAL PEARLS

▶ The most common cause of anemia in pregnancy is iron deficiency.

▶ The two most common causes of microcytic anemia are iron deficiency and thalassemia.

▶ An elevated A2 hemoglobin level is suggestive of β-thalassemia disorder, whereas an elevated hemoglobin F level is suggestive of α-thalassemia.

▶ For mild anemias, it is acceptable to initiate a trial of iron supplementation and reassess the hemoglobin level.

▶ The most common cause of megaloblastic anemia in pregnancy is folate deficiency.

- ▶ Hemolysis in individuals with glucose-6-phosphate dehydrogenase deficiency may be triggered by sulfonamides, nitrofurantoin, or antimalarial agents.

- ▶ Patients with sickle cell anemia may develop vaso-occlusive crisis. Acute chest syndrome affects the lungs and is diagnosed by a new pulmonary infiltrate, dyspnea, hypoxia after ruling out pulmonary embolism or pneumonia.

- ▶ Acute chest syndrome, a complication of sickle cell disease, when severe is best treated with partial exchange transfusion.

REFERENCES

American College of Obstetricians and Gynecologists. Anemia in pregnancy. *ACOG Practice Bulletin* 95. Washington, DC; 2008.

Castro LC, Ognyemi D. Common medical and surgical conditions complicating pregnancy. In: Hacker NF, Gambone JC, Hobel CJ, eds. *Essentials of Obstetrics and Gynecology*. 5th ed. Philadelphia, PA: Saunders; 2009:191-218.

Cunningham FG, Leveno KJ, Bloom SL, Hauth JC, Gilstrap LC III, Wenstrom KD. Hematological disorders. In: *Williams Obstetrics*. 23rd ed. New York, NY: McGraw-Hill Education; 2010:1043-1167.

Cunningham FG, Leveno KJ, Bloom SL, Hauth JC, Gilstrap LC III, Wenstrom KD. Teratology, drugs, and medications. In: *Williams Obstetrics*. 24th ed. New York, NY: McGraw-Hill Education; 2014:1021.

CASE 3

After a 4-hour labor, a 31-year-old G4P3 woman undergoes an uneventful vaginal delivery of a 7 lb 8 oz infant over an intact perineum. During her labor, she is noted to have mild variable decelerations and accelerations that increase 20 beats per minute (bpm) above the baseline heart rate. At delivery, the male baby has Apgar scores of 8 at 1 minute, and 9 at 5 minute. Slight lengthening of the cord occurs after 28 minutes along with a small gush of blood per vagina. As the placenta is being delivered, a shaggy, reddish, bulging mass is noted at the introitus around the placenta.

▶ What is the most likely diagnosis?
▶ What is the most likely complication to occur in this patient?

ANSWERS TO CASE 3:
Uterine Inversion

Summary: A 31-year-old G4P3 woman has a normal vaginal delivery of her baby; after slight lengthening of the cord, a reddish mass is noted bulging in the introitus.

- **Most likely diagnosis:** Uterine inversion.
- **Most likely complication:** Postpartum hemorrhage.

ANALYSIS

Objectives

1. Know the signs of spontaneous placental separation.
2. Recognize the clinical presentation of uterine inversion.
3. Understand that the most common cause of uterine inversion is undue traction of the cord before placental separation.

Considerations

This patient's history reveals that the first and second stages of labor are normal. The third stage of labor (placental delivery) reaches close to the upper limits of normal. There is evidence for **partial** placental separation, but there were not clear signs of **complete** placental separation such as lengthening of the cord. The four signs of placental separation are (1) gush of blood, (2) lengthening of the cord, (3) globular and firm shape of the uterus, and (4) the uterus rises up to the anterior abdominal wall. In this case, although there is not good evidence for placental separation, traction on the cord is exerted, which results in an inverted uterus. The reddish bulging mass noted adjacent to the placenta is the endometrial surface; hence, the mass will have a shaggy appearance and be all around the placenta. Other masses and/or organs may at times prolapse, such as vaginal or cervical tissue, but these will have a smooth appearance.

APPROACH TO:
Inverted Uterus

DEFINITIONS

ACTIVE MANAGEMENT OF THIRD STAGE OF LABOR: Maneuvers that attempt to facilitate delivery of the placenta to promote uterine contractions and reduce blood loss.

PHYSIOLOGIC MANAGEMENT OF THIRD STAGE OF LABOR: Allowing the natural separation of the placenta before taking any intervention.

THIRD STAGE OF LABOR: From delivery of infant to the delivery of the placenta (upper limit of normal is 30 minutes).

ABNORMALLY RETAINED PLACENTA: Third stage of labor that has exceeded 30 minutes.

UTERINE INVERSION: A "turning inside out" of the uterus; whereupon the fundus of the uterus moves through the cervix, into the vagina (Figure 3–1).

SIGNS OF PLACENTAL SEPARATION: Cord lengthening, gush of blood, globular uterine shape, and uterus lifting up to the anterior abdominal wall.

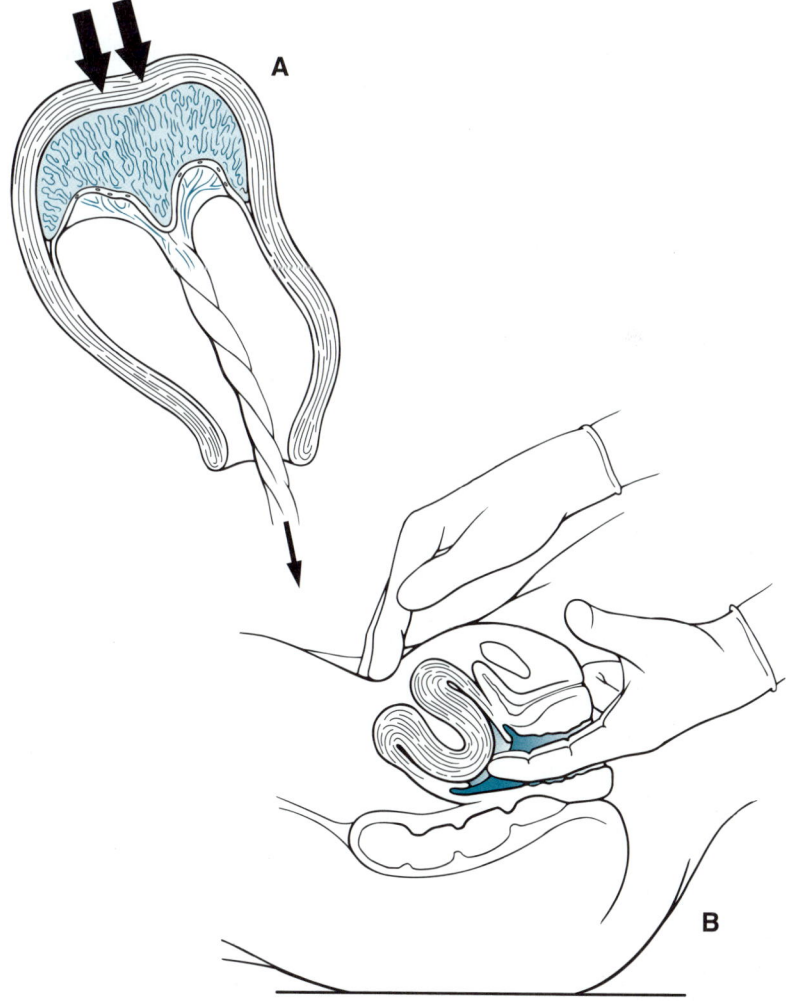

Figure 3–1. Inverted uterus. Uterine inversion can occur when excessive umbilical cord traction is exerted on a fundally implanted, unseparated placenta (**A**). Upon recognition, the operator attempts to reposition the inverted uterus using cupped fingers (**B**).

CLINICAL APPROACH

After a vaginal delivery, 95% of women experience spontaneous placenta separation within 30 minutes. Because the uterus and placenta are no longer joined, the placenta is usually in the lower segment of the uterus, just inside the cervix, and the uterus is often contracted. The umbilical cord lengthens due to the placenta having dropped into the lower portion of the uterus. The gush of blood represents bleeding from the placental bed, usually coinciding with placental separation. If the placenta has not separated, excessive force on the cord may lead to uterine inversion. Massive hemorrhage usually results; thus, in this situation, the practitioner must be prepared for rapid volume replacement. Although it was classically taught by some that the shock was out of proportion to the actual amount of blood loss, this is not the case. In other words, the shock is due to massive hemorrhage.

The best method of averting a uterine inversion is to await spontaneous separation of the placenta from the uterus before placing traction on the umbilical cord. Even after one or two signs of placental separation are present, the operator should be cautious not to put undue tension on the cord. At times, part of the placenta may separate, revealing the gush of blood, but the remaining attached placenta may induce a uterine inversion or traumatic severing of the cord. The grand-multiparous patient with the placenta implanted in the fundus (top of uterus) is at particular risk for uterine inversion. A placenta accreta, an abnormally adherent placenta, is also a risk factor.

TREATMENT

With the diagnosis of an inverted uterus, immediate assistance—including that of an anesthesiologist—is essential because a uterine relaxation anesthetic agent, such as halothane (for uterine replacement), and/or emergency surgery may be necessary. If the placenta has already separated, the recently inverted uterus may sometimes be replaced by using the gloved palm and cupped fingers. Two intravenous lines should be started as soon as possible and preferably prior to placental separation, since **profuse hemorrhage** may follow placental removal. Terbutaline or magnesium sulfate can also be utilized to relax the uterus if necessary prior to uterine replacement. Upon replacing the uterine fundus to the normal location, the relaxation agents are stopped, and then uterotonic agents, such as oxytocin, are given to prevent re-inversion and also to slow down the bleeding. Placement of the clinician's fist inside the uterus to maintain the normal structure of the uterus may help to prevent re-inversion.

Note: Even with optimal treatment of uterine inversion, hemorrhage is almost a certainty.

CURRENT CONTROVERSY

There is robust debate about whether active management or physiologic management of the third stage of labor is best. Table 3–1 shows the differences between these two interventions. In several studies, active management slightly reduces the incidence of postpartum hemorrhage, probably due to early use of uterotonic agents (usually after delivery of the baby's anterior shoulder). Examples of

Table 3–1 • ACTIVE MANAGEMENT VERSUS PHYSIOLOGIC MANAGEMENT OF THE THIRD STAGE OF LABOR

	Active Management	Physiologic Management
Uterotonic agents	None, or after placenta has delivered	With delivery of the anterior shoulder
Cord traction	None until clear signs of placental separation	Controlled cord traction when uterus contracted
Assessment of uterus	Uterine size and tone	Uterine size and tone

uterotonic agents include oxytocin, misoprostol, or ergotamine. Proponents of physiologic management of labor argue that there is less risk of entrapment of a retained placenta (due to difficulty with manual separation when uterotonic agents are given), and less chance of uterine inversion. There is currently no consensus of the best method.

COMPREHENSION QUESTIONS

3.1 A 23-year-old G1P0 woman at 38 weeks' gestation delivered a 7 lb 4 oz baby boy vaginally. Upon delivery of the placenta, there was noted to be an inverted uterus, which was successfully managed including replacement of the uterus. Which of the following placental implantation sites would most likely predispose to an inverted uterus?

A. Fundal
B. Anterior
C. Posterior
D. Lateral
E. Lower segment

3.2 A 24-year-old woman underwent a normal vaginal delivery of a term infant female. After the delivery, the placenta does not deliver even after 30 minutes. Which of the following would be the next step for this patient?

A. Initiate oxytocin
B. Wait for an additional 30 minutes
C. Hysterectomy
D. Attempt a manual extraction of the placenta
E. Misoprostol estrogen intravaginally

3.3 A 32-year-old G1P0 woman at 40 weeks' gestation undergoes a normal vaginal delivery. Delivery of the placenta is complicated by an inverted uterus, with subsequent hemorrhage leading to 1500 mL of blood loss. She is managed with a transfusion of erythrocytes. Which of the following is the best explanation of the mechanism of hemorrhage?
   A. Inverted uterus stretches the uterus, causing trauma to blood vessels leading to bleeding.
   B. Inverted uterus leads to inability for an adequate myometrial contraction effect.
   C. Inverted uterus causes a local coagulopathy reaction to the uterus and endometrium.
   D. Inverted uterus causes muscular abrasions and lacerations leading to bleeding.

3.4 A 33-year-old G5P5 woman, who is being induced for preeclampsia, delivers a 9 lb baby. Upon delivery of the placenta, uterine inversion is noted. The physician attempts to replace the uterus, but the cervix is tightly contracted, preventing the fundus of the uterus from being repositioned. Which of the following is the best therapy for this patient?
   A. Vaginal hysterectomy
   B. Dührssen incisions of the cervix
   C. Halothane anesthesia
   D. Discontinue the magnesium sulfate
   E. Infuse oxytocin intravenously

3.5 A 25-year-old G1P0 woman delivers a 33-week infant vaginally. The delivery is uncomplicated. If the obstetrician wishes to optimize outcome for the infant, the cord should be clamped:
   A. Immediately
   B. Between 30 and 60 seconds
   C. After 60 seconds
   D. Leave the cord unclamped until delivery of the placenta

ANSWERS

3.1 **A.** A fundally implanted placenta predisposes to uterine inversion. A placenta implanted in either the anterior, posterior, lateral, or lower segment of the uterus does not have the direct angle that a fundally implanted placenta has through the cervix and out the vagina. The best method for preventing inversion is to await spontaneous separation of the placenta from the uterus before placing traction on the umbilical cord.

3.2 **D.** After 30 minutes, the placenta is abnormally retained, and a manual extraction is generally attempted. Waiting for another 30 minutes may lead to maternal hemorrhage, which may then lead to an indication for a hysterectomy. However, a hysterectomy would not be the initial step after 30 minutes have passed during the third stage of labor. Oxytocin should not be administered until the placenta has been delivered and the uterine fundus (when inverted) is placed back to its normal location. Oxytocin is a uterotonic agent that aids in allowing the uterus to contract down on itself in an effort to stop bleeding after the placenta has been removed. Intravaginal estrogen is not indicated for this scenario and is typically prescribed to patients with vaginal atrophy.

3.3 **B.** An inverted uterus makes it impossible for the uterus to establish its normal tone, and to contract. Thus, the myometrial fibers do not exert their normal tourniquet effect on the spiral arteries. The endometrial placental bed pours out blood, which previously had been perfusing the intervillous space. Thus, uterine atony is the most common reason for hemorrhage in inverted uterus. The muscle of the uterus and the vasculature is seldom damaged. Replacing the uterus to its normal position and assisting tonicity of the uterus will alleviate the bleeding.

3.4 **C.** A uterine relaxing agent (such as halothane anesthesia) is the best initial therapy for a nonreducible uterus. Terbutaline and magnesium sulfate can also be used to relax the uterus if necessary. Oxytocin is a uterotonic agent and may be used following replacement of the uterine fundus to its normal location. Dührssen incisions are used to treat the entrapped fetal head of a breech vaginal delivery and would not be indicated for uterine inversion. A vaginal hysterectomy would not be the best treatment option for this patient either.

3.5. **B.** Delayed cord clamping of between 30 and 60 seconds is beneficial for preterm infants due to increasing total iron stores and hemoglobin levels, and decreasing the risk of intraventricular hemorrhage in the infants. Immediate birth outcomes such as Apgar scores, umbilical cord pH, or respiratory distress is unaffected by the timing of cord clamping. Delayed cord clamping also improves iron stores in term infants, but may also lead to a higher risk of hyperbilirubinemia.

CLINICAL PEARLS

▶ Although it can occur spontaneously, one of the most common causes of inverted uterus is undue traction on the cord when the placenta has not yet separated.

▶ The signs of placental separation are (1) gush of blood, (2) lengthening of the cord, (3) globular-shaped uterus, and (4) the uterus rising to the anterior abdominal wall.

▶ Hemorrhage is a common complication of an inverted uterus due to uterine atony associated with inversion.

▶ The upper limit of normal for the third stage of labor (time between delivery of the infant and delivery of the placenta) is 30 minutes.

▶ When the placenta does not deliver spontaneously after 30 minutes, then a manual extraction of the placenta should be attempted.

▶ There is current controversy about whether active management or physiologic management of the third stage of labor is best.

▶ Active management of the third stage of labor seems to decrease the risk of postpartum hemorrhage.

REFERENCES

American College of Obstetricians and Gynecologists. Postpartum hemorrhage. *ACOG Practice Bulletin 76*. Washington, DC; American College of Obstetricians and Gynecologists; 2006. (Reaffirmed 2011.)

Baskett TF. Acute uterine inversion: a review of 40 cases. *J Obstet Gyneacol Can*. 2002;24:953-57.

Cunningham FG, Leveno KJ, Bloom SL, Gilstrap LC III, Hauth JC, Wenstrom KD. Obstetrical hemorrhage. In: *Williams Obstetrics*. 24th ed. New York, NY: McGraw-Hill; 2014:809-854.

Kim M, Hyashi RH, Gambone JC. Obstetrical hemorrhage and puerperal sepsis. In: Hacker NF, Gambone JC, Hobel CJ, eds. *Essentials of Obstetrics and Gynecology*. 5th ed. Philadelphia, PA: Saunders; 2009:128-138.

You WB, Zahn CM. Postpartum hemorrhage, abnormally adherent placenta, uterine inversion, and puerperal hematomas. *Clin Obstet Gynecol*. 2006;49:184.

CASE 4

A 25-year-old G2P1 woman is delivering at 42 weeks' gestation. The woman is noted to have a body mass index of 42 kg/m². The fetal weight clinically appears to be about 3700 g. After a 4-hour first stage of labor and a 2-hour second stage of labor, the fetal head delivers but is noted to be retracted back toward the patient's introitus. The fetal shoulders do not deliver, even with maternal pushing.

- What is your next step in management?
- What is a likely complication that can occur because of this situation?
- What maternal condition would most likely put the patient at risk for this condition?

ANSWERS TO CASE 4:
Shoulder Dystocia

Summary: A 25-year-old obese G2P1 woman is delivering at 42 weeks' gestation; the fetus appears clinically to be 3700 g (average weight). After a 4-hour first stage of labor and a 2-hour second stage of labor, the head delivers but the shoulders do not easily deliver.

- **Next step in management:** McRoberts maneuver (hyperflexion of the maternal hips onto the maternal abdomen and/or suprapubic pressure).
- **Likely complication:** A likely maternal complication is postpartum hemorrhage; a common neonatal complication is a brachial plexus injury such as an Erb palsy.
- **Maternal condition:** Gestational diabetes, which increases the fetal weight on the shoulders and abdomen.

ANALYSIS

Objectives

1. Understand the risk factors for shoulder dystocia.
2. Understand that shoulder dystocia is an obstetric emergency, and be familiar with the initial maneuvers used to manage this condition.
3. Know the neonatal complications that can occur with shoulder dystocia.

Considerations

The patient is multiparous and obese, both of which are risk factors although not the strongest risk factors, for shoulder dystocia. The prenatal risk factors in order of significance are (1) prior shoulder dystocia, (2) fetal macrosomia, and (3) maternal gestational diabetes. There is no indication of gestational diabetes in this patient. The patient is post-term at 42 weeks, which increases the likelihood of fetal macrosomia. The patient's prolonged second stage of labor (upper limits for a multiparous patient is 1 hour without and 2 hours with epidural analgesia) may be a nonspecific indicator of impending shoulder dystocia. Nevertheless, the diagnosis is straightforward, in that the fetal shoulders are described as not easily delivering. The fetal head is retracted back toward the maternal introitus, the "turtle sign." Because most shoulder dystocia events are unpredictable, as in this case, the clinician must be proficient in the management of this entity, particularly because of the potential for fetal injury.

SECTION II: CASES 61

APPROACH TO:
Shoulder Dystocia

DEFINITIONS

SHOULDER DYSTOCIA: Inability of the fetal shoulders to deliver spontaneously, usually due to the impaction of the anterior shoulder behind the maternal symphysis pubis.

McROBERTS MANEUVER: The maternal thighs are sharply flexed against the maternal abdomen to straighten the sacrum relative to the lumbar spine and rotate the symphysis pubis anteriorly toward the maternal head (Figure 4-1).

SUPRAPUBIC PRESSURE: The operator's hand is used to push on the suprapubic region in a downward or lateral direction in an effort to push the fetal shoulder into an oblique plane and from behind the symphysis pubis.

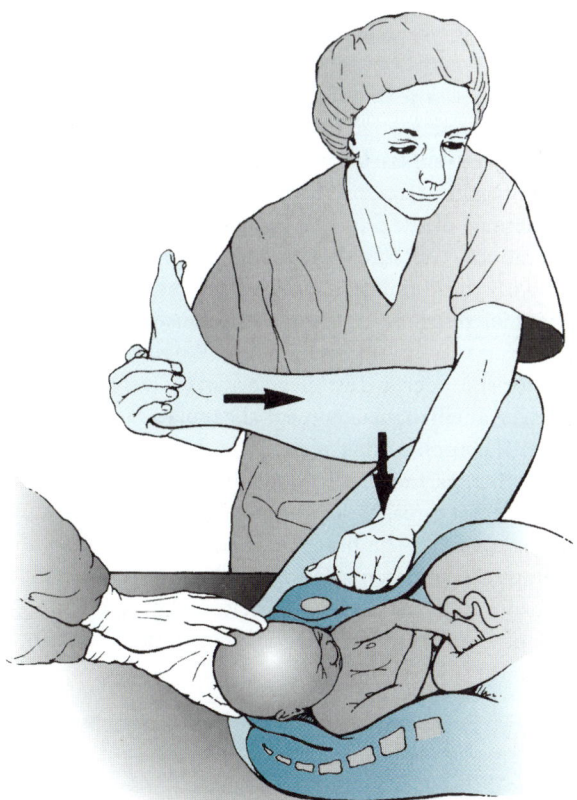

Figure 4–1. Maneuvers for shoulder dystocia. The McRoberts maneuver involves flexing the maternal thighs against the abdomen. Suprapubic pressure attempts to push the fetal shoulders into an oblique plane. (Reproduced with permission from Cunningham FG, et al. *Williams Obstetrics*. 22nd ed. New York, NY: McGraw-Hill; 2005:515.)

ERB PALSY: A brachial plexus injury involving the C5–C6 nerve roots, which may result from the downward traction of the anterior shoulder; the baby usually has weakness of the deltoid and infraspinatus muscles as well as the flexor muscles of the forearm. The arm often hangs limply by the side and is internally rotated.

CLINICAL APPROACH

Because of the unpredictability and urgency of shoulder dystocia, the clinician should rehearse its management and be ready when the situation is encountered. Shoulder dystocia should be suspected with **prior history of shoulder dystocia, fetal macrosomia, gestational diabetes**, excessive weight gain (>35 lbs) in pregnancy, maternal obesity, and prolonged second stage of labor. With gestational diabetes, the elevated fetal insulin levels are associated with increased weight centrally (shoulders and abdomen). However, it must be noted that almost one-half of all cases occur in babies weighing less than 4000 g, and shoulder dystocia is frequently unsuspected. Significant fetal hypoxia may occur with undue delay from the delivery of the head to the body. Moreover, excessive traction on the fetal head may lead to a brachial plexus injury to the baby. It should be recognized that brachial plexus injury can occur with vaginal delivery not associated with shoulder dystocia, or even with cesarean delivery. Shoulder dystocia is not resolved with more traction, but by maneuvers to relieve the impaction of the anterior shoulder (Table 4–1).

The diagnosis is suspected when external rotation of the fetal head is difficult, and the fetal head may retract back toward the maternal introitus, the "turtle sign." The diagnosis is confirmed when the baby fails to deliver with normal symmetric traction. The first actions of the fetus are nonmanipulative, such as the McRoberts maneuver and suprapubic pressure. Fortunately, the majority of shoulder dystocia cases are relieved with these nonmanipulative actions. Fundal pressure should be avoided when shoulder dystocia is diagnosed because of the increased associated neonatal injury. Other maneuvers include the Wood's corkscrew (progressively rotating the posterior shoulder in 180° in a corkscrew fashion), delivery of the posterior arm, and the Zavanelli maneuver (cephalic replacement with immediate cesarean section). Maternal complications of shoulder dystocia include both postpartum hemorrhage and vaginal/perineal lacerations. Fetal complications include brachial plexus injuries, clavicle fractures, hypoxic-ischemic encephalopathy, and even death.

One area of controversy is the practice of cesarean delivery in certain circumstances in an attempt to avoid shoulder dystocia; indications include macrosomia diagnosed on ultrasound, particularly with maternal gestational diabetes. Because of the imprecision of estimated fetal weights and prediction of shoulder dystocia,

Table 4–1 • COMMON MANEUVERS FOR TREATMENT OF SHOULDER DYSTOCIA
McRoberts maneuver (hyperflex maternal thighs)
Suprapubic pressure
Wood's corkscrew maneuver
Delivery of the posterior arm
Zavanelli maneuver (cephalic replacement and cesarean)

there is no uniform agreement regarding this practice. Operative vaginal delivery, such as vacuum- or forceps-assisted deliveries in the face of possible fetal macrosomia, may possibly increase the risk of shoulder dystocia.

COMPREHENSION QUESTIONS

4.1 A 25-year-old G1P0 woman delivers a 4000 g infant, and encounters a shoulder dystocia. Which of the following is a risk factor for this condition?
  A. Maternal gestational diabetes
  B. Fetal hydrocephalus
  C. Fetal prematurity
  D. Precipitous (fast) labor

4.2 A 30-year-old woman is noted to be in active labor at 40 weeks' gestation. Delivery of the fetal head occurs, but the fetal shoulders do not deliver with the normal traction. The fetal head is retracted toward the maternal introitus. Which of the following is a useful maneuver for this situation?
  A. Internal podalic version
  B. Suprapubic pressure
  C. Fundal pressure
  D. Intentional fracture of the fetal humerus
  E. Delivery of the anterior arm

4.3 A 3800 g male infant is delivered vaginally. A shoulder dystocia was encountered. If a neonatal injury is suspected, what is the likely finding in the infant?
  A. Arm that is fixed and flexed and hypertonic
  B. Arm that is at its side and internally rotated
  C. Clavicle fracture
  D. Depressed skull fracture
  E. Dislocated elbow

Match the following mechanisms (A-E) to the stated maneuver (4.4-4.6):
  A. Anterior rotation of the symphysis pubis
  B. Decreases the fetal bony diameter from shoulder–shoulder to shoulder–axilla
  C. Fracture of the clavicle
  D. Displaces the fetal shoulder axis from anterior–posterior to oblique
  E. Separates the maternal symphysis pubis

4.4 The clinician performs a delivery of the posterior fetal arm.

4.5 The McRoberts maneuver is utilized.

4.6 The nurse is instructed to apply the suprapubic pressure maneuver.

ANSWERS

4.1 **A.** Gestational diabetes is a risk factor because the fetal shoulders and abdomen are disproportionately bigger than the head, therefore the head may pass through with no problems, yet it is quite difficult to deliver the anterior shoulder since it is lodged behind the maternal symphysis pubis. The McRoberts maneuver and application of suprapubic pressure are two techniques that attempt to relieve the impaction of the anterior shoulder. Unlike gestational diabetes, the complication with hydrocephalus is that the fetal head is greater than the body. The head itself may have a difficult time passing through the pelvis, but if it does pass, the shoulders would have no problem passing through since their width would be smaller than the width of the fetal head. The premature fetus typically has a well-proportioned body, but is overall smaller in size than the average-sized baby. No part of a premature fetus' body should typically get impacted anywhere along the birth canal. With precipitous labor, there is a decreased chance that a shoulder dystocia will occur, whereas a prolonged second stage of labor should raise suspicion that a dystocia is present.

4.2 **B.** The patient in this question has shoulder dystocia. The McRoberts maneuver or suprapubic pressure is generally the first maneuver used. The McRoberts maneuver involves sharply flexing the maternal thighs against the maternal abdomen to straighten the sacrum relative to the lumbar spine and rotate the symphysis pubis anteriorly toward the maternal head. Applying suprapubic pressure, or pushing on the suprapubic region, relieves the fetal shoulder from being impacted behind the symphysis pubis. The internal podalic version is an obstetric procedure in which the fetus, typically in a transverse position, is rotated inside the womb to where the feet or a foot is the presenting part during labor and delivery. This method would not be applicable in this situation because the fetus is presenting in the proper cephalic position. Fracturing of the fetal humerus is a complication that can occur with shoulder dystocia if one of the fetal arms is pulled or tugged on too forcefully. Attempting to deliver the anterior shoulder in the setting of shoulder dystocia can result in a brachial plexus injury involving the C5–C6 nerve roots. As a result, the baby could have weakness of the deltoid and infraspinatus muscles as well as the flexor muscles of the forearm (Erb palsy/"Waiter's tip").

4.3 **B.** An Erb palsy is the most common injury of the neonate in a shoulder dystocia. The arm is typically limp and at its side with the arm internally rotated. If the palsy is severe, then the infant may not be able to move its fingers. Eighty percent of the time, brachial plexus injuries will improve with physical therapy. However, if the nerve roots are avulsed rather than simply injured, the neuropathy usually will not resolve.

4.4 **B.** With delivery of the posterior arm, the shoulder girdle diameter is reduced from shoulder-to-shoulder to shoulder-to-axilla, which usually allows the fetus to deliver. The danger with this maneuver is potential injury to the infant's humerus, such as a fracture. Fortunately, it is typically a simple fracture of the midshaft which heals well.

4.5 **A.** The McRoberts maneuver causes anterior rotation of the symphysis pubis and flattening of the lumbar spine. This relieves the anterior shoulder from impaction and allows for delivery of the fetus. Separating the symphysis pubis is not associated with any kind of mechanism or maneuver for relieving shoulder dystocia. Fracturing the humerus is never indicated either, and may also lead to brachial plexus injury.

4.6 **D.** The rationale of suprapubic pressure is to move the fetal shoulders from the anteroposterior to an oblique plane, allowing the shoulder to slip out from under the symphysis pubis. Applying fundal pressure would only supply a greater force of the fetal shoulder against the symphysis pubis and possibly cause a more complex and serious situation such as brachial plexus injury to the fetus.

CLINICAL PEARLS

▶ Shoulder dystocia cannot be predicted nor prevented in the majority of cases.

▶ The biggest risk factor for shoulder dystocia is fetal macrosomia, particularly in a woman who has gestational diabetes.

▶ The estimation of fetal weight is most often inaccurate, as is the diagnosis of macrosomia.

▶ The most common injury to the neonate in a shoulder dystocia is brachial plexus injury, such as Erb palsy.

▶ The first actions for shoulder dystocia are generally the McRoberts maneuver or suprapubic pressure.

▶ Fundal pressure should not be used once shoulder dystocia is encountered.

REFERENCES

American College of Obstetricians and Gynecologists. Shoulder dystocia. *ACOG Practice Bulletin 40.* Washington, DC; 2002. (Reaffirmed 2015).

Bashore RA, Ogunyemi D, Hayashi RH. Uterine contractility and dystocia. In: Hacker NF, Gambone JC, Hobel CJ, eds. *Essentials of Obstetrics and Gynecology.* 5th ed. Philadelphia, PA: Saunders; 2009:139-145.

Cunningham FG, Leveno KJ, Bloom SL, et al. Vaginal delivery—shoulder dystocia. In: *Williams Obstetrics.* 24th ed. New York, NY: McGraw-Hill Education; Chap. 27, 2014.

CASE 5

A 22-year-old G3P2 woman at 40 weeks' gestation complains of strong uterine contractions. She denies leakage of fluid per vagina. She denies medical illnesses. Her antenatal history is unremarkable. On examination, the blood pressure (BP) is 120/80 mm Hg, heart rate (HR) is 85 beats per minute (bpm), and temperature is 98°F (36.6°C). The fetal heart rate is in the 140 to 150 bpm range. The cervix is dilated at 5 cm and the vertex is at −3 station. Upon artificial rupture of membranes, fetal bradycardia to the 70 to 80 bpm range is noted for 3 minutes without recovery.

▶ What is your next step?

ANSWER TO CASE 5:
Fetal Bradycardia (Cord Prolapse)

Summary: A 22-year-old G3P2 woman at term is in labor with a cervical dilation of 5 cm; the vertex is at −3 station. Upon artificial rupture of membranes, persistent fetal bradycardia to the 70 to 80 bpm range is noted for 3 minutes.

- **Next step:** Vaginal examination to assess for umbilical cord prolapse.

ANALYSIS
Objectives

1. Understand that the first step in the evaluation of fetal bradycardia in the face of rupture of membranes should be to rule out umbilical cord prolapse.
2. Understand that the treatment for cord prolapse is emergent cesarean delivery.
3. Know that an unengaged presenting part, or a transverse fetal lies with rupture of membranes, predisposes to cord prolapse.

Considerations

This patient has had two prior deliveries. She is currently in labor and her cervix is 5 cm dilated. The fetal vertex is at −3 station, indicating that the fetal head is unengaged. With artificial rupture of membranes, fetal bradycardia is noted. This situation is very typical for a cord prolapse, where the umbilical cord protrudes through the cervical os. Usually, the fetal head will fill the pelvis and prevent the cord from prolapsing. However, with an unengaged fetal presentation, such as in this case, umbilical cord accidents are more likely. Thus, as a general rule, artificial rupture of membranes should be avoided with an unengaged fetal part. Situations such as a transverse fetal lie or a footling breech presentation are also predisposing conditions. It is not uncommon for a multiparous patient to have an unengaged fetal head during early labor. The lesson in this case is not to rupture membranes with an unengaged fetal presentation. With fetal bradycardia, the next step would be a digital examination of the vagina to assess for the umbilical cord, which would feel like a rope-like structure through the cervical os. If the umbilical cord is palpated and the diagnosis of cord prolapse confirmed, the patient should be taken for immediate cesarean delivery. The physician should place the patient in Trendelenburg position (head down), and keep his or her hand in the vagina to elevate the presenting part, thus keeping pressure off the cord.

APPROACH TO:
Fetal Bradycardia

DEFINITIONS

ENGAGEMENT: Largest transverse (biparietal) diameter of the fetal head has negotiated the bony pelvic inlet.

FETAL BRADYCARDIA: Baseline fetal heart rate <110 bpm for >10 minutes.

UMBILICAL CORD PROLAPSE: Umbilical cord enters through the cervical os presenting in front of the presenting part.

ARTIFICIAL RUPTURE OF MEMBRANES: Maneuver used to cause a perforation in the fetal chorioamniotic membranes.

CLINICAL APPROACH

The onset of fetal bradycardia should be confirmed either by internal fetal scalp electrode or ultrasound, and distinguished from the maternal pulse rate. The initial steps should be directed at improving maternal oxygenation and delivery of cardiac output to the uterus. These maneuvers include (1) placement of the patient on her side to move the uterus from the great vessels, thus improving blood return to the heart, (2) intravenous (IV) fluid bolus if the patient is possibly volume depleted, (3) administration of 100% oxygen by face mask, and (4) stopping oxytocin if it is being given (Table 5–1).

Simultaneously with these maneuvers, the practitioner should try to identify the cause of the bradycardia, such as hyperstimulation with oxytocin. With this process, the uterus will be tetanic, or the uterine contractions will be frequent (every 1 minute); often a β-agonist, such as terbutaline, given intravenously will be helpful to relax the uterine musculature. Hypotension due to an epidural catheter is another common cause. Intravenous hydration is the first remedy, and if unsuccessful, then support of the blood pressure with ephedrine, a pressor agent, is often useful. A vaginal examination, when the membranes are ruptured, is "a must" to identify overt umbilical cord prolapse. A rope-like cord will be palpated, often with pulsations (Figure 5–1). The best treatment is elevation of the presenting part digitally and emergent cesarean delivery. In women with prior cesarean delivery, uterine rupture may manifest as fetal bradycardia.

Table 5–1 • STEPS TO TAKE WITH FETAL BRADYCARDIA
Confirm fetal heart rate (vs maternal heart rate)
Vaginal examination to assess for cord prolapse
Positional changes
Oxygen
Intravenous fluid bolus and pressors if hypotension persists
Discontinue oxytocin, consider beta-agonist if tachysystole

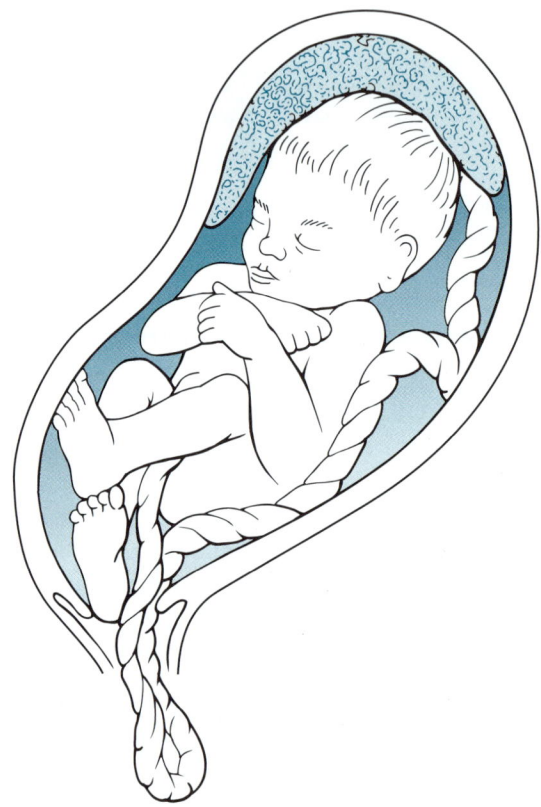

Figure 5-1. Umbilical cord prolapse. A footling breech presentation predisposes to umbilical cord prolapse.

FETAL HEART RATE ASSESSMENT

The baseline fetal heart rate is normally between 110 and 160 bpm, with fetal bradycardia <110 bpm and tachycardia >160 bpm. The fetal heart rate typically has moderate variability, whereas diminished variability may be caused by sedating medications or more rarely fetal acidosis. Accelerations are abrupt increases in fetal heart rate of at least 15 bpm lasting for 15 seconds, and typically are indicative of adequate fetal oxygenation. Decelerations may be early, late, or variable depending on its configuration and timing with the uterine contraction.

> **CASE CORRELATION**
> - See also Case 1, Normal Labor and Decelerations to review definitions of bradycardia, and types of decelerations.

COMPREHENSION QUESTIONS

5.1 An 18-year-old woman, who had undergone a previous low-transverse cesarean delivery, is admitted for active labor. During labor, an intrauterine pressure catheter displays normal uterine contractions every 3 minutes with intensity up to 60 mm Hg. Fetal bradycardia ensues. Which of the following statements is most accurate?

   A. The normal intrauterine pressure catheter display makes uterine rupture unlikely.
   B. The most common sign of uterine rupture is a fetal heart rate abnormality.
   C. If the patient has a uterine rupture, the practitioner should wait to see whether the heart tones return to decide on route of delivery.
   D. The intrauterine pressure catheter has been found to be helpful in preventing uterine rupture.

5.2 A 32-year-old G1P0 woman is at 42 weeks' gestation and being induced for post-term pregnancy. She has had an uncomplicated prenatal course. Her BP is 100/60 mm Hg. The fundal height is 40 cm. Her cervix is closed, 3 cm long, and firm on consistency. The obstetrician decides on using a cervical ripening agent with misoprostol in the vagina. Approximately 2 hours after placing the misoprostol, the patient has an episode of fetal prolonged deceleration to 80 bpm for 6 minutes. Which of the following is the most likely etiology of the prolonged deceleration?

   A. Placental abruption
   B. Sepsis
   C. Umbilical cord prolapse
   D. Uterine hyperstimulation

5.3 A 28-year-old G1P0 woman at 35 weeks' gestation is in the obstetrical (OB) triage area with spontaneous rupture of membranes. The fetal heart rate baseline is 150 bpm with normal variability. There are accelerations seen, and numerous late decelerations noted. In an effort to improve oxygenation to the fetus, which of the following maneuvers would most likely help in this circumstance?

   A. Supine position
   B. Epidural anesthesia
   C. Morphine sulfate
   D. Stop the oxytocin

5.4 A 33-year-old G2P1 woman at 39 weeks' gestation in active labor is noted to have a 10-minute episode of bradycardia on the external fetal heart rate tracing in the range of 100 bpm, which has not resolved. Her cervix is closed. Which of the following is the best initial step in management of this patient?

A. Fetal scalp pH assessment
B. Emergency cesarean delivery
C. Intravenous atropine
D. Intravenous terbutaline
E. Assess maternal pulse

5.5 A 25-year-old G1P0 woman at 38 weeks' gestation is in active labor. The patient is noted to be 5 cm dilated/100% effaced/−1 station. She is in severe pain. She received meperidine intravenously and after an hour, her pain is still severe. The patient has an epidural catheter for pain control. Her BP is 90/50 mm Hg and HR is 90 bpm. The fetal heart rate reveals a baseline of 140 bpm with persistent late decelerations. Which of the following is the best next step in managing this patient?

A. Emergency cesarean
B. Ephedrine intravenously
C. Naloxone intravenously
D. Transfusion with packed erythrocytes

ANSWERS

5.1 **B.** The most common finding in a uterine rupture is a fetal heart rate abnormality, such as fetal bradycardia, deep variable decelerations, or late decelerations. The intrauterine pressure catheter has not been found to be helpful and sometimes confuses the picture and may delay the diagnosis of uterine rupture. Immediate cesarean section is indicated for suspected uterine rupture.

5.2 **D.** Prolonged fetal decelerations or fetal bradycardia associated with misoprostol cervical ripening is typically associated with uterine hyperstimulation, defined as greater than five uterine contractions in a 10-minute window. Although any of the prostaglandin cervical ripening agents may induce uterine hyperstimulation, misoprostol generally is associated with a higher risk. Its benefit is the very low cost.

5.3 **D.** The supine position causes uterine compression on the vena cava, which decreases the venous return of blood to the heart, leading to supine hypotension. One important maneuver when encountering fetal heart rate abnormalities is a positional change, such as the lateral decubitus position. Oxytocin and epidural anesthesia both can decrease oxygen delivery to the placental bed. Oxytocin may hyperstimulate the uterus and cause frequent contractions; this then results in frequent vasoconstriction of the uterine vessels which decreases the amount of blood arriving to the placenta and fetus over time. Thus, **stopping the oxytocin may help improve oxygenation.** An epidural can cause hypotension in the mother which may then lead to fetal bradycardia by also decreasing the amount of blood profusing the fetus per given time. Morphine sulfate can cause respiratory depression in the fetus, so it would not be a method of choice for increasing delivery of oxygen to the fetus.

5.4 **E.** The first step in the assessment of apparent fetal bradycardia is differentiating the fetal heart rate from the maternal pulse. This may be done with the use of a fetal scalp electrode or ultrasound. A fetal scalp pH is a maneuver to assess whether or not the fetus is receiving sufficient oxygen during labor, but cannot be done with a closed cervix. It requires at least 4-cm dilation to get a sample of blood from the fetal scalp. It is rarely performed today. If fetal bradycardia is confirmed, various maneuvers may be implemented to improve maternal oxygenation (placement of mother on her left side, IV fluid bolus, 100% O_2 face mask, and stopping oxytocin). Simultaneously, IV terbutaline may be given to help relax the uterine musculature in an effort to increase blood flow and O_2 supply to the fetus. If none of these methods work, a vaginal examination may reveal a cord prolapse, in this case the best treatment is elevation of the presenting part digitally and emergent cesarean delivery. Atropine may be used in a nonpregnant patient to treat bradycardia or arrhythmias, but is not indicated for fetal bradycardia.

5.5 **B.** This patient likely has late decelerations because of hypotension caused by the epidural. Sympathetic blockade from the epidural leads to vasodilation. The first treatment is intravenous fluids, and if the hypotension and/or late decelerations are persistent, then a vasopressive agent such as ephedrine is used. Meperidine (Demerol) is associated with decreased fetal heart rate variability but not hypotension. Cesarean may be required if the fetal heart rate tracing does not improve, but typically epidural-induced hypotension will respond to therapy.

CLINICAL PEARLS

▶ The first steps in assessing fetal bradycardia after artificial rupture of membranes are distinguishing the heart rate from the maternal pulse rate and examining the vagina to assess for cord prolapse.

▶ The best therapy for umbilical cord prolapse is elevation of the presenting part and emergency cesarean delivery.

▶ The risk of cord prolapse with a vertex presentation or frank breech presentation is very low; the risk with a footling breech or transverse lie is substantially higher.

▶ The most common finding with uterine rupture is a fetal heart rate abnormality such as deep variable decelerations or bradycardia.

▶ The best treatment for suspected uterine rupture is immediate cesarean delivery.

REFERENCES

American College of Obstetricians and Gynecologists. Management of intrapartum fetal heart rate tracings. *ACOG Practice Bulletin 116.* Washington, DC; 2010.

Bayshore RA, Koos BJ. Fetal surveillance during labor. In: Hacker NF, Gambone JC, Hobel CJ, eds. *Essentials of Obstetrics and Gynecology.* 5th ed. Philadelphia, PA: Saunders; 2009:119-127.

Cunningham FG, Leveno KJ, Bloom SL, Hauth JC, Gilstrap LC III, Wenstrom KD. Intrapartum assessment. In: *Williams Obstetrics.* 23rd ed. New York, NY: McGraw-Hill; 2010:447-456.

CASE 6

A 29-year-old parous (G5P4) woman at 39 weeks' gestation with preeclampsia delivers vaginally. Her prenatal course has been uncomplicated except for asymptomatic bacteriuria caused by *Escherichia coli* in the first trimester treated with oral cephalexin. She denies a family history of bleeding diathesis. After the placenta is delivered, there is appreciable vaginal bleeding estimated at 1000 cc.

- What is the most likely diagnosis?
- What is the next step in therapy?

ANSWERS TO CASE 6:
Postpartum Hemorrhage

Summary: A 29-year-old parous (G5P4) woman at 39 weeks' gestation with preeclampsia delivers vaginally. She denies a family history of a bleeding diathesis. After the placenta is delivered, there is appreciable vaginal bleeding, estimated at 1000 cc.

- **Most likely diagnosis:** Uterine atony.
- **Next step in therapy:** Dilute intravenous (IV) oxytocin, bedside uterine massage and compression, and if this is ineffective, then intramuscular prostaglandin F_2-alpha (Hemabate) or rectal misoprostol.

ANALYSIS
Objectives

1. Know the definition of postpartum hemorrhage.
2. Understand that the most common cause of postpartum hemorrhage is uterine atony.
3. Know the treatment for uterine atony and the contraindications for the various agents.

Considerations

This 29-year-old woman delivers at 39 weeks' gestation and has an estimated blood loss of 1000 cc after the placenta delivers. This meets the definition of postpartum hemorrhage for a vaginal delivery, which is a loss of 500 mL or more. The most common etiology is uterine atony, in which the myometrium has not contracted to cut off the uterine spiral arteries that are supplying the placental bed. Bladder emptying, uterine massage, and dilute oxytocin are the first therapies. If these are ineffective, then prostaglandin F_2-alpha or rectal misoprostol is the next agent to be used in this patient. Because she is hypertensive, methylergonovine maleate (Methergine) is contraindicated. It should be noted that if the uterus is palpated and found to be firm and yet bleeding continues, a laceration to the genital tract should be suspected. Her risk factors for uterine atony include preeclampsia since she is likely to be treated with magnesium sulfate.

APPROACH TO:
Postpartum Hemorrhage

DEFINITIONS

POSTPARTUM HEMORRHAGE (PPH): Classically defined as greater than 500 mL of blood loss at a vaginal delivery and greater than 1000 mL during a cesarean delivery. Practically speaking, it means significant bleeding that may result in hemodynamic instability if unabated.

Also, a decline in hematocrit levels of 10% has been used to define postpartum hemorrhage, but it is not a satisfactory definition because determinations of hemoglobin or hematocrit concentrations may not reflect the current hematologic status.

UTERINE ATONY: Lack of myometrial contraction, clinically manifested by a boggy uterus.

METHYLERGONOVINE MALEATE (METHERGINE): An ergot alkaloid agent that induces myometrial contraction as a treatment of uterine atony, contraindicated in hypertension.

PROSTAGLANDIN F_2-ALPHA: A prostaglandin compound that stimulates myometrial contraction, contraindicated in asthmatic patients.

CLINICAL APPROACH

Postpartum hemorrhage is defined as primary (early) and secondary (late) according to whether it occurs within the first 24 hours or after that period. **The most common cause of early PPH is uterine atony**, with bleeding arising from the placental implantation site. (See Table 6–1 for risk factors.)

The physical examination reveals a boggy uterus. Table 6–2 summarizes the stepwise approach to PPH. Because of the large proportion of cardiac output that perfuses the uterus and placental bed, a postpartum woman can exsanguinate in 10 to 15 minutes without intervention.

Uterotonic agents include intramuscular methylergonovine (Methergine), intramuscular prostaglandin F_2-alpha, and rectal misoprostol. Ergot alkaloids should not be given in women with hypertensive disease because of the risk of stroke. Prostaglandin F_2-alpha should not be administered in those with asthma due to the potential for bronchoconstriction. Among these three agents, rectal misoprostol has emerged in many centers as the preferred agent due to high efficacy, low cost,

Table 6–1 • RISK FACTORS FOR UTERINE ATONY
Magnesium sulfate
Oxytocin use during labor
Rapid labor and/or delivery
Overdistention of the uterus (macrosomia, multifetal pregnancy, and hydramnios)
Intraamniotic infection (chorioamnionitis)
Prolonged labor
High parity

Table 6–2 • TREATMENT FOR POSTPARTUM HEMORRHAGE		
Assessment Steps	Intervention	Comment
Assess hemorrhage by vital signs and blood in collection (recall that Hgb not accurate)	Support ABCs	Continue to monitor ABCs and support BP
Palpate uterine fundus	If firm, consider lacerations (surgical management) or coagulopathy (replace clotting factors) If boggy, then bimanual massage and IV dilute oxytocin	Bimanual compression with abdominal hand and vaginal hand concurrently
Pharmacological agents	Ergot alkaloids, prostaglandin F_2-alpha and/or misoprostol × 2–3 doses	Contraindications to ergot alkaloid = hypertension; contraindication to PG F2-alpha = asthma
If continues to bleed	Two large-bore IVs, Foley catheter placement to empty bladder, call for blood, monitor vitals, move the patient to the OR	Do not continue interventions in the labor and delivery room if no response to medications
If somewhat stable, consider nonsurgical intervention	Intrauterine balloon or uterine artery embolization	Intrauterine balloon can tamponade bleeding
If unstable or bleeding rapidly, then laparotomy	If future childbearing is desired, consider compression stitches such as B-lynch, ligation of blood supplies such as O'Leary sutures for ligating bilateral uterine arteries If no childbearing desired, then hysterectomy	

and low side effects. If medical therapy is ineffective, two large-bore intravenous lines should be placed, the blood bank should be notified, and anesthesiologist alerted. Intrauterine tamponade such as with a balloon can be performed while preparing for surgical therapy. Surgical therapy may include exploratory laparotomy with interruption of the blood vessels to the uterus such as uterine artery ligation or internal iliac artery ligation. More recently, suture methods that attempt to compress the uterus, such as the B-lynch stitch, have been described. If these fail, hysterectomy may be lifesaving.

Other causes of early PPH include **genital tract lacerations**, which should be suspected with a **firm contracted uterus while bleeding persists.** The vaginal side walls and cervix should be especially carefully inspected. Repair of the complete extent of the laceration is important. **Uterine inversion** (see Case 3), whether partial or complete, must also be considered. Placental causes include **accreta** or **retained placenta.** If the uterus is firm and there are no lacerations, one must also consider **coagulopathy.**

Secondary (late) PPH, defined as occurring after the first 24 hours, may be caused by **subinvolution of the placental site,** usually occurring at 10 to 14 days after delivery. In this disorder, the eschar over the placental bed usually falls off and the lack of myometrial contraction at the site leads to bleeding. Classically, the patient will not have bleeding until about 2 weeks after delivery and is not significantly anemic. Oral ergot alkaloid and careful follow-up is the standard treatment; other options include intravenous dilute oxytocin or intramuscular prostaglandin F_2-alpha compounds.

Other causes of secondary postpartum hemorrhage include uterine atony (perhaps secondary to retained products of conception) and infection. Ultrasound examination helps to confirm the diagnosis. If uterus is atonic, uterotonic agents are the first-line therapy. If suspecting retained products of conception, suction dilation and curettage can be performed. Women with retained products of conception (POCs) generally have uterine cramping and bleeding. If suspecting infection (endometritis), broad-spectrum antibiotics are indicated. Endometritis is suspected with uterine fundal tenderness, fever, and foul-smelling lochia.

Emerging Concepts

Recent studies have indicated that active management of the third stage of labor reduces the incidence and severity of PPH. This includes oxytocin given immediately upon delivery of the infant, late cord clamping, and gentle cord traction with uterine countertraction with a well-contracted uterus. Several randomized trials found a 25% to 50% decrease in the incidence of PPH. Although retained placenta is a theoretical risk with early oxytocin administration, studies have not found this complication.

> ### CASE CORRELATION
> - See also Case 3, Uterine Inversion, which is strongly associated with postpartum hemorrhage; see also Section I—Approach to Reading and What Is the Most Likely Diagnosis—for the clinical approach.

COMPREHENSION QUESTIONS

6.1 A 24-year-old G1P0 woman at 39 weeks' gestation had induction of labor due to gestational hypertension. She was placed on magnesium sulfate for seizure prophylaxis. She was placed on oxytocin for 15 hours and reached a cervical dilation of 6 cm. After being at 6-cm dilation for 3 hours despite adequate uterine contractions as judged by 240 Montevideo units, she underwent a cesarean delivery. The baby was delivered without difficulty through a low-transverse incision. Upon delivery of the placenta, profuse bleeding was noted from the uterus, reaching 1500 mL. Which of the following is the most likely cause of hemorrhage in this patient?

   A. Uterine atony
   B. Uterine laceration
   C. Coagulopathy
   D. Uterine inversion
   E. Retained placenta

6.2 A 26-year-old G2P1001 woman underwent a normal vaginal delivery. A viable 7 lb 4 oz male infant was delivered. The placenta delivered spontaneously. The obstetrician noted significant blood loss from the vagina, totaling approximately 700 mL. The uterine fundus appeared to be well contracted. Which of the following is the most common etiology for the bleeding in this patient?
A. Retained placenta
B. Genital tract laceration
C. Uterine atony
D. Coagulopathy
E. Endometrial ulceration

6.3 A 32-year-old woman has severe postpartum hemorrhage that does not respond to medical therapy. The obstetrician states that surgical management is the best therapy. The patient desires future childbearing. Which of the following is most appropriate to achieve the therapeutic goals?
A. Utero-ovarian ligament ligation
B. Hypogastric artery ligation
C. Supracervical hysterectomy
D. Ligation of the external iliac artery
E. Cervical cerclage

6.4 A 34-year-old woman is noted to have significant uterine bleeding after a vaginal delivery complicated by placenta abruption. She is noted to be bleeding from multiple venipuncture sites. Which of the following is the best therapy?
A. Immediate hysterectomy
B. Packing of the uterus
C. Hypogastric artery ligation
D. Ligation of utero-ovarian ligaments
E. Correction of coagulopathy

6.5 A 26-year-old G2P2 woman underwent a normal vaginal delivery 10 days previously. She comes into the doctor's clinic complaining of a large amount of bright red bleeding beginning since 5 PM the previous day. Which of the following is the most likely diagnosis?
A. Uterine atony
B. Cervical laceration
C. Vaginal laceration
D. Subinvolution of the uterus
E. Normal menses

ANSWERS

6.1 **A.** Uterine atony is the most common cause of PPH, even after cesarean delivery. With a prolonged labor, such as with arrest of active phase, a patient is at risk for uterine atony. The finding of a boggy uterus would be confirmatory. Certainly, lacerations or injury to uterine vessels are potential issues and should be visible on examination. The treatment for uterine atony during cesarean is similar to a patient who underwent vaginal delivery, including intravenous dilute Pitocin, prostaglandin compounds (such as intramuscular PG F_2-alpha or rectal misoprostol). If these measures are unsuccessful, surgical management of uterine atony includes ligation of blood supply to the uterus to decrease the pulse pressure (suture ligation of the ascending branch of the uterine artery or the utero-ovarian ligament or internal iliac artery) or placement of compression stitches (B-lynch stitch) that try to compress the uterus with external suture "netting." Sometimes hysterectomy needs to be performed when the patient is unresponsive to these conservative surgical techniques.

6.2 **B.** Genital tract laceration is the most common cause of PPH in a well-contracted uterus. This is most likely arising from a cervical laceration, commonly laterally into or adjacent to the arterial supply of the cervix. Upon recognition of PPH, the physician should address the ABCs, assess the patient's blood pressure (BP) and heart rate (HR), and have IV isotonic crystalloid infusing quickly. A second large-bore IV infusion should be started. The most common cause of PPH is uterine atony and so attention should be directed toward fundal massage and infusion of oxytocin (Pitocin). If the fundus is firm and the uterus well contracted, the next step should be to assess for a genital tract laceration. Inspection for whether the bleeding is coming supracervical (uterus) versus cervical or lower in the genital tract is critical. Supracervical bleeding speaks for coagulopathy, retained POC, or atypical uterine atony. The cervix and then vagina should be carefully inspected for lacerations. Often, if the patient is in a regular labor and delivery room, moving the patient to the operating room with adequate lighting and anesthesia can be helpful. Blood products should be on hand if bleeding persists. At times, a genital tract laceration may extend high into the vaginal fornix; careful assessment of the full extent of the laceration and judicious surgical repair is warranted.

6.3 **B.** Ligation of the ascending branch of the uterine arteries and the internal iliac (hypogastric) artery are methods for decreasing the pulse pressure to the uterus and can help in PPH. Ligation of utero-ovarian ligaments can be performed in addition to ligation of uterine arteries, which can diminish further blood flow to the uterus. Ligation of the external iliac artery would lead to lower extremity necrosis. A cervical cerclage is not a treatment option for hemorrhage; instead, it is a procedure performed in order to prevent preterm labor and delivery in a pregnant woman with cervical insufficiency.

6.4 **E.** Bleeding from multiple venipuncture sites together with abruption suggests a coagulopathy. This is a systemic response, so no type of localized treatment (such as hypogastric artery ligation or utero-ovarian ligament ligation) will fix the problem. A patient with disseminated intravascular coagulation can present with a simultaneously occurring thrombotic and bleeding problems, which makes it difficult to choose a treatment option.

6.5 **D.** The most common cause of late postpartum hemorrhage is subinvolution of the uterus, in which the placental implantation site does not decrease in size as expected; thus, when the eschar overlying the placental site falls off (7–10 days after delivery), there is more bleeding than expected. The treatment is uterotonic agents such as ergot alkaloids or misoprostol. The bleeding almost always decreases quickly, such as within 12 hours.

CLINICAL PEARLS

▶ The most common cause of postpartum hemorrhage is uterine atony.

▶ The most common cause of early PPH with a firm, well-contracted uterus is a genital tract laceration.

▶ The most common cause of late postpartum hemorrhage (after the first 24 hours) is subinvolution of the uterus.

▶ Hypertensive disease is a contraindication for ergot alkaloids, and asthma is a contraindication for prostaglandin F_2-alpha.

▶ The evaluation and treatment of PPH should be systematic and efficient and involves two aspects: stabilization of the circulatory status and addressing the hemorrhage.

▶ Stabilization of the patient begins by addressing the ABCs, ensuring a second large-bore IV infusion of isotonic crystalloid and availability of blood products if needed, and constantly monitoring key hemodynamic parameters (mental status, BP, HR, urinary output, bleeding, and capillary refill).

▶ The systematic search for the etiology of PPH should begin with uterine atony, then genital tract lacerations with careful inspection to discern whether the bleeding is supracervical, cervical, or lower genital tract.

REFERENCES

American College of Obstetricians and Gynecologists. Postpartum hemorrhage. *ACOG Practice Bulletin* 76. Washington, DC; 2006. (Reaffirmed 2013.)

Cunningham FG, Leveno KJ, Bloom SL, Hauth JC, Gilstrap LC III, Wenstrom KD. Obstetrical hemorrhage. In: *Williams Obstetrics*. 24th ed. New York, NY: McGraw-Hill; 2014:619-670.

Kim M, Hyashi RH, Gambone JC. Obstetrical hemorrhage and puerperal sepsis. In: Hacker NF, Gambone JC, Hobel CJ, eds. *Essentials of Obstetrics and Gynecology*. 5th ed. Philadelphia, PA: Saunders; 2009:128-138.

WHO Recommendations for the Prevention and Treatment of Postpartum Haemorrhage. Geneva: World Health Organization; 2012.

CASE 7

A 20-year-old G1P0 woman at 16 weeks' gestation by last menstrual period (LMP) has received a serum maternal α-fetoprotein (AFP) test that returned as 2.8 multiples of the median (MOM). She is fairly sure of her last menstrual period and has regular menses. She denies a family history of congenital anomalies or chromosomal abnormalities. On examination, she is afebrile, her blood pressure (BP) is 100/70 mm Hg, and her heart rate (HR) is 70 beats per minute (bpm). The heart and lung examinations are normal. The fundal height is midway between the symphysis pubis and the umbilicus. Fetal heart tones are in the range of 140 bpm.

▶ What is your next diagnostic step?
▶ What is the purpose of the maternal serum α-fetoprotein (msAFP) test?

# ANSWER TO CASE 7:
Serum Screening in Pregnancy

Summary: A 20-year-old G1P0 woman at 16 weeks' gestation by a fairly certain last menstrual period has received a serum maternal α-fetoprotein test that returned as 2.8 MOM.

- **Next diagnostic step:** Basic obstetric ultrasound examination to assess for dates and multiple gestations.
- **Purpose of msAFP:** The purpose is to assess the risk for a fetal open neural tube defect, and can also be used to assess for the risk of aneuploidy, such as fetal Down syndrome or trisomy 18.

ANALYSIS
Objectives

1. Understand that the most common causes of abnormal serum screening are wrong dates and multiple gestations.
2. Know that an elevated maternal serum α-fetoprotein level may be associated with an open neural tube defect.
3. Know that a low msAFP level may be associated with fetal Down syndrome.
4. Be aware of the large number of noninvasive and invasive tests for fetal anomalies and aneuploidy.
5. Be aware of some of the teratogens and their fetal effects.

Considerations

This patient is at 16 weeks' gestation by a fairly certain last menstrual period, which is consistent with the clinical examination. The gestational age window of 16 to 20 weeks is the appropriate time to screen with serum testing. The msAFP returned as 2.8 MOM, which exceeds the usual cutoff of 2.0 or 2.5 MOM. The interpretation of the msAFP depends on gestational age and number of fetuses. The components of a certain last menstrual period are (1) patient sure of date of last menstrual period, (2) regular menses, (3) LMP was normal, and (4) patient has had no spotting or bleeding after LMP. The uterine size correlates with the dates. At 16 weeks' gestation, the fundus is usually midway between the symphysis pubis and the umbilicus. At 20 weeks' gestation, the fundal height is generally at the level of the umbilicus. Although this patient has a sure LMP and size and date consistency, there is still a significant risk of a dating abnormality or a multifetal gestation. Hence, the next appropriate step is the basic ultrasound examination. If there is a dating error, the msAFP result would be recalculated based on the corrected gestational age. If the msAFP is still abnormally elevated, then at an early gestational age such as 16 weeks, repeating the serum test is an option. For women with abnormally elevated msAFP at a later gestational age, such as 20 weeks, genetic counseling and referral for amniocentesis may be considered.

APPROACH TO:
Abnormal Serum Screening in Pregnancy

DEFINITIONS

ALPHA-FETOPROTEIN: A glycoprotein made by the fetal liver, analogous to the adult albumin.

FIRST-TRIMESTER SCREENING: Use of biochemical markers (PAPP-A and β-hCG) and/or transvaginalsonography measuring the aspect in the posterior neck region called the "nuchal translucency" giving a risk of Down syndrome and trisomy 18. This is performed between 10 and 13 weeks' gestation.

NEURAL TUBE DEFECT: Failure of closure of the embryonic neural folds leading to an absent cranium and cerebral hemispheres (anencephaly) or nonclosure of the vertebral arches (spina bifida).

OPEN NEURAL TUBE DEFECT: A neural tube defect that is not covered by skin.

MATERNAL SERUM α-FETOPROTEIN: α-Fetoprotein level drawn from maternal blood; this may be elevated due to increased amniotic fluid α-fetoprotein.

TRISOMY SCREEN: Three or four serum markers that may indicate an increased risk of chromosomal abnormalities, drawn in the second trimester (typically between 15 and 21 weeks' gestation). A common combination includes maternal serum α-fetoprotein, human chorionic gonadotropin (hCG), inhibin-A, and unconjugated estriol.

TERATOGEN: An agent or factor that causes a malformation in the embryo.

CLINICAL APPROACH

The triple (or trisomy) screen is used in pregnant women between 15 and 21 weeks' gestation to identify those pregnancies that may be complicated by neural tube defects, Down syndrome, or trisomy 18. It is a multiple marker test, and the term "triple" is often used to denote that it analyzes three chemicals in the maternal serum to determine the risk for neural tube defects or fetal aneuploidy: α-fetoprotein, human chorionic gonadotropinhCG, and unconjugated estriol. Although the triple screen may be offered to women over the age of 35 years, or advanced maternal age, genetic amniocentesis provides more diagnostic information.

α-Fetoprotein is a glycoprotein synthesized initially by the fetal yolk sac and then later by the fetal gastrointestinal tract and liver. It passes into the maternal circulation by diffusion through the chorioamniotic membranes. When there is an opening in the fetus not covered by skin, levels of AFP increase in the amniotic fluid and maternal serum. Maternal serum AFP is measured in MOM. Different laboratories have different cutoff levels for abnormal AFP; in general, **levels >2.0 to 2.5 MOM are suspicious for neural tube defects and warrant further evaluation.** However, an abnormally elevated serum AFP level does not

Table 7–1 • CAUSES OF ELEVATED AND LOW msAFP
Elevated msAFP
Underestimation of gestational age Multiple gestations Neural tube defects Abdominal wall defects Cystic hygroma Fetal skin defects Sacrococcygealteratoma Decreased maternal weight Oligohydramnios
Decreased msAFP
Overestimation of gestational age Chromosomal trisomies Molar pregnancy Fetal death Increased maternal weight

necessarily coincide with fetal neural tube defects. Other causes of elevated and decreased maternal serum AFP are listed in Table 7–1.

In contrast to neural tube defects, which have an abnormally elevated maternal serum AFP, those pregnancies complicated by Down syndrome have a low maternal serum AFP.

Unconjugated estriol is also decreased in fetuses with Down syndrome. Human chorionic gonadotropin, however, is elevated in these fetuses. By combining these serum chemicals into a multiple marker screening test, approximately 60% of all Down syndrome pregnancies can be identified. With trisomy 18, all of the serum markers are abnormally low. Different variations of the multiple marker test exist, such as one that adds inhibin A as a fourth analyte to further improve detection rates. (Table 7–2 lists the noninvasive and invasive tests).

First-trimester Down syndrome screening has also become available to women. This allows prediction of abnormal pregnancies at an earlier gestational age. First-trimester screening combines two serum analytes: pregnancy-associated plasma protein (PAPP-A) and free β-hCG with sonographic measurement of nuchal

Table 7–2 • OVERVIEW OF PRENATAL GENETIC TESTS
Noninvasive Techniques
For fetal structural anomalies (ultrasound, magnetic resonance imaging) For neural tube defects (msAFP) For fetal Down syndrome (msAFP, maternal uE3, hCG, inhibin A) For various aneuploidy (cell-free fetal DNA)
Invasive Techniques
Fetal visualization (fetoscopy) Fetal tissue sampling (amniocentesis, chorionic villus sampling, percutaneous umbilical blood sampling) Preimplantation blastocyst biopsy (with IVF)

Table 7–3 • SERUM ANALYTES ASSOCIATED WITH FETAL ANOMALIES

Genetic Disorder	AFP	uE3	hCG	Inhibin A	PAPP-A	Beta hCG
Trisomy 21	↓	↓	↑	↑	↓	↑
Trisomy 18	↓	↓	↓	N/A	↓	↓
Trisomy 13	N/A	N/A	N/A	N/A	↓	↓

translucency (see Table 7–3). The nuchal translucency is an echolucent area seen at the back of the fetal neck. In abnormal pregnancies, the levels of PAPP-A and free β-hCG tend to be decreased, whereas the nuchal translucency is thickened. When performed between 10 and 13 weeks' gestation, 85% of Down syndrome may be identified and 90% of trisomy 18 may be identified. Furthermore, first-trimester screening may be combined with second-trimester screening to improve the detection rate of Down syndrome to 90%.

The first step in the management of an abnormal triple screen is a basic ultrasound to determine the correct gestational age, to identify the possibility of multiple gestation, and to exclude fetal demise. The most common cause of abnormal serum screening is wrong dating. If the risk of trisomy or neural tube defects is still increased after a basic sonogram, amniocentesis or targeted ultrasound is offered. A targeted examination can correctly identify fetuses with neural tube defects by direct visualization of the fetal head and spine. Furthermore, ultrasound may also detect those fetuses suspicious for having Down syndrome by identification of a thickened nuchal fold, shortened femur length, or echogenic bowel. Other conditions associated with an abnormally high or low maternal serum AFP, such as abdominal wall defects, oligohydramnios, and fetal skin defects, can be identified with ultrasound.

Because high-resolution sonography can detect up to 95% of neural tube defects, some practitioners will not proceed with invasive testing for an elevated msAFP. However, when amniocentesis is chosen for an elevated msAFP, the amniotic fluid is tested for AFP levels. Fetal karyotype is also obtained through amniocentesis, which will identify fetal aneuploidy, such as the trisomies. Fetal loss rate from an amniocentesis is about 0.5%. Other complications include rupture of membranes and chorioamnionitis.

The identification of a fetus affected by a neural tube defect or a chromosomal abnormality can be an ethical and moral dilemma for the parents, whose previous hopes and dreams for having a "normal" child are now extinguished. The parents should not be forced into any decision, but should be provided information in an unbiased fashion.

Emerging Concepts

At the writing of this chapter, the use of noninvasive blood test on maternal blood assays fetal DNA for trisomy 21, 18, and 13, and several other aneuplopiodes, and is for use between 10 and 22 weeks' gestation. Approximately 13% of cell-free fetal DNA (cfDNA) in the maternal serum is fetal in origin. The technology known as massively parallel shotgun sequencing analyzes and amplifies cfDNA to detect

Table 7–4 • SELECT LISTING OF TERATOGENS	
Agent	Effect on Embryo
Androgens	Masculinization of female fetus, labial fusion
Alcohol	Fetal alcohol syndrome, IUGR, microcephaly
Phenytoin (Dilantin)	Fetal hydantoin syndrome, IUGR, microcephaly, facial defects
Lithium carbonate	Heart and great vessel defects (Epstein anomaly)
Methotrexate	Skeletal defects, limb defects
Retinoic acid (vitamin A)	Facial defects, neural tube defects
ACE inhibitors	Skull anomalies, limb defects, miscarriage; renal tubule dysgenesis, renal failure in neonate, oligohydramnios
Warfarin	CNS and skeletal defects
Valproic acid, carbamazepine	Neural tube defects

excessive fetal chromosomes. Initial studies indicate a 97% sensitivity and near 99% specificity rate for Down syndrome, but the study populations were small. Other algorithms are being developed to likewise incorporate age-related risk together with laboratory cfDNA results. This technology has not been well studied in large populations yet; and its role at the time of printing was delegated to those women at high risk for Down syndrome. Both the American College of Obstetricians and Gynecologists and the Society for Maternal Fetal Medicine cautioned against the use of cfDNA as a definitive diagnostic test (acting on results), but still as a screening test, since there were false positive results noted.

Teratogens

Every baby has a 3% to 5% baseline risk of a birth defect. Specific exposures to agents during organogenesis—days 15 to 60—may lead to malformations. During the first 2 weeks of gestation, a teratogen usually has an "all or nothing" effect. In other words, the embryo is killed or recovers from the exposure. For some prescribed medications, the benefits may outweigh the risks. There is a consensus, however, that some agents should never be used during pregnancy (retinoic acid derivatives). See Table 7–4 for a partial listing of common teratogens.

COMPREHENSION QUESTIONS

7.1 A 23-year-old G1P0 woman at 20 weeks' gestation undergoes an ultrasound examination for size greater than her dates. The ultrasound reveals hydramnios with an amniotic fluid index of 30 cm. The fetal abdomen reveals a cystic mass in the right abdominal region and a cystic mass in the left abdominal area. Which of the following is the most likely associated condition?

   A. Gestational diabetes
   B. Congenital ovarian tumors
   C. Down syndrome
   D. Rh isoimmunization

7.2 A 28-year-old woman delivers a baby with a cleft palate and cleft lip. The baby is otherwise healthy. The patient asks about whether there is a genetic reason for this anomaly. Which of the following is the best explanation of the genetics of this condition?

A. Autosomal dominant
B. Autosomal recessive
C. X-linked dominant
D. X-linked recessive
E. Multifactorial

7.3 A 22-year-old G2P1 woman at 25 weeks' gestation with a sure last menstrual period asks for serum screening. The patient's sister has one child with Down syndrome and, otherwise, there is no family history of anomalies or genetic disorders. Which of the following is the most appropriate response?

A. Amniocentesis is the appropriate test.
B. Serum screening should be performed.
C. Explain to the patient that it is too late for serum screening, but that her risk for Down syndrome is not much higher than her age-related risk.
D. The patient being only 22 years of age does not need serum screening.
E. The patient has a 25% chance of her baby having Down syndrome.

7.4 A 28-year-old G1P0 woman at 16 weeks' gestation is noted to have an elevated msAFP at 2.9 MOM. She underwent a targeted ultrasound examination which did not reveal a neural tube defect. Her physician also undertakes a diligent search for an etiology for the elevated msAFP without identifying an etiology. Which of the following conditions is this patient at increased risk?

A. Increased incidence of stillbirth
B. Gestational diabetes
C. Placenta previa
D. Molar pregnancy
E. Down syndrome

7.5 A 22-year-old woman is seen for her first prenatal visit at 16 weeks' gestation with a family history of congenital deafness and neonatal renal disease. The patient's hearing is normal. Which of the following is the best next step?

A. Amniocentesis for karyotype
B. Amniocentesis for rubella PCR
C. Genetic counseling
D. Glucose challenge testing

7.6 A 34-year-old woman is noted to be at 34 weeks' gestation. The size is less than her dates. An ultrasound is performed which reveals oligohydramnios with an AFI of 2.1 cm. Which of the following agents may be responsible for this condition?
   A. Lithium exposure
   B. Angiotensin converting enzyme (ACE) inhibitor
   C. Oral hypoglycemic agent
   D. Phenytoin (Dilantin)

ANSWERS

7.1 **C.** This baby has the "double bubble" of duodenalatresia. The hydramnios results from the inability of the baby to swallow. Duodenal atresia is strongly associated with fetal Down syndrome. Gestational diabetes is associated with hydramnios occasionally; however, duodenal atresia is not related. Rh isoimmunization can also lead to hydramnios and hydrops but not duodenal atresia.

7.2 **E.** The genetics for cleft palate and cleft lip in the absence of other anomalies is multifactorial, and not a clear genetic transmission. The risk of recurrence is generally about 5%. The risk is higher if one of the parents also has a cleft lip/palate. Other disorders that are multifactorial include cardiac malformations and neural tube defects.

7.3 **C.** The window for serum screening is usually between 15 and 21 weeks, so that her gestational age of 25 weeks is too late. The history of her sister having a baby with Down syndrome confers a very small, if any, increased risk for her own pregnancy. If the patient herself had a prior baby with Down syndrome, the risk would be substantially increased, and genetic counseling with possible amniocentesis for karyotype would be appropriate.

7.4 **A.** Pregnancies with elevated msAFP, which after evaluation are unexplained, are at increased risk for stillbirth, growth restriction, preeclampsia, and placental abruption. Thus, many practitioners will perform serial ultrasound examinations, monitor for these complications, and perform fetal antenatal testing such as biophysical profile testing.

7.5 **C.** Genetic counseling is appropriate with a family history of possible heritable syndromes. A glucose challenge test would not be helpful in evaluating heritable syndromes because it is used as a screen for gestational diabetes. Genetic counseling is recommended before a risky procedure, such as an amniocentesis, is performed because based on the family history, it may not be indicated in this situation.

7.6 **B.** Oligohydramnios is found with fetal exposure to ACE inhibitors. Neonatal renal failure may also be noted. Lithium is associated with Epstein anomaly (a fetal heart malformation); Dilantin is associated with a fetal hydantoin syndrome of intrauterine growth retardation, microcephaly, and facial defects.

CLINICAL PEARLS

► The most common cause of abnormal triple screening is wrong dates.

► The next step in the evaluation of abnormal triple screening is the basic ultrasound.

► Up to 95% of neural tube defects are detectable by targeted sonography.

► About 60% of Down syndrome cases are detected with the triple screen with an elevated human chorionic gonadotropin level, low msAFP, and low unconjugated estriol.

► An elevated msAFP suggests a neural tube defect, but there are many other etiologies.

► Cell-free DNA testing may be very useful especially in high-risk individuals, but should not be used in general in low-risk individuals.

► Cell-free DNA testing should not be viewed as a diagnostic test and does have false positives and negatives, especially in low-risk patients.

► Teratogenic exposure prior to 2 weeks' gestation leads to an "all or nothing effect." Organogenesis occurs between days 15 and 60 of embryonic life.

REFERENCES

American College of Obstetricians and Gynecologists. Screening for fetal chromosomal abnormalities. *ACOG Practice Bulletin 77*. Washington, DC; 2007. (Reaffirmed 2011.)

American College of Obstetricians and Gynecologists. Cell-free DNA screening for fetal aneuploidy. *ACOG Committee Opinion 640*. Washington, DC; 2015.

Cunningham FG, Leveno KJ, Spong CY. Prenatal diagnosis and fetal therapy. In: *Williams Obstetrics*. 24th ed. New York, NY: McGraw-Hill; 2014:313-339.

Lu MC, Williams J III, Hobel CJ. Antepartum care: preconception and prenatal care, genetic evaluation and teratology, and antenatal fetal assessment. In: Hacker NF, Gambone JC, Hobel CJ, eds. *Essentials of Obstetrics and Gynecology*. 5th ed. Philadelphia, PA: Saunders; 2009:71-90.

Sifakis S, Papantoniou N, Kappou D, Antsaklis A. Noninvasive prenatal diagnosis of Down syndrome: current knowledge and novel insights. *J Perinat Med*. 2012;40:319-327.

CASE 8

A 31-year-old G4P3003 woman at 36 weeks' gestation is admitted to the labor and delivery unit for evaluation of uterine contractions. She has a known twin pregnancy, and throughout the pregnancy, she had significant nausea and vomiting, but otherwise her prenatal course has been unremarkable. Serial ultrasound examinations have been performed showing concordant growth of the twins. She takes prenatal vitamins, an iron supplement, and folic acid. On examination, blood pressure (BP) is 110/70 mm Hg, pulse is 80 beats per minute (bpm), and respiratory rate is 18 breaths per minute. Fundal height is 41 cm. Her cervix is 4 cm dilated and 90% effaced. Ultrasound examination reveals a twin pregnancy with a dividing membrane, and adequate amniotic fluid. The twins are presenting vertex/vertex. After 2 hours of labor, the patient dilates to 6 cm. Artificial rupture of membranes is undertaken to allow for a fetal scalp electrode of twin A. A moderate amount of vaginal bleeding is noted after rupture of membranes. Twin A's fetal heart rate tracing initially was in the 140 bpm baseline, and then increases to 170 bpm, and now has a sinusoidal appearance.

- ▶ What is the most likely diagnosis?
- ▶ What is the cause of this condition?
- ▶ What is the next step in management?

ANSWERS TO CASE 8:
Twin Gestation with Vasa Previa

Summary: A 31-year-old G4P3 woman at 36 weeks' gestation with a twin pregnancy presents in labor. Upon rupture of membranes, there is moderate vaginal bleeding noted. Twin A has fetal tachycardia and now a sinusoidal heart rate pattern.

- **Most likely diagnosis:** Twin gestation with vasa previa.

- **Cause of this condition:** The exact pathophysiologic mechanism of vasa previa is not known, but it is associated with a velamentous cord insertion (explained below), accessory placental lobes, and second trimester placenta previa. The incidence of vasa previa is increased in pregnancies conceived by in vitro fertilization (IVF).

- **Next step:** Stat cesarean and alert pediatricians for likelihood of anemia in twin A.

ANALYSIS
Objectives

1. Become familiar with the mechanisms responsible for twinning.
2. Understand the implications of twin gestation for a pregnancy (both maternal and fetal effects).
3. Recognize risk factors for and complications of vasa previa.

Considerations

This 31-year-old woman presents with a known twin gestation and ultrasound findings consistent with a vasa previa, where a fetal vessel overlies the internal cervical os. This presents a danger to the fetus when rupture of membranes occurs, as the fetus can rapidly exsanguinate. Prenatal diagnosis of this condition is of the utmost importance, as there is *nearly a two-fold increased chance of survival with prenatal diagnosis*; unfortunately, it is difficult to diagnose prenatally. The twin gestation has its own set of possible complications that must be considered. These include the increased risk of congenital anomalies, preterm labor, preeclampsia, postpartum hemorrhage, and maternal death. Finally, the sinusoidal heart rate pattern is a rare finding (a category III ominous pattern), and usually associated with severe fetal anemia.

APPROACH TO:
Multiple Gestation

DEFINITIONS

VELAMENTOUS CORD INSERTION: Umbilical vessels separate before reaching the placenta, protected only by a thin fold of amnion, instead of by the cord or the placenta itself; these vessels are susceptible to tearing after rupture of membranes.

VASA PREVIA: Umbilical vessels that are not protected by cord or membranes, which cross the internal cervical os in front of the fetal presenting part; this most commonly occurs with a velamentous cord insertion or a placenta with one or more accessory lobes.

BILOBED OR SUCCENTURIATE-LOBED PLACENTA: A placenta with either one or more accessory lobes.

MONOZYGOTIC TWINS: Twins formed by the fertilization of one egg by one sperm.

DIZYGOTIC TWINS: Twins formed by the fertilization of two eggs by two sperm.

CHORIONICITY: The number of placentas in a twin or higher order gestation; in monozygotic twins, can either be monochorionic or dichorionic. Dizygotic twins are always dichorionic.

AMNIONICITY: The number of amniotic sacs in a twin or higher order gestation; monozygotic twins may be monoamnionic or diamniotic whereas dizygotic twins are always diamniotic.

CLINICAL APPROACH

The incidence of twin gestation has dramatically increased in the United States over the last two or three decades. This is a result of the increasing use of infertility treatments, including ovulation induction and in vitro fertilization. This dramatic increase has created a new public health concern, as twin pregnancies are associated with a higher rate of preterm delivery and all of the complications associated with it. The other complications of twin gestation include a higher rate of congenital malformations, a two-time increased risk of preeclampsia and postpartum hemorrhage, and twin–twin transfusion (TTT) syndrome.

There are two types of twinning: monozygotic and dizygotic. Monozygotic twins are formed when one egg is fertilized by one sperm followed by an error in cleavage; the incidence is not related to race, heredity, age, or parity. The exact mechanism of monozygotic twinning is not known, but may be caused by a delay in normal events, such as when tubal motility is decreased. Oral contraceptives (OCPs) slow tubal motility, so it is important to know if a mother has used OCPs within 3 months of becoming pregnant. This is associated with an increased incidence of twinning.

Table 8–1 • CHORIONICITY AND AMNIONICITY OF MONOZYGOTIC TWINS

Timing of Division (after Fertilization)	Resulting Chronicity and Amnionicity
First 72 hours	Dichorionic/diamniotic
Day 4-8	Monochorionic/diamniotic
Day 8-12	Monochorionic/monoamniotic
After day 12	Conjoined twins

The second way to categorize twins is by their membranes: the chorionicity and amnionicity of monozygotic twins is determined by the timing of division of the embryos (see Table 8–1, and Figures 8–1 and 8–2). Relative to dizygotic twins, monozygotic twins are associated with a higher incidence of discordant growth and malformations, with monochorionic twins being associated with a much higher rate of spontaneous abortion.

Dizygotic twins are formed by the fertilization of two eggs by two sperms. The incidence is influenced by race, heredity, maternal age, parity, and fertility drugs. The incidence is 1:100 in white women and 1:80 in black women. The rate of dizygotic twinning increases with maternal age and peaks at 37 years. There is an increased incidence of a twin pregnancy when the mother is a dizygotic twin. Fertility treatments are responsible for many twin gestations. Clomiphene induces ovulation and promotes the maturation of multiple follicles, therefore increasing the number of eggs released during ovulation and available for fertilization. In vitro fertilization involves the transfer of two to four embryos to the uterus. If more than one implants, a twin or higher order gestation occurs. All dizygotic twins are dichorionic/diamniotic.

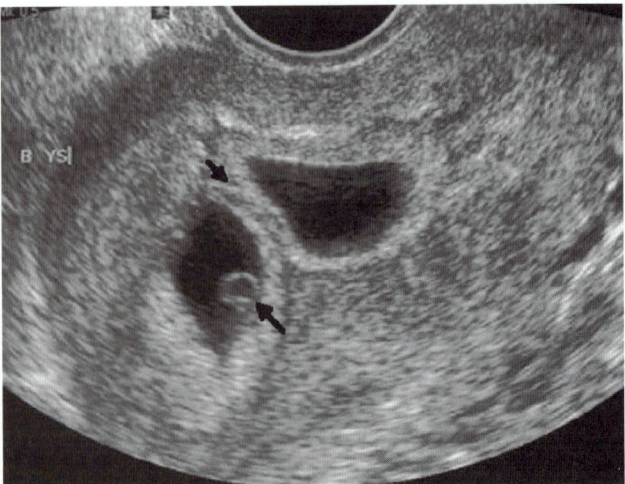

Figure 8–1. Twin gestation with thick dividing membrane indicating dichorionic, diamniotic membrane. The bottom arrow points to yolk sac and the top arrow points to dividing membrane. (*Reproduced, with permission, from Cunningham FG, Leveno KJ, Bloom SL, et al.* Williams Obstetrics. *23rd ed. New York, NY: McGraw-Hill; 2010, Figure 39–7a.*)

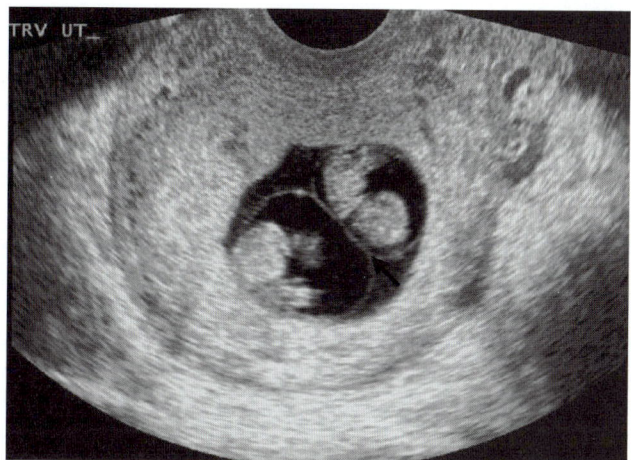

Figure 8–2. Twin gestation with thin dividing membrane indicating monochorionic, diamniotic membrane. This is a monozygotic twin. (*Reproduced, with permission, from Cunningham FG, Leveno KJ, Bloom SL, et al. Williams Obstetrics. 23rd edition. Figure 39–7b.*)

In any kind of twin gestation, it is important to remember that maternal screening and physiology may be different from that in a singleton pregnancy. Increased maternal serum α-fetoprotein (msAFP) may be misleading, especially in the case of a vanishing twin where only one fetus is seen on ultrasound. Nausea and vomiting can be increased in a twin gestation, due to higher serum levels of hCG. Hemodynamically, blood volume and stroke volume are increased more than in a singleton pregnancy. However, the red cell mass increases proportionately less, so there is greater physiologic anemia. Blood pressure at 20 weeks is usually lower than in a singleton pregnancy, but is higher by delivery. Finally, there is a greater increase in size and weight of the uterus, as might be expected.

Maternal complications more common with multiple gestations include preeclampsia, gestational diabetes, anemia, deep venous thrombosis, postpartum hemorrhage, and the need for cesarean delivery. Fetal or placental complications include preterm delivery, intrauterine growth retardation (IUGR), polyhydramnios, stillbirth, fetal anomalies, placenta previa, abruption, and twin–twin transfusion syndrome. In TTT syndrome, one twin is the donor and the other the recipient such that one twin is larger with more amniotic fluid and the other twin smaller with oligohydramnios. Treatment includes laser ablation of the shared anastomotic vessels at special centers, or serial amniocentesis for decompression. When there is no dividing membrane between the twins, cord entanglement can occur, leading to a 50% perinatal mortality rate. Thus, an important part of the ultrasound evaluation of twin gestations is identification of a dividing membrane.

When a multiple gestation is diagnosed, the patient should be followed in a high-risk clinic with serial ultrasound examinations for growth and comparison weight, and careful monitoring for the above complications. Delivery can be vaginal when both twins are presenting as vertex. When the first twin is nonvertex, cesarean delivery is usually performed. When the first twin is vertex, delivery of the nonvertex second twin is individualized.

Vasa previa is a serious condition that can cause fetal death rapidly after rupture of membranes. Survival is increased more than two-fold by prenatal diagnosis, from 44% to 97%. However, prenatal diagnosis is difficult. It is difficult to identify on vaginal examination, especially before membrane rupture, and ultrasound may give some hint. Currently, accepted risk factors are a bilobed, succenturiate-lobed, or low-lying placenta, multifetal pregnancy, and pregnancy resulting from in vitro fertilization. Women with these risk factors or suggestive ultrasound findings should have a color Doppler ultrasound. If vasa previa is identified, a planned cesarean delivery should take place before rupture of membranes, around 35 to 36 weeks of gestation. Digital vaginal examination is contraindicated in cases of vasa previa.

Because fetal blood volume at term is only 250 to 500 cc, it is not hard to imagine that the fetus may exsanguinate within minutes of an umbilical vessel being torn. Fetal heart rate abnormalities such as tachycardia, recurrent decelerations, prolonged bradycardia, and a sinusoidal pattern can indicate serious fetal compromise and should prompt evaluation for its cause. If fetal bleeding is uncertain, the Apt test and Kleihauer–Betke test can be used to differentiate fetal from maternal blood.

COMPREHENSION QUESTIONS

8.1 A 28-year-old G1P0 woman is diagnosed as having a twin gestation at 15 weeks' gestation. Careful examination of the membranes reveals that there is a very thin membrane between the two fetuses. Which of the following statements is most accurate?

A. It is likely that one fetus is a male and the other a female.
B. It is likely that this is a dizygotic gestation.
C. It is likely that this is a monozygotic gestation.
D. It is likely that there are two separate placentas.

8.2 A 25-year-old G2P1001 woman at 27 weeks' gestation has been followed for twin gestation. She is undergoing her third ultrasound examination today. Her ultrasound findings are as follows:

	Twin A	Twin A
Estimated weight	500 g	1100 g
Amniotic fluid	2 cm	26 cm

Which of the following is the best next step for this patient?

A. Chorionic villus sampling
B. Repeat ultrasound in 3 weeks
C. Laser ablation of vessels
D. Revision of dates for twin B

8.3 A 32-year-old G1P0 woman undergoes an IVF pregnancy cycle and becomes pregnant with triplets. She has been followed in a high-risk obstetrics clinic with an uncomplicated pregnancy course. She arrives to the hospital labor and delivery unit at 30 weeks' gestation with a blood pressure of 150/100 mm Hg, and 2+ proteinuria. Additionally, she complains of dyspnea. Her oxygen saturation is 82% on room air. She is contracting every 4 minutes. The patient is diagnosed with preeclampsia. Which of the following statements is most accurate?

A. Await spontaneous labor
B. Induce labor immediately
C. Cesarean at 34 weeks' gestation
D. Cesarean at 39 weeks' gestation

ANSWERS

8.1 **C.** The ultrasound findings are consistent with monochorionic, diamniotic twins, since there is only a thin membrane between the two gestations. Since a dizygotic gestation always gives rise to a dichorionic diamniotic gestation, this patient must have a monozygotic pregnancy which split at 4 to 8 days after fertilization. A monozygotic pregnancy is at greater risk for IUGR, stillbirth, and TTT syndrome.

8.2 **C.** The large discrepancy of fetal weight and amniotic fluid volume between the two gestations is consistent with TTT syndrome. The best treatment is laser ablation of the shared vessels, but this procedure is only available at select centers. Another option is serial amniotic fluid reduction. In TTT syndrome, one twin acts as the donor (smaller) and the other as the recipient (larger). A high stillbirth risk exists with this condition.

8.3 **B.** This patient likely has pulmonary edema due to preeclampsia as well as the increased plasma volume due to multiple gestations. The higher the number of pregnancies, the more the plasma volume, and greater the risk of pulmonary edema. This patient should be placed on intravenous furosemide to decrease intravascular volume, magnesium sulfate for seizure prophylaxis, and plans made for delivery. Although deep venous thrombosis (DVT) and pulmonary embolism is always a consideration in a pregnant woman with dyspnea and hypoxemia, pulmonary edema would be more likely. The chest radiograph would be helpful to differentiate the two conditions (infiltrates with pulmonary edema, clear in pulmonary embolism). Tocolysis and corticosteroids would be useful in isolated preterm labor, although many experts avoid their use in multiple gestations because of the risk of pulmonary edema.

CLINICAL PEARLS

▶ The two types of twin gestations are mono- and dizygotic. Monozygotic twins are associated with a higher rate of anomalies and maternal complications.

▶ Maternal effects of pregnancy are enhanced in twin gestation—increased nausea and vomiting, greater "physiologic" anemia, greater increase in blood pressure after 20 weeks, and greater increase in size and weight of the uterus.

▶ TTT syndrome should be suspected with a substantial discordance of the twins and discrepancy of the distribution of the amniotic fluid volume.

▶ Twin gestation without a dividing membrane is associated with a high stillbirth rate due to cord entanglement.

▶ Vasa previa is a serious condition that can cause rapid fetal demise after rupture of membranes.

▶ Prenatal diagnosis of a vasa previa is best made by ultrasound with color Doppler, and management is planned cesarean delivery before rupture of membranes.

REFERENCES

Chasen, ST, Chervenak, FA. Twin pregnancy: prenatal issues; 2012, Accessed 10.02.2012.

Cunningham FG, Leveno KJ, Bloom SL, Spong CY, Dashe J. Abnormalities of the placenta, umbilical cord, and membranes. In: *Williams Obstetrics*. 24th ed. New York, NY: McGraw-Hill; 2014: 577-587.

Cunningham FG, Leveno KJ, Bloom SL, Spong CY, Dashe J. Multifetal gestation. In: *Williams Obstetrics*. 23rd ed. New York, NY: McGraw-Hill; 2014:859-889.

Lockwood, CJ, Russo-Stieglitz, K. Vasa previa and velamentous cord; 2014 Accessed 10.06.2014.

Oyelese Y, Sulian JC. Placenta previa, placenta accreta, and vasa previa. *ACOG Clinical Expert Series*. *Obstet Gynecol*. 2006;107:927-941.

Strehlow S, Uzelac P. Complications of labor & delivery. In: DeCherney AH, Nathan L, eds. *Current Diagnosis & Treatment of Obstetrics & Gynecology*. 11th ed. New York, McGraw-Hill; 2012.

CASE 9

A 31-year-old G3P2 woman at 39 weeks' gestation arrives at the labor and delivery area complaining of strong uterine contractions of 4-hour duration; her membranes ruptured 2 hours ago. She has a history of herpes simplex virus (HSV) infections. She denies any blisters, and her last herpetic outbreak was 4 months ago. She is taking oral acyclovir. She notes a 1-day history of tingling in the perineal area. On examination, her blood pressure (BP) is 110/60 mm Hg, temperature is 99°F (37.2°C), and heart rate (HR) is 80 beats per minute (bpm). Her lungs are clear to auscultation. Her abdomen reveals a fundal height of 40 cm. The fetal heart rate is 140 bpm, reactive, and without decelerations. The uterine contractions are every 3 minutes. The external genitalia are normal without evidence of lesions. The vagina, cervix, and perianal region are normal in appearance. The vaginal fluid is consistent with rupture of membranes, showing ferning and an alkalotic pH.

▶ What is your next step?
▶ What is the most likely diagnosis?

ANSWERS TO CASE 9:
Herpes Simplex Virus Infection in Labor

Summary: A 31-year-old G3P2 woman at 39 weeks' gestation is in labor and her membranes ruptured 2 hours ago. She has a history of herpes simplex virus (HSV) infections and is taking oral acyclovir suppressive therapy. She has a 1-day history of tingling in the perineal area.

- **Next step:** Counsel patient about risks of neonatal HSV infection and offer a cesarean delivery.
- **Most likely diagnosis:** Herpes simplex virus recurrence with prodromal symptoms.

ANALYSIS
Objectives

1. Understand the indications for cesarean delivery due to HSV infection in pregnancy.
2. Know that HSV may cause neonatal encephalitis.
3. Understand that symptoms of prodromal infection may indicate viral shedding.

Considerations

The patient is in labor and has experienced rupture of membranes. She has a history of HSV infections. Although she has no lesions visible and is taking acyclovir suppressive therapy, she complains of tingling of the perineal region. These symptoms are sufficient to suggest an HSV outbreak. With HSV shedding of the genital tract, there is risk of neonatal infection, especially encephalitis, which can lead to severe permanent CNS compromise. The patient should be counseled about the neonatal risks, and offered cesarean delivery to decrease the risk of neonatal exposure to the HSV.

APPROACH TO:
Herpes Simplex Virus in Pregnancy

DEFINITIONS

HERPES SIMPLEX VIRUS PRODROMAL SYMPTOMS: Prior to the outbreak of the classic vesicles, the patient may complain of burning, itching, or tingling.

NEONATAL HERPES INFECTION: HSV can cause disseminated infection with major organ involvement; be confined to encephalitis, eyes, skin, or mucosa; or be asymptomatic. The vast majority of neonatal herpes infections occur via exposure to virus in fluids and secretions of the genital tract, although 5% to 10% may occur in the antepartum period transplacentally. Infants born to women who acquire a new HSV infection near delivery have a 30% to 50% risk of infection, due mostly to increased viral load in the mother.

CLINICAL APPROACH

Herpes cultures or polymerase chain reaction (PCR) are not useful in the acute management of pregnant women who present in labor or with rupture of membranes. They are helpful in making the diagnosis during the prenatal course, when the patient may develop lesions and the diagnosis is in question. Once a woman has been diagnosed with HSV, the practitioner uses his or her best clinical judgment to assess for the presence of HSV in the genital tract during the time of labor. A meticulous inspection of the external genitalia, vagina, cervix (including by speculum examination), and perianal area should be undertaken for the typical herpetic lesions, such as vesicles or ulcers (Figure 9–1). Additionally, the patient

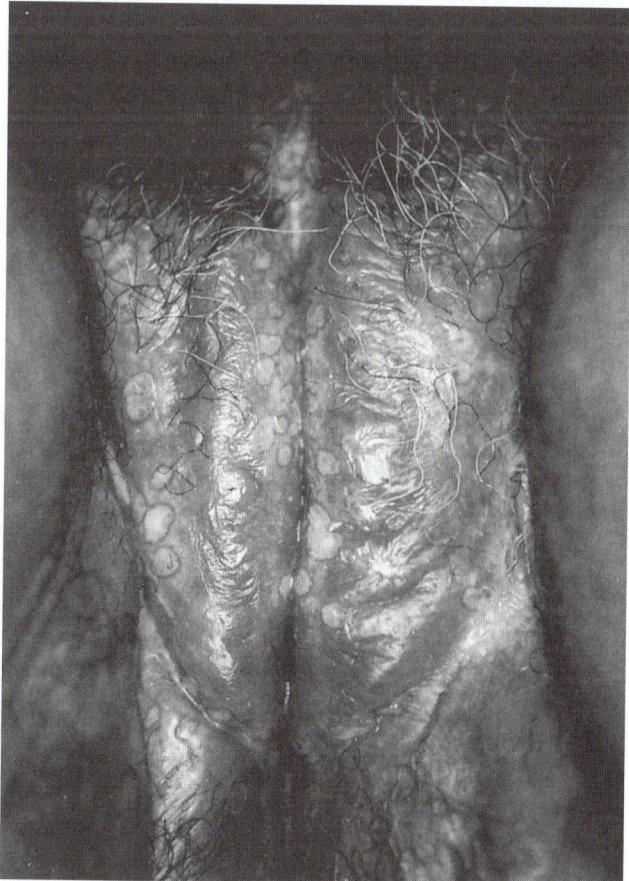

Figure 9–1. First episode of primary genital herpes simplex virus infection. (*Reproduced with permission from Wendel GD, Cunningham FG. Sexually transmitted diseases in pregnancy. In: Williams Obstetrics. 18th ed. (Suppl. 13). Norwalk, CT: Appleton & Lange.*)

should be queried thoroughly about the presence of prodromal symptoms. When there are no lesions or prodromal symptoms, the patient should be counseled that she is at low risk for viral shedding and likely has a small but possible risk of neonatal herpes infection. Usually the patient will opt for vaginal delivery under these circumstances. In contrast, **the presence of prodromal symptoms or genital lesions suspicious for HSV is sufficient to warrant a recommendation for cesarean delivery to prevent neonatal infection.**

The highest risk factor for neonatal infection is acquisition of new HSV infection near the time of delivery, anywhere from a 30% to 50% risk. For this reason, the Centers for Disease Control and Prevention (CDC) recommends that women who have not been infected with HSV abstain from sex with partners with known HSV infection in the third trimester.

Two subtypes of HSV have been identified: HSV-1 and HSV-2. HSV-1 is responsible for most nongenital disease; however, HSV-1 has been increasingly implicated in up to 50% of new onset genital infections in adolescents and young adults. HSV-2 is found almost exclusively in the genital region, and the vast majority of recurrences are due to HSV-2. Although there is cross-reactivity between HSV-1 and HSV-2 proteins, prior HSV-1 exposure often fails to prevent infection with HSV-2, though it may reduce severity of symptoms (see Table 9–1). Acyclovir has activity against both HSV-1 and HSV-2. In a primary herpes outbreak, oral

Table 9–1 • CATEGORIES OF GENITAL HSV INFECTIONS

Terminology	Definition	Clinical Manifestation	Transmission Rate
Primary infection	HSV infection in an individual who has no HSV IgG antibodies (no prior exposure to HSV; HSV-1 and HSV-2 negative)	Systemic symptoms include fever, malaise, fever, nausea Local symptoms: burning, itching, lesions (last about 21 days) NOTE: Up to 75% of women have asymptomatic primary HSV infections	50%
Nonprimary first episode infection	A first HSV infection in a woman who has the heterologous IgG antibody (Example: The first HSV-2 outbreak in a woman with HSV-1 IgG antibody, but no HSV-2 antibody)	Systemic symptoms and local symptoms usually milder and less duration that primary infection (lesions last about 14 days)	33%
Recurrent infection	A genital HSV infection in a woman who has homologous IgG antibody (Example: HSV-2 outbreak in a woman who has HSV-2 IgG)	No systemic symptoms; local symptoms (lesions last about 9 days, and viral shedding about 4 days and lower viral load than primary or nonprimary first episode)	0%-4%
Asymptomatic viral shedding	Presence of HSV virus in the genital region in the absence of symptoms	Usually brief periods (24-48 hours) of viral shedding, affecting about 1%-2% of pregnant women	0%-4%

acyclovir reduces viral shedding, pain symptoms, and is associated with faster healing of the lesions. Newer medications such as valacyclovir or famciclovir require less frequent dosing due to their increased bioavailability, but are more expensive.

The use of oral suppressive antiviral therapy at 36 weeks for women who have had a recurrence or first episode during pregnancy has been shown to decrease viral shedding and the frequency of outbreaks at term, and decrease the need for cesarean delivery. It is unclear whether this prophylaxis is useful for those without a recurrence during pregnancy, yet many practitioners will recommend prophylaxis. If there is no HSV involvement of the breast, the patient may breastfeed. Use of acyclovir for suppression has also been found to be safe in breastfeeding mothers.

Controversies

Some experts recommend serologic screening for HSV-2 antibodies for couples so that antiviral suppression and safer sex practices as well as counseling of women can be performed. For instance, in the circumstance where the pregnant woman is HSV-2 antibody negative, and the partner is HSV-2 antibody positive, safer sex practices may be adopted. However, there is no evidence that this practice is cost-effective or would reduce neonatal HSV infection. At this time, routine screening for antibodies and suppressive therapy for seropositive partners is not recommended.

COMPREHENSION QUESTIONS

9.1 A 32-year-old G1P0 woman at 24 weeks' gestation is seen by her obstetrician for painful vesicles on the vulva. PCR is performed and returns as HSV-2. The obstetrician counsels the patient about the possibility of needing cesarean when she goes into labor. Which of the following is an indication for cesarean section due to maternal HSV?

   A. Vesicular lesions noted on the cervix
   B. History of lesions noted on the vagina 1 month previously, now not visible
   C. Lesions noted on the posterior thigh
   D. Tingling of the chest wall with lesions consistent with herpes zoster

9.2 A 29-year-old G2P1 woman is seen in the office for her pregnancy at 16 weeks' gestation. She complains of some burning of the vulvar area. Two blisters are noted on the labia majora. PCR is performed on the lesions, which returns as HSV-1. Which of the following statements is most accurate in the counseling of this patient?

   A. Because this result is HSV-1, the finding is likely a false-positive result and the patient does not likely have a herpes infection.
   B. Because of the finding of HSV-1, the neonate is not at risk for herpes encephalitis.
   C. The patient should be treated the same whether the infection is HSV-1 or HSV-2.
   D. The patient likely has an HIV infection since HSV-1 was isolated in the vulvar area.

9.3 A 35-year-old healthy G2P1 woman at 20 weeks' gestation presents with primary episode of herpes simplex virus, confirmed by PCR. Oral acyclovir is given for a 10-day course. Which of the following is the rationale for the acyclovir therapy?
A. Decrease the likelihood of recurrence and need for cesarean
B. Decrease the likelihood of transplacental transmission to the fetus
C. Decrease the duration of viral shedding and duration of the current infection
D. Increase the patient's immunity and IgG levels to HSV

9.4 A 34-year-old woman is seen at her internist's office complaining of vulvar pain. On examination, three ulcers are noted on the right labia majora. The lesions have ragged edges, a necrotic base, and there is adenopathy noted on the right inguinal region. Which of the following is the most likely diagnosis?
A. Syphilis
B. Herpes simplex virus
C. Chancroid
D. Squamous cell carcinoma
E. Bartholin gland abscess

9.5 A 3-day-old 3500-g neonate is seen in the neonatal intensive care unit with suspected congenital herpes simplex virus infection. The infant has had several seizures and is on antiviral therapy. Which of the following is the most likely scenario of infection to this infant?
A. Primary infection during the time of labor
B. Nonprimary first episode infection at the time of labor
C. Recurrent infection at the time of labor
D. Asymptomatic shedding in a patient with a history of HSV
E. Asymptomatic shedding in a patient without a history of HSV

ANSWERS

9.1 **A.** The presence of prodromal symptoms or lesions along the genital tract (ie, cervix) suspicious for HSV is sufficient to warrant a cesarean delivery to prevent neonatal infection. When there are no lesions or prodromal symptoms, the patient should be counseled that she is at low risk for viral shedding and has an unknown risk of neonatal herpes infection; typically, the patient will opt for vaginal delivery. The posterior thigh is unlikely to inoculate the baby during delivery, and is not an indication for cesarean delivery. Lesions on the chest wall consistent with herpes zoster would not necessitate cesarean delivery; however, the baby should still not come in contact with these lesions, and breast feeding should be avoided. Herpes zoster infection in a neonate can have fatal consequences.

9.2 **C.** Although HSV-1 is usually found above the waist and HSV-2 below the waist, there are often exceptions. PCR is highly sensitive and specific, and it is unlikely that the viral subtype is erroneous. HSV-1 can also cause neonatal encephalitis, and the patient should be counseled and treated the same as if HSV-2 were isolated. A finding of HSV-1 in the vulvar region does not suggest HIV infection; nevertheless, the patient should have screening for sexually transmitted infections.

9.3 **C.** The rationale for oral acyclovir therapy at the primary outbreak is to decrease viral shedding and the duration of infection. The acyclovir does not affect the likelihood of future recurrence and does not change the patient's immune response. Oral suppressive antiviral therapy beginning at 36 weeks should also be considered in this patient to reduce the chance of viral shedding and recurrence near the time of delivery. There is no evidence that oral acyclovir alters transplacental transmission to the fetus, although reducing the viremia may help.

9.4 **C.** Chancroid is a rare cause of infectious vulvar ulcers in the United States, although worldwide it is quite common; thus, cases occurring in the United States are related to ports of entry. **Chancroid** is a sexually transmitted disease (STD) caused by the gram-negative bacterium *Haemophilusducreyi* and, like HSV, is characterized by painful genital lesions. HSV is the most common cause of infectious vulvar ulcers in the United States, and individuals are typically infected with the HSV-2 virus that is sexually transmitted. Genital herpes can cause recurrent painful genital sores, and herpes infection can become severe in people who are immunosuppressed. **Syphilis** typically presents during the first stage of the disease as a small, round, and painless chancre in the area of the body exposed to the spirochete. The Bartholin glands, responsible for vaginal secretions, are located at the entrance of the vagina; they may enlarge into painless abscesses when they become clogged and infected. Vulvar carcinoma typically is nontender, ulcerative, and is more common in postmenopausal women.

9.5 **E.** Currently in the United States, the vast majority of neonatal HSV infections occur due to asymptomatic viral shedding during a primary infection or nonprimary first episode at term. In 75% to 90% of situations involving neonatal HSV infection, the women have had no history of an HSV infection. Thus, strategies for prevention are challenging. Some investigators have advocated for serologic screening of all pregnant women, and advising those who are seronegative for one or both HSV subtypes to refrain from genital/genital or oral/genital exposure in the third trimester.

CLINICAL PEARLS

▶ Cesarean delivery should be offered to a woman with a history of HSV who has prodromal symptoms or suspicious lesions of the genital tract.

▶ Herpes simplex virus is the most common cause of infectious vulvar ulcers in the United States.

▶ Most neonatal herpes infections occur from HSV from genital tract secretions and fluids, although 5% of neonatal infections are acquired in utero. These are usually due to primary or nonprimary first episode infections.

▶ The cervix, vagina, and vulva must be inspected carefully for lesions in a patient in labor with a history of herpes simplex virus.

▶ Acyclovir and analogous agents given in pregnancy during primary episodes can decrease the duration of viral shedding and duration of lesions.

▶ Acyclovir suppression, when a primary HSV infection or recurrence occurs in pregnancy, can decrease the likelihood of recurrence and need for cesarean.

REFERENCES

American College of Obstetricians and Gynecologists. Gynecologic herpes simplex virus infections. *ACOG Practice Bulletin 57*. Washington, DC; 2004. (Reaffirmed 2014.)

American College of Obstetricians and Gynecologists. Management of herpes in pregnancy. *ACOG Practice Bulletin 82*. Washington, DC; 2007. (Reaffirmed 2014.)

Castro LC, Ognyemi D. Common medical and surgical conditions complicating pregnancy. In: Hacker NF, Gambone JC, Hobel CJ, eds. *Essentials of Obstetrics and Gynecology*. 5th ed. Philadelphia, PA: Saunders; 2009:191-218 [no updated reference].

Centers for Disease Control and Prevention (CDC). Sexually-Transmitted Diseases Treatment Guidelines; 2015. http://www.cdc.gov/std/tg2015/herpes.htm; Accessed 30.06.15.

Cunningham F, Leveno KJ, Bloom SL, et al. Sexually transmitted infections. In: *Williams Obstetrics*. 24th ed. New York, NY: McGraw-Hill; 2013:1271-1274.

CASE 10

A 30-year-old G5P4 woman at 32 weeks' gestation complains of significant bright red vaginal bleeding. She denies uterine contractions, leakage of fluid, or trauma. The patient states that 4 weeks previously, after she had engaged in sexual intercourse, she experienced some vaginal spotting. On examination, her blood pressure is 110/60 mm Hg, heart rate (HR) is 80 beats per minute (bpm), and temperature is 99°F (37.2°C). The heart and lung examinations are normal. The abdomen is soft and uterus nontender. Fetal heart tones are in the range of 140 to 150 bpm.

- ▶ What is your next step?
- ▶ What is the most likely diagnosis?
- ▶ What will be the long-term management of this patient?

ANSWERS TO CASE 10:
Placenta Previa

Summary: A 30-year-old G5P4 woman at 32 weeks' gestation complains of painless vaginal bleeding. Four weeks previously, she experienced some postcoital vaginal spotting. The abdomen is soft and uterus nontender. Fetal heart tones are in the range of 140 to 150 bpm.

- **Next step:** Ultrasound examination.
- **Most likely diagnosis:** Placenta previa.
- **Long-term management:** Expectant management as long as the bleeding is not excessive. Cesarean delivery at 34 weeks' gestation (see new reference later in this case).

ANALYSIS
Objectives

1. Know the differential diagnosis of antepartum bleeding.
2. Understand that painless vaginal bleeding is consistent with placenta previa.
3. Understand that the ultrasound examination is a good method for assessing placental location.

Considerations

This patient is experiencing antepartum vaginal bleeding (bleeding after 20 weeks' gestation). Because of the painless nature of the bleeding and lack of risk factors for placental abruption, this case is more likely to be placenta previa, defined as the placenta overlying the internal os of the cervix. Placental abruption (premature separation of the placenta) usually is associated with painful uterine contractions or excess uterine tone. The history of postcoital spotting earlier during the pregnancy is consistent with previa because vaginal intercourse may induce bleeding. The ultrasound examination is performed before a vaginal examination because vaginal manipulation (even a speculum examination) may induce bleeding. Because the patient is hemodynamically stable, and the fetal heart tones are normal, expectant management is the best therapy at 32 weeks' gestation (due to the prematurity risks). If the same patient were at 35 to 36 weeks' gestation, delivery by cesarean section would be prudent.

SECTION II: CASES   113

APPROACH TO:
Antepartum Vaginal Bleeding

DEFINITIONS

ANTEPARTUM VAGINAL BLEEDING: Vaginal bleeding occurring after 20 weeks gestation.

PLACENTA PREVIA: The placenta completely covers the internal os of the uterine cervix (Figure 10–1).

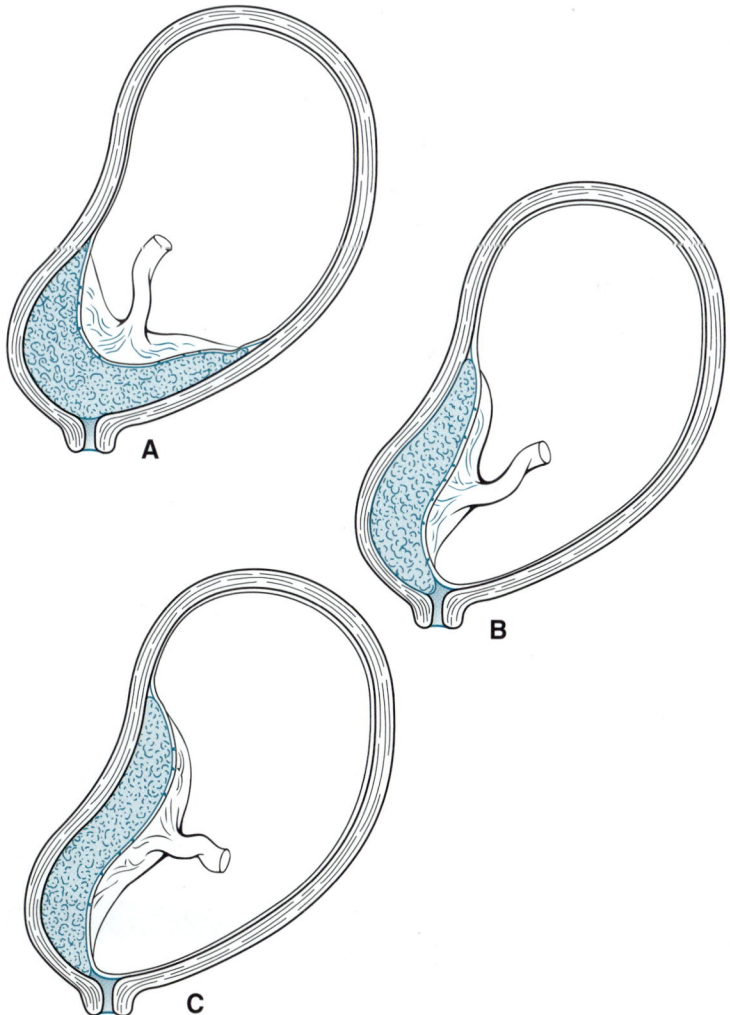

Figure 10–1. Types of placenta previa. Complete placenta previa (**A**), marginal placenta previa (**B**), and low-lying placentation (**C**) are depicted.

MARGINAL PLACENTA PREVIA: The placenta lies within 2 cm of the internal os of the cervix, but does not fully cover it.

LOW-LYING PLACENTA: The edge of the placenta is within 2 cm of the internal cervical os.

PLACENTAL ABRUPTION: Premature separation of a normally implanted placenta.

VASA PREVIA: Umbilical cord vessels that insert into the membranes with the vessels overlying the internal cervical os, thus being vulnerable to fetal exsanguination upon rupture of membranes.

CLINICAL APPROACH

Antepartum hemorrhage is defined as significant vaginal bleeding after 20 weeks' gestation. The two most common causes of significant antepartum bleeding are **placental abruption** and **placenta previa** (Table 10–1). The main differentiator based on a patient's history is that the vaginal bleeding is painless in a previa and painful in an abruption secondary to contractions. Placenta previa affects approximately 0.4% of deliveries, of which 70% to 80% will have at least one episode of bleeding. When the patient complains of antepartum hemorrhage, the physician should first rule out placenta previa by ultrasound even before a speculum or digital examination, since these maneuvers may induce bleeding. Ultrasound is an accurate method of assessing placental location. At times, transabdominal sonography may not be able to visualize the placenta, and transvaginal ultrasound is necessary and is more reliable for visualizing the internal cervical os.

The natural history of placenta previa is such that the first episode of bleeding does not usually cause sufficient concern as to necessitate delivery. Hence, a woman with a preterm gestation and placenta previa is usually observed on bed rest and complete pelvic rest in an effort to prolong gestation and avoid morbidity of fetal prematurity. Often, the second or third episode of bleeding forces delivery. The bleeding from previa rarely leads to coagulopathy, as opposed to that of placental abruption. Because the lower uterine segment is poorly contractile, postpartum bleeding may ensue. Several risk factors have been cited including parity, increased maternal age, smoking, multiple gestations, prior curettage, and prior cesarean delivery. Of note, **placenta accreta** (invasion of the placenta into the uterus) is more common with placenta previa, particularly in the presence of a uterine scar such as after a cesarean delivery. Timing of delivery depends on clinical circumstances for placenta previa and placenta accreta. A persistent hemorrhage mandates cesarean delivery regardless of gestational age. In asymptomatic patients, cesarean section as early as 34 weeks' gestation appears to balance the fetal risk of prematurity and the

Table 10-1 • RISK FACTORS FOR PLACENTA PREVIA
Grand multiparity
Prior cesarean delivery
Prior uterine curettage
Previous placenta previa
Multiple gestation

maternal benefit of a scheduled delivery. The National Institutes of Health concluded that elective delivery is ideal at 36-37 completed weeks for these patients, but practices still vary. There is no demonstrated benefit to performing amniocentesis for fetal lung maturity prior to delivery at any gestational age.

COMPREHENSION QUESTIONS

10.1 A 28-year-old woman at 32 weeks' gestation is seen in the obstetrical (OB) triage area for vaginal bleeding described as significant with clots. She denies cramping or pain. An ultrasound is performed revealing that the placenta is covering the internal os of the cervix. Which of the following is a risk factor for this patient's condition?

   A. Prior salpingitis
   B. Hypertension
   C. Multiple gestations
   D. Polyhydramnios

10.2 A 21-year-old patient at 28 weeks' gestation has vaginal bleeding and is diagnosed with placenta previa. Which of the following is a typical feature of this condition?

   A. Painful bleeding
   B. Commonly associated with coagulopathy
   C. First episode of bleeding is usually profuse
   D. Associated with postcoital spotting

10.3 A 33-year-old woman at 37 weeks' gestation, confirmed by first-trimester sonography, presents with moderately severe vaginal bleeding. She is noted on sonography to have a placenta previa. Which of the following is the best management for this patient?

   A. Induction of labor
   B. Tocolysis of labor
   C. Cesarean delivery
   D. Expectant management
   E. Intrauterine transfusion

10.4 A 22-year-old G1P0 woman at 34 weeks' gestation presents with moderate vaginal bleeding and no uterine contractions. Her blood pressure (BP) is 110/60 mm Hg and heart rate (HR) 103 beats per minute (bpm). The abdomen is nontender. Which of the following sequence of examinations is most appropriate?

   A. Speculum examination, ultrasound examination, digital examination
   B. Ultrasound examination, digital examination, speculum examination
   C. Digital examination, ultrasound examination, speculum examination
   D. Ultrasound examination, speculum examination, digital examination

10.5 An 18-year-old adolescent female is noted to have a marginal placenta previa on an ultrasound examination at 22 weeks' gestation. She does not have vaginal bleeding or spotting. Which of the following is the most appropriate management?

A. Schedule cesarean delivery at 39 weeks
B. Schedule an amniocentesis at 34 weeks and deliver by cesarean if the fetal lungs are mature
C. Schedule an MRI examination at 35 weeks to assess for possible percreta involving the bladder
D. Reassess placental position at 32 weeks' gestation by ultrasound
E. Recommend termination of pregnancy

ANSWERS

10.1 **C.** Multiple gestation, with the increased surface area of placentation, is a risk factor for placenta previa. Hypertension is not a risk factor for placenta previa; however, it is one of the main risk factors for placental abruption. Polyhydramnios, due to the excess amount of amniotic fluid in the amniotic sac, is also a risk factor for placenta abruption. Salpingitis involves inflammation and infection of the fallopian tubes and over time may lead to permanent scarring of the tubes. Since this particular process is limited to the tubes, there is not an increased risk of placenta previa; rather there is an increased risk of ectopic pregnancy.

10.2 **D.** Postcoital spotting is a common complaint in a patient with placenta previa. Unlike placenta abruption, placenta previa is not commonly associated with coagulopathy, painful bleeding, or having a profuse first episode of bleeding. The main distinguishing factor between a previa and abruption is the presence or absence of pain. With abruption, painful uterine contractions are typically the chief complaint, whereas previa is painless. Although the first episode of bleeding with a previa usually does not raise enough concern to deliver immediately, the second or third bleeding episodes will send the patient to the operation room (OR) for a cesarean delivery.

10.3 **C.** The best plan for placenta previa at term is cesarean delivery. There is no need to place the patient at risk for hemorrhage when the fetus' lungs are mature enough for life outside the womb; therefore, expectant management would not be the best choice for this scenario. A patient with a scheduled cesarean delivery does not need to be induced for labor, nor does she need tocolysis since the status of the patient's labor is typically insignificant in a cesarean delivery. A patient with previa should not deliver vaginally since the lower uterine segment is poorly contractile, and postpartum bleeding may ensue. An intrauterine transfusion is also not indicated for this patient because the baby is going to be delivered and will be independent of the mother's blood supply. Even in the setting of an Rh− mother with an Rh+ fetus, an intrauterine transfusion before delivery would pose a significantly greater risk to the mother and baby than waiting to evaluate the situation after birth.

10.4 **D.** Ultrasound should be performed first to rule out previa, speculum examination second to assess the cervix and look for lacerations, and finally digital examination. Performing either a speculum examination or digital examination before evaluating the patient with ultrasound puts the patient at risk for hemorrhage. In the setting of a previa, the lower uterine segment and cervix are highly vascularized, and varices of the cervix may be visualized on speculum examination in some situations; however, the speculum itself may cause trauma to these varices and induce bleeding. A blind digital examination may result in further separation of the placenta from the uterus, which could also cause significant bleeding.

10.5 **D.** Very often, a marginal or low-lying placenta previa at the early second trimester will resolve by transmigration of the placenta. It is too early to discuss scheduling a cesarean delivery since the placenta previa may resolve and allow for vaginal delivery. An ultrasound should be repeated in the third trimester to see whether or not the placenta has migrated. There would be no reason to be concerned about a percreta if the placenta migrates to a more favorable position; therefore, scheduling a magnetic resonance imaging (MRI) is not indicated at this time. In addition, an MRI is expensive, but it may be useful in the case of ultrasound-negative antepartum vaginal bleeding. If there is suspicion that a percreta exists, a previa has most likely already been diagnosed in the late second trimester or third trimester, so a scheduled cesarean delivery would most likely already be in the plan. During the cesarean, the physician will be able to assess the extent of the placental implantation and base management on how far the placenta has penetrated through the uterine wall. Placenta percreta and increta are usually diagnosed during a cesarean delivery and not radiographically. Amniocentesis for fetal lung maturity is not necessary in the setting of placenta previa at any gestational age. Recommending termination of pregnancy would be inappropriate in this case. Even if the patient has a placenta previa at the time of delivery, both the mother and baby have an excellent prognosis if a cesarean delivery is performed.

CLINICAL PEARLS

- Painless antepartum vaginal bleeding suggests the diagnosis of placenta previa.
- Ultrasound is the diagnostic test of choice in assessing placenta previa and should be performed before digital or speculum examination.
- Cesarean section is the best route of delivery for placenta previa.
- Placenta previa, in the face of prior cesarean deliveries, increases the risk of placenta accreta.
- When placenta previa is diagnosed at an early gestation, such as second trimester, repeat sonography is warranted since many times the placenta will move away from the cervix (transmigration).

REFERENCES

American College of Obstetricians and Gynecologists. Postpartum hemorrhage. *ACOG Practice Bulletin* 76. Washington, DC; 2006. (Reaffirmed 2015.)

Balayla J, Wo BL, Bedard MJ. A late-preterm, early-term stratified analysis of neonatal outcomes by gestational age in placenta previa: defining the optimal timing for delivery. *J Matern Fetal Neonatal Med.* 2015 January;8:1-6.

Cunningham FG, Leveno KJ, Bloom SL, et al. Obstetrical hemorrhage. In: *Williams Obstetrics.* 24th ed. New York, NY: McGraw-Hill; 2014:780-828.

Gabbe SG, Niebyl JR, Simpson JL, et al. Antepartum and postpartum hemorrhage. In: *Obstetrics Normal and Problem Pregnancies.* 6th ed. Philadelphia, PA: Elsevier; 2012:415-444.

Kim M, Hyashi RH, Gambone JC. Obstetrical hemorrhage and puerperal sepsis. In: Hacker NF, Gambone JC, Hobel CJ, eds. *Essentials of Obstetrics and Gynecology.* 5th ed. Philadelphia, PA: Saunders; 2009:128-138.

Masselli G, Brunelli R, Parasassi T, Perrone G, Gualdi G. Magnetic resonance imaging of clinically stable late pregnancy bleeding: beyond ultrasound. *Eur Radiol.* 2011;21:1841-1849.

Robinson BK, Grobman WA. Effectiveness of timing strategies for delivery of individuals with placenta previa and accreta. *Obstet Gynecol.* 2010 October;116(4):835-842.

Spong CY, Mercer BM, D'Alton M, Kilpatrick S, Blackwell S, Saade G. Timing of indicated late-preterm and early-term birth. *Obstet Gynecol.* 2011 August;118(2 Pt 1):323-333.

CASE 11

A 22-year-old G2P1 woman at 35 weeks' gestation, who admits to cocaine abuse, complains of abdominal pain. She states that she has been experiencing moderate vaginal bleeding, no leakage of fluid per vagina, and has no history of trauma. On examination, her blood pressure is 150/90 mm Hg, and heart rate (HR) is 110 beats per minute (bpm). The fundus reveals tenderness, and a moderate amount of dark vaginal blood is noted in the vaginal vault. The ultrasound examination shows no placental abnormalities. The cervix is 1 cm dilated. The fetal heart tones are in the range of 160 to 170 bpm. The urine protein to creatinine ratio is 0.1 (normal < 0.3).

- ▶ What is the most likely diagnosis?
- ▶ What are complications that can occur due to this situation?
- ▶ What is the best management for this condition?

ANSWERS TO CASE 11:
Placental Abruption

Summary: A 22-year-old G2P1 cocaine user at 35 weeks' gestation complains of abdominal pain and moderate vaginal bleeding. On examination, her blood pressure is 150/90 mm Hg, and HR is 110 bpm. The fundus reveals tenderness. The ultrasound is normal. The fetal heart tones are in the range of 160 to 170 bpm.

- **Most likely diagnosis:** Placental abruption.
- **Complications that can occur:** Hemorrhage, fetal to maternal bleeding, coagulopathy, and preterm delivery.
- **Best management for this condition:** Delivery (at 35 weeks, the risks of abruption significantly outweigh the risks of prematurity).

ANALYSIS
See also answers to Case 10.

Objectives

1. Understand that placental abruption and placenta previa are major causes of antepartum hemorrhage.
2. Know the clinical presentation of abruptio placentae.
3. Understand that coagulopathy is a complication of placental abruption.

Considerations

The patient complains of painful antepartum bleeding, which is consistent with placental abruption. Also, she has several risk factors for abruptio placentae, such as hypertension and cocaine use (Table 11–1). The best treatment for pregnancies near term (>34 weeks) when abruption is strongly suspected is delivery. The natural history of placental abruption is extension of the separation, leading to complete shearing of the placenta from the uterus. As opposed to the diagnosis of placenta previa (see Case 10), ultrasound examination is a poor method of assessment for abruption. This is because the freshly developed blood clot behind the placenta has the same sonographic texture as the placenta itself. The urine protein to creatinine (P/C) ratio of 0.1 is normal and consistent with gestational hypertension or hypertensive due to cocaine; however, a P/C ratio ≥0.3 would be consistent with abnormal proteinuria and preeclampsia.

Table 11–1 • RISK FACTORS FOR ABRUPTIO PLACENTAE
Hypertension (Chronic and Preeclampsia)
Previous abruption in a prior pregnancy
Cocaine use
Short umbilical cord
Trauma (direct or indirect)
Uteroplacental insufficiency
Submucosal leiomyomata
Sudden uterine decompression (hydramnios)
Cigarette smoking
Preterm premature rupture of membranes

APPROACH TO:
Suspected Placental Abruption

DEFINITIONS

CONCEALED ABRUPTION: When the bleeding occurs completely behind the placenta and no external bleeding is noted, this condition is less common than overt hemorrhage but more dangerous.

FETOMATERNAL HEMORRHAGE: Fetal blood that enters into the maternal circulation.

COUVELAIRE UTERUS: Bleeding into the myometrium of the uterus giving a discolored appearance to the uterine surface.

CLINICAL APPROACH

As compared to placenta previa (see Case 10), **abruptio placentae is more dangerous and unpredictable.** Furthermore, the diagnosis is much more difficult to establish. Ultrasound examination is not helpful in the majority of cases; a normal ultrasound examination does not rule out placental abruption. There is no one test that is diagnostic of placental abruption, but rather the clinical picture must be taken as a whole. Thus, a patient at risk for abruptio placentae (a hypertensive patient or one who has recently been involved in a motor vehicle accident), who complains of vaginal bleeding after 20 weeks' gestation, must be suspected of having a placental abruption. Furthermore, the bleeding is often associated with uterine pain or hypertonus. The blood may seep into the uterine muscle and cause a reddish discoloration also known as the "Couvelaire uterus." Uterine atony and postpartum hemorrhage after delivery may occur. Upon delivery, a blood clot adherent to the placenta is often seen. Another complication of abruption is coagulopathy. When the **abruption is of sufficient severity to cause fetal death, coagulopathy is found in one-third or more of cases.** The coagulopathy is secondary to hypofibrinogenemia, and clinically evident bleeding is usually not encountered unless the fibrinogen level is below 100 to 150 mg/dL.

The diagnosis of placental abruption is difficult because the clinical presentation is variable. Although painful vaginal bleeding is the hallmark, preterm labor, stillbirth, and/or fetal heart rate abnormalities may also be seen. Ultrasound diagnosis is not sensitive. A concealed abruption can occur when blood is trapped behind the placenta, so that external hemorrhage is not seen. Serial hemoglobin levels, following the fundal height and assessment of the fetal heart rate pattern, are often helpful. As compared to placenta previa, fetal-to-maternal hemorrhage is more common with placental abruption, and some practitioners recommend testing for fetal erythrocytes from the maternal blood. One such test of acid elution methodology is called the Kleihauer–Betke test, which takes advantage of the different solubilities of maternal versus fetal hemoglobin.

The management of placental abruption is dependent on the fetal gestational age, fetal status, and the hemodynamic status of the mother. **Delivery is the usual management!** However, in a woman with a premature fetus (<34 weeks) and a diagnosis of "chronic abruption," expectant management may be exercised if the patient is stable with no active bleeding or signs of fetal compromise. Although there is no contraindication to vaginal delivery, cesarean section is often the chosen route of delivery for fetal indications. In cases of abruptions that are associated with fetal death and coagulopathy, the vaginal route is most often the safest for the mother. In the latter scenario, blood products and intravenous fluids are given to maintain the hematocrit above 25% to 30% and a urine output of at least 30 mL/h. These women generally have very rapid labors. Many of these women will manifest hypertension or preeclampsia following volume replacement, and it may be necessary to start magnesium sulfate for eclampsia prophylaxis.

Future Pregnancies

There is a high recurrence risk of abruption, ranging from 5% to 10%. If a patient experiences abruptio placentae with two consecutive abruptions, the recurrence rate is as high as 25%. Smoking is the biggest modifiable risk factor (40-fold increased risk in smokers).

Women with prior abruption is an indication for early delivery for future pregnancies.

CASE CORRELATION

- See also Case 8 (Twin Gestation with Vasa Previa) and Case 10 (Placenta Previa) for other presentations of antepartum hemorrhage. Among these causes, placental abruption is slightly more common than placenta previa, with vasa previa being more rare.

COMPREHENSION QUESTIONS

11.1 An 18-year-old pregnant woman is noted to have vaginal bleeding. She is bleeding from venipuncture sites, IV sites, and from her gums. Which of the following is the most likely underlying diagnosis?
   A. Placental abruption
   B. Placenta previa
   C. Gestational diabetes
   D. Multifetal gestation
   E. Gestational trophoblastic disease

11.2 A 32-year-old woman is seen in the obstetrical unit at the hospital. She is at 29 weeks' gestation, with a chief complaint of significant vaginal bleeding. She had a stillbirth with her prior pregnancy due to placental abruption. The patient asks the physician about the accuracy of ultrasound in the diagnosis of abruption. Which of the following statements is most accurate?
   A. Fetal ultrasound is more accurate in diagnosing placental abruption than placenta previa.
   B. Fetal ultrasound is quite sensitive in diagnosing placental abruption.
   C. Ultrasound is sensitive in diagnosing abruption that occurs in the lower aspect of the uterus.
   D. Fetal ultrasound is not sensitive in diagnosing placental abruption.

11.3 Which of the following is the most significant risk factor for abruptio placentae?
   A. Prior cesarean delivery
   B. Breech presentation
   C. Trauma
   D. Marijuana use
   E. Placenta accreta

11.4 A 35-year-old woman presents with bright red vaginal bleeding at 30 weeks' gestation. Her urine drug screen is positive. Which of the following is most likely to be present in her drug screen?
   A. Marijuana
   B. Alcohol
   C. Barbiturates
   D. Cocaine
   E. Benzodiazepines

11.5 A 28-year-old G1 P0 woman at 34 weeks' gestation with chronic hypertension is admitted to the hospital for bright red bleeding per vagina. Her BP is 150/90, HR 90 and urine protein/creatinine ratio of 0.1. She is estimated to have lost 900 mL, and is actively bleeding. Her cervix is 2 cm dilated. The ultrasound shows a normal placenta. The fetal monitor reveals a hypertonic uterus and no fetal heart tones. Fetal demise is confirmed by ultrasound. Laboratories show hemoglobin of 9.5 g/dL, platelet count of 90,000/fL, and prothrombin time (PT) international normalized ratio (INR) of 2.0, and PTT of 50 seconds. Which of the following is the best management for this patient?
A. Admission and careful observation in the ICU
B. Induction of labor with plan for vaginal delivery
C. Partial exchange transfusion
D. Urgent cesarean delivery
E. Intravenous terbutaline

ANSWERS

11.1 **A.** Placental abruption is a common cause of coagulopathy. Consumptive coagulopathy, also known as disseminated intravascular coagulation (DIC), involves the overactivation of the procoagulant pathways and can be a fatal complication of a placental abruption or other causes of hemorrhage. Placenta previa rarely results in consumptive coagulopathy, since there is usually a significantly less amount of bleeding involved in comparison with abruption. Gestational diabetes is more commonly associated with fetal macrosomia, and places the fetus at risk for shoulder dystocia at the time of delivery. Coagulopathy is not likely to be seen in gestational diabetes. A multifetal gestation puts a patient at a higher risk for a placenta previa due to the larger surface area required for the placenta(s), but as mentioned before, coagulopathy is not common in previa. The multifetal gestation itself does not increase maternal risk of coagulopathy. Gestational trophoblastic disease can be a benign or malignant cancer that develops in a woman's womb and is commonly associated with a molar pregnancy. Bleeding from a site of metastasis may lead to hemorrhagic shock, but this is not very common, and therefore the chance of developing DIC from this complication is even less likely.

11.2 **D.** Sonography is accurate in identifying previa, but not sensitive in diagnosing placental abruption. An ultrasound examination is a poor method for assessment of abruption because the freshly developed blood clot behind the placenta has the same sonographic texture as the placenta itself. A high index of suspicion for abruption must be exercised when evaluating the clinical picture as a whole. An extra challenging situation exists in the setting of a concealed abruption, in which the bleeding occurs behind the placenta and no external bleeding is noted. This is extremely dangerous since a greater amount of time will most likely pass before the abruption is diagnosed.

11.3 **C.** Trauma is the most significant risk factor for abruption in comparison to the other answer choices. Extreme forces can shear the placenta away from the uterus in these situations. Marijuana, as opposed to cocaine, is not associated with abruption since it does not cause maternal hypertension and vasoconstriction like cocaine. A prior cesarean delivery may predispose a patient to placenta previa with an associated accreta in future pregnancies, but neither a prior cesarean delivery nor an accreta is a significant risk factor for abruption. The most significant fetal risk associated with breech presentation is cord prolapse, which can lead to significant oxygen deprivation to the fetus. Other risk factors for placental abruption include: uterine leiomyomata (especially submucosal type), hypertension, cocaine use, short umbilical cord, uteroplacental insufficiency, hydramnios, smoking, and preterm premature rupture of membranes (PPROM).

11.4 **D.** Cocaine use is strongly associated with the development of placental abruption due to its effect on the vasculature (vasospasm).

11.5 **B.** Fetal demise complicates 15% of clinically evident abruptions. When the abruption is severe enough to be associated with fetal demise, the patient will have clinical DIC in 25% of cases. Whereas, the management of placental abruption with a live fetus many times includes cesarean, with a fetal demise, the management focuses on vaginal delivery. This patient has findings consistent with DIC, and so clotting factors such as fresh frozen plasma, red blood cells, and also platelets should be transfused.

CLINICAL PEARLS

▶ Painful antepartum bleeding should make one suspicious of placental abruption.

▶ The diagnosis of abruptio placentae is a clinical one since it can present in many different ways.

▶ The major risk factors for abruptio placentae are hypertension, trauma, and cocaine use, with hypertension being most common.

▶ A concealed abruption may hide significant bleeding without external hemorrhage.

▶ The most common cause of antepartum bleeding with coagulopathy is abruptio placentae.

▶ Placental abruption may lead to fetal-to-maternal hemorrhage.

▶ The risk of recurrence with abruption is significant, and may necessitate early delivery with subsequent pregnancies.

REFERENCES

Cunningham FG, Leveno KJ, Bloom SL, et al. Obstetrical hemorrhage. In: *Williams Obstetrics*. 24th ed. New York, NY: McGraw-Hill; 2014:757-803.

Kim M, Hyashi RH, Gambone JC. Obstetrical hemorrhage and puerperal sepsis. In: Hacker NF, Gambone JC, Hobel CJ, eds. *Essentials of Obstetrics and Gynecology*. 5th ed. Philadelphia, PA: Saunders; 2009:128-138.

CASE 12

A 35-year-old G5P4 woman at 39 weeks' gestation is undergoing a vaginal delivery. She has a history of previous myomectomy and one prior low-transverse cesarean delivery. She was counseled about the risks, benefits, and alternatives of vaginal birth after cesarean, and elected a trial of labor. She proceeded through a normal labor. The delivery of the baby is uneventful. The placenta does not deliver after 30 minutes, and a manual extraction of the placenta is undertaken. The placenta seems to be firmly adherent to the uterus.

▶ What is the most likely diagnosis?
▶ What is your next step in management for this patient?

ANSWERS TO CASE 12:
Placenta Accreta

Summary: A 35-year-old G5P4 woman at term with a prior history of a myomectomy and cesarean delivery is undergoing a vaginal delivery. The retained placenta is firmly adherent to the uterus when there is an attempt at manual extraction.

- **Most likely diagnosis:** Placenta accreta.
- **Next step in management for this patient:** Hysterectomy.

ANALYSIS
Objectives

1. Know the risk factors for and the clinical diagnosis of placenta accreta.
2. Understand that hysterectomy is usually the best treatment for placenta accreta.

Considerations

This patient has had two previous uterine incisions, which increases the risk of placenta accreta. The placenta is noted to be very adherent to the uterus, which is the clinical definition of placenta accreta, although the histopathological diagnosis requires a defect of the decidua basalis layer. The usual management of true placental accreta is hysterectomy since attempts to remove a firmly attached placenta often lead to torrential hemorrhage and/or maternal exsanguination. Conservative management of placenta accreta, such as removal of as much placenta as possible and packing the uterus, often leads to excess mortality as compared to immediate hysterectomy. Nevertheless, in the rare case of a younger patient who strongly desires more children, this option may be entertained.

APPROACH TO:
Placenta Accreta

DEFINITIONS

PLACENTA ACCRETA: Abnormal adherence of the placenta to the uterine wall due to an abnormality of the decidua basalis layer of the uterus. The placental villi are attached directly to the myometrium.

PLACENTA INCRETA: The abnormally implanted placenta penetrates into the myometrium.

PLACENTA PERCRETA: The abnormally implanted placenta penetrates entirely through the myometrium into the serosa. Often invasion into adjacent organs (eg, bladder, bowel) is noted.

CLINICAL APPROACH

Risk factors for placental adherence include low-lying placentation or placenta previa, prior cesarean delivery or uterine curettage, or prior myomectomy. Antepartum bleeding may occur, especially when associated with placenta previa (see also Cases 10 [previa] and 11 [abruption] for more common causes of antepartum hemorrhage). With complete placenta accreta, there may be no antepartum bleeding and only a retained placenta. Excessive traction on the cord may lead to uterine inversion. With a retained placenta, clinicians will usually attempt a manual extraction of the placenta, in an effort to find a cleavage plane between the placenta and the uterus (Nitabuch's layer). With placenta accreta, no cleavage plane is found. Prompt puerperal hysterectomy is usually the optimal choice in this circumstance. Because the placenta is so firmly adherent, attempts to conserve the uterus, such as leaving the placenta in situ, curettage of the placenta or removing the placenta "piecemeal," are often unsuccessful, and may lead to torrential hemorrhage and maternal exsanguination. Recent research has pointed out the importance of a multidisciplinary team approach when placenta accreta is known or is suspected prenatally to optimize perinatal outcomes.

Placenta accreta should be suspected in circumstances of placenta previa, particularly with a history of a prior cesarean delivery (Table 12–1). **The greater the number of prior cesareans in the face of current placenta previa, the higher the risk of accreta, exponentially.** For example, a woman with three or more prior cesarean deliveries and a low-lying anterior placenta suggestive of partial previa or a known placenta previa has up to a 40% to 50% chance of having placenta accreta. Some practitioners advise performing ultrasound examinations to assess the placental location in those women who have had a prior cesarean delivery. Studies examining the accuracy of magnetic resonance imaging (MRI) to diagnose placenta accreta prior to delivery reveal a sensitivity of only 38%. When the placenta is anterior or low-lying in position, there is a greater risk of accreta. One caution is that a low-lying placenta or placenta previa diagnosed in the first/second trimester typically

Table 12–1 • RISK FACTORS FOR PLACENTA ACCRETA

Placenta previa or low-lying—with or without prior uterine scar
Prior cesarean scar or other uterine scar (eg, transmural myomectomy, metroplasty, resection of cornual ectopic)—with or without previa
Cesarean scar implantation of gestational sac
Prior uterine curettage
Advanced maternal age
IVF pregnancy
Multifetal pregnancy
Exponentially increasing risk with increasing number of prior cesareans *and* current placenta previa
Prior Asherman syndrome
Prior endometrial ablation
Uterine leiomyomata
Prior pelvic irradiation
Smoking

resolves by the third trimester, as the lower uterine segment develops, a phenomenon known as trophotropism. When an antenatal diagnosis of placenta accreta/previa is suspected, a planned cesarean hysterectomy should be arranged prior to the onset of labor, preferably. In this instance, the infant is delivered between 34 and 35 weeks (after betamethasone administration, without amniocentesis to check fetal lung maturity indices) without disturbing the trophoblast implantation site, and the placenta is left in situ as the hysterectomy is performed immediately after delivery of the infant.

> ### CASE CORRELATION
> - See also Case 3 (Uterine Inversion) as placenta accreta is a risk factor for uterine inversion.

COMPREHENSION QUESTIONS

12.1 A 33-year-old G3P2002 woman who had two prior cesareans is currently at 38 weeks' gestation. She is noted to have a posterior placenta. On ultrasound, there is evidence of possible placenta accreta. The patient is counseled about the possible risk of need for hysterectomy. Which of the following is the most accurate statement?

A. Having two prior cesareans is associated with a 50% risk for placenta accreta.

B. Placenta accreta is associated with a defect in the myometrial layer of the uterus.

C. If the patient had gestational diabetes, the risk for placenta accreta would be even higher.

D. The posterior placenta may be associated with less of a risk for accreta than an anterior placenta.

12.2 A 25-year-old woman at 34 weeks' gestation is noted to have a placenta previa, after she presented with vaginal bleeding and has undergone sonography. At 37 weeks, she has a scheduled cesarean. Upon cesarean section, bluish tissue densely adherent between the uterus and maternal bladder is noted. Which of the following is the most likely diagnosis?

A. Placenta accreta

B. Placenta melanoma

C. Placenta percreta

D. Placental polyp

12.3 A 29-year-old G1P0 woman at 39 weeks' gestation delivered vaginally. Her placenta does not deliver easily. A manual extraction of the placenta is attempted and the placenta seems to be adherent to the uterus. A hysterectomy is contemplated, but the patient refuses due to strongly desiring more children. The cord is ligated with suture as high as possible. The patient is given the option of methotrexate therapy. Which of the following is the most likely complication after this intervention?

A. Coagulopathy
B. Utero-vaginal fistula
C. Infection
D. Malignant degeneration

12.4 A 32-year-old woman undergoes myomectomy for symptomatic uterine fibroids, all of which are subserosal. The endometrial cavity was not entered during the procedure. Which of the following statements is most likely to be correct regarding the risk of placental accreta?

A. Her risk of accreta is most likely to be increased due to the myomectomy.
B. Her risk of accreta is most likely to be decreased due to the myomectomy.
C. Her risk of accreta is most likely not affected by the myomectomy.
D. If the myomectomy incisions are anterior, then she has an increased risk of a placental polyp.

ANSWERS

12.1 **D.** Placenta accreta is more common with increasing number of cesareans and placenta previa. Three prior cesareans *with* placenta previa are associated with up to a 50% risk for placenta accreta, in which the decidua basalis layer is defective. It is the endometrial layer that is defective and not the myometrial layer. Nevertheless, the placenta may grow into the myometrium or even through the entire uterus to the serosa.

12.2 **C.** The blue tissue densely adherent between the uterus and bladder is very characteristic of percreta, where the placenta penetrates entirely through the myometrium to the serosa and adheres to the bladder. Hematuria may be present in this situation. These findings are not typically found with placenta accreta or polyps. Malignant melanoma can metastasize to the placenta, but this is much less common under these circumstances.

12.3 **C.** The best management of placenta accreta is hysterectomy due to the great risk of hemorrhage if the placenta is attempted to be removed. When the patient refuses hysterectomy, then ligation of the umbilical cord as high as possible and attempt at IV methotrexate therapy has been attempted with limited success. Other than hemorrhage, the other complication to be concerned about is infection. The necrosis of the placental tissue can be a nidus for infection.

12.4 **C.** In general, myomectomy incisions on the serosal (outside) surface of the uterus do not predispose to accreta because the endometrium is not disturbed. However, the risk of accreta is not decreased due to the myomectomy either. Placental polyps result from retained products after either a term pregnancy or incomplete abortion, and occur inside the uterus. Therefore, the location of the incisions for a myomectomy will not influence whether or not a patient develops polyps. Placental implantation over a submucosal uterine fibroid may increase the risk of focal accreta.

CLINICAL PEARLS

▶ The usual management of placenta accreta/previa (abnormal adherence of the placenta to the uterus) is prelabor cesarean hysterectomy around 34 to 35 weeks, after betamethasone administration (without amniocentesis for fetal lung maturity indices).

▶ Placenta accreta is associated with a defect in the decidua basalis (Nitabuch's) layer and a significant increase in maternal mortality risk

▶ The risk of placenta accreta increases in a woman with a prior uterine incision and placenta previa. The greater the number of cesareans, the higher the risk of accreta, exponentially.

▶ Low-lying or placenta previa diagnosed in the first/second trimester will often resolve later in pregnancy, so repeat sonography is required.

▶ Expert prenatal sonography and MRI are required for prenatal suspicion of placenta accreta.

▶ Multidisciplinary approach to prenatally suspected cases of morbidly adherent placentation is paramount for optimal perinatal outcomes—involving obstetrics, maternal-fetal medicine, gynecologic oncology, urology, radiology, vascular surgery, anesthesia, neonatology, blood bank, and/or intensive care specialists.

REFERENCES

American College of Obstetricians and Gynecologists. Postpartum hemorrhage. *ACOG Practice Bulletin 76.* Washington, DC; 2006. (Reaffirmed 2013.)

American College of Obstetricians and Gynecologists. Placenta accreta. *ACOG Committee Opinion 529.* Washington, DC; 2012.

Bailit JL, Grobman WA, Rice MM, et al. Morbidly adherent placenta treatments and outcomes. *Obstet Gynecol.* 2015;125:683-689.

Cunningham FG, Leveno KJ, Bloom SL, et al. Obstetrical hemorrhage. In: *Williams Obstetrics.* 24th ed. New York, NY: McGraw-Hill; 2014:830-832.

Eller AG, Bennett, MA, Sharshiner M, et al. Maternal morbidity in cases of placenta accreta managed by a multidisciplinary care team compared with standard obstetric care. *Obstet Gynecol.* 2011 February;117 (2 Pt 1):331-337.

Eller AG, Porter TF, Soisson P, Silver RM. Optimal management strategies for placenta accreta. *BJOG*. 2009 April;116(5):648-654. Epub 2009 February 4.

Kim M, Hyashi RH, Gambone JC. Obstetrical hemorrhage and puerperal sepsis. In: Hacker NF, Gambone JC, Hobel CJ, eds. *Essentials of Obstetrics and Gynecology*. 5th ed. Philadelphia, PA: Saunders; 2009:128-138.

Robinson BK, Grobman WA. Effectiveness of timing strategies for delivery of individuals with placenta previa and accreta. *Obstet Gynecol*. 2010 October;116(4):835-842.

Silver RM, Fox KA, Barton JR, et al. Center of excellence for placenta accreta. *Am J Obstet Gynecol*. 2015:561-567.

Silver RM, Landon MB, Rouse DJ, et al. National Institute of Child Health and Human Development Maternal–Fetal Medicine Units Network. Maternal morbidity associated with multiple repeat cesarean deliveries. *Obstet Gynecol*. 2006 June;107(6):1226-1232.

Warshak CR, Ramos GA, Eskander R, et al. Effect of predelivery diagnosis in 99 consecutive cases of placenta accreta. *Obstet Gynecol*. 2010 January;115(1):65-69.

CASE 13

A 23-year-old G2P1 woman at 16 weeks' gestation complains of a 12-hour history of colicky, right lower abdominal pain, and nausea with vomiting. She denies vaginal bleeding or leakage of fluid per vagina. She denies diarrhea or eating stale foods. She has a history of an 8-cm ovarian cyst, and otherwise has been in good health. She denies dysuria or fever, and has had no surgeries. Her vital signs include a blood pressure (BP) of 100/70 mm Hg, heart rate (HR) of 105 beats per minute (bpm), respiratory rate (RR) of 12 breaths per minute, and temperature of 99°F (37.2°C). On abdominal examination, her bowel sounds are hypoactive. The abdomen is tender in the right lower quadrant region with significant involuntary guarding. The cervix is closed. The fetal heart tones are in the range of 140 bpm.

▶ What is the most likely diagnosis?
▶ What is the best treatment for this condition?

ANSWERS TO CASE 13:
Abdominal Pain in Pregnancy (Ovarian Torsion)

Summary: A 23-year-old G2P1 woman at 16 weeks' gestation with an 8-cm ovarian cyst complains of a 12-hour history of colicky, right lower abdominal pain, and nausea with vomiting. The abdomen is tender in the right lower quadrant region with significant involuntary guarding.

- **Most likely diagnosis:** Torsion of the ovary.
- **Best treatment for this condition:** Surgery (laparotomy due to the pregnancy).

ANALYSIS
Objectives

1. Know the clinical presentation of some of the common causes of abdominal pain in pregnancy (acute appendicitis, acute cholecystitis, ovarian torsion, placental abruption, and ectopic pregnancy).
2. Understand that surgery is the best treatment for ovarian torsion.
3. Know that oophorectomy does not necessarily need to be performed in ovarian torsion.

Considerations

This woman, who is pregnant at 16 weeks' gestation, has a history of an 8-cm ovarian cyst. The ovarian mass is most likely a dermoid cyst because of her young age. The acute onset of colicky, lower abdominal pain, and nausea with vomiting are consistent with ovarian torsion, which is the twisting of the ovarian vessels leading to ischemia. Gastrointestinal complaints are common. She does not have a history of abdominal surgeries and the abdomen is not markedly distended, making bowel obstruction less likely. The treatment for ovarian torsion is surgical. Because her gestational age is 16 weeks, laparoscopy is an option. Sometimes, the size of the mass makes exploratory laparotomy the best choice. Upon opening the abdomen, the surgeon would examine the ovary for viability. Sometimes, untwisting of the ovarian pedicle can lead to reperfusion of the ovary. An ovarian cystectomy, that is, removing only the cyst and leaving the remainder of the normal ovarian tissue intact, is the best treatment. This patient is somewhat atypical regarding the gestational age, since the majority of pregnant women with ovarian torsion present either at 14 weeks' gestation when the uterus rises above the pelvic brim, or immediately postpartum when the uterus rapidly involutes.

APPROACH TO:
Abdominal Pain in Pregnancy

CLINICAL APPROACH

Diseases related to and unrelated to the pregnancy must be considered. Additionally, the pregnancy state may alter the risk factors for the different causes of abdominal pain, and change the presentation and symptoms. Common causes of abdominal pain in pregnant women include appendicitis, acute cholecystitis, ovarian torsion, placental abruption, and ectopic pregnancy. Less common is carneous or red degeneration of a uterine fibroid, caused by the rapid growth due to high estrogen levels. Affected patients will complain of point tenderness at the uterine fibroid, confirmed on ultrasound. Often, it is difficult to differentiate from among these different etiologies, but a careful history and physical and re-examination are the most important steps (Table 13–1).

Table 13–1 • DIFFERENTIAL DIAGNOSIS OF ABDOMINAL PAIN IN PREGNANCY

	Time during Pregnancy	Location	Associated Symptoms	Treatment
Appendicitis	Any trimester	Right lower quadrant →right flank or right upper quadrant	Nausea and vomiting Anorexia Leukocytosis Fever	Surgical
Cholecystitis	After first trimester	Right upper quadrant	Nausea and vomiting Anorexia Leukocytosis Fever	Surgical
Torsion	More commonly at 14 weeks' gestation or after delivery	Unilateral, abdominal, or pelvic	Nausea and vomiting; colicky pain	Surgical
Pancreatitis	Any trimester	Epigastric pain radiating to the back	Constant, boring pain, nausea and vomiting	Nothing by mouth, ERCP if common bile duct stone suspected
Placental abruption	Second and third trimesters	Midline persistent uterine	Vaginal bleeding Abnormal fetal heart tracings	Delivery
Ectopic pregnancy	First trimester	Pelvic or abdominal pain, usually unilateral	Nausea and vomiting Syncope Spotting	Surgical or medical
Ruptured corpus luteum	First trimester	Lower abdomen, sometimes unilateral	Acute onset of sharp pain, sometimes associated with syncope	Observation if self-limited; sometimes requires surgery if persistent bleeding

Acute Appendicitis

The diagnosis of appendicitis can be difficult to make because many of the presenting symptoms are common complaints in pregnancy. Furthermore, a delay in diagnosis (especially in the third trimester) frequently leads to maternal morbidity and perinatal problems, such as preterm labor and abortion. Patients typically present with nausea, emesis, fever, and anorexia. The location of the abdominal pain is not typically in the right lower quadrant (as is classic for nonpregnant patients), but instead is superior and lateral to the McBurney point. This is due to the effect of the **enlarged uterus pushing on the appendix to move it upward and outward toward the flank**, at times mimicking pyelonephritis. Diagnosis is made clinically, and because of the morbidity involved in a missed diagnosis, it is generally better to err on the side of overdiagnosing than underdiagnosing this disease. When appendicitis is suspected, the treatment is surgical regardless of gestational age, along with intravenous antibiotics.

Acute Cholecystitis

A common physiologic effect of pregnancy is an increase in gallbladder volume and biliary sludge (especially after the first trimester). The biliary sludge then serves as a precursor to gallstones. While gallstones are often asymptomatic, the most common symptoms are right upper quadrant pain following a meal, nausea, a "bloated sensation," and, possibly, emesis. In the absence of infection or fever, this is called **biliary colic**. Less commonly, when obstruction of the cystic or common bile duct occurs, the pain may be severe and unrelenting, and the patient may become icteric. When fever and leukocytosis are present, the patient with gallstones likely has cholecystitis. Other complications of gallstones include pancreatitis and ascending cholangitis, a serious life-threatening infection. The diagnosis of cholelithiasis is often established by an abdominal ultrasound revealing gallstones and dilation and thickening of the gallbladder wall. Simple biliary colic in pregnancy is usually treated with a low-fat diet and observed until postpartum. However, in the face of **cholecystitis, biliary obstruction, or pancreatitis in pregnancy, surgery is the treatment of choice**; generally, supportive medical management is used initially during the acute phase.

Ovarian Torsion

Patients with known or newly diagnosed large ovarian masses are at risk for ovarian torsion. **Ovarian torsion is the most frequent and serious complication of a benign ovarian cyst.** Pregnancy is a risk factor, especially around 14 weeks and after delivery. Symptoms include unilateral abdominal and pelvic colicky pain associated with nausea and vomiting. **The acute onset of colicky pain is typical.** Treatment is surgical with ovarian conservation if possible. If untwisting the adnexa results in reperfusion, an ovarian cystectomy may be performed. However, if perfusion cannot be restored, oophorectomy is indicated.

Placental Abruption

Abruption is a common cause of third-trimester bleeding and is usually associated with abdominal pain. Risk factors include a history of previous abruption, hypertensive disease in pregnancy, trauma, cocaine use, smoking, or preterm premature rupture of membranes. Patients typically present with vaginal bleeding with persistent crampy midline uterine tenderness and at times abnormal fetal heart tracings. Diagnosis is made clinically and ultrasound is not very reliable. The treatment is generally delivery, often by cesarean.

Ectopic Pregnancy

The leading cause of maternal mortality in the first and second trimesters is ectopic pregnancy. Patients usually have amenorrhea with some vaginal spotting and lower abdominal and pelvic pain. The pain is typically sharp and tearing and may be associated with nausea and vomiting. Physical findings include a slightly enlarged uterus and perhaps a palpable adnexal mass. In the case of ectopic ruptures, the patient may experience syncope or hypovolemia. Transvaginal sonography and serum human chorionic gonadotropin (hCG) levels can help with the diagnosis of ectopic pregnancy in >90% of cases. Treatment options include surgery (especially with hemodynamically unstable patients) and, in appropriately selected patients, methotrexate.

Ruptured Corpus Luteum

Corpus luteum cysts develop from mature Graafian follicles and are associated with normal endocrine function or prolonged secretion of progesterone. They are usually <3 cm in diameter. There can be intrafollicular bleeding because of thin-walled capillaries that invade the granulosa cells from the theca interna. **When the hemorrhage is excessive, the cyst can enlarge and there is an increased risk of rupture.** Cysts tend to rupture more during pregnancy, probably due to the increased incidence and friability of corpus lutea in pregnancy. Anticoagulation therapy also predisposes to cyst rupture, and these women should receive medication to prevent ovulation. Patients with hemorrhagic corpus lutea usually present with the sudden onset of severe lower abdominal pain. This presentation is especially common in women with a hemoperitoneum. Some women will complain of unilateral cramping and lower abdominal pain for 1 to 2 weeks before overt rupture. Corpus luteum cysts rupture more commonly between days 20 and 26 of the menstrual cycle.

The differential diagnosis of a suspected hemorrhagic corpus luteum should include ectopic pregnancy, ruptured endometrioma, adnexal torsion, appendicitis, and splenic injury or rupture. Ultrasound examination may show free intraperitoneal fluid, and perhaps fluid around an ovary. The diagnosis is confirmed by laparoscopy. The first step in the treatment of a ruptured corpus luteal cyst is to secure hemostasis. Once the bleeding stops, no further therapy is required; if the bleeding continues, however, a cystectomy should be performed with preservation of the remaining normal portion of ovary.

Progesterone is largely produced by the corpus luteum until about 10 weeks' gestation. Until approximately the seventh week, the pregnancy is dependent on the progesterone secreted by the corpus luteum. Human chorionic gonadotropin serves to maintain the luteal function until placental steroidogenesis is established. There is shared function between the placenta and corpus luteum from the seventh to tenth week; after 10 weeks, the placenta emerges as the major source of progesterone. Therefore, if the corpus luteum is removed surgically prior to 10 to 12 weeks' gestation, exogenous progesterone is needed to sustain the pregnancy. If the corpus luteum is excised after 10 to 12 weeks' gestation, no supplemental progesterone is required.

CASE CORRELATION

- See also Case 11 (Placental Abruption), which typically presents as painful vaginal bleeding in the third trimester. Less commonly, a concealed abruption may not present with visible bleeding.

COMPREHENSION QUESTIONS

13.1 A 28-year-old G1P0 woman at 28 weeks' gestation presents to the hospital with fever, nausea and vomiting, and anorexia of 2 days' duration. On examination, her temperature is 100.7°F (38.16°C), HR is 104 bpm, and BP is 100/60 mm Hg. Her abdomen reveals tenderness on the right lateral aspect at the level of the umbilicus. There is mild right flank tenderness. A urinalysis is normal. In consideration of the diagnostic possibilities, which of the following is most accurate regarding this patient?

A. Appendicitis should be considered since the appendix location changes during pregnancy.

B. Cholecystitis is best diagnosed by CT scan of the abdomen.

C. Pyelonephritis commonly presents with normal urinalysis findings.

D. Inflammatory bowel disease should strongly be considered in this patient.

13.2 Upon performing laparoscopy for a suspected ovarian torsion on an 18-year-old nulliparous woman, the surgeon sees that the ovarian vascular pedicle has twisted 1 to 1.5 times and that the ovary appears somewhat bluish. Which of the following is the best management at this point?

A. Oophorectomy with excision close to the ovary

B. Oophorectomy with excision of the vascular pedicle to prevent possible embolization of the thrombosis

C. Unwind the vascular pedicle to assess the viability of the ovary

D. Bilateral salpingo-oophorectomy

E. Intravenous heparin therapy

13.3 A 32-year-old G1P0 woman at 29 weeks' gestation presents with a 1-day history of severe midepigastric abdominal pain radiating to the back, and multiple episodes of nausea and vomiting. On examination, her BP is 100/60 mm Hg, HR is 110 bpm, and temperature is 99°F (36.6°C). Her abdominal examination has tenderness and diffuse rebound. The serum amylase level is markedly elevated. Which of the following is the next step?

A. Initiate a high-protein, low-fat diet

B. Immediate surgical excision of the inflamed aspect of the pancreas

C. Ultrasound imaging of the abdomen

D. Delivery of the infant

13.4 An 18-year-old G1P0 woman complains of a 2-month history of colicky, right abdominal pain when she eats. It is associated with nausea and emesis. She states that the pain radiates to her right shoulder. The patient has a family history of diabetes. Which of the following is the most likely diagnosis?
   A. Peptic ulcer disease
   B. Cholelithiasis
   C. Appendicitis
   D. Ovarian torsion

13.5 A 19-year-old G1P0 woman at 28 weeks' gestation arrives to the obstetric (OB) triage area complaining of a 12-hour history of abdominal pain. She denies trauma, vaginal bleeding, or fever. On examination, her temperature is 99°F (37.2°C), HR is 100 bpm, and BP is 100/70 mm Hg. Her abdominal examination reveals hypoactive bowel sounds, diffuse abdominal pain with guarding. Which of the following statements regarding the abdominal pain is most accurate?
   A. The absence of vaginal bleeding rules out abruption as an etiology.
   B. Ovarian torsion is typically characterized by constant pain.
   C. The gallbladder typically moves superior and laterally with pregnancy.
   D. Degenerating leiomyoma typically presents with localized tenderness over the fibroid.

13.6 A 20-year-old G1P0 woman at 12 weeks' gestation is noted to have a suspected ruptured ectopic pregnancy. On sonography, there is a moderate amount of free fluid in the abdominal cavity. The medical student assigned to evaluate the patient is amazed by the apparent stability of the patient. Which of the following is the earliest indicator of hypovolemia?
   A. Tachycardia
   B. Hypotension
   C. Positive tilt
   D. Lethargy and confusion
   E. Decreased urine output

ANSWERS

13.1 **A.** The growing uterus pushes the appendix superior and lateral. The diagnosis of appendicitis during pregnancy can be difficult since patients frequently present with symptoms common in pregnancy. A delay in diagnosis, on the other hand, can lead to maternal morbidity and perinatal problems. Typically, patients present with nausea, emesis, fever, and anorexia. Abdominal pain is not located in the right lower quadrant as in nonpregnant patients because the growing uterus pushes on the appendix in an upward and outward direction, toward the flank and sometimes mimicking pyelonephritis. Regardless of gestational age, the treatment is surgical with intravenous (IV) antibiotics. Cholecystitis is also common in pregnancy, but usually presents with right abdominal pain in the subcostal region and may radiate to the right shoulder. Gallstones are best diagnosed with ultrasound rather than computed tomography (CT) scan. Pyelonephritis almost always is associated with pyuria (white blood cell [WBC] in urine), and usually causes fever and flank tenderness. Inflammatory bowel disease presents in young patients with bloody diarrhea and abdominal pain. This patient does not have diarrhea or loose stools.

13.2 **C.** Unless the ovary appears necrotic, the ovarian pedicle can be untwisted and the ovary observed for viability. An oophorectomy would not be indicated in this patient unless the ovaries were necrotic from the prolonged lack of perfusion, or if after untwisting the ovary, reperfusion cannot be established. It is important to try and conserve the ovary especially in such a young patient. Previously, it was thought that a torsioned ovarian vasculature with thrombus needed excision due to the possibility of embolization. This has been disproved and neither excision of the clotted vessels or heparin is required.

13.3 **C.** With the diagnosis of pancreatitis, the next diagnostic steps include assessing the severity of the condition (such as with Ranson criteria of hypoxia, hemorrhagic complications, renal insufficiency, etc), and looking for an underlying etiology for the pancreatitis. In pregnancy, the most common cause of pancreatitis is gallstones, although alcohol use, hyperlipidemia, and medications are sometimes implicated. Thus, the best next step is ultrasound to assess for gallstones. If gallstones are found, then consideration may be given to eventual cholecystectomy once the patient is stabilized. Endoscopic retrograde cholangiopancreatography (ERCP) with endoscopic stone extraction can be performed if a common bile duct stone is suspected. A patient with pancreatitis should have nothing by mouth. Surgery on the inflamed pancreas is harmful. Delivery of the pregnancy is not indicated.

13.4 **B.** This patient has a classic presentation of symptomatic cholelithiasis (biliary colic). In pregnancy, this condition is usually treated with a low-fat diet and observed until postpartum. However, if the patient were to develop cholecystitis (gallstones with fever and leukocytosis), biliary obstruction, or pancreatitis in pregnancy, surgery is the treatment of choice; generally, supportive medical management is used initially during the acute phase.

13.5 **D.** Fibroids of the uterus can be associated with red or carneous degeneration during pregnancy due to the estrogen levels leading to rapid growth of the fibroid. The fibroid outgrows its blood supply leading to ischemia and pain. Typically, the pain of a degenerating fibroid is localized over the leiomyoma. Abruption can be concealed with bleeding behind the placenta. The gallbladder usually does not move during pregnancy, whereas the appendix will move superiorly and laterally. Ovarian torsion is associated with colicky abdominal pain and comes and goes.

13.6 **E.** Renal blood flow is decreased with early hypovolemia as reflected by decreased urine output. This is a compensatory mechanism to make blood volume available to the body. Typically before tachycardia or hypotension occurs, a positive tilt test is noted. By the time hypotension is noted at rest in a young, healthy patient, 30% of blood volume is lost.

CLINICAL PEARLS

- In pregnancy, the appendix moves superiorly and laterally from the normal location.
- The acute onset of colicky abdominal pain is typical of ovarian torsion.
- With ovarian torsion, the clinician can untwist the pedicle and observe the ovary for viability.
- Ectopic pregnancy should be suspected in any woman with abdominal pain.
- The most common cause of hemoperitoneum in early pregnancy is ectopic pregnancy.
- A ruptured corpus luteum can mimic an ectopic pregnancy.
- Hemorrhagic corpus lutea can occur more commonly in patients with bleeding tendencies either congenital (von Willebrand) or iatrogenic (Coumadin induced).
- When the corpus luteum is excised in a pregnancy of less than 10 to 12 weeks gestation, progesterone should be supplemented.

REFERENCES

Castro LC, Ognyemi D. Common medical and surgical conditions complicating pregnancy. In: Hacker NF, Gambone JC, Hobel CJ, eds. *Essentials of Obstetrics and Gynecology*. 5th ed. Philadelphia, PA: Saunders; 2009:191-218.

Katz VL. Benign gynecologic lesions. In: Katz VL, Lentz GM, Lobo RA, Gersenson DM, eds. *Comprehensive Gynecology*. 5th ed. St. Louis, MO: Mosby-Year Book; 2007:419-470.

CASE 14

A 24-year-old G1P0 woman at 28 weeks' gestation complains of a 2-week duration of generalized pruritus. She denies rashes, exposures to insects, or allergies. Her medications include prenatal vitamins and iron supplementation. On examination, her blood pressure (BP) is 100/60 mm Hg, heart rate (HR) is 80 beats per minute (bpm), and weight is 140 lb. She is anicteric. The skin is without rashes. The fetal heart tones are in the range of 140 bpm. The patient says the itching is intense and she cannot sleep at night.

- What is the most likely diagnosis?
- What is the best treatment for this condition?
- What is the best management of the pregnancy?

ANSWER TO CASE 14:
Pruritus (Cholestasis) of Pregnancy

Summary: A 24-year-old G1P0 at 28 weeks' gestation complains of a 2-week duration of generalized pruritus. She is anicteric and normotensive. The skin is without rashes. The fetal heart tones are in the range of 140 bpm.

- **Most likely diagnosis:** Intrahepatic cholestasis of pregnancy (ICP).
- **Best treatment:** Ursodeoxycholic acid (UDCA).
- **Management of the pregnancy:** Fetal testing such as a biophysical profile once a week with consideration of delivery at 37 to 38 weeks due to the increased risk of stillbirth associated with ICP.

ANALYSIS
Objectives

1. Know the differential diagnosis of pruritus in pregnancy.
2. Understand the clinical presentation of intrahepatic cholestasis of pregnancy.
3. Know that the first line of treatment of cholestasis of pregnancy is ursodeoxycholic acid.
4. Be aware of the increased risk of stillbirth with ICP, and the rationale for fetal testing.

Considerations

This 24-year-old woman, who is at 28 weeks' gestational age, complains of generalized pruritus in the absence of a rash, which is consistent with ICP. The diffuse location of the itching and lack of rash makes a contact dermatitis unlikely. Another cause of pruritus unique to pregnancy is pruritic urticarial papules and plaques of pregnancy (PUPPP), which are erythematous papules and hives beginning in the abdominal area and often spreading to the buttocks. This is unlikely, as the patient does not have a rash. This patient's clinical picture does not resemble herpes gestationis, a condition causing intense itching but associated with erythematous blisters on the abdomen and extremities. Thus, the most likely etiology in this case is intrahepatic cholestasis, a process in which bile salts are incompletely cleared by the liver, accumulate in the body, and are deposited in the dermis, causing pruritus. This disorder usually begins in the third trimester. There are no associated skin rashes, other than excoriations from patient scratching. The diagnosis is one of exclusion, but serum bile acid levels are usually elevated. Oral UDCA is the treatment of choice, which decreases total serum bile acid levels and help to relieve the itching. Fetal testing such as biophysical profile or nonstress test examinations are usually started, with the plan for early delivery such as between 37 and 38 weeks' gestation due to the increased risk of stillbirth.

APPROACH TO:
Pruritus in Pregnancy

DEFINITIONS

INTRAHEPATIC CHOLESTASIS OF PREGNANCY (ICP): Intrahepatic cholestasis of unknown etiology in pregnancy whereby the patient usually complains of pruritus with or without jaundice and no skin rash.

PRURITIC URTICARIAL PAPULES AND PLAQUES OF PREGNANCY (PUPPP): A common skin condition of unknown etiology unique to pregnancy characterized by intense pruritus and erythematous papules on the abdomen and extremities.

HERPES GESTATIONIS: Rare skin condition only seen in pregnancy; it is characterized by intense itching and vesicles on the abdomen and extremities.

FETAL TESTING: Examinations such as biophysical profile, nonstress tests, and umbilical Doppler velocity testing to assess the health of the fetus (likelihood of fetal death, usually within 1 week).

CLINICAL APPROACH

Intrahepatic Cholestasis of Pregnancy

Pruritus in pregnancy may be caused by many disorders, of which one of the most common is **intrahepatic cholestasis of pregnancy (ICP)**, a condition that usually begins in the third trimester. It begins as mild pruritus without lesions, usually at night, and gradually increases in severity. The itching is usually more severe on the extremities than on the trunk, with predilection for the palms and soles. It may recur in subsequent pregnancies and with the ingestion of oral contraceptives, suggesting a hormone-related pathogenesis. The disease is common in some ethnic populations such as Swedes and Chileans, suggesting a genetic basis for the disease process. Approximately 15% are associated with adenosine triphosphate binding cassette gene, which transports phospholipids across hepatocyte membranes. Thus, a family history of ICP may suggest this defect.

Increased levels of circulating bile acids can help to confirm the diagnosis, but ICP is a clinical diagnosis. Elevated liver function tests can be seen and there are no hepatic sequelae in the mother. ICP is associated with significant adverse risk for the fetus, such as spontaneous preterm birth, meconium stained amniotic fluid and stillbirth. **The risk of fetal demise and adverse fetal outcomes increases with higher bile acid concentrations and increasing gestational age.** There is also an increased incidence of gallstones associated with the pruritus of pregnancy. The first line of treatment for ICP is a synthetic bile acid, ursodeoxycholic acid (UDCA). It reduces circulating bile acid in mother and baby. It improves pruritus in mother and reduces the risk of preterm labor, nonreassuring fetal status and respiratory depression in the baby. Other treatments for ICP include antihistamines, cornstarch baths, and cholestyramine (a bile salt binder). There is not complete agreement about the management of the pregnancy, but many practitioners will utilize weekly fetal testing such as biophysical profile, and delivery at 37 weeks to try to prevent stillbirth. Cholestasis of pregnancy must be distinguished from viral hepatitis and other causes of pruritus or liver disease. Women with a history of ICP may have a recurrence of cholestasis and pruritus with the use of oral contraceptives or other estrogen containing medications; alternative contraception should be recommended.

Herpes gestationis, which has no relationship to herpes simplex virus, is a pruritic bullous disease of the skin. It usually begins in the second trimester of pregnancy and the reported incidence is less than 1 in 1000 pregnancies. The etiology is thought to be autoimmune related. The presence of IgG autoantibody directed at the basement membrane has been demonstrated and may result in activation of the classic complement pathway by autoantibodies directed against the basement membrane zone. The clinical features are characterized by intense pruritus followed by extensive patches of cutaneous erythema and subsequent formation of small vesicles and tense bullae. The limbs are affected more often than the trunk. Definitive diagnosis is made by immunofluorescent examination of biopsy specimens. There have been reports of an increased incidence of fetal growth retardation and stillbirth. Transient neonatal herpes gestationis has also been reported at birth. Treatment has primarily been the use of oral corticosteroids.

The lesions of PUPPP usually begin on the abdomen and spread to the thighs and sometimes the buttocks and arms. The lesions, as their name describes, consist of erythematous urticarial plaques and small papules surrounded by a narrow, pale halo. The incidence of PUPPP is <1% of pregnant women. Immunofluorescent studies are negative for both immunoglobulin G (IgG) and complement levels. Histologic findings consist of normal epidermis accompanied by a superficial perivascular infiltrate of lymphocytes and histiocytes associated with edema of the papillary dermis. There are no studies to suggest an adverse effect on fetal and maternal outcome. Therapy includes topical steroids and antihistamines.

Acute Fatty Liver of Pregnancy

Acute fatty liver of pregnancy (AFLP) is a rare, serious condition involving microvesicular steatosis of the liver thought to be due to mitochondrial dysfunction in the oxidation of fatty acids, which leads to its accumulation in liver cells. Affected women often are heterozygous for long chain 3-hydroxyacyl-coenzyme A dehydrogenase (LCHAD) deficiency. This presents as right upper quadrant pain, malaise, nausea and vomiting, acute renal failure, hypoglycemia, coagulopathy, and acute and fulminant liver failure. Hyperbilirubinemia and jaundice are common. Delivery of the infant is the only definitive treatment and should be performed immediately due to the high maternal and fetal mortality with this condition.

TESTS TO MONITOR FETAL HEALTH

When conditions affect fetal well being, and increase the risk of stillbirth (such as hypertension or fetal growth restriction), a test for fetal health is often employed. These are usually started at 32 to 34 weeks' gestation, but may be started as early as viability. Table 14–1 lists various fetal tests.

Table 14-1 • SELECTED TESTS OF FETAL WELL BEING

Test	Description	Results	Rationale
Nonstress test (NST)	Fetal heart rate and uterine contraction monitor for 20 minutes	Two accelerations in 20 minutes is considered reactive or reassuring (significant decelerations may be nonreassuring)	A well-oxygenated fetus will have the capacity to develop accelerations; however, a nonreactive NST may be a sleep cycle and further testing such as with BPP is the usual next step
Contraction stress test	Fetal heart rate and uterine contraction monitor with the inducement of uterine contractions such as with oxytocin	Two accelerations in 20 minutes, with the absence of late decelerations with considered reassuring	A reactive NST is reassuring, but a fetus without late decelerations "under stress" is even more reassuring. However, there can be false positive CST results. Also in preterm gestations, CST can be problematic since it may cause a preterm delivery
Biophysical profile (BPP)	Five components each scored with 0 or 2 points: • NST • Fetal breathing • Fetal tone • Fetal movement • Amniotic fluid volume*	Scores of 8/10 with normal amniotic fluid, or 10/10 are considered reassuring. Scores of 6/10 is equivocal, and 4/10 or lower is considered nonreassuring (high risk of fetal death)	Acute placental insufficiency affects the NST, breathing, tone, and movement; chronic uteroplacental insufficiency affects the amniotic fluid volume. Together, there is a more complete picture of fetal status
Modified biophysical profile	Taking only part of the BPP components, usually the NST and amniotic fluid volume	A reactive NST without decelerations with normal amniotic fluid volume is considered reassuring	A reassuring modified BPP has been shown to be as predictive as the full BPP
Umbilical Doppler velocity	Assessment of umbilical artery blood flow	Velocity of flow during systole and diastole	Reverse end-diastolic flow is ominous and usually means fetal death in 24-48 hours; absent end-diastolic flow also worrisome

*Normal amniotic fluid volume is either the summation of four quadrant vertical measures (amniotic fluid index >5 cm or deepest vertical pocket of at least 2 cm × 2 cm).

COMPREHENSION QUESTIONS

14.1 A 31-year-old G2P1001 woman at 28 weeks' gestation presents with generalized pruritus. She has no rashes on her body and is diagnosed as having probable intrahepatic cholestasis of pregnancy. Which of the following is most accurate?

A. Hepatic transaminase levels are usually in the 2000 U/L range.
B. Is associated with hypertension.
C. May be associated with an increased perinatal morbidity.
D. Often is associated with thrombocytopenia.

14.2 A 30-year-old G1P0 woman presents for her routine prenatal care appointment at 36 weeks' gestation with pruritic skin rash over her abdomen. She is diagnosed as having pruritic urticarial papules and plaques of pregnancy (PUPPP). Which of the following best describes the pregnancy outcome with her diagnosis?

A. Somewhat increased perinatal morbidity and mortality
B. Increased preterm delivery rate
C. Increased preeclampsia
D. No effect on pregnancy

14.3 A 33-year-old G1P0 woman at 39 weeks' gestation is in labor. She has been diagnosed with herpes gestationis with the characteristic pruritus and vesicular lesions on the abdomen. Which of the following precautions is best advised for this patient?

A. Cesarean delivery is indicated.
B. Neonatal lesions may be noted and will resolve.
C. Vaginal delivery is permissible if the lesions are not in the introitus region and provided that oral acyclovir is given to the baby.
D. Tocolysis and oral steroid use is advisable until the lesions are healed.

14.4 A 24-year-old G2P1001 woman is at 34 weeks' gestation and noted to be icteric. She also has nausea and vomiting and malaise. A diagnosis of acute fatty liver of pregnancy is made, and the obstetrician recommends immediate delivery. Which of the following is most consistent with acute fatty liver of pregnancy?

A. Elevated serum bile acid levels
B. Hypoglycemia requiring multiple D50 injections
C. Proteinuria of 500 mg over 24 hours
D. Oligohydramnios noted on ultrasound

14.5 A 34-year-old G2P1 woman at 36 weeks' gestation with a diagnosis of ICP is undergoing fetal testing. If the BPP shows the following, what is your next step?

- NST is reactive without decelerations.
- Fetal breathing is present.
- Fetal movement is present.
- Fetal tone is present.
- Amniotic fluid index is 4 cm.

A. Contraction stress testing
B. Induce labor
C. Repeat BPP in 1 week
D. Umbilical Doppler velocity testing

ANSWERS

14.1 **C.** Intrahepatic cholestasis in pregnancy may be associated with increased perinatal morbidity, especially when accompanied by jaundice. It is rare for liver enzymes to be elevated or for there to be any hepatic sequelae in the mother; however, every patient who is suspected of having cholestasis of pregnancy should have their liver enzymes checked to avoid fetal morbidity and mortality. Hepatic enzyme levels are normally <3 U/L; women with intrahepatic cholestasis may have slightly elevated levels but almost never in the thousands. On presentation, no rash typically accompanies the pruritus. Thrombocytopenia is not involved in this disorder; however, it is involved in a life-threatening condition of pregnancy known as HELLP (hemolysis, elevated liver enzymes, low platelets) syndrome.

14.2 **D.** PUPPP is not thought to be associated with adverse pregnancy outcomes. The diagnosis is made presumptively based on clinical presentation, with the rash almost always starting on or near the abdominal striae of the abdomen. They are usually small red "bumps" that are intensely pruritic. The treatment is symptomatic. Interestingly, this condition usually occurs with the first pregnancy and usually does not recur, with the most common onset at 35 to 36 weeks' gestation.

14.3 **B.** Neonatal lesions are sometimes seen with herpes gestationis caused by the IgG antibodies crossing the placenta, and these lesions will resolve. Herpes gestationis is not the same as herpes simplex virus. The latter would necessitate cesarean delivery to avoid infection to the baby.

14.4 **B.** Hypoglycemia is relatively unique to acute fatty liver of pregnancy. Because of the liver insufficiency, glycogen storage is compromised leading to low serum glucose levels, which often require multiple doses of dextrose. Proteinuria is more consistent with preeclampsia, oligohydramnios is nonspecific, and bile acids are more consistent with ICP.

14.5. **B.** The biophysical profile in this case is 8/10 but with low amniotic fluid volume (oligohydramnios). The oligohydramnios is concerning and is associated with a 20 to 40× increase in fetal death as compared to normal amniotic fluid. Thus, the best management in this setting is induction of labor. Contraction stress testing or umbilical Doppler flow testing would not add much, or be reassuring. Repeat BPP in 1 week would be appropriate if the BPP were reassuring.

CLINICAL PEARLS

▶ The most common cause of generalized pruritus in pregnancy in the absence of skin lesions is cholestasis of pregnancy.

▶ Cholestatic jaundice in pregnancy may be associated with increased adverse pregnancy outcomes.

▶ The lesions of PUPPP usually begin on the abdomen and spread to the thighs and sometimes the buttocks and arms.

▶ ICP is associated with adverse fetal outcomes, which PUPPP is not.

▶ Acute fatty liver of pregnancy is a rare but serious condition that can lead to fulminant liver failure. Immediate delivery is warranted.

▶ Fetal testing for well being include NST, CST, BPP, and umbilical Doppler velocity assessment, and are used in circumstances of increased risk of stillbirth.

REFERENCES

Bacq Y, Sentilhes L, Reyes HB, et al. Efficacy of ursodeoxycholic acid in treating intrahepatic cholestasis of pregnancy: a meta-analysis. *Gastroenterology*. 2012;143:1492.

Castro LC, Ognyemi D. Common medical and surgical conditions complicating pregnancy. In: Hacker NF, Gambone JC, Hobel CJ, eds. *Essentials of Obstetrics and Gynecology*. 5th ed. Philadelphia, PA: Saunders; 2009:191-218.

Cunningham F, Leveno K, Bloom S, Spong CY, Dashe J. *Williams Obstetrics 24/E*. McGraw-Hill Professional; 2014.

Geenes V, Chappell LC, Seed PT, et al. Association of severe intrahepatic cholestasis of pregnancy with adverse pregnancy outcomes: a prospective population-based case-control study. *Hepatology*. 2014;59:1482.

Lee RH, Goodwin TM, Greenspoon J, Incerpi M. The prevalence of intrahepatic cholestasis of pregnancy in a primarily Latina Los Angeles population. *J Perinatol*. 2006;26:527.

Rajasri AG, Srestha R, Mitchell J. Acute fatty liver of pregnancy (AFLP)—an overview. *J Obstet Gynecol*. 2007;27(3):237-240.

Williamson F, Geenes V. Intrahepatic cholestasis of pregnancy. *Obstet Gynecol*. 2014;124(1):120-133.

CASE 15

A 19-year-old G1P0 woman at 20 weeks' gestation complains of the acute onset of pleuritic chest pain and severe dyspnea. She denies a history of reactive airway disease or cough. She has no history of trauma. On examination, her temperature is 98°F (36.6°C), heart rate (HR) is 120 beats per minute (bpm), blood pressure (BP) is 130/70 mm Hg, and respiratory rate (RR) is 40 breaths per minute. The lung examination reveals clear lungs bilaterally. The heart examination shows tachycardia. The fetal heart tones are in the range of 140 to 150 bpm. The oxygen saturation level is 89%. Supplemental oxygen is given.

- What test would most likely lead to the diagnosis?
- What is your concern?

ANSWERS TO CASE 15:
Pulmonary Embolus in Pregnancy

Summary: A 19-year-old G1P0 woman at 20 weeks' gestation complains of the acute onset of pleuritic chest pain and severe dyspnea. On examination, her HR is 120 bpm and RR is 40 breaths per minute. The lung examination reveals clear lungs bilaterally. The oxygen saturation is low.

- **Test most likely to lead to the diagnosis:** Spiral computed tomography or ventilation/perfusion (V/Q) imaging of the lungs.
- **Concern:** Pulmonary embolism.

ANALYSIS
Objectives

1. Understand that pleuritic chest pain and severe dyspnea are common presenting symptoms of pulmonary embolism.
2. Know that the pregnant woman is predisposed to deep venous thrombosis due to venous obstruction and a hypercoagulable state.
3. Understand that the spiral computed tomography (CT) or V/Q imaging scan is an initial diagnostic test for pulmonary embolism.

Considerations

This 19-year-old woman at 20 weeks' gestation complains of the acute onset of severe dyspnea and pleuritic chest pain. The physical examination confirms respiratory distress due to tachycardia and tachypnea. The lungs are clear on auscultation, and the patient does not complain of cough or fever, which rules out reactive airway disease or significant pneumonia. Clear lungs also speak against pulmonary edema. The patient has significant hypoxia with oxygen saturation of 89%, which translates to a partial pressure of 58 mm Hg (life-threatening). Thus, the most likely diagnosis is pulmonary embolism. Although many diagnostic tests should be considered in the initial evaluation of a patient with respiratory distress (such as arterial blood gas, chest radiograph, electrocardiograph), in this case, a CT pulmonary angiogram (CTPA), also referred to as spiral/helical CT, or ventilation-perfusion (V/Q) scan would likely lead to the diagnosis. The D-dimer assay may also be used in nonpregnant patients with a low pretest probability for pulmonary embolism (PE). The test has been shown to have a good negative predictive value, making it useful in ruling out pulmonary embolism if negative. However, since an elevated D-dimer level is normally found in pregnant patients, the assay would have limited value in this case.

If the imaging confirms pulmonary embolism, then the patient should receive anticoagulation to help stabilize the clot and decrease the likelihood of further venous thromboembolism. Pregnancy itself leads to an increased risk for thromboembolism by causing venous stasis and decreased outflow due to the mechanical effect of the uterus on the vena cava; additionally, the high estrogen levels induce a hypercoagulable state due to the increase in clotting factors, particularly fibrinogen.

APPROACH TO:
Respiratory Distress in Pregnancy

DEFINITIONS

DEEP VENOUS THROMBOSIS: Blood clot involving the deep veins of the lower extremity, rather than just the superficial involvement of the saphenous system.

PULMONARY EMBOLUS: Blood clot that is lodged in the pulmonary arterial circulation, usually arising from a thrombus of the lower extremity or pelvis.

HELICAL COMPUTED TOMOGRAPHY PULMONARY ANGIOGRAM: High-resolution imaging using intravenous (IV) contrast with multiple sections to allow for three-dimensional analysis and examination for vascular filling defects in the pulmonary vasculature.

MAGNETIC RESONANCE ANGIOGRAPHY: High-resolution magnetic resonance imaging using IV contrast to assess for vascular defects, typically not used in pregnancy due to the gadolinium.

VENTILATION-PERFUSION SCAN IMAGING PROCEDURE: Using a small amount of intravenous, radioactively tagged albumin, such as technetium, in conjunction with a ventilation imaging, with inhaled xenon or technetium, in an effort to find large ventilation-perfusion mismatches suggestive of pulmonary embolism.

DUPLEX ULTRASOUND FLOW STUDY: Ultrasound technique using both real-time sonography and Doppler flow to assess for deep venous thrombosis (DVT).

CLINICAL APPROACH

Respiratory distress is an acute emergency and necessitates rapid assessment and therapy. **Oxygen is the most important substrate for the human body**, and even 5 or 10 minutes of severe hypoxemia can lead to devastating consequences. Hence, a quick evaluation of the patient's respiratory condition, including the respiratory rate and effort; use of accessory muscles, such as intercostal and supraclavicular muscles; anxiety; and cyanosis; may indicate mild or severe disease. (See Figure 15–1 for one algorithm to evaluate dyspnea in pregnancy.) The highest priority is to identify impending respiratory failure, since this condition would require immediate intubation and mechanical ventilation. Pulse oximetry and arterial blood gas studies should be ordered while information is gathered during the history and physical. A cursory and targeted history directed at the pulmonary or cardiac organs, such as a history of reactive airway disease, exposure to anaphylactoid stimuli such as penicillin or bee sting, chest trauma, cardiac valvular disease, chest pain, or palpitations,

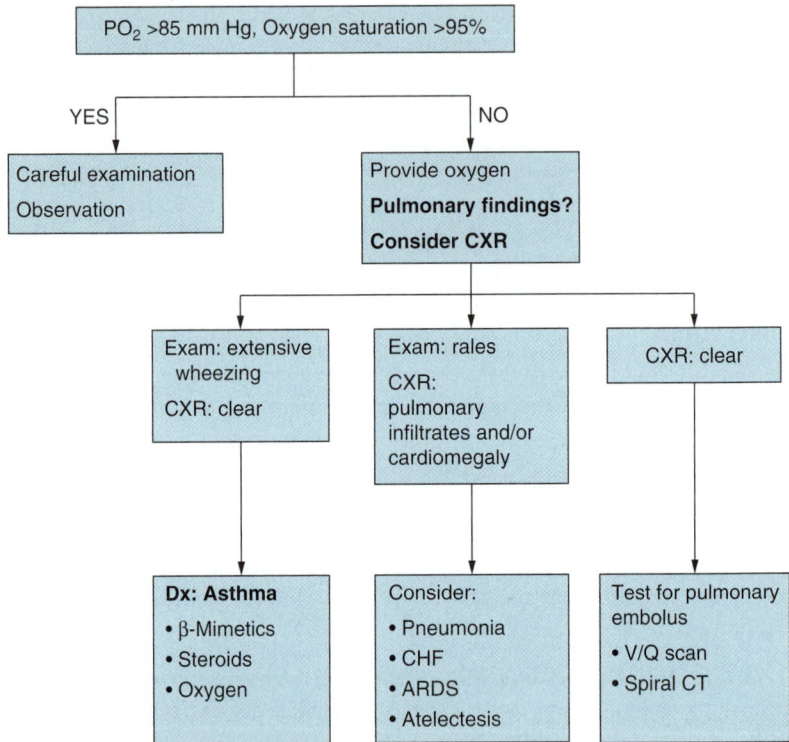

Figure 15–1. Algorithm for evaluation of dyspnea in pregnancy.

are important. Meanwhile, the physical examination should be directed at the heart and lung evaluation. The heart should be assessed for cardiomegaly and valvular disorders. The lungs should be auscultated for wheezes, rhonchi, rales, or absent breath sounds. The abdomen, back, and skin should also be examined.

A pulse oximetry reading of <90% corresponds to an oxygen tension of <60 mm Hg. Supplemental oxygen should immediately be given. An arterial blood gas should be obtained to assess for hypoxemia, carbon dioxide retention, and acid–base status. These findings should be evaluated in the context of the physiological changes in pregnancy (see Table 15–1). A chest radiograph should be performed rather expeditiously to differentiate cardiac versus pulmonary causes of hypoxemia. A large cardiac silhouette may indicate peripartum cardiomyopathy, which is treated by diuretic and inotropic therapy; pulmonary infiltrates may indicate pneumonia or pulmonary edema. A clear chest radiograph in the face of hypoxemia suggests pulmonary embolism, although early in the course of pneumonia, the chest x-ray may appear normal.

The diagnosis of pulmonary embolism may be made presumptively on the basis of high clinical suspicion, hypoxemia, and a clear chest x-ray. In some cases, intravenous heparin is initiated prophylactically while confirmatory testing is ordered. Diagnostic algorithms differ, but chest x-ray followed by either CTPA or V/Q scan has been shown to be an effective strategy in pregnant patients. Although controversial, CTPA and V/Q scan appear to provide comparable accuracy in diagnosis

Table 15-1 • NORMAL ARTERIAL BLOOD GAS CHANGES IN PREGNANCY

Parameter	Nonpregnant Value	Pregnant Value	Comment
pH	7.40	7.45	Respiratory alkalosis with partial metabolic compensation
PO_2 (mm Hg)	90–100	95–105	Increased tidal volume leads to increased minute ventilation and higher oxygen level
PCO_2 (mm Hg)	40	28	Higher tidal volume leads to increased minute ventilation and lower PCO_2
HCO_3 (mEq/L)	24	19	Renal excretion of bicarbonate to partially compensate for respiratory alkalosis, leads to lower serum bicarbonate, making the pregnant woman more prone to metabolic acidosis

as well as similar levels of radiation. The choice of imaging modality will depend on physician preference, patient contraindications, and the speed at which the test can be obtained. Many institutions have CTPA more readily available compared to V/Q scan. If the patient presents with symptoms of concurrent DVT, compression ultrasonography of the proximal veins should be ordered first.

Once the diagnosis of acute thromboembolism is confirmed, the pregnant woman is usually placed on full intravenous anticoagulation therapy for 5 to 7 days. Later, the therapy is generally switched to subcutaneous therapy to maintain the aPTT at 1.5 to 2.5 times control (if unfractionated heparin is used) for at least 3 months after the acute event. Heparin, which is a potent thrombin inhibitor that blocks conversion of fibrinogen to fibrin, combines with antithrombin III to stabilize the clot and inhibit its propagation. Both unfractionated heparin and low molecular weight heparin (LMWH) are safe to use in pregnancy as they do not cross the placenta. LMWH has the advantages of fewer bleeding complications and freedom from aPTT monitoring to assess therapeutic anticoagulation. After 3 months, either full heparinization or "prophylactic heparinization" doses can be utilized for the remainder of the pregnancy and for 6 weeks postpartum. Warfarin is associated with teratogenicity and is rarely used in pregnancy.

Estrogen products, such as oral contraceptive agents, are relatively contraindicated in women diagnosed with pulmonary embolism. Prophylactic anticoagulation for future pregnancies is more controversial, but is often used. Although pregnancy itself may induce thrombosis, many experts advise obtaining tests for other causes of thrombosis such as **protein S and protein C deficiency, prothrombin gene G20210A, antithrombin III activity, Factor V Leiden (FVL) mutation, hyperhomocysteinemia, and antiphospholipid antibodies.** Aside from antiphospholipid syndrome, which is typically treated with aspirin and heparin during pregnancy, the remaining thrombophilias without prior history of VTE are usually not given anticoagulation during pregnancy. Specifically, heterozygous Factor V Leiden mutation in the absence of prior VTE is usually not given anticoagulation; however, homozygous FVL or a prior history of VTE confers a much higher thrombosis risk and generally requires anticoagulation.

Deep Venous Thrombosis

Deep venous thrombosis (DVT) occurs in slightly <1% of pregnancies. The pregnant state increases the risk fivefold due to the venous stasis with the large gravid uterus pressing on the vena cava and the hypercoagulable state due to the increase in clotting factors. Cesarean delivery further increases the risk of DVT. Although clots involving the superficial venous system pose virtually no danger and may be treated with analgesia, DVT is associated with pulmonary embolism in 40% of untreated cases. The risk of death is increased tenfold when pulmonary embolism is unrecognized and untreated. Therefore, early diagnosis and anticoagulation treatment are crucial.

Signs and symptoms of DVT include deep leg pain, linear cords palpated along the calf, and tenderness and swelling of the lower extremity. A 2-cm difference in leg circumferences is also highly suggestive. Unfortunately, none of these findings are very specific for DVT, and in fact, the examination is normal in half of patients with DVT. Hence, imaging tests are necessary for confirmation.

In pregnancy, the diagnostic test of choice is Doppler ultrasound imaging, which usually employs a 5- to 7.5-MHz Doppler transducer to measure venous blood flow with and without compression of the deep veins. This modality is nearly as sensitive and specific as the time-honored method of contrast venography.

Management of DVT is primarily anticoagulation with bed rest and extremity elevation. Anticoagulation therapy is the same as pulmonary embolism treatment with full intravenous doses for 5 to 7 days, followed by subcutaneous therapy for at least 3 months after the acute event. After 3 months, either full or prophylactic heparin doses can be utilized for the remainder of the pregnancy and for 6 weeks postpartum. Patients who have additional risk factors for thromboembolism outside of pregnancy may need long-term anticoagulation.

AMNIOTIC FLUID EMBOLISM

Another clinical scenario that can present similarly to pulmonary embolism is **amniotic fluid embolism (AFE)**. This occurs when amniotic fluid enters the maternal circulation and subsequently causes obstruction and vasoconstriction of the pulmonary vessels due to fetal debris and vasoactive substances in the fluid. The patient may present with sudden dyspnea, hypoxia, hypotension, and coagulopathy. Fetal heart tones often become nonreassuring secondary to hypoperfusion. AFE most often occurs during labor or immediately postpartum. It is considered an exceedingly rare event, which is difficult to predict, but there are some risk factors associated with AFE: caesarian delivery, instrumental vaginal delivery, induction of labor, traumatic delivery, placental abruption, placenta accreta, advanced maternal age, and grandmuliparity. The rate of maternal mortality ranges from 20% to 60% and is typically due to cardiovascular collapse. Treatment is largely supportive with immediate delivery if there is rapid maternal or fetal decompensation.

MATERNAL MORTALITY

Recent studies on maternal death have shown a pregnancy-related mortality ratio of 16 per 100 000 live births in the United States, with a slight upward trend over the years. Ratios are higher in African-American women and tend to increase with maternal age. **The most common overall etiology for maternal mortality is embolism of all types,** followed by cardiovascular conditions and infection. Recent rates of mortality due to hemorrhage, hypertensive disorders, embolism, and anesthesia complications have declined, whereas **cardiovascular conditions and infectious causes have increased**. This suggests that the increasing number of pregnant women with comorbid health conditions may be playing a role in maternal adverse outcomes.

COMPREHENSION QUESTIONS

15.1 A 32-year-old woman pregnant at 29 weeks' gestation is noted to have symptoms concerning for a pulmonary embolism. The evaluation included chest radiograph, arterial blood gas, EKG, and CT pulmonary angiogram. A diagnosis of pulmonary embolism is made. Which of the following is most likely to be present in this patient?

   A. Dyspnea
   B. Chest pain
   C. Palpitations
   D. Hemoptysis
   E. Sudden death

15.2 A third-year medical student is assigned to perform a chart review of the cases of maternal mortality occurring in a hospital over the past 20 years. When the cases are collated, the student organizes the deaths by etiology. Which of the following is most likely to be the common underlying mechanism of death?

   A. Uterine atony
   B. Hypercoagulable state
   C. Hypertensive disease
   D. Sepsis
   E. Rupture of pregnancy through the fallopian tube

15.3 A 28-year-old otherwise healthy woman is found incidentally to have a factor V Leiden mutation (heterozygous). She is pregnant at 14 weeks' gestation. Which of the following is the best management of this patient?

   A. Aspirin therapy
   B. Expectant management
   C. Coumadin (Warfarin) therapy
   D. Heparin therapy

15.4 A 29-year-old G1P0 woman at 14 weeks' gestation is seen in the emergency room for possible diabetic ketoacidosis. The emergency room physician is evaluating the arterial blood gas which has been performed, and the findings are listed below. Based on these findings, which of the following is the most accurate statement?

pH 7.45; PO_2 103 mm Hg; PCO_2 31 mm Hg; HCO_3 18 mEq/L

A. The markedly decreased bicarbonate level indicates that the patient likely has DKA.
B. The decreased PCO_2 indicates that the patient is likely having a panic attack.
C. This arterial blood gas result is normal for pregnancy.
D. The elevated arterial pH reading likely indicates a metabolic alkylosis condition.

15.5 A 19-year-old G1P0 woman at 29 weeks' gestation has reactive airway disease. She has received two nebulized albuterol inhalant treatments with still some wheezing. Her arterial blood gas findings are listed below. Based on these findings, which of the following is the most accurate statement?

pH 7.40; PO_2 94 mm Hg; PCO_2 35 mm Hg; HCO_3 20 mEq/L

A. The low PO_2 level indicates significant exacerbation of the reactive airway disease.
B. The PCO_2 level indicates significant retained PCO_2 and a worrisome respiratory failure.
C. The arterial blood gas is normal in pregnancy.
D. The serum bicarbonate level is elevated for pregnancy and indicates metabolic alkalosis.

15.6 A 27-year-old G1P0 is at 31 weeks' gestation. She is seen by her physician for right leg pain and calf tenderness. A Doppler flow study indicates a deep venous thrombosis of the right lower extremity. Which of the following is a reason for the increased incidence of venous thromboembolism in pregnancy?

A. Venous stasis
B. Decreased clotting factors levels
C. Elevated platelet count
D. Endothelial damage

15.7 A 38-year-old G2P1 woman had been diagnosed with a deep venous thrombosis of the right leg when she was at 8 weeks' gestational age. She has been on subcutaneous heparin therapy for 6 months. Which of the following is the most likely result of long-term heparin therapy?

A. Osteoporosis
B. Thrombophilia
C. Fetal intracranial hemorrhage
D. Diabetes mellitus

ANSWERS

15.1 **A.** Dyspnea is the most common symptom of pulmonary embolus, whereas tachypnea is the most common sign. Another common symptom is pleuritic chest pain. A person with a pulmonary embolus may also experience palpitations or feel like they are having an anxiety attack. Few patients will have hemoptysis. However, these symptoms are not nearly as common as dyspnea. Sudden death is uncommon, but is more likely in a massive embolus. Patients with a pre-existing heart or lung condition are at increased risk of mortality. When a patient presents with dyspnea, the clinician should prioritize the examination and assessment toward the possibility of significant hypoxia.

15.2 **B.** Embolism (both thrombotic and amniotic) is the most common cause of maternal mortality. Pregnant women are predisposed to deep venous thromboses due to the obstructive effects the growing uterus has on the great vessels (ie, vena cava) and the hypercoagulable state of pregnancy, which persists for about 6 weeks postpartum. Hemorrhage typically occurs postpartum, usually due to uterine atony. The readily available blood products decrease the likelihood of death. Hypertensive disease is not typically deadly at the time of diagnosis and can be medically managed before, during, and after pregnancy. Ectopic pregnancies are usually not deadly unless rupture occurs and the patient goes into shock. Though this can occur, it is less common than embolism. Patients usually present with early signs (ie, vaginal bleeding) and symptoms (ie, adnexal pain) of an ectopic pregnancy before rupture occurs. Sepsis can also send a patient into shock; however, there are usually signs and symptoms of a bacterial infection (ie, fever, chills, vomiting) that will prompt medical intervention before there is progression to shock.

15.3 **B.** A patient who is heterozygous for FVL mutation and never had a VTE episode is at low risk for developing VTE in pregnancy. Generally, these patients are expectantly managed and not given anticoagulation. However, if she had a prior DVT or pulmonary embolism, or was homozygous for FVL mutation, then heparin (usually low molecular weight) would be advisable.

15.4 **C.** This arterial blood gas is normal in a pregnant woman. Pregnancy induces a respiratory alkalosis with partial metabolic compensation. This is the reason the serum bicarbonate level is decreased as compared to the nonpregnant patient.

15.5 **B.** This arterial blood gas reveals a PCO_2 of 35 mm Hg, which is elevated. In the face of reactive airway disease, this retained PCO_2 is worrisome, and may indicate respiratory failure. Initially, with asthma, hyperventilation should be associated with a decreased PCO_2. When the PCO_2 increases, fatigue, ineffective ventilation, or respiratory failure are possibilities.

15.6 **A.** Venous stasis is one of the main factors contributing to the hypercoagulable state in pregnancy. Venous stasis is present due to the uterus compressing the vena cava. Usually, the platelet count is slightly lower in the pregnant state. The lower limit of normal is 150 000/mm^3 in the nonpregnant patient and 120 000/mm³ in the pregnant woman. There is an increased level of clotting factors in pregnancy, and this along with venous stasis are the two factors that increase the risk of DVT in a pregnant woman fivefold. Endothelial damage is part of Virchow's triad (stasis, hypercoagulability, and endothelial damage) that contributes to thrombosis. It typically does not play a role during the pregnancy, but rather in the postpartum period when delivery, especially if surgical, may have caused some vascular damage.

15.7 **A.** The most common side effect of long-term heparin use in pregnancy is osteoporosis, usually not apparent unless on the agent for at least a month. The mechanism is thought to be overactive osteoclast activity as well as decreased osteoblast activity. Thrombocytopenia and bleeding episodes are other adverse effects. Heparin-induced thrombocytopenia occurs in <0.5% of pregnant women on subcutaneous heparin, and is less common than in nonpregnant individuals. Thrombocytopenia usually is manifest within the first 10 days of heparin use. Both unfractionated heparin and LMWH are associated with thrombocytopenia. Although there is conflicting evidence, LMWH may have a lower incidence of osteoporosis.

CLINICAL PEARLS

▶ The diagnosis of pulmonary embolism is suspected in a patient with dyspnea, a clear chest radiograph, and hypoxemia. It is confirmed with imaging tests such as ventilation-perfusion scan or CT pulmonary angiogram.

▶ The most common presenting symptom of pulmonary embolism is dyspnea.

▶ Amniotic fluid embolism may present during delivery with sudden hypoxia, hypotension, coagulopathy, and fetal distress.

▶ The most common cause of maternal mortality is embolism (both thromboembolism and amniotic fluid embolism).

▶ A PO_2 of <80 mm Hg in a pregnant woman is abnormal.

▶ The physical examination is not very useful in assessing for deep venous thrombosis (DVT).

▶ Venous duplex Doppler sonography is an accurate method to diagnose DVT.

▶ After a DVT or pulmonary embolus is diagnosed, anticoagulation is indicated for at least 3 months.

▶ The most common locations for DVT after gynecologic surgery are the lower extremities and the pelvic veins.

▶ Heterozygous Factor V Leiden mutation in the absence of prior VTE usually does not require anticoagulation during pregnancy.

REFERENCES

American College of Obstetricians and Gynecologists. Prevention of deep vein thrombosis and pulmonary embolism. *ACOG Practice Bulletin 84*. Washington, DC; 2007.

American College of Obstetricians and Gynecologists. Thromboembolism in pregnancy. *ACOG Practice Bulletin 123*. Washington, DC; November 2011.

Castro LC, Ognyemi D. Common medical and surgical conditions complicating pregnancy. In: Hacker NF, Gambone JC, Hobel CJ, eds. *Essentials of Obstetrics and Gynecology*. 5th ed. Philadelphia, PA: Saunders; 2009:191-218.

Clark SR. Amniotic fluid embolism. *Obstetrics and Gynecology*. 2014;123(2 Pt 1):337-348.

Creanga AA, Berg CJ, Syverson C, Seed K, Bruce FC, Callaghan WM. Pregnancy-related mortality in the United States, 2006-2010. *Obstetrics and Gynecology*. 2015;125(1):5-12.

Cunningham FG, Leveno KJ, Bloom SL, Hauth JC, Gilstrap LC III, Wenstrom KD. Pulmonary disorders. In: *Williams Obstetrics*. 22nd ed. New York, NY: McGraw-Hill; 2005:1055-1072.

Leung AN, Bull TM, Jaeschke R, et al. American Thoracic Society documents: an official American Thoracic Society/Society of Thoracic Radiology Clinical Practice Guideline—evaluation of suspected pulmonary embolism in pregnancy. *Radiology*. 2012;262(2):635-646.

CASE 16

A 19-year-old G1P0 woman at 29 weeks' gestation arrives to the hospital because of severe dyspnea of 6 hours' duration. Her prenatal course has been unremarkable, and she denies any medical problems. Her blood pressure (BP) is 160/114 mm Hg, heart rate (HR) is 105 beats per minute (bpm), respiratory rate (RR) is 40 breaths per minute and labored, and oxygen saturation is 90%. The fetal heart tones are in the range of 140 bpm. A urine protein to creatinine ratio is 0.6. The serum alanine transaminase (ALT) is 84 IU/L (normal < 35) and aspartate transaminase (AST) is 90 IU/L (normal < 35). The prenatal records show the following:

Gestational Age	BP (mm Hg)	Urine Protein	FHT (bpm)	Fundal Height (cm)
8 weeks	100/60	0	140	
12 weeks	110/70	0	148	
16 weeks	100/76	0	150	
20 weeks	105/58	0	138	20
26 weeks	130/89	1+	142	25

▶ What is the most likely diagnosis?
▶ What is your immediate next step?
▶ What are your priority laboratory tests?
▶ What is your management plan?

ANSWERS TO CASE 16:
Preeclampsia with Severe Features

Summary: A 19-year-old G1P0 woman at 29 weeks' gestation has acute onset of severe dyspnea, RR of 40 breaths per minute and labored, new onset severely elevated BP of 160/114 and elevated protein/creatinine ratio, and elevated liver function tests. The prenatal records show normal BPs in the pregnancy with a borderline elevated BP and 1+ proteinuria at the last visit (26 weeks).

- **Most likely diagnosis:** Preeclampsia with severe features

- **Immediate next step:** The highest priority must be to improve oxygenation. Sufficient oxygen must be provided to raise the O_2 saturation >94%, and if the patient is tiring, ventilator support may be required. The second priority is to lower the BP with intravenous (IV) antihypertensive agents. If pulmonary edema is confirmed, IV diuresis such as furosemide should be given.

- **Priority Lab tests: Complete blood count** (CBC) with platelet count and renal function test (creatinine).

- **Management:** Stabilize maternal status (optimize oxygenation, lower BP to safe level below 160/110 mm Hg), stabilize fetal status, administer corticosteroids for fetal lung maturity, start magnesium sulfate for seizure prophylaxis, and move toward delivery.

ANALYSIS

Objectives

1. Know the clinical presentation and diagnostic criteria for four categories of hypertensive disorders of pregnancy.
2. Know the serious sequelae of severe features of preeclampsia, including pulmonary edema.
3. Understand the management of preeclampsia with severe features at the preterm and term gestations.

Considerations

The patient is nulliparous, which is a risk factor for preeclampsia. She has preeclampsia based on new onset BP exceeding 140/90 mm Hg with proteinuria (urine protein/creatinine ratio exceeding 0.3). The patient has a record of normal BPs in her first 24 weeks of pregnancy (with borderline BP and 1+ proteinuria at 26 weeks), which is evidence that she does not have chronic hypertension. She has **preeclampsia with severe features** based on any one of three criteria: **blood pressure, elevated liver function tests, and likely pulmonary edema.** An O_2 saturation of 60% correlates to a pO_2 level of 60 mm Hg. Thus, the most immediate next step would be to improve oxygenation. The patient should be given 100% oxygen by face mask and if lung auscultation confirms pulmonary edema, then IV furosemide should be given. Concurrently, the BP needs to be lowered from the severe level (≥160/110 mm Hg) to prevent stroke. The physical exam and an urgent portable chest x-ray can help to assess for cardiomyopathy, pulmonary embolism, or asthma. Stabilization of maternal status has priority over fetal status; however, there should not be undue delay to evaluate the fetal status: fetal heart rate pattern and ultrasound for fetal weight, and amniotic fluid measurement. **Deciding whether to deliver a preeclamptic patient with severe features depends on the risk to maternal/fetal well being, the stability of the patient, and the gestational age.** In the face of pulmonary edema, delivery must be enacted, since the pregnant woman's life is in immediate jeopardy. In the face of marked prematurity, some severe features such as mildly elevated but stable liver function tests may be observed carefully without delivery. The **key laboratories to draw are the CBC with platelet count, LFTs, and the serum creatinine.** The **management of this patient includes magnesium sulfate for seizure prophylaxis and delivery.** Because of the preterm gestation, antenatal **corticosteroid administration** is important to promote lung maturity, and **GBS prophylaxis** such as with IV penicillin.

APPROACH TO:
Hypertensive Disease in Pregnancy

DEFINITIONS

CHRONIC HYPERTENSION: Blood pressure of 140/90 mm Hg before pregnancy or at less than 20 weeks' gestation, or persisting more than 12 weeks' postpartum.

GESTATIONAL HYPERTENSION: Hypertension without proteinuria (or other features of preeclampsia) at >20 weeks' gestation persistent for at least 4 hours.

PREECLAMPSIA: Hypertension (140 systolic or 90 diastolic) measured twice 6 hours apart with the new onset of proteinuria (>300 mg over 24 hours, or a urine protein to creatinine ratio >0.3) usually at a gestational age greater than 20 weeks. In the absence of proteinuria, hypertension and one of the following findings may suffice: thrombocytopenia, impaired liver function tests, renal insufficiency, pulmonary edema, cerebral disturbances, or visual impairment.

ECLAMPSIA: Seizure disorder associated with preeclampsia.

HELLP SYNDROME: Hemolysis, elevated liver function tests, low platelets, possibly a subset of severe preeclampsia, associated with significant fetal/maternal morbidity and mortality.

POSTERIOR REVERSIBLE ENCEPHALOPATHY SYNDROME (PRES): A cliniconeuroradiological syndrome with headache, encephalopathy, seizures, cortical visual disturbances, usually diagnosed with clinical features and magnetic resonance imaging (MRI) (showing enhancement in the posterior parietal areas). Prompt recognition and treatment of PRES with antihypertensives, antiepileptics, and intensive care unit (ICU) monitoring is important to prevent long-term neurological sequelae.

SEVERE FEATURE OF PREECLAMPSIA: Vasospasm associated with preeclampsia of such extent that maternal end organs are threatened, usually necessitating delivery of the baby regardless of gestational age.

SUPERIMPOSED PREECLAMPSIA: Development of preeclampsia in a patient with chronic hypertension, often diagnosed by an increased blood pressure and/or new onset proteinuria, which can be with or without severe features.

SUPERIMPOSED PREECLAMPSIA WITH SEVERE FEATURES: Development of preeclampsia in a patient with chronic hypertension with severe hypertension despite maximum therapy, cerebral/visual symptoms, pulmonary edema, low platelets, elevated LFT, or new onset renal insufficiency (Cr ≥ 1.1 mg/dL).

CLINICAL APPROACH

Hypertensive disorders complicate 3% to 4% of pregnancies and can be organized into several categories:

- Gestational hypertension
- Preeclampsia with or without severe features
- Chronic hypertension
- Superimposed preeclampsia with or without severe features
- Eclampsia

Gestational Hypertensive patients have only increased blood pressures without proteinuria or other features of preeclampsia. Up to 1/3 of those who are thought to have gestational hypertension are later found to have preeclampsia.

Preeclampsia is characterized by hypertension and proteinuria; less commonly, there is absence of proteinuria but evidence of vasospastic disease via other end-organ manifestations (see Table 16–1). Although not a criterion, nondependent edema is also usually present. An elevated blood pressure is diagnosed with a systolic blood pressure at or >140 mm Hg or diastolic blood pressure at or >90 mm Hg. Two elevated BPs, measured 6 hours apart (BP taken in the seated position), are needed for the formal diagnosis of preeclampsia, although at term, presumptive diagnoses with persistent hypertension over a shorter interval often guides management. Proteinuria is usually based on timed urine collection, defined as equal to or greater than 300 mg of protein in 24 hours, although a P/Cr ratio ≥0.3 is accurate.

Table 16–1 • DIAGNOSIS OF PREECLAMPSIA

New onset hypertension (140 systolic or 90 diastolic) twice over 6 hours with any one of:
- Proteinuria (≥300 mg/24 hours, or protein/Cr ≥ 0.3 mg/dL, or dipstick ≥ 1 + or greater)
- Thrombocytopenia (platelets < 100 000/mm³)
- Impaired LFT (2× normal)
- Renal insufficiency (Cr ≥ 1.1 mg/dL)
- Pulmonary edema
- New onset cerebral disturbance or visual impairment

Table 16–2 • SEVERE FEATURES OF PREECLAMPSIA (ANY ONE OF THE FOLLOWING)
• Systolic BP ≥ 160 mm Hg or diastolic BP ≥ 110 mm Hg on two occasions 4 hours apart • Platelets < 100 000/mm³ • Impaired LFT (2× normal) or severe persistent epigastric or RUQ pain • Progressive renal insufficiency (Cr ≥ 1.1 mg/dL) • Pulmonary edema • New onset cerebral or visual disturbance

Preeclampsia is further categorized as **with or without severe features.** See Table 16–2. With severe vasospasm to the brain, headache or visual disturbances can occur. Capillary leakage can lead to pulmonary edema. Right upper quadrant or epigastric pain or elevated LFTs result from hepatic injury.

Chronic hypertension includes preexisting hypertension or hypertension that develops prior to 20 weeks' gestation. These patients are at risk for intrauterine growth restriction (IUGR), fetal demise, or placental abruption. A patient with chronic hypertension is at risk for developing preeclampsia and, if this develops, her diagnosis is labeled as **superimposed preeclampsia**; this diagnosis is made on the basis of new onset of severe and uncontrollable hypertension, or new onset proteinuria, or a severe feature (Table 16–2). **Eclampsia** occurs when the patient with preeclampsia develops convulsions or seizures, but can occur without elevated blood pressure or proteinuria.

Pathophysiology

The underlying pathophysiology of preeclampsia is vasospasm and "leaky vessels," but its origin is unclear. It is cured only by termination of the pregnancy, and the disease process almost always resolves after delivery. Vasospasm and endothelial damage result in leakage of serum between the endothelial cells and cause local hypoxemia of tissue. Hypoxemia leads to hemolysis, necrosis, and other end-organ damage. The **vasospasm leads to increased systemic vascular resistance (hypertension), decreased intravascular volume, and decreased oncotic pressure;** these changes place a patient more susceptible to pulmonary edema and sensitive to fluid shifts (fluid overload with IV fluids, and hypotension with blood loss).

Clinical Evaluation

Patients are usually unaware of the hypertension and proteinuria, and typically the presence of symptoms indicates severe disease. Hence, one of the important roles of prenatal care is to identify patients with hypertension and proteinuria prior to severe disease. Complications of preeclampsia include placental abruption, eclampsia (with possible intracerebral hemorrhage), coagulopathies, renal failure, hepatic subcapsular hematoma, hepatic rupture, and uteroplacental insufficiency. Fetal growth restriction, poor Apgar scores, and fetal acidosis are also more often seen.

Risk factors for preeclampsia include nulliparity, extremes of age, African-American race, personal history of severe preeclampsia, family history of preeclampsia, chronic hypertension, chronic renal disease, obesity, antiphospholipid syndrome, diabetes, and multifetal gestation. The history and physical examination is focused on end-organ disease.

It is important to review and evaluate the blood pressures prior to 20 weeks' gestation (to assess for chronic hypertension). Patients with chronic hypertension may sometimes already have mild proteinuria, so it is important to establish a baseline to later document superimposed preeclampsia (substantial increase in proteinuria). Also one should document any sudden increase in weight (indicating possible edema). On physical examination, serial blood pressures should be checked along with a urinalysis.

Laboratory tests should include a complete blood count (CBC; check platelet count and hemoconcentration), urinalysis and 24-hour urine protein collection or protein/creatinine ratio (check for proteinuria), liver function tests, LDH (elevated with hemolysis), and creatinine. Fetal testing (such as biophysical profile) is also usually performed to evaluate uteroplacental insufficiency.

Management

After the diagnosis of preeclampsia is made, the management will depend on the gestational age of the fetus and the severity of the disease (see Table 16–3 and Figure 16–1 for one management scheme). **Gestational hypertensive or preeclamptic patients without severe features** can be observed and delivered at term (37 weeks), and magnesium sulfate use is individualized. **Chronic hypertensive patients who are well controlled** and uncomplicated can be observed and delivered at **38 to 39 weeks.** When severe features complicate preeclampsia or superimposed preeclampsia, the risks of the preeclampsia must be weighed against the risk of prematurity. When the fetus is premature, the following issues are considered:

1. What are the immediate threats to maternal status, how stable is the patient, and can these threats be ameliorated?

2. What are the immediate threats to fetal status, how stable is the fetus, and can these threats be ameliorated?

3. What is the gestational age? If <34 weeks' gestation, can delivery be safely delayed for 48 hours to allow corticosteroids to have maximum efficacy?

4. What is the natural history of the severe feature and does it seem to be worsening rapidly?

Observation of a patient with severe features should be performed in a tertiary center, since the risks to both the woman and the fetus are substantial. **With an unstable patient, delivery is always warranted regardless of gestational age. NSAIDs may elevate the BP in postpartum preeclamptic patients and should be avoided.**

Acute Management of Severe Hypertension

The acute-onset of severe hypertension (160 systolic or 110 diastolic, NOTE "or") that persists >15 minutes is considered a hypertensive emergency. **Therapy should be initiated quickly to avoid stroke.** Systolic hypertension is as important or even more important as a predictor of cerebral injury. **First line agents include IV labetolol, IV hydralazine, or oral nifedipine;** typically after an initial dose, the BP is retaken 20 minutes later and further higher dose therapy is given if the BP is still in the severe range.

Table 16–3 • MANAGEMENT OF HYPERTENSION IN PREGNANCY

Category	Assessment	Management
Gestational hypertension or preeclampsia without severe features	1. Check for symptoms 2. Check BP 2×/week 3. Check platelet count, LFT, Cr 1×/week 4. Check serial US for fetal growth* 5. BPP once a week for fetal well being	No bed rest needed No anti-BP meds needed Delivery at 37 0/7 weeks (magnesium sulfate use individualized)
Chronic hypertension without severely elevated BP (uncomplicated)	1. Oral antihypertensive agent if BP ≥ 150/100, or on agent prepregnancy 2. Check BP and urine protein at prenatal visits 3. Serial US to assess for fetal growth 4. BPP starting at 30–32 weeks	Delivery at 38-39 weeks

Preeclampsia or superimposed preeclampsia with severe features	1. Stabilize maternal status, such as control BP if ≥ 160 systolic or 110 diastolic
	2. Assess for maternal and/or fetal threats (CBC, LFT, Cr)
	3. Assess fetal weight, FHR pattern, and/or BPP
		• If ≥34 weeks, administer magnesium sulfate and deliver
		• If <34 weeks, corticosteroids, magnesium sulfate, and assess maternal/fetal stability
		  a. <34 weeks and maternal/fetal status stable= wait at least 48 hours, then delivery (with magnesium sulfate)
		  b. With greater prematurity, if delivery delayed, monitor carefully and reassess daily in tertiary center
		  c. If fetal or maternal status unstable, deliver immediately (with magnesium sulfate)
		• Regardless of gestation age, deliver for uncontrollable severe hypertension (max meds), eclampsia, pulmonary edema, abruption, DIC, nonreassuring fetal status
		• NOTE: If IUGR, use BPP and umbilical art Dopplers to guide

Acutely elevated BP (160 systolic or 110 diastolic)		Use IV labetolol or IV hydralazine or oral nifedipine immediately (reassess 20 minutes later) and escalate dose or alternate agent to bring BP to safe level

*If IUGR found, then BPP and umbilical artery Doppler testing.

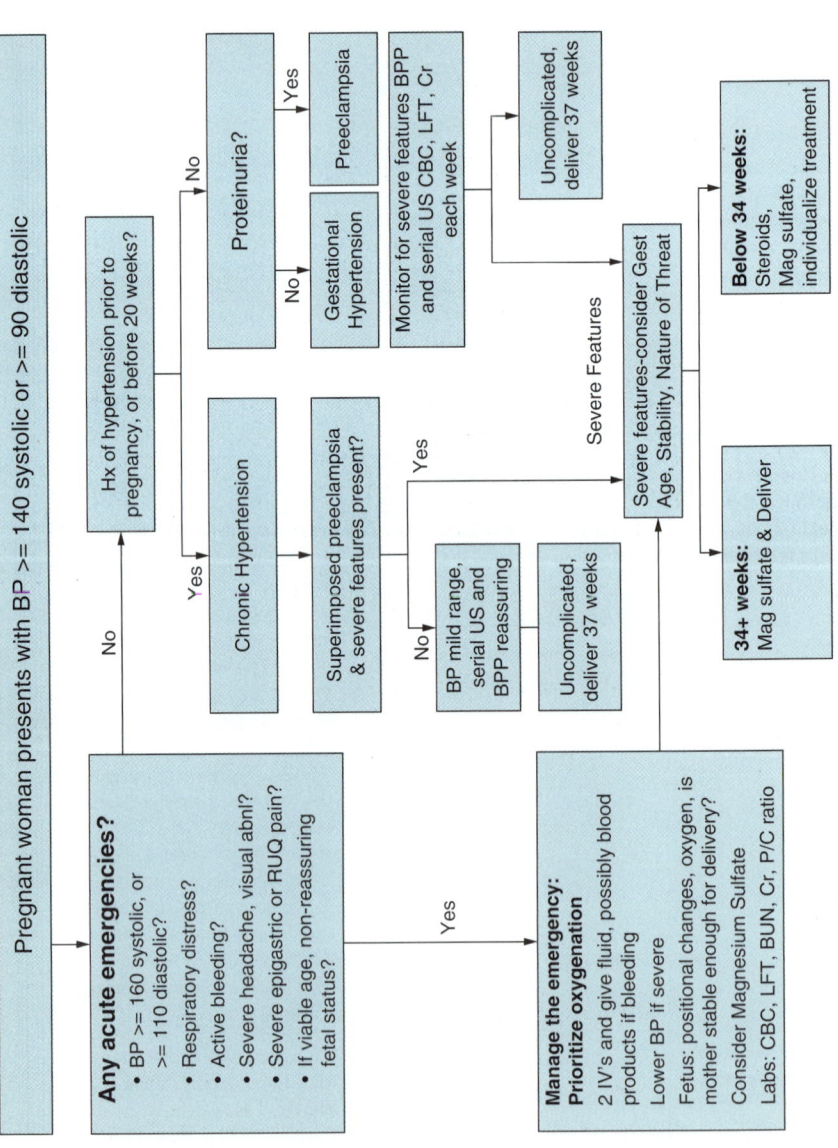

Figure 16–1 Algorithm for management of hypertension in pregnancy.

Eclampsia

Eclampsia is one of the most feared complications of preeclampsia, and the greatest risk for occurrence is just prior to delivery, during labor (intrapartum), and within the first 24 hours' postpartum. During labor, the preeclamptic patient should be started on the anticonvulsant magnesium sulfate. Since magnesium is excreted by the kidneys, it is important to monitor urine output, respiratory depression, dyspnea (side effect of magnesium sulfate is pulmonary edema), and abolition of the deep tendon reflexes (first sign of toxic effects is hyporeflexia). Hypertension is not affected by the magnesium. Severe hypertension needs to be controlled with antihypertensive medications such as hydralazine or labetalol. After delivery, magnesium sulfate is discontinued approximately 24 hours' postpartum. The hypertension and proteinuria frequently will resolve. Occasionally, the patient's blood pressure remains high and an antihypertensive medication is needed after delivery. After discharge, the patient usually follows up in 1 to 2 weeks to check blood pressures and proteinuria.

Emerging Concepts

There may be different mechanisms of preeclampsia. There is evidence that early disease (prior to 34 weeks) may be due to placental factors, such as inadequate or abnormal trophoblastic invasion into the spiral arteries. Investigators have noted abnormal "notching" uterine artery Doppler waveforms in patients prior to the clinical development of preeclampsia; these individuals seem to have worse and earlier-onset disease. In contrast, women with late-onset preeclampsia may be predisposed due to "constitutional" factors such as obesity. These patients tend to have a more favorable course. Also, there is some evidence that in significantly obese patients, bariatric surgery prior to pregnancy may reduce the risk of preeclampsia (and the risks of obesity). **Low dose aspirin** (started in late first trimester) may slightly reduce the recurrence of preeclampsia. Women who have had one or more pregnancies complicated by severe features <34 weeks' gestation are candidates. **Women with preeclampsia may have an increased risk of cardiovascular disease** in later life, and may benefit from screening for hypertension and cardiovascular risk factors throughout their life.

CASE CORRELATION

- See also Case 14 on intrahepatic cholestasis of pregnancy (ICP) and the discussion of acute fatty liver of pregnancy.

    A common differential diagnosis of abnormal liver function tests in pregnancy includes preeclampsia, AFLP, HELLP syndrome, and ICP. The following features can help differentiate:

- AFLP—nausea and vomiting, icteric, hypoglycemia, coagulopathy
- Preeclampsia—LFTs 100 to 300 IU/L range, hypertension, proteinuria
- HELLP—hemolysis, LFTs can be up to 1000 IU/L, platelet <100 000/μL
- ICP—generalized itching, mildly elevated LFTs, elevated bile salts

COMPREHENSION QUESTIONS

16.1 A 29-year-old G1P0 woman at 28 weeks' gestation is admitted to the hospital for preeclampsia. Her blood pressure (BP) is 150/100 mm Hg and protein excretion is 500 mg in 24 hours. On day 7 in the hospital, she is diagnosed with severe features of preeclampsia and the decision is made to administer magnesium sulfate and deliver the baby. Which of the following findings is most likely present in this patient to necessitate delivery?

A. Elevated uric acid levels
B. 5 g of proteinuria excreted in a 24-hour period
C. 4+ pedal edema
D. Platelet count of 115 000/μL
E. PT INR of 1.9 and PTT of 50 s

16.2 Which of the following is the best management of an 18-year-old G1P0 woman at 28 weeks' gestation with a blood pressure of 160/110 mm Hg, elevated liver function tests, and a platelet count of 60 000/μL?

A. Oral antihypertensive therapy
B. Platelet transfusion
C. Magnesium sulfate therapy and induction of labor
D. Intravenous immunoglobulin therapy

16.3 A 19-year-old G1P0 woman at 39 weeks' gestation is diagnosed with preeclampsia based on a blood pressure in the range of 150/90 mm Hg and 2+ proteinuria on urine dipstick. She complains of a severe headache. The patient is placed on magnesium sulfate and develops flushing and fatigue. She asks about the need for the magnesium sulfate. You explain that it is to prevent the seizures that may complicate preeclampsia and may even cause death. The patient asks how seizures associated with preeclampsia can cause mortality. Which of the following is the most common mechanism?

A. Intracerebral hemorrhage
B. Myocardial infarction
C. Electrolyte abnormalities
D. Aspiration

16.4 A 33-year-old woman at 29 weeks' gestation is noted to have a blood pressure of 150/90 mm Hg and a protein/creatinine ratio of 0.6. The platelet count, liver function tests, and creatinine are normal. Which of the following is the best management for this patient?

A. Induction of labor
B. Cesarean section
C. Antihypertensive therapy
D. Expectant management

16.5 A 25-year-old G1P0 woman at 28 weeks is diagnosed with severe preeclampsia based on a BP of 160/100 mm Hg and a platelet count of 98 000/mm^3. The patient is treated with hydralazine for the hypertension. Which of the following is the most appropriate reason for delivery?

A. Blood pressures persist in the range of 150/95 mm Hg
B. Urine protein increases to 5 g over 24 hours
C. The patient reaches 32 weeks' gestation
D. Patient develops pulmonary edema
E. Repeat platelet count is 95 000/mm^3

16.6 On postpartum day 1, a 28-year-old G1P1 woman reports some headache and problems with her vision bilaterally. Her BP is 150/95 mm Hg and P/C ratio is 0.5. Her neurological examination is normal but her vision is impaired in both eyes. Which of the following is the best next step?

A. Antihypertensive agent
B. IV Mannitol
C. MRI of the brain
D. CT imaging of the brain
E. Ophthalmic eye drops to both eyes

Choose the best management plan (A-E) for each of the clinical scenarios (16.7-16.10):

A. Corticosteroids
B. Antihypertensive agent
C. Biophysical profile
D. Magnesium sulfate and delivery
E. Continued observation

16.7 A 32-year-old G2P1 woman is at 35 weeks with chronic hypertension. The BP is in the 140/95 range.

16.8 A 28-year-old G1P0 woman is at 30 weeks' gestation with superimposed preeclampsia. The BP is 150/100. The platelet count is 95 000 and LFT is 2× normal. BPP is 10/10.

16.9 A 30-year-old G2P1 woman is at 31 weeks with chronic hypertension, using oral labetolol. Her BP in the office is 160/95 and 162/90. The urine protein is negative.

16.10 A 24-year-old G3P2 woman at 34 weeks' gestation is noted to have preeclampsia. The BP is 150/90 and P/C ratio is 0.5. A fetal ultrasound shows the estimated fetal weight is at the 8th percentile.

ANSWERS

16.1 **E.** A severe feature of preeclampsia (Table 16–2) may or may not necessitate immediate delivery. In this case, DIC is the most concerning condition and requires delivery at any gestational age. Pedal edema is not pathologic; nondependent edema, such as of the face and hands, may be consistent with preeclampsia but does not indicate severity of disease. Low platelets are associated with HELLP syndrome, a form of hemolytic anemia in pregnancy, and are very worrisome. Uric acid levels are known to be elevated with preeclampsia; however, it is not a criterion for severe preeclampsia. In general, the criteria for severe preeclampsia indicate end-organ threat, and generally require delivery for gestational age at or >34 weeks, and depending on the nature of the threat and the stability of the patient, perhaps delivery at an earlier gestational age.

16.2 **C.** Although the pregnancy is only 28 weeks, in light of the severe feature of preeclampsia with marked thrombocytopenia, the best treatment is magnesium sulfate and delivery. When preeclampsia with severe features is diagnosed, delivery depends on the nature of the threat, the stability of the patient/fetus, and the gestational age. If the platelet count was higher (90 000), expectant management may be entertained at a tertiary center. Oral antihypertensive therapy, such as labetalol, may be given to the patient to control blood pressure; however, it should not be used as the "treatment" for severe preeclampsia. The platelet levels are not low enough to require transfusion; intravenous immunoglobulin (IVIG) is used for various autoimmune diseases, but not indicated in this patient.

16.3 **A.** The most common cause of maternal death due to eclampsia is intracerebral hemorrhage. Eclampsia is one of the most feared complications of preeclampsia, and the greatest risk for occurrence is just prior to delivery, during labor (intrapartum), and within the first 24 hours' postpartum. Patients with gestational hypertension or preeclampsia without severe features do not necessarily require magnesium sulfate for seizure prophylaxis. This patient has a severe headache which is a severe feature. Magnesium sulfate has been proven to be superior to other anticonvulsants such as valium, Dilantin, or phenobarbital. One dictum that is useful in the emergency room or obstetrical unit is that "a pregnant patient greater than 20 weeks' gestation without a history of epilepsy who presents with seizures has eclampsia until otherwise proven."

16.4 **D.** In the preterm patient with mild preeclampsia, expectant management is generally employed until severe features are noted or the pregnancy reaches 37 weeks. In other words, the risks of prematurity usually outweigh the risks of the preeclampsia until end-organ threat is manifest. Had this patient been at term, the best step in management would be to induce labor; this is because at term, the risks of prematurity are minimal. Severe, but not mild hypertension associated with preeclampsia, should be controlled with hypertensive medication. Antihypertensive agents are useful in chronic hypertension but not in preeclampsia unless the BP is in the severe range; lowering these BPs can help avoid stroke. For the patient in this scenario, neither induction nor cesarean section is indicated since she is not yet at term. It is not a requirement for a preeclamptic patient to deliver by cesarean. This patient can be followed as an outpatient with twice weekly BP checks and once a week platelet count, Cr, and LFTs.

16.5 **D.** Pulmonary edema is an indication for delivery at a preterm gestation. Proteinuria of 5 g over 24 hours is no longer criteria of a severe feature of preeclampsia and does not correspond to maternal or fetal outcome. Mild thrombocytopenia (80 000-100 000) that is stable may be judiciously observed in this patient (in a tertiary care center). A DIC panel should be performed to ensure there is not a coagulopathy, since that would be an indication for immediate delivery.

16.6 **C.** This patient is postpartum and likely has preeclampsia based on the elevated BP and the proteinuria. The symptoms may be due to PRES syndrome, which needs to be quickly diagnosed by MR imaging, since aggressive therapy must be enacted to prevent long-term brain dysfunction. An antihypertensive agent does not generally need to be used unless the BP is severe (160 systolic or 110 diastolic). CT imaging can discern an intracranial bleed, and is useful if the patient had an eclamptic episode. Eye drops would be indicated with a conjunctivitis.

16.7 **C.** A biophysical profile should be performed. A patient with chronic hypertension that is well controlled should be monitored carefully for superimposed preeclampsia, complications such as abruption, serial ultrasound examinations to assess for IUGR, fetal testing such as BPP weekly, and delivered at 38 to 39 weeks.

16.8 **A.** Corticosteroid therapy is the single most important intervention to impact on the neonatal outcome in a pregnancy <34 weeks when delivery is expected imminently (within 7 days). Magnesium sulfate is often given during this time of carefully monitoring the platelet count and liver function tests, but not necessarily delivery. This change in carefully observing patients with stable mild thrombocytopenia and stable elevated LFTs is based on the knowledge of antenatal corticosteroid impact on neonatal outcome.

16.9 **B.** This patient has severely elevated BP and must receive an antihypertensive agent ASAP to reduce the risk of stroke. This may be IV labetolol, IV hydralazine, or oral nifedipine. Although corticosteroids and BPP are viable answer choices, the highest priority is to lower the BP.

16.10 **C.** This patient likely has IUGR. The next step would be to evaluate possible fetal compromise with BPP and umbilical artery Doppler studies. At 34 weeks, corticosteroid therapy is not effective. Magnesium sulfate and delivery is an option, but more information such as assessment of fetal status would give a more complete picture. The BPs are in the mild range, and so an antihypertensive agent is not needed.

CLINICAL PEARLS

▶ In general, the treatment of gestational hypertension or preeclampsia without severe features at or beyond 37 weeks' gestation is delivery. Use of magnesium sulfate is individualized.

▶ The management of preeclampsia without severe features in a preterm pregnancy is observation until severe features are noted, or term gestation is reached.

▶ Severe features complicating preeclampsia or superimposed preeclampsia at a gestational age of 34 weeks or higher should be given magnesium sulfate and delivered. Those <34 weeks may be judiciously observed in specialized facilities.

▶ The most common cause of significant proteinuria in pregnancy is preeclampsia.

▶ Magnesium sulfate is the best anticonvulsant to prevent eclampsia.

▶ The first sign of magnesium toxicity is loss of deep tendon reflexes.

▶ Chronic hypertension is diagnosed when a pregnant woman has hypertension prior to 20 weeks' gestation, or if the hypertension persists beyond 12 weeks' postpartum.

▶ Gestational hypertension is when a pregnant woman has hypertension after 20 weeks of gestation without proteinuria or other evidence of preeclampsia.

▶ Acute onset severe hypertension (160 systolic or 110 diastolic) persisting > 15 minutes is considered a hypertensive emergency. IV labetolol, IV hydralazine, or oral nifedipine are first line agents.

REFERENCES

American College of Obstetricians and Gynecologists. Diagnosis and management of preeclampsia and eclampsia. *ACOG Practice Bulletin 33*. Washington, DC; 2012.

Castro LC. Hypertensive disorders of pregnancy. In: Hacker NF, Gambone JC, Hobel CJ, eds. *Essentials of Obstetrics and Gynecology*. 5th ed. Philadelphia, PA: Saunders; 2009:173-182.

Cunningham FG, Leveno KJ, Bloom SL, et al. Pregnancy hypertension. In: *Williams Obstetrics*. 24th ed. New York, NY: McGraw-Hill; 2014:706-756.

Task Force on Hypertension in Pregnancy. American College of Obstetricians and Gynecologists. *Hypertension in Pregnancy*; 2013.

CASE 17

A healthy 19-year-old G1P0 woman at 29 weeks' gestation presents to the labor and delivery area complaining of intermittent abdominal pain. She denies leakage of fluid or bleeding per vagina. Her antenatal history has been unremarkable. She has been eating and drinking normally. On examination, her blood pressure (BP) is 110/70 mm Hg, heart rate (HR) is 90 beats per minute (bpm), and temperature is 99°F (37.2°C). The fetal heart rate tracing reveals a baseline heart rate of 120 bpm and a reactive pattern. Uterine contractions are occurring every 3 to 5 minutes. On pelvic examination, her cervix is 3 cm dilated, 90% effaced, and the fetal vertex is presenting at −1 station.

- What is the most likely diagnosis?
- What is your next step in management?
- What test of the vaginal fluid prior to digital examination may indicate risk for preterm delivery?
- What medication can be given to decrease the risk of neurological impairment in the baby?

ANSWERS TO CASE 17:
Preterm Labor

Summary: A healthy 19-year-old G1P0 woman at 29 weeks' gestation complains of intermittent abdominal pain. Her vital signs are normal. The fetal heart rate tracing reveals a baseline heart rate of 120 bpm and is reactive. Uterine contractions are noted every 3 to 5 minutes. Her cervix is 3 cm dilated, 90% effaced, and the fetal vertex is presenting at −1 station.

- **Most likely diagnosis:** Preterm labor.
- **Next step in management:** Tocolysis, try to identify a cause of the preterm labor, antenatal steroids, and antibiotics for GBS prophylaxis.
- **Test of vaginal fluid:** Fetal fibronectin assay.
- **Medication for neuroprotection:** Magnesium sulfate may be given for pregnancies of <32 weeks when there is imminent delivery.

ANALYSIS
Objectives

1. Understand how to diagnose preterm labor.
2. Understand that the basic approach to preterm labor is tocolysis, identification of an etiology, steroids, and magnesium sulfate (if appropriate).
3. Know the common causes of preterm delivery.

Considerations

This 19-year-old nulliparous woman is at 29 weeks' gestation and complains of intermittent abdominal pain. The monitor indicates uterine contractions every 3 to 5 minutes, and her cervix is dilated at 3 cm and effaced at 90%. This is sufficient to diagnose preterm labor in a nulliparous woman. If she had a previous vaginal delivery, the diagnosis may not be so clear cut. Because of the significant prematurity, many practitioners may elect to treat for preterm labor. A single examination revealing 2-cm dilation and 80% effacement in a nulliparous woman would be sufficient to diagnose preterm labor. Prior to digital examination, one should swab the posterior vaginal fornix for fetal fibronectin (fFN), which, if positive, may indicate risk of preterm birth. In contrast, a negative fFN assay is strongly associated with no delivery within 1 week. Another objective test for preterm delivery risk is transvaginal cervical length ultrasound measurements. A shortened cervix, especially with lower uterine segment changes (funneling or beaking of the amniotic cavity into the cervix), is worrisome. Tocolysis should be initiated, unless there is a contraindication (such as intra-amniotic infection or severe preeclampsia). Also, since the pregnancy is <34 weeks' gestation, **intramuscular (IM) antenatal steroids should be given to enhance fetal pulmonary maturity.** In fact, the use of antenatal corticosteroids is the single most important obstetrical intervention available that positively impacts on neonatal morbidity and survival. A careful search should also be undertaken to identify an underlying cause of preterm labor, such as urinary tract infection, cervical infection, bacterial vaginosis, generalized infection, trauma or abruption, hydramnios, or multiple gestations. Finally, intravenous (IV) antibiotics, such as penicillin, are helpful in case the tocolysis is unsuccessful to reduce the likelihood of GBS sepsis in the neonate. Last, recent studies have shown that if the pregnancy is <31 6/7 weeks, starting magnesium could help the neurodevelopment of the preterm baby, reducing cases of cerebral palsy in preterm infants.

APPROACH TO:
Preterm Labor

DEFINITIONS

PRETERM LABOR: Cervical change associated with uterine contractions prior to 37 complete weeks and after 20 weeks' gestation. In a nulliparous woman, uterine contractions and a single cervical examination revealing 2-cm dilation and 80% effacement or greater are sufficient to make the diagnosis.

TOCOLYSIS: Pharmacologic agents used to delay delivery once preterm labor is diagnosed. The most commonly used agents are indomethacin, nifedipine, terbutaline, and ritodrine. Recent evidence has indicated that magnesium sulfate may be ineffective as a tocolytic agent but has been shown to decrease the risk of cerebral palsy in surviving infants if birth is anticipated before 32 weeks' gestation.

ANTENATAL STEROIDS: Betamethasone or dexamethasone is given intramuscularly to the pregnant woman in an effort to decrease some of the complications of prematurity, particularly respiratory distress syndrome (intraventricular hemorrhage in the more extremely premature babies).

FETAL FIBRONECTIN ASSAY: A basement membrane protein that helps bind placental membranes to the decidua of the uterus. A vaginal swab is used to detect its presence. Its best utility is a negative result, which is associated with a 99% chance of not delivering within 1 week.

CERVICAL LENGTH ASSESSMENT: Transvaginal ultrasound to measure the cervical length. Cervical length of <25 mm results in an increased risk of preterm delivery. Also an impinging of the amniotic cavity into the cervix, so-called funneling, increases the risk of preterm delivery. However, a short cervix or a positive fetal fibronectin alone should not be used exclusively to diagnose preterm labor in an acute situation, as the positive predictive value is poor.

LATE PRETERM GESTATION: Delivery that occurs between 34+0 weeks and 36+6 weeks. This is the subset of preterm births that are most rapidly increasing and comprises most preterm deliveries.

CLINICAL APPROACH

Preterm labor is defined as cervical change in the midst of regular uterine contractions occurring between 20 and 37 weeks' gestation. The incidence in the United States is approximately 11% of pregnancies, and it is the cause of significant perinatal morbidity and mortality. There are many risk factors associated with preterm delivery, but the most significant one is a history of a prior spontaneous preterm birth (see Table 17–1).

The main symptoms of preterm labor are uterine contractions and abdominal tightening. Sometimes, pelvic pressure or increased vaginal discharge may also be present. The diagnosis is established by confirming cervical change over time by the same examiner, if possible, or finding the cervix to be 2-cm dilated and 80% effaced in a nulliparous woman. Once the diagnosis has been made, an etiology should be sought. Tocolysis is considered if the gestational age is less than 34 to 35 weeks, and steroids are administered if the gestational age is <34 weeks. The work-up for preterm labor is summarized in Table 17–2.

Recent randomized controlled trials have suggested that magnesium sulfate is not effective as a tocolytic agent but may be useful for fetal neuroprotection. Other medications include terbutaline, ritodrine, nifedipine, and indomethacin. The speculated mechanism of action of magnesium is competitive inhibition of calcium to decrease its availability for actin–myosin interaction, thus decreasing myometrial activity (see Table 17–3).

Nifedipine reduces intracellular calcium by inhibiting voltage-activated calcium channels. Side effects include pulmonary edema, respiratory depression, neonatal depression, and, if given for a long term, osteoporosis. **Pulmonary edema** is often the most serious side effect, and is seen more often with the β-agonist agents. A complication of indomethacin is closure of the ductus arteriosus, leading to severe neonatal pulmonary hypertension; oligohydramnios may also be seen.

Antenatal steroids should be given between 23 and 34 weeks' gestation when there is no evidence of overt systemic infection. Only one course of corticosteroids is utilized. However, if 7 to 14 days or more have elapsed and the patient re-enters preterm labor and is still <34 weeks, one additional "rescue" course of corticosteroids may be considered. Repeat rescue doses are contraindicated. Antenatal corticosteroids are associated with improved neonatal survival, and lower severity and incidence of respiratory distress syndrome (RDS). In the early gestational ages, the effect is to

Table 17–1 • RISK FACTORS FOR PRETERM LABOR
Preterm premature rupture of membranes
Multiple gestations
Previous preterm labor or birth
Hydramnios
Uterine anomaly
History of cervical cone biopsy
Cocaine abuse
African–American race
Abdominal trauma
Pyelonephritis
Abdominal surgery in pregnancy

Table 17–2 • WORK-UP FOR PRETERM LABOR

History to assess for risk factors
Physical examination with speculum examination to assess for ruptured membranes
Serial digital cervical examinations
Complete blood count
Urine drug screen (especially for cocaine metabolites)
Urinalysis, urine culture, and sensitivity
Cervical tests for gonorrhea (possibly *Chlamydia*)
Vaginal culture for group B streptococcus
Ultrasound examination for fetal weight and fetal presentation

lower the risk of intraventricular hemorrhage; at gestations >28 weeks, the primary goal is to lower the incidence of respiratory distress syndrome.

Weekly injections of 17 α-hydroxyprogesteronecaproate from 16 to 36 weeks' gestation have been shown to help reduce the incidence of preterm birth in women at high risk. These include a history of previous spontaneous preterm delivery.

Table 17–3 • COMMON TOCOLYTIC AGENTS

Tocolytic Agents	Drug Class	Method of Action	Side Effects/ Complications	Contraindications
Magnesium sulfate	Minerals	Competitively inhibits calcium	**Pulmonary edema,** respiratory depression	Myocardial damage, heart block, diabetic coma (do not use with calcium channel blockers)
Terbutaline; Ritodrine	β-agonists	Selective for β$_2$ receptors; relaxes smooth muscles	**Pulmonary edema, increased pulse pressure, *hyper*glycemia, *hypo*kalemia, and tachycardia**	Arrhythmia, hypertension, seizure disorder
Nifedipine	Calcium channel blocker	Inhibits calcium ion influx into vascular smooth muscle	CHF, MI, pulmonary edema, and severe hypotension; flushing	**Hypotension;**
Indomethacin	NSAID	Decreased prostaglandin synthesis	**Closure of fetus' ductus arteriosus, which would lead to pulmonary hypertension, oligohydramnios**	Third trimester of pregnancy due to possible effects on ductus arteriosus
17-α-hydroxyprogesteronecaproate	Synthetic progesterone, hormone replacement therapy	Inhibits pituitary gonadotropin release; maintains a pregnancy	Breast pain and tenderness, dizziness, abdominal pain, intermittent bleeding	Undiagnosed vaginal bleeding

Emerging Research

The use of vaginal ultrasound to assess the cervical length and characteristics and the use of progesterone or cerclage in those patients with a short cervix are being intensively studied. The most efficacious progesterone preparation (IM injections versus vaginal gel) is unclear. Another area of research is the use of antenatal corticosteroids in pregnancies beyond 34 weeks. At the time of this writing, there is some evidence about its efficacy up to 36 weeks gestation.

COMPREHENSION QUESTIONS

17.1 A 26-year-old woman is noted to be at 29 weeks' gestation. Her last pregnancy ended in delivery at 30 weeks' gestation. In screening for various types of infection, which of the following is most likely to be associated with preterm delivery?

A. Herpes simplex virus
B. *Candida* vaginitis
C. Chlamydia cervicitis
D. Gonococcal cervicitis
E. Group B streptococcus of the vagina

17.2 A 25-year-old G1P0 woman is at 28 weeks' gestation. She is noted to have regular uterine contractions, and her cervix is dilated at 2 cm and 80% effaced. Preterm labor is diagnosed. The physician reviews the record and notes that the patient should not have tocolytic therapy. Which one of the following is a contraindication for tocolysis?

A. Suspected placental abruption
B. Group B streptococcal bacteriuria
C. Recent laparotomy
D. Uterine fibroids

17.3 A 35-year-old G1P0 woman at 32 weeks' gestation was seen in the obstetric (OB) triage unit the previous day with uterine contractions. On admission, the fetal heart rate is 140 bpm with accelerations and no decelerations. A fetal fibronectin assay is performed, which was positive. Over the course of the next 24 hours, the patient was examined and noted to have cervical dilation from 1 to 2 cm and effacement from 30% to 90%. A tocolytic agent is used. A repeat fetal heart rate pattern reveals a baseline of 140 bpm with moderate repetitive variable decelerations. Which of the following is the most likely tocolytic agent used?

A. Nifedipine
B. Indomethacin
C. Magnesium sulfate
D. Terbutaline

17.4 A 28-year-old woman G1P0 at 29 weeks' gestation is treated with terbutaline for preterm labor. Her cervix had dilated to 3 cm and was 90% effaced. She also received betamethasone intramuscularly to enhance fetal lung maturity. The following day, the patient develops dyspnea, tachypnea, and an oxygen saturation level of 80%. Oxygen is given. Which of the following is the best therapeutic agent?
   A. IV antibiotic therapy for probable pneumonia
   B. IV heparin therapy for probable deep venous thrombosis
   C. IV furosemide for probable pulmonary edema
   D. Oral digoxin for probable cardiomyopathy

ANSWERS

17.1 **D.** Infections of various types are associated with preterm delivery. Gonococcal cervicitis is strongly associated with preterm delivery, whereas chlamydial infection is not as strongly associated. Urinary tract infections, particularly pyelonephritis, are associated with preterm delivery. Bacterial vaginosis may be linked with preterm delivery, although treatment of this condition does not seem to affect the risk.

17.2 **A.** Suspected abruption is a relative contraindication for tocolysis because the abruption may extend. The natural history of abruption is extension of the separation, leading to complete shearing of the placenta from the uterus. If this happens, delivery would be the best treatment with the administration of antenatal steroids to decrease the chance of respiratory distress syndrome in the preterm baby; expectant management may be exercised if the patient is stable with no active bleeding or no sign of fetal compromise since this is a premature fetus. Nevertheless, giving tocolytics would increase the chance of hemorrhage in mothers after delivery because it will be more difficult to get the uterus to contract on itself, since tocolytics also act as a uterine relaxant. Infection with Group B streptococcal bacteriuria is not a contraindication for tocolysis; however, the mother should be placed on antibiotic prophylaxis in the event that she delivers or has preterm premature rupture of membranes (PPROM). A recent laparotomy and uterine fibroid may increase the risk of preterm labor, but would not be a contraindication for administration of tocolytics, assuming that both the mother and the fetus are stable.

17.3 **B.** This patient has a change in her fetal heart rate tracing after tocolysis is used. Now, she has significant variable decelerations, which are caused by cord compression. A sudden worsening in the frequency and/or severity of variable decelerations can be caused by oligohydramnios (less amniotic fluid to buffer the cord from compression), rupture of membranes, or descent of the fetal head, such as in labor, so that a nuchal cord (around the neck) may tighten. Indomethacin is associated with decreased amniotic fluid and oligohydramnios, and this is the most likely etiology.

17.4 **C.** In a patient on tocolytic therapy, pulmonary edema is a hazard, particularly when on β-agonists. The tachycardia that often occurs decreases the diastolic filling time, leading to increased end-diastolic pressure. Besides oxygen, IV furosemide is effective in decreasing intravascular fluid and thus decreasing hydrostatic pressure, hopefully relieving the fluid from the interstitial spaces of the lungs. Of course, the terbutaline should also be discontinued. A β-agonist therapy is associated with an increased pulse pressure, hyperglycemia, hypokalemia, and tachycardia.

CLINICAL PEARLS

▶ Dyspnea occurring in a woman with preterm labor and tocolysis is usually due to pulmonary edema.

▶ The goal in treating preterm labor is to identify the cause, give steroids (if gestation is at 24 to 34 weeks), tocolysis, and magnesium sulfate for neuroprotection.

▶ The most common cause of neonatal morbidity in a preterm infant is respiratory distress syndrome.

▶ β-Agonist therapy has multiple side effects including tachycardia, widened pulse pressure, hyperglycemia, and hypokalemia.

▶ A negative cervical fetal fibronectin assay virtually guarantees no delivery within 1 week.

▶ Transvaginal sonography indicating a shortened cervix especially with funneling and/or beaking is suggestive of risk for preterm delivery.

▶ Progesterone (17 OHP) injections given weekly from 16 to 36 weeks' gestation in women with a history of prior spontaneous preterm births decreases the risk of preterm birth by one-third.

REFERENCES

American College of Obstetricians and Gynecologists. Management of preterm labor. *ACOG Practice Bulletin 127*. Washington, DC; 2012.

American College of Obstetrics and Gynecologists. Prediction and prevention of preterm birth. *ACOG Practice Bulletin 130*. Washington, DC; 2012.

American College of Obstetricians and Gynecologists. Use of progesterone to reduce preterm birth. *ACOG Committee Opinion 419*. Washington, DC; 2008.

American College of Obstetrics and Gynecologists. Magnesium sulfate use in obstetrics. *ACOG Committee Opinion 573*. Washington, DC; 2013.

American College of Obstetricians and Gynecologists. Magnesium sulfate before anticipated preterm birth for neuroprotection. *Committee Opinion 455*. Washington, DC; 2010.

Cunningham FG, Leveno KJ, Bloom SL, Hauth JC, Gilstrap LC III, Wenstrom KD. Preterm birth. In: *Williams Obstetrics*. 22nd ed. New York, NY: McGraw-Hill; 2005:855-880.

Hobel CJ. Obstetrical complications: preterm labor, PROM, IUGR, postterm pregnancy, and IUFD. In: Hacker NF, Gambone JC, Hobel CJ, eds. *Essentials of Obstetrics and Gynecology*. 5th ed. Philadelphia, PA: Saunders; 2009:146-159.

Norwitz ER, Caughey AB. Progesterone supplementation and the prevention of preterm birth. *Rev Obstetr Gynecol*. 2011;4(2):60-72.

CASE 18

A 24-year-old G2P1 woman at 30 weeks' gestation was admitted to the hospital 2 days ago for premature rupture of membranes. Her antenatal history has been unremarkable. Today, she states that her baby is moving normally, and she denies any fever or chills. Her past medical and surgical histories are unremarkable. On examination, her temperature is 100.8°F (38.2°C), blood pressure (BP) is 100/60 mm Hg, and heart rate (HR) is 90 beats per minute (bpm). Her lungs are clear to auscultation. No costovertebral angle tenderness is found. The uterine fundal height is 30 cm, and the uterus is slightly tender to palpation. No lower extremity cords are palpated. The fetal heart tones are persistently in the range of 170 to 175 bpm without decelerations. There are no uterine contractions.

▶ What is the most likely diagnosis?
▶ What is the best management for this patient?
▶ What is the most likely etiology of this condition?

ANSWERS TO CASE 18:
Preterm Premature Rupture of Membranes (PPROM) and Intra-Amniotic Infection

Summary: A 24-year-old G2P1 woman at 30 weeks' gestation was admitted 2 days ago for premature rupture of membranes. Her temperature is 100.8°F (38.2°C). The uterine fundus is slightly tender. There is persistent fetal tachycardia in the range of 170 to 175 bpm.

- **Most likely diagnosis:** Intra-amniotic infection (chorioamnionitis).
- **Best management for this patient:** Intravenous (IV) antibiotics (ampicillin and gentamicin) and induction of labor.
- **Etiology of this condition:** Ascending infection from vaginal organisms.

ANALYSIS
Objectives

1. Know that infection and labor are the two most common acute complications of preterm premature rupture of membranes.
2. Know the clinical presentation of intra-amniotic infection, and that fetal tachycardia is an early sign of this infection.
3. Understand that broad-spectrum antibiotic therapy and delivery are the appropriate treatment of intra-amniotic infection.

Considerations

This 24-year-old woman at 30 weeks' gestation has preterm premature rupture of membranes. Upon presentation to the hospital, the practitioner should assess for infection; in the absence of signs of overt systemic infection, corticosteroid therapy should be administered to reduce the risk of respiratory distress syndrome in the infant if delivery occurs. Additionally, broad-spectrum antibiotic therapy is given to help reduce the incidence of intra-amniotic infection, delay delivery, and reduce the risk of maternal uterine infection. The scenario does not indicate whether antibiotics were initiated upon admission to the hospital. At a gestational age of <34 weeks, the risks of prematurity outweigh the risks of infection, so expectant management was chosen. After 2 days in the hospital, the patient develops fever, uterine tenderness, and fetal tachycardia, which are all signs consistent with intra-amniotic infection. Upon recognition of this diagnosis, the patient should be given intravenous antibiotic therapy, such as ampicillin and gentamicin. Neonates are most commonly affected by group B streptococci and gram-negative enteric organisms such as *Escherichia coli*. Since delivery is also an important aspect of therapy for both neonatal and maternal well-being, induction of labor and vaginal delivery is the best course of action in this case. See Figure 18–1 for a management scheme.

SECTION II: CASES   191

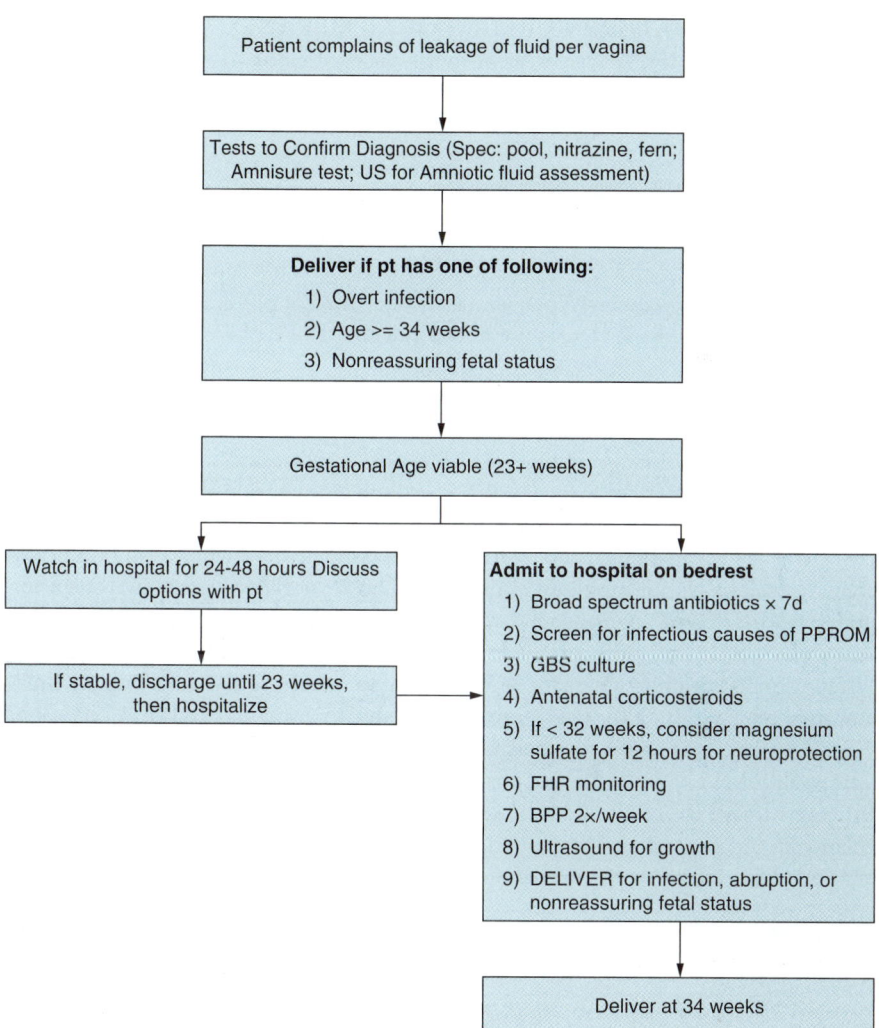

Figure 18–1. Algorithm for the management of PPROM.

APPROACH TO:
Preterm PROM

DEFINITIONS

PREMATURE RUPTURE OF MEMBRANES: Rupture of membranes prior to the onset of labor.

PRETERM PREMATURE RUPTURE OF MEMBRANES: Rupture of membranes in a gestation <37 weeks, prior to the onset of labor.

LATENCY PERIOD: The duration of time from rupture of membranes to onset of labor.

CLINICAL APPROACH

Preterm premature rupture of membrane is defined as rupture of membranes prior to the onset of labor and at <37 weeks of pregnancy. This complication occurs in about 1% of all pregnancies. Approximately one-third of preterm births are associated with PPROM. Risk factors are noted in Table 18–1.

Clinical Evaluation

The history consistent with PPROM is that of a loss or "gush" of fluid per vagina followed by a constant leakage of fluid, which is very accurate and should be taken seriously. The diagnosis is confirmed with a speculum examination showing the pooling of amniotic fluid in the posterior vaginal vault, positive nitrazine test showing alkaline changes of the vaginal fluid, and a ferning pattern of the fluid when seen on microscopy. Occasionally, the speculum examination may be negative, but clinical suspicion is high; in these cases, an ultrasound examination revealing oligohydramnios is consistent with PPROM. AmniSure is an immunoassay test recently approved by the Food Drug Administration to assess for ROM; it tests for placental alpha macroglobulin-1, a protein which is 10,000 times more concentrated in amniotic fluid than cervical or vaginal secretions. The sensitivity is noted to be 96% and specificity of nearly 100%. The swab should be placed in the posterior vaginal prior to any vaginal examination. Etiologies for PPROM should be undertaken such as: urine culture, genital assay for chlamydia and gonorrhea. Ultrasound examination for fetal weight, presentation, and amniotic fluid volume is performed. GBS cultures are usually performed.

Outcome

The outcome is dependent on the gestational age. Approximately half of patients with PPROM will go into labor within 48 hours, and 90% within 1 week. Complications of preterm delivery, such as respiratory distress syndrome, are common. Other complications include chorioamnionitis (intra-amniotic infection), placental abruption, and necrotizing enterocolitis.

Chorioamnionitis affects about 1% of all pregnancies, and 7% to 10% of those with PPROM with prolonged rupture of membranes. Maternal fever, maternal

Table 18–1 • RISK FACTORS FOR PPROM
Lower socioeconomic status
Sexually transmitted diseases
Cigarette smoking
Cervical conization
Emergency cerclage
Multiple gestations
Hydramnios
Placental abruption

tachycardia, uterine tenderness, and malodorous vaginal discharge are some clinical indicators. An **early sign is fetal tachycardia**, a baseline heart rate of >160 bpm.

Treatment

The treatment of PPROM is controversial. Prior to 34 weeks' gestation, antenatal steroids are given to enhance fetal lung maturity in the absence of overt infection. Broad-spectrum antibiotic therapy (usually ampicillin and erythromycin, initially IV for 48 hours and then orally for 5 days to complete a 7-day course) has been shown to delay delivery and decrease the incidence of chorioamnionitis. Patients are placed on bed rest and expectantly managed when the risk of infection is thought to be less than the risk of prematurity, which is usually at 34 weeks' gestation. Occasionally (<10%) of patients with PPROM will have resealing of membranes and may be discharged home; to confirm that the membrane has resealed, there should be absence of leakage of fluid, several negative speculum examinations, and normal amniotic fluid volume.

With previable PPROM, particularly at <22 weeks' gestation, the patient and family should be given informed consent about the risks of pulmonary hypoplasia and outcomes. Corticosteroids and antibiotics are not recommended at this gestational age.

After a **gestational age of 34 to 35 weeks, the treatment is usually delivery.** Some of the risks of expectant management include stillbirth, cord accident, infection, and abruption. When infection is apparent, broad-spectrum antibiotics, such as intravenous ampicillin and gentamicin, should be initiated and labor should be induced. Also, the infant should be delivered when there is evidence of fetal lung maturity, such as by the presence of phosphatidyl glycerol (PG) in the vaginal pool amniotic fluid.

Controversies

Some practitioners will use tocolytic agents with PPROM to delay delivery for 48 hours, allowing the corticosteroids to have its effect. Others argue that preterm labor likely indicates subclinical infection and tocolysis causes harm. There is no clear consensus on this issue. Progesterone may be proven to be useful in women who have had PPROM in a prior pregnancy or who currently have PPROM; studies are ongoing at the writing of this chapter.

> ### CASE CORRELATION
> - See also Case 17 (Preterm Labor) since premature PROM accounts for a significant fraction of preterm delivery.

COMPREHENSION QUESTIONS

18.1 A 31-year-old G1P0 at 33 weeks' gestation is admitted for preterm premature rupture of membranes. Which of the following statements is correct?
   A. Magnesium sulfate should be given for neuroprotection.
   B. Broad-spectrum antibiotic therapy is indicated only with maternal fever.
   C. Labor is the most common acute complication to be expected.
   D. Vaginal candidiasis is a risk factor for preterm premature rupture of membranes.

18.2 A 30-year-old G2P1 woman at 28 weeks' gestation with preterm premature rupture of membranes is suspected of having intra-amniotic infection based on fetal tachycardia. The maternal temperature is 98.8°F. Which of the following is the most accurate method to confirm the intra-amniotic infection?
   A. Serum maternal leukocyte count
   B. Speculum examination of the vaginal discharge
   C. Amniotic fluid Gram stain by amniocentesis
   D. Palpation of the maternal uterus
   E. Height of oral temperature

18.3 An 18-year-old Hispanic G1P0 woman has a clinical presentation of intra-amniotic infection. She denies any leakage of fluid per vagina, and repeated speculum examinations fail to identify rupture of membranes. Which of the following organisms is most likely to be the underlying etiology?
   A. Group B streptococci
   B. *Listeria monocytogenes*
   C. *Clostridia difficile*
   D. *Chlamydia trachomatis*
   E. *Escherichia coli*

18.4 A 32-year-old woman at 33 weeks' gestation notes leakage of clear vaginal fluid. She denies uterine contractions. The estimated fetal weight on sonography is 2000 g. Vaginal fluid shows the presence of phosphatidyl glycerol. Which of the following is the next step?
   A. Expectant management
   B. Intramuscular corticosteroids
   C. Induction of labor
   D. Ultrasound-guided amniocentesis

18.5 A 30-year-old woman G2P1001 is at 32 weeks' gestation and is diagnosed with PPROM. She is placed on bed rest and reports continued leakage of clear fluid each day. There are no signs of infection. A fetal heart rate tracing is performed twice weekly. Today, there is an abnormality of the fetal heart rate tracing. Which of the following is most likely to be seen?

A. Early decelerations
B. Late decelerations
C. Variable decelerations
D. Sinusoidal heart rate pattern

ANSWERS

18.1 **C.** Labor is the most common complication associated with PROM. Antibiotics should be given to prolong the pregnancy and decrease the risk of infection. The gestational age is **<34 weeks, so antenatal steroids** should be given. Magnesium sulfate is given for neuroprotection for pregnancies <32 weeks. Vaginal candidiasis is not a risk factor for PPROM; however, a lower socioeconomic status, STDs, cigarette smoking, cervical conization, emergency cerclage, multiple gestation, hydramnios, and placental abruption are risk factors.

18.2 **C. Amniocentesis-revealing organisms on Gram stain are diagnostic of infection.** A high serum maternal leukocyte count may be suggestive of infection, but it would not be specific for an intra-amniotic infection. Similarly, a speculum examination may reveal an infectious-appearing vaginal discharge; however, this would neither confirm that an infection is present or that a specific type of infection is present, especially since increased vaginal discharge is common in pregnancy. Palpation of the maternal uterus and height of an oral temperature would also not be diagnostic.

18.3 **B.** *Listeria* may induce **chorioamnionitis without rupture of membranes**; the mechanism is transplacental spread. A history of ingesting unpasteurized milk products (eg, some varieties of goat cheese) should raise clinical suspicion of *Listeria*. **Group B streptococci and gram-negative enteric organisms such as *E. coli* are the most common organisms to affect neonates.**

18.4 **C.** When **fetal lung maturity** is demonstrated on vaginal amniotic fluid by the **presence of PG, delivery is the best next step** when there is leakage of fluid. Expectant management and intramuscular corticosteroids place the mother at an increased risk of developing an intra-amniotic infection. Corticosteroids suppress the immune system, and expectant management prolongs the time frame that an ascending infection from the vagina can cause an intra-amniotic infection. Expectant management is undertaken when the risk of infection is thought to be less than the risk of prematurity, but this is not the case for this scenario with a fetus that shows signs of lung maturity. There is no indication for an ultrasound-guided amniocentesis.

18.5 **C.** The most common finding with PPROM would be variable decelerations likely due to oligohydramnios from the rupture of membranes. With ROM, there is insufficient fluid to "buffer the cord" from compression, and variable decelerations are common. A change of the patient's position often alleviates the decelerations.

CLINICAL PEARLS

▶ Pregnancies complicated by premature rupture of membranes after 34 to 35 weeks' gestation are usually managed by induction of labor.

▶ Pregnancies with PPROM <34 weeks' gestation are usually managed expectantly.

▶ The earliest sign of chorioamnionitis (intra-amniotic infection) is usually fetal tachycardia.

▶ Pregnancies complicated by PPROM and chorioamnionitis should be treated with broad-spectrum antibiotics (like ampicillin and gentamicin) and delivery.

▶ Antenatal corticosteroids should be given to patients with PPROM up to 34 weeks' gestation, unless there is overt infection.

REFERENCES

American College of Obstetricians and Gynecologists. Premature rupture of membranes. *ACOG Practice Bulletin 139*. Washington, DC; 2013.

Cunningham FG, Leveno KJ, Bloom SL, Hauth JC, Rouse DJ, Spong CY. Preterm birth. In: *Williams Obstetrics*. 24th ed. New York, NY: McGraw-Hill; 2014:804-831.

Hobel CJ. Obstetrical complications: preterm labor, PROM, IUGR, postterm pregnancy, and IUFD. In: Hacker NF, Gambone JC, Hobel CJ, eds. *Essentials of Obstetrics and Gynecology*. 5th ed. Philadelphia, PA: Saunders; 2009:146-159.

CASE 19

A 24-year-old G2P1 woman at 22 weeks' gestation complains of an episode of myalgias and low-grade fever 1 month ago. Her 2-year-old son had high fever and "red cheeks." On examination, her blood pressure is 110/60 mm Hg, heart rate is 82 beats per minute (bpm), and she is afebrile. The heart and lung examinations are normal. The fundal height is 28 cm and fetal parts are difficult to palpate.

▶ What is the most likely diagnosis?
▶ What is the most likely mechanism?

ANSWERS TO CASE 19:
Parvovirus Infection in Pregnancy

Summary: A 24-year-old G2P1 woman at 22 weeks' gestation complains of an episode of myalgias and low-grade fever 1 month ago. Her 2-year-old son had high fever and "red cheeks." The fundal height is 28 cm and fetal parts are difficult to palpate.

- **Most likely diagnosis:** Hydramnios, with probable fetal hydrops due to parvovirus B19 infection.

- **Most likely mechanism:** Fetal anemia due to neonatal parvovirus infection, which inhibits bone marrow erythrocyte production.

ANALYSIS
Objectives

1. Know the clinical presentation of parvovirus infection in children and adults.
2. Understand the possible effects of parvovirus B19 infection on pregnancy.
3. Know the clinical presentation of hydramnios.

Considerations

This 22-year-old woman presents with a history of myalgias and low-grade fever. Her 2-year-old son had "red cheeks" and high fever. This illustrates the difference in the clinical presentation of parvovirus B19 infection in an adult versus that of a child. Adults rarely have high fever, but more often have malaise, arthralgias, and myalgias, and a reticular (lacy) faint rash that comes and goes. Up to 20% of adults will have no symptoms. In contrast, children often develop the classic "slapped cheek" appearance and high fever, which is the manifestation of "fifth disease." Parvovirus infections in pregnancy may cause a fetal infection, which may lead to suppression of the erythrocyte precursors of the bone marrow. Severe fetal aplastic anemia may result, leading to fetal hydrops. One of the earliest signs of fetal hydrops is hydramnios or excess amniotic fluid. This patient's uterine size is greater than that predicted by her dates, and fetal parts are difficult to palpate, which are classic findings of hydramnios. An ultrasound examination would confirm the fetal and amniotic fluid effects. The diagnosis of parvovirus B19 infection is made by serology (see Table 19–1).

Table 19–1 • PREGNANT PATIENT EXPOSED TO PARVOVIRUS B19

IgM	IgG	Diagnosis	Management
Negative	Positive	Prior infection, immune	Reassurance
Negative	Negative	If more than incubation time (20 days) from exposure, then susceptible, not infected	Counsel about perhaps staying away from infected setting
Negative	Negative	If less than 20 days from exposure, then possible early infection^a vs not infected	Repeat IgG and IgM in 4 weeks
Positive	Negative	Probable acute infection^a but possible false-positive IgM	Repeat IgG and IgM in 1-2 weeks, expect both to be positive indicating acute infection

^aOnce acute infection is diagnosed, then weekly ultrasounds assessing for hydrops.

APPROACH TO:
Parvovirus Infection in Pregnancy

DEFINITIONS

FIFTH DISEASE: Illness caused by a single-stranded deoxyribonucleic acid (DNA) virus, parvovirus B19, also known as erythema infectiosum.

FETAL HYDROPS: A serious condition of excess fluid in body cavities, such as ascites, skin edema, pericardial effusion, and/or pleural effusion.

HYDRAMNIOS (OR POLYHYDRAMNIOS): Excess amniotic fluid.

SINUSOIDAL HEART RATE PATTERN: A fetal heart rate pattern that resembles a sine wave with cycles of 3 to 5 per minute, indicative of severe fetal anemia or fetal asphyxia.

CLINICAL APPROACH

Parvovirus B19 infection is common, and up to 50% of adults have been infected during childhood or adolescence. It usually causes minimal or no symptoms in the adult, but may lead to devastating consequences for the fetus. A small, single-stranded DNA virus, parvovirus B19, causes a red "slapped cheek" appearance and fever in children; adults usually are less symptomatic and often have peripheral arthopathy, and a characteristic lacy reticular rash, which comes and goes (Figure 19–1). The disease is transmissible 5 to 10 days after exposure, and this infectious period ends once symptoms appear.

School-aged children are commonly affected, and frequently transmit the virus to adults. Exposure to an infected household member carries a 50% risk of infection, and the risk is 20% to 50% in child care settings. Specific immunoglobulin M (IgM) antibody confirms the diagnosis. Although there is no universal consensus

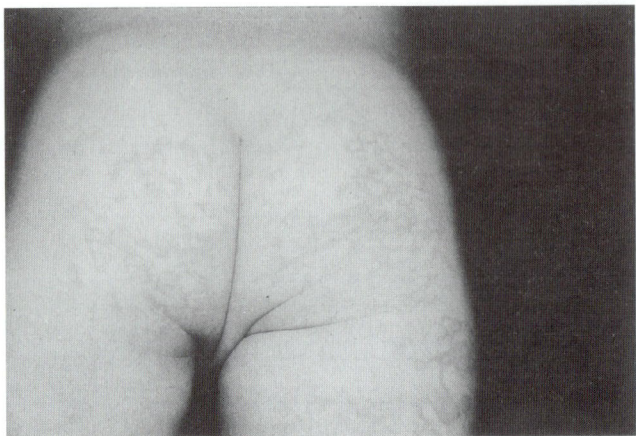

Figure 19–1. Fifth disease. Lacy reticular rash of erythema infectiosum. (Reproduced with permission from Kasper DL, et al. *Harrison's Principles of Internal Medicine.* 16th ed. New York: McGraw-Hill; 2005:1056.)

about how to follow pregnant women who are infected with parvovirus B19, one commonly used strategy includes fetal ultrasounds every 1 to 2 weeks for 8 to 12 weeks after a positive IgM assay. Because the virus may cause an aplastic anemia by destroying erythroid precursors in the bone marrow, Doppler assessment is used to assess for severe fetal anemia. If evidence of hydrops or severe anemia is present, fetal blood should be sampled to obtain a hematocrit for fetal transfusion.

Approximately half of pregnant women will have had parvovirus infection and be immune. IgG and IgM serologies are helpful (see Table 19–1). Less than 5% of those susceptible pregnant women who are infected after 20 weeks' gestation will have fetuses complicated by anemia, but pregnancies at <20 weeks have a higher risk of fetal loss. There is no vaccine available for parvovirus.

Parvovirus infection may lead to spontaneous abortion, stillbirth, and hydrops. **Hydrops fetalis** is defined as excess fluid located in two or more fetal body cavities, and many times is associated with hydramnios (see Table 19–2 for causes of hydramnios); pregnancies <20 weeks' gestation are at particular risk. Parvovirus is the most common infectious cause of nonimmune hydrops (fetal cardiac arrhythmias are the most common cause of nonimmune hydrops overall). Theories about

Table 19–2 • CAUSES OF HYDRAMNIOS
Fetal central nervous system anomalies
Fetal gastrointestinal tract malformations
Fetal chromosomal abnormalities
Fetal nonimmune hydrops
Maternal diabetes
Isoimmunization
Multiple gestation
Syphilis

the mechanism of the hydrops include the observation that severe anemia may cause heart failure, or induction of the hematopoietic centers in the liver to replace normal liver tissue, leading to low serum protein. The anemia is usually transient. If hydrops does not develop within 8 weeks of maternal infection, it is unlikely to occur.

Middle cerebral artery (MCA) Doppler waveforms can be used to assess for possible fetal anemia with elevated systolic velocity. For those patients who are susceptible and are exposed to parvovirus, serology is obtained to assess for possible infection, and serial ultrasound and MCA Doppler examinations are recommended until about 10 weeks postexposure.

For severely affected fetuses, intrauterine transfusion is one option, while mild cases may sometimes be observed. Other causes of fetal anemia are isoimmunization, such as an Rh-negative woman who is sensitized to develop anti-D antibodies, a large fetal-to-maternal hemorrhage, or thalassemia. An unusual fetal heart rate pattern, called a **sinusoidal pattern**, is associated with severe fetal anemia or asphyxia.

The possibility of exposure to parvovirus B19 may be a source of anxiety for pregnant women. Exclusion from the workplace (eg, school or daycare) during endemic periods is not recommended, however, pregnant women may be advised to avoid people exposed to fifth disease. Routine serologic screening is not recommended, and such screening should be reserved for pregnant women with symptoms of parvovirus B19 infection, recent exposure to people with confirmed or suspected fifth disease.

Other Congenital Infections

Cytomegalovirus (CMV) is a DNA virus and is the most common congenital infection in the United States, affecting 1% of neonates; most are asymptomatic. Affected infants can have microcephaly, periventricular calcifications, deafness, chorioretinitis (blindness), seizures, and interstitial pneumonia. Exposure is from blood, urine, or saliva and especially from school-aged children. Vertical transmission can occur with primary or secondary infections. **Transmission is highest in the third trimester, but neonatal effects are worse in the first trimester.** Serology and PCR are helpful in diagnosis. Ultrasound may show abdominal/liver calcifications, cerebral ventriculomegaly, intracranial calcifications, microcephaly, and IUGR. Since there is no treatment, prevention remains the mainstay: **careful handwashing, avoid sharing utensils especially with children (see also Table 19–3).**

Toxoplasmosis is caused by the intracellular parasite *Toxoplasma gondii*. Exposure can be from undercooked meat or oocysts from the feces of infected cats. Vertical transmission increases with gestational age, but severity is worse in early pregnancy. Serology is not consistent and PCR is the best method for diagnosis. Ultrasound may show ventriculomegaly, intracranial calcifications, microcephaly, ascites, hepatosplenomegaly, and IUGR. Pregnant women infected with toxoplasmosis are treated with spiramycin to reduce transplacental transfer; although recommended by the CDC, spiramycin is not commercially available, but can be obtained through the FDA. Fetal infection is treated with pyrimethamine and sulfadiazine. Most neonates are asymptomatic at birth, but can later develop chorioretinitis (85% by an age of 20 years) and hearing loss. **The classic triad is hydrocephalus, intracranial calcifications, and chorioretinitis.** The keys in prevention are pet care precautions (avoid changing cat litter), handwashing, and meat preparation.

Table 19–3 • INTRAUTERINE INFECTIONS

Infectious Agent	Presentation	Transmission	Diagnosis	Treatment
Parvovirus	Fetal anemia, hydrops, miscarriage	Fetal loss high <20 weeks' gestation; 5% anemia if >20 weeks	Serology	Delivery if near term; intrauterine transfusion
Cytomegalovirus	Microcephaly, periventricular calcifications, deafness, chorioretinitis, seizures	Highest in third trimester; worse effects in first trimester	Serology and PCR	None; prevention is key
Toxoplasmosis	Classic triad: hydrocephalus, intracranial calcifications, chorioretinitis; hearing loss	Any gestational age but worse outcome in first trimester	PCR	Pyrimethamine and sulfadiazine
Rubella	Classic triad: cataracts, sensorineural deafness, and cardiac defects; also microcephaly and thrombocytopenia	Severe effects when <8 weeks' gestation; 50% risk 9-20 weeks, no effects after 20 weeks	Serology and PCR	None; prevention via immunization

Rubella

Rubella is caused by a ribonucleic acid (RNA) togavirus. Maternal infection in the first 8 weeks of pregnancy confers an 80% risk of major congenital defects, between 9 and 12 weeks' gestation of 50%, and virtually no risk at 20+ weeks. The classic triad of congenital rubella is **cataracts, sensorineural deafness (60%), and cardiac defects (pulmonary artery stenosis and patent ductus arteriosus). Microcephaly, thrombocytopenic purpura, and IUGR** can be seen. Prevention is through immunization of susceptible patients.

COMPREHENSION QUESTIONS

19.1 A 24-year-old G1P0 woman at 27 weeks' gestation is noted to have a fetal size greater than her dates. A fetal ultrasound performed reveals fetal hydrops. The fetal heart tones are in the range of 140 bpm. Middle cerebral artery Doppler studies indicate increased flow. Which of the following is the most likely etiology?

A. Fetal cardiac tachyarrhythmia
B. Immune thrombocytopenia purpura
C. Rh isoimmunization
D. Intrauterine growth restriction
E. Gestational diabetes

19.2 A 32-year-old G2P1 woman at 32 weeks' gestation is seen in consultation at the maternal fetal medicine center of a hospital. A diagnosis of hydramnios is made on the basis of an amniotic fluid volume of 32 cm (normal 5 to 25 cm). Which of the following is the most likely cause of the patient's condition?
   A. Fetal duodenal atresia
   B. Fetal renal disease
   C. Uteroplacental insufficiency
   D. Hemolysis elevated liver enzymes, low platelets (HELLP) syndrome
   E. Immune thrombocytopenia purpura

19.3 A 22-year-old school teacher at 28 weeks' gestation has a history of a faint rash and low-grade fever. She states that fifth disease is spreading in her school. Serology is obtained for parvovirus B19 revealing that the IgM is negative, and the IgG is negative. Which of the following statements is most accurate?
   A. This patient is immune to parvovirus B19 and does not need to be concerned.
   B. This patient is not infected with parvovirus B19, and is susceptible.
   C. This patient is infected with parvovirus B19 and is at risk for fetal hydrops.
   D. There is insufficient information to draw a conclusion about whether this patient is infected.

Please match the most likely infectious agent (A-E) to the clinical scenario (19.4-19.7):
   A. CMV
   B. Parvovirus B19
   C. Rubella
   D. Syphilis
   E. Toxoplasmosis

19.4 A 25-year-old G1P0 woman at 30 weeks' gestation is noted on ultrasound to have fetal IUGR with estimated fetal weight of 2nd percentile. There microcephaly and periventricular calcifications are noted.

19.5 A 30-year-old G2P1 woman delivers an infant at term. The neonate is noted to have an abnormal light reflex. Also a machine like murmur is noted on auscultation.

19.6 A 36-year-old G3P2 woman undergoes ultrasound examination for size greater than dates. The ultrasound shows fetal ascites, increased amniotic fluid, hydrocephalus, and intracranial calcifications.

19.7 A 19-year-old G1P0 woman is at 7 weeks' gestation and develops a perinatal infection. The obstetrician explains that this particular infection has a very high transmission rate and fetal effects in the first trimester.

ANSWERS

19.1 **C.** Rh isoimmunization can lead to significant fetal anemia if the baby is Rh positive. With the use of RhoGAM, this is a rare event today. Other causes of isoimmunization, such as anti-Kell disease, are still a concern. Middle cerebral artery Doppler studies indicating increased velocity of flow are consistent with significant fetal anemia. This is due to cerebral autoregulation. Fetal cardiac arrhythmias, especially supraventricular tachycardia, are associated with non-immune hydrops, but this would not affect the bone marrow and cause anemia. ITP is associated with maternal thrombocytopenia, and rarely fetal thrombocytopenia. IUGR is usually associated with polycythemia. Gestational diabetes does not typically affect the hemoglobin level.

19.2 **A.** Hydramnios is associated with problems with fetal swallowing or intestinal atresias, or associated with hydrops. Fetal duodenal atresia, diagnosed by the "double bubble" on ultrasound, is associated with hydramnios. Fetal renal disease or placental insufficiency is associated with oligohydramnios. With ITP in pregnancy, antiplatelet antibodies may cross the placenta and cause neonatal thrombocytopenia. HELLP syndrome is a serious, possibly deadly syndrome associated with preeclampsia. Rather than polyhydramnios, **oligohydramnios** is associated with HELLP.

19.3 **D.** IgM and IgG serology is the most common method to diagnose acute fifth disease. Typically, in the acute setting, if the IgG is positive and IgM is negative, it indicates that the patient has been exposed to parvovirus previously and is immune. When the IgG is negative and IgM is positive, then it usually means acute parvovirus infection; sometimes a false-positive IgM can occur, so the IgG and IgM are repeated in 1 to 2 weeks at which time the IgG should be positive with a true infection. When the IgG and IgM are both negative, then the patient typically will not be infected and susceptible, provided sufficient time has elapsed past incubation period. In this case, the patient has some symptoms of parvovirus infection in a high-risk setting, so although both IgG and IgM are negative, it would be wise to repeat it in 4 weeks to ensure that the incubation period (up to 20 days) has elapsed and antibodies have formed.

19.4 **A.** CMV affected infants can have microcephaly, periventricular calcifications, deafness, chorioretinitis (blindness), seizures, and interstitial pneumonia.

19.5 **C.** The classic triad of congenital rubella is congenital cataracts, cardiac defects, and deafness. The abnormal light reflex suggests cataracts. The machine-like murmur which is continuous is consistent with PDA.

19.6 **E.** The classic triad of congenital toxoplasmosis is cerebral ventriculomegaly, chorioretinitis, and intracranial calcifications.

19.7 **C.** Rubella has a very high transmission rate in the first trimester (50%) and high rate of fetal anomalies.

CLINICAL PEARLS

▶ Parvovirus infection in pregnancy can cause fetal anemia leading to hydrops fetalis.

▶ Hydramnios is one of the earliest manifestations of fetal hydrops.

▶ A parvovirus infection in the adult commonly leads to subtle findings of myalgias, malaise, and the reticular rash, whereas an infected child often has high fever and a "slapped cheek" appearance.

▶ Some causes of hydramnios include gestational diabetes, isoimmunization, syphilis, fetal cardiac arrhythmias, and fetal intestinal atresias.

▶ A pregnant woman who is diagnosed with a parvovirus infection will have weekly ultrasound examinations for 12 weeks to assess for fetal hydrops/hydramnios.

▶ The classic triad of congenital rubella is heart defects, cataracts, and deafness. The rate of vertical transmission in the first trimester is 50%.

▶ Congenital CMV is the most common perinatal infection worldwide. Affected infants have IUGR, microcephaly, periventricular calcifications, and hepatosplenomegaly.

▶ Careful handwashing is important in the prevention of CMV infection.

▶ The classic triad of congenital toxoplasmosis is cerebral ventriculomegaly, chorioretinitis, and intracranial calcifications.

REFERENCES

American College of Obstetricians and Gynecologists. Cytomegalovirus, parvovirus B19, varicella zoser, and toxoplasmosis in pregnancy. *ACOG Practice Bulletin 151.* Washington, DC; 2015.

Castro LC, Ognyemi D. Common medical and surgical conditions complicating pregnancy. In: Hacker NF, Gambone JC, Hobel CJ, eds. *Essentials of Obstetrics and Gynecology.* 5th ed. Philadelphia, PA: Saunders; 2010:191-218.

Centers for Disease Control and Prevention. Pregnancy and fifth disease. Atlanta, GA: CDC; 2012. http://www.cdc.gov/parvovirusb19/pregnancy.html; Accessed 15.07.2015.

Cunningham F, Leveno KJ, Bloom SL, et al. Amnionic fluid. In: Cunningham F, Leveno KJ, Bloom SL, et al. *Williams Obstetrics.* 24th ed. New York, NY: McGraw-Hill Education; 2013. http://accessmedicine.mhmedical.com; Accessed 15.06.2015.

CASE 20

An 18-year-old G1P0 woman at 22 weeks' gestation has a positive *Chlamydia* deoxyribonucleic acid (DNA) assay of the endocervix. She denies vaginal discharge, lower abdominal pain, or fever. On examination, her blood pressure is 110/70 mm Hg, heart rate is 70 beats per minute (bpm), and she is afebrile. Her heart and lung examinations are normal. Her abdomen is nontender and gravid. The fundal height is 20 cm and fetal heart tones are in the 140 bpm range. The gonococcal culture is negative and the Pap smear result is normal. Her human immunodeficiency virus (HIV) test by enzyme-linked immunosorbent assay (ELISA) is also positive.

- ▶ What is your next step in therapy of the chlamydial test?
- ▶ What is the next diagnostic step for the positive HIV test?
- ▶ What is the optimal treatment for a pregnant woman who has an HIV infection?

ANSWERS TO CASE 20:
Chlamydial Cervicitis and HIV in Pregnancy

Summary: An 18-year-old G1P0 woman at 22 weeks' gestation has a positive *Chlamydia* DNA assay of the endocervix, and a positive HIV ELISA test. She denies lower abdominal pain and is afebrile. Her abdomen is nontender and gravid. The gonococcal culture is negative.

- **Next step in therapy:** Oral erythromycin, azithromycin, or amoxicillin.
- **Next diagnostic step for HIV:** Either Western blot confirmation, or polymerase chain reaction (PCR) confirmation.
- **Optimal treatment of HIV infection in pregnancy:** Assessment of stage of HIV infection, initiation of highly active antiretroviral therapy (HAART), offer elective cesarean delivery, oral zidovudine to the neonate.

ANALYSIS
Objectives

1. Understand that *Chlamydia trachomatis* is a common cause of cervicitis, and options of treatment in pregnancy.
2. Know that chlamydial infections may lead to neonatal pneumonia or conjunctivitis if untreated.
3. Understand the approach to screening for and treating HIV infection in pregnancy.
4. Be aware of the relationship of HIV viral load on vertical transmission.
5. Understand the approach to hepatitis B and C perinatal infection.

Considerations

This 18-year-old nulliparous woman at 22 weeks' gestation has a positive DNA test for *Chlamydia*. These types of tests are often utilized because of their high sensitivity and specificity, yet lower cost as compared with chlamydial cultures. This patient has a chlamydial infection, which is more common than gonorrheal involvement; accordingly, her gonorrheal culture was negative. Chlamydial endocervical infection has not been proven to cause adverse problems with pregnancy, such as preterm labor or preterm premature rupture of membranes. It has been implicated in neonatal conjunctivitis and pneumonia. Interestingly, the erythromycin eye ointment given at birth does not prevent chlamydial conjunctivitis, although it does protect against gonococcal eye infection. Babies with documented chlamydial ophthalmic infections are given oral erythromycin for 14 days. Because it is mainly neonatal disease, that is the issue, an important time to screen for the organism would be the third trimester, close to the time of delivery. Treatment for the pregnant patient includes erythromycin or amoxicillin for 7 days or azithromycin as a one-time dose.

APPROACH TO:
Cervicitis and HIV in Pregnancy

DEFINITIONS

CHLAMYDIAL NEONATE INFECTION: Conjunctivitis or pneumonia acquired by inoculation during the birth process.

TETRACYCLINE EFFECT: Tetracycline compounds, such as doxycycline, taken by pregnant women can lead to yellow staining of the fetal teeth.

CLINICAL APPROACH

Chlamydia and Gonorrhea

Chlamydia trachomatis is an obligate intracellular organism with several serotypes. It is one of the most common sexually transmitted organisms in the United States, causing urethritis, mucopurulent cervicitis, and late postpartum endometritis. The majority of women, however, are asymptomatic. Vertical transmission may occur during the labor and delivery process, leading to neonatal conjunctivitis or pneumonia. It is unclear whether chlamydial infection of the cervix is associated with preterm labor or preterm rupture of membranes; thus, the main concern is for the neonate. Eye prophylaxis is effective for preventing gonococcal conjunctivitis but not chlamydial involvement. **Chlamydial conjunctivitis** is now the **most common cause of conjunctivitis** in the **first month of life**. Late postpartum endometritis, occurring 2 to 3 weeks after delivery, is associated with chlamydial disease.

Some risk factors for chlamydial infections include unmarried status, age under 25 years, multiple sexual partners, and late or no prenatal care. The discharge is often difficult to detect because of the increased cervical mucus in pregnancy. Direct fluorescent antibody tests and DNA detection tests using PCR are highly sensitive and specific, and less costly than culture. Treatment includes oral erythromycin, amoxicillin, or azithromycin. Tetracycline and doxycycline are contraindicated in pregnancy because of the possibility of staining of the neonatal teeth. Because reinfection is common, repeat testing is recommended in the third trimester.

Gonococcal infection may complicate pregnancy, especially in teens or those with a history of sexually transmitted disease. Gonococcal cervicitis is associated with abortion, preterm labor, preterm premature rupture of membranes, chorioamnionitis, neonatal sepsis, and postpartum infection. Disseminated gonococcal disease is more common in the pregnant women (especially the second or third trimester), presenting as pustular skin lesions, arthralgias, and septic arthritis. Untreated gonococcal ophthalmia can progress to corneal scarring and blindness. *Chlamydia* commonly is present in a patient who is infected with gonorrhea. Thus, the usual treatment for gonococcal cervicitis is ceftriaxone intramuscularly and an additional antibiotic for *C. trachomatis*, such as erythromycin.

HIV Infection

Efforts in public health in the United States have reduced the vertical transmission from 27% to less than 2%. The basic components include **widespread HIV testing, counseling, antiretroviral therapy, viral load assessment, cesarean delivery when appropriate, and counseling to avoid breast feeding.**

Heterosexual spread of HIV is the most common mode of transmission accounting for 72% of HIV transmission among women in the United States. Women of color account for 80% of HIV infections in women. HIV infection leads to progressive debilitation of the immune system, rendering infected individuals susceptible to opportunistic infections and neoplasias that rarely afflict patients with intact immune systems. Furthermore, the unborn fetus may become infected either by transplacental passage or during the delivery process. The neonate may also acquire HIV from infected breast milk. Because measures in pregnancy, during delivery, and postpartum can dramatically **decrease the risk of vertical transmission** to the fetus, HIV serostatus should be obtained on every pregnant woman as early as possible in pregnancy and repeated at the time of labor or delivery.

Up to 20% of HIV-infected pregnant women do not have prenatal care, and may present to labor and delivery units without treatment. Recently, the CDC has recommended that labor and delivery units consider using rapid HIV testing (results ready within 45 minutes) for those women with unknown HIV status, so that HIV infection can be identified and measures may be taken to reduce the risk of vertical transmission.

Initially, patients may either be asymptomatic or have symptoms that mimic a mononucleosis-like illness. Antibodies to the HIV virus are usually detectable 1 month after infection and are almost always detectable within 3 months. Antibody testing begins with a screening test, either an ELISA or a rapid test. A positive screening test is followed with a confirmatory test, either a Western blot or an immunofluorescence assay. A person is only considered positive for HIV after a confirmatory test has been performed. The standard antibody tests may take 3 to 5 days, while the rapid tests return results in minutes to hours. Fourth-generation assays for the simultaneous detection of HIV-1 p24 antigen and anti-IgG and IgM antibodies for HIV-1/HIV-2. Because p24 antigen can be detected 2 to 4 weeks after HIV exposure, the window period for accurately diagnosing HIV status is significantly reduced. A reactive HIV-1/2 antigen/antibody combination immunoassay requires further testing to differentiate HIV-1 versus HIV-2 antibodies; an HIV-1 negative or indeterminate antibody test should be followed up by an HIV-1 nucleic acid test (for antigen).

Studies have been unable to determine, with certainty, the effect of pregnancy on HIV disease progression. There continues to be correlation between maternal disease stage at the time of diagnosis with the viral load and transmission rates. When loads are reduced to undetectable levels, transmission to the fetus becomes uncommon. Viral load and CD4 T-cell testing are ways to monitor a woman's health status. In pregnancy, the viral load should be evaluated monthly until it is no longer detectable. The goal in pregnancy is to maintain a viral load under 1000 ribonucleic acid

(RNA) copies per milliliter. **In women with viral loads exceeding 1000 RNA copies/mL, scheduled cesarean (prior to labor or ROM) has been shown to significantly reduce the risk of vertical infection.**

Combination retroviral therapy decreases the risk of perinatal transmission to <2%, and the best route of delivery is not clear. There is some evidence that cesarean delivery can further decrease vertical transmission, but cesarean delivery increases maternal risks of infection and hemorrhage. Thus, HIV-positive women with viral load counts below 1000 copies/mL should be carefully counseled. Those HIV-infected women who choose to deliver vaginally should receive intravenous zidovudine (ZDV) during labor. Breast feeding should be discouraged. The neonate should also receive oral ZDV syrup.

Antiviral Therapy

Treatment regimens include polytherapy (usually consisting of nucleoside reverse transcriptase inhibitor [NRTI] such as zidovudine, and a protease inhibitor [PI] or less commonly non-nucleoside reverse transcriptase inhibitor [NNRTI]) to decrease resistance. NRTIs cross the placenta and are classes B and C. Patients should have regular monitoring of liver function tests and blood counts to detect toxicity. The use of protease inhibitors may slightly increase the risk of prematurity, and there may be a slight association of HAART and preeclampsia. Nevertheless, the benefits generally far outweigh the risks. Antiviral therapy shows no increase in congenital anomalies with the exception of **efavirenz**, an NNRTI, which is associated with neural tube defects.

Hepatitis Testing

Hepatitis B surface antigen testing is recommended for all pregnant patients. Those with co-infection should be treated with antiviral agent such as tenofovir and lamivudine. Infants should receive hepatitis B immunoglobulin (Ig) at birth and start the vaccination within 12 hours of birth. Up to 50% of HIV-infected individuals are coinfection with hepatitis C (HCV); confirmation is by hepatitis C antibody by ELISA. Deciding whether to treat hepatitis C with interferon and/or ribavirin in pregnancy is complicated; ribavirin is associated with fetal anomalies when given around the time of conception of both men and women (category X). Coinfection with HIV increases the risk of neonatal infection with hepatitis C, and multidrug antiviral therapy may reduce this risk. Women who are not HIV infected with either hepatitis B or hepatitis C may breast feed. Cesarean has not been shown to affect transmission.

CASE CORRELATION

- See also Case 9 (Herpes Simplex Virus).

COMPREHENSION QUESTIONS

20.1 Which of the following is a characteristic of chlamydial infection?
   A. It has a characteristic appearance on Gram stain.
   B. It has a propensity for transitional and columnar epithelia.
   C. It causes neonatal pneumonia, usually with a high fever and sepsis.
   D. It is one of the leading causes of deafness worldwide.

20.2 Which of the following statements is True regarding C. trachomatis infections?
   A. The organism has a fairly rapid replication cycle, about 6 hours.
   B. It is an obligate intracellular organism.
   C. Erythromycin eyedrops are an effective means of preventing chlamydial conjunctivitis.
   D. It is associated with acute early endometritis.
   E. it is a cause of infectious arthritis.

20.3 A 28-year-old parous woman at 16 weeks' gestation is noted to have a positive Chlamydia assay of the endocervix. She is asymptomatic. Which of the following is an acceptable treatment?
   A. Intramuscular azithromycin
   B. Intramuscular ceftriaxone
   C. Oral amoxicillin
   D. Oral ciprofloxacin
   E. Oral doxycycline

20.4 An 18-year-old G1P0 woman at 38 weeks' gestation comes into the obstetrical unit in active labor. She denies leakage of fluid. She states that she is HIV infected, but had not received any medications or prenatal care. She is 5-cm dilated. Which of the following is the most appropriate step?
   A. Immediate cesarean delivery
   B. Intravenous acyclovir and allow labor
   C. Intravenous zidovudine and allow labor
   D. Rupture of membranes, placement of fetal scalp electrode, and uterine contraction monitor

20.5 A 27-year-old woman has been diagnosed with an HIV infection based on a positive ELISA and confirmed by the Western blot analysis. Which of the following is the most likely method that the patient became infected?

A. Exposure to infected blood via splash contamination
B. Heterosexual intercourse
C. Homosexual intercourse
D. Intravenous drug use
E. Renal dialysis center

20.6 A 34-year-old G1P0 woman at 16 weeks' gestation comes in for her first prenatal visit. Her hepatitis B surface antigen is positive. Which of the following is the best next step?

A. Advise to terminate pregnancy
B. Start multidrug antiviral therapy
C. Administer hepatitis B immune globulin
D. Ultrasound of the liver
E. Liver function tests and further hepatitis serology

20.7 A 32-year-old G2P1 woman who is at 8 weeks' pregnant states that she has hepatitis C. Her HIV test is negative. She asks what can be done to reduce the risk of hepatitis C to her unborn baby. You recommend:

A. Avoid breast feeding
B. Initiate ribavirin antiviral therapy
C. Avoid invasive procedures
D. Recommend cesarean delivery

ANSWERS

20.1 **B.** *Chlamydia* is not typically seen on Gram stain because it is an intracellular organism. It does have a propensity for columnar and transitional epithelia, and it is a leading cause of preventable blindness worldwide. It can cause neonatal pneumonia or conjunctivitis. However, the presentation of the pneumonia is not typically associated with high fever or sepsis.

20.2 **B.** *Chlamydia* is an obligate intracellular organism associated with **late postpartum endometritis** and has a long replication cycle. Erythromycin eyedrops are an effective means of preventing gonococcal eye infection but chlamydial infection must be treated systemically with erythromycin. Gonococcal cervicitis is more likely to disseminate during pregnancy, and a patient may present with septic arthritis, arthralgias, and pustular skin lesions.

20.3 **C.** Oral amoxicillin is well tolerated and effective treatment of chlamydial cervicitis in pregnancy. Oral azithromycin can be tolerated as well. Erythromycin estolate can lead to liver dysfunction in pregnancy; thus, the estolate salt is contraindicated in pregnant women. Intramuscular ceftriaxone is used to treat gonococcal cervicitis. Doxycycline, or tetracycline, is contraindicated in pregnancy because of the possibility of staining neonatal teeth. Ciprofloxacin is also contraindicated in pregnancy because it may lead to neonatal musculoskeletal problems.

20.4 **C.** Because labor has already begun, elective cesarean delivery will not affect vertical transmission. In other words, the cesarean would need to be performed prior to rupture of membranes or labor to effectively decrease vertical transmission. **Intravenous ZDV** and minimizing trauma to the baby, such as avoiding fetal scalp electrode, intrauterine pressure catheters, forceps, and vacuum delivery, is advisable. Acyclovir is used to prevent viral shedding in patients infected with HSV. The neonate generally also receives oral ZDV syrup.

20.5 **B.** The most common method of HIV transmission to women in the United States is currently heterosexual intercourse.

20.6 **E.** When a patient has a positive hepatitis B surface antigen result, it means the individual has replicating virus; the next step is to determine the stage: acute, chronic, or chronic carrier. Liver function tests and IgM hepatitis B core Ab, and hepatitis B e antigen and antibody can help to make this determination.

20.7 **C.** Vertical transmission increases with high viral load, prolonged rupture of membranes, and invasive procedures. Cesarean does not affect the risk of neonatal infection. Fetal scalp electrodes should be avoided if possible. Breast feeding does not seem to increase the risk of transmission unless there is cracked or bleeding nipples. Antiviral therapy is usually not used in pregnancy due to the side effects; ribavirin in particular is category X and usually avoided in pregnancy.

CLINICAL PEARLS

▶ The best treatments for chlamydial cervicitis in pregnancy are erythromycin, azithromycin, and amoxicillin.

▶ *Chlamydia* can cause conjunctivitis or pneumonia in the neonate.

▶ Ophthalmic antibiotics administered to the neonate help to prevent gonococcal disease but not chlamydial conjunctivitis.

▶ The most common mode of HIV transmission in women is through heterosexual contact.

▶ Women account for the majority of cases of HIV transmission in the United States.

▶ With widespread prenatal testing for HIV, use of HAART, cesarean delivery when viral load is high, zidovudine to the neonate, and avoiding breast feeding, vertical transmission is now below 2% in the United States.

▶ When born to a mother with hepatitis B surface antigen positive, hepatitis B immunoglobulin and vaccine should be given to a neonate within several hours of birth.

▶ The vertical transmission of hepatitis C vertical depends on viral load especially in the third trimester, coinfection with HIV, prolonged rupture of membranes, and invasive procedure.

▶ Cesarean delivery does not affect the perinatal transmission of hepatitis C.

REFERENCES

American College of Obstetricians and Gynecologists. Gynecologic care of women with HIV. *The ACOG Practice Bulletin 117*. Washington, DC; 2010. (Reaffirmed 2015.)

American College of Obstetricians and Gynecologists. Routine human immunodeficiency virus screening. ACOG *Committee Opinion 411*. Washington, DC; 2008.

American College of Obstetricians and Gynecologists. Scheduled cesarean delivery and the prevention of vertical transmission of HIV infection. *ACOG Committee Opinion 234*. Washington, DC; 2000. (Reaffirmed 2010.)

Castro LC, Ognyemi D. Common medical and surgical conditions complicating pregnancy. In: Hacker NF, Gambone JC, Hobel CJ, eds. *Essentials of Obstetrics and Gynecology*. 5th ed. Philadelphia, PA: Saunders; 2009:191-218.

Cunningham FG, Leveno KJ, Bloom SL, Hauth JC, Gilstrap LC III, Wenstrom KD. Sexually transmitted diseases. In: *Williams Obstetrics*. 24th ed. New York, NY: McGraw-Hill; 2014:1235-1258.

Gibbs RS, Sweet RI, Duff PW. Maternal and fetal infectious disorders. In: Creasy RK, Resnik R, Iams JD, eds. *Maternal–Fetal Medicine*. 6th ed. Philadelphia, PA: Saunders; 2009:362-384.

Minkoff HL. Human immunodeficiency virus. In: Creasy RK, Resnik R, Iams JD, eds. *Maternal–Fetal Medicine*. 6th ed. Philadelphia, PA: Saunders; 2009:803-813.

CASE 21

An 18-year-old G2P1 at 35 weeks' gestation has a history of Graves disease and is under treatment with oral methimazole (MMI). She states that over the last day, she has been feeling as though her "heart is pounding." She also complains of nervousness, sweating, and diarrhea. On examination, her blood pressure (BP) is 150/110 mm Hg, heart rate (HR) is 140 beats per minute (bpm), respiratory rate is (RR) 25 breaths per minute, and temperature is 100.8°F (38.2°C). The patient appears anxious, disoriented, and somewhat confused. The thyroid gland is mildly tender and enlarged. The cardiac examination reveals tachycardia with III/VI systolic murmur. The fetal heart rate tracing shows a baseline in the 160 bpm range without decelerations. Deep tendon reflexes are 4+ with clonus. Her leukocyte count is 20 000/mm^3.

- What is the most likely diagnosis?
- What is the best management for this condition?

ANSWERS TO CASE 21:
Thyroid Storm in Pregnancy

Summary: An 18-year-old G2P1 at 35 weeks' gestation is taking MMI for Graves disease. She has a 1-day history of palpitations, nervousness, sweating, and diarrhea. On examination, her BP is 150/110 mm Hg, HR is 140 (bpm), RR is 25 breaths per minute, and temperature is 100.8°F (38.2°C). The patient appears anxious, disoriented, and somewhat confused. The thyroid is mildly tender and enlarged. Deep tendon reflexes are 4+ with clonus. She has a leukocytosis.

- **Most likely diagnosis:** Thyroid storm.
- **Best management for this condition:** A β-blocker (such as propranolol), corticosteroids, and propylthiouracil (PTU) or methimazole.

ANALYSIS

Objectives

1. Know that the most common cause of hyperthyroidism in the United States is Graves disease.
2. Recognize the clinical presentation and danger of thyroid storm.
3. Be aware of postpartum thyroiditis and its three-part presentation.

Considerations

This 18-year-old woman at 35 weeks' gestation has a history of hyperthyroidism due to Graves disease. In the United States, the majority of hyperthyroidism is due to Graves disease; the clinical presentation is typically that of a painless, uniformly enlarged thyroid gland with occasional proptosis. She is being treated with MMI, which is the most commonly used medication for hyperthyroidism in pregnancy. For whatever reason, which is not stated, the patient has symptoms of increased thyrotoxicosis of 1-day duration. Some possible reasons include noncompliance with the medication, or a stressor, such as surgery or an illness. This woman not only has the nervousness and palpitations of hyperthyroidism, but also autonomic instability, which is the hallmark of thyroid storm. Her blood pressure is 150/110 mm Hg and her temperature is elevated. She is disoriented and markedly confused. Thyroid storm must be recognized because it carries a significant risk of mortality. The therapy consists of a β-blocking agent, such as propranolol, corticosteroids, and anti-thyroid medications. The preferred agent in this setting is PTU because of its faster onset of action and ability to inhibit peripheral conversion of T4 to T3. In a nonpregnant patient or a pregnant patient who is sufficiently ill, a saturated solution of potassium iodide oral drops may also be used; however, this agent may affect the fetal thyroid gland. Notably, the patient has a high white blood cell count. Methimazole has been rarely linked with possible fetal scalp defects and aplasia, so it is not used in the first trimester. Recently, the

Food and Drug Administration issued a blackbox warning regarding PTU because of the severe liver toxicity it can cause, as well as bone marrow aplasia, leading to leukopenia, and sepsis.

APPROACH TO:
Thyrotoxicosis in Pregnancy

DEFINITIONS

HYPERTHYROIDISM: A syndrome caused by excess thyroid hormone, leading to nervousness, tachycardia, palpitations, weight loss, diarrhea, and heat intolerance.

THYROID STORM: Extreme thyrotoxicosis leading to central nervous system dysfunction (coma or delirium) and autonomic instability (hyperthermia, hypertension, or hypotension).

GRAVES DISEASE: An autoimmune disease characterized by the production of abnormal antibodies which act on the thyroid-stimulating hormone receptor causing overstimulation of the thyroid. It is the most common cause of thyrotoxicosis in the United States, associated with a diffusely enlarged goiter.

FREE THYROXINE (T_4): Unbound or biologically active thyroxine hormone.

THIONAMIDE ANTITHYROID MEDICATIONS: Propylthiouracil and MMI, medications that inhibit thyroid hormone synthesis, are the two thionamide medications approved for use in the United States.

CLINICAL APPROACH

Hyperthyroidism is rare in pregnancy, occurring in about 1 in 2000 pregnancies. Symptoms of thyrotoxicosis include tachycardia, heat intolerance, nausea, weight loss or failure to gain weight despite adequate food intake, thyromegaly, thyroid bruit, tremor, exophthalmos, and systolic hypertension. The most common cause of hyperthyroidism in pregnancy is Graves disease, an autoimmune disorder in which antibodies are produced which mimic the function of thyroid-stimulating hormone (TSH). These antibodies stimulate the thyroid gland to produce more thyroid hormone, leading to the symptoms responsible for thyrotoxicosis. The diagnosis of hyperthyroidism is confirmed in the presence of elevated free thyroxine and low serum TSH levels. Treatment during pregnancy may be medical or surgical; however, generally, hyperthyroidism in pregnancy is managed medically. Propylthiouracil is generally accepted as the drug of choice in pregnancy. PTU inhibits the peripheral conversion of T_4 to T_3 but may cross the placenta somewhat. Methimazole is another option. Both PTU and MMI cross the placenta and can lead to some transient neonatal hypothyroidism. Because MMI has been possibly associated with aplasia cutis (congenital skin or scalp defects), PTU is usually the drug of choice in the first trimester of pregnancy, due to the possible fetal effects of MMI; after the first trimester, the pregnant woman is usually switched to MMI due to the reported hepatic toxicity of PTU. Radioactive iodine is contraindicated in pregnancy due to fetal effects. Thyroidectomy is reserved for those patients who are noncompliant with or cannot tolerate medical therapy. Risks from surgery include vocal cord paralysis and hypoparathyroidism.

Thyroid storm is a rare but life-threatening complication of hyperthyroidism. Symptoms suggestive of storm include **altered mental status, hyperthermia, cardiac arrhythmia, hypertension, vomiting, and diarrhea.** Infection, surgery, labor or delivery, or other stressors may trigger thyroid storm in patients with hyperthyroidism. Congestive heart failure can result from the effects of thyroxine on the myocardium. Because the mortality rate associated with thyroid storm is high, accurate early identification is crucial. These patients are best monitored in an intensive care unit. High-dose propylthiouracil is administered by mouth or nasogastric tube. β-Blockers are used to control the symptoms of tachycardia; however, they should be used with caution in those patients with congestive heart failure. Acetaminophen or cooling blankets are used for hyperthermia. Corticosteroids may also be used to prevent the peripheral conversion of T_4 to T_3.

Maternal hyperthyroidism may result in either fetal hyper- or hypothyroidism. When identified antenatally, the fetus should be treated either with maternal administration of PTU or injection of intra-amniotic thyroxine (fetal hypothyroidism). Failure to identify fetal thyrotoxicosis can result in nonimmune hydrops and fetal demise.

Postpartum Thyroiditis

About 5% of postpartum women will have postpartum thyroiditis with the peak onset at 6 months post delivery. There are three phases: hyperthyroid, hypothyroid, and euthyroid (although some will remain hypothyroid). The pathophysiology is similar to Hashimoto's thyroiditis (lymphocytic infiltration) and is associated with antimicrosomal antibodies and antiperoxidase antibodies. Risk factors include type I diabetes (25% risk) and previous postpartum thyroiditis (20% risk). Treatment is antithyroid medications during the hyperthyroid phase, and monitoring carefully to switch to thyroid replacement during the hypothyroid phase.

Hypothyrodism

Recently, subclinical maternal hypothyroidism has gained interest, since this condition may be associated with adverse effects on neurological development and childhood intelligence. There is some evidence that levothyroxine replacement in the first trimester may lead to better outcomes. Currently, there is no consensus on universal screening for maternal hypothyroidism; however, those patients at increased risk or with symptoms should certainly undergo screening.

Hyperparathyroidism

Rarely, hyperparathyroidism can affect pregnant women. The patient may have kidney stones, or lethargy or pain. The diagnosis is made by an elevated serum calcium level, low serum phosphate, and elevated parathyroid hormone level (primary hyperparathyroidism). In the first and second trimesters, surgery (parathyroidectomy) is the treatment of choice. In the third trimester, oral phosphate, a low calcium diet, and expectant management are generally preferred unless symptoms are significant. Surgery is usually performed after delivery.

COMPREHENSION QUESTIONS

21.1 A 25-year-old third-year G1P0 medical student had been diagnosed with borderline hypothyroidism 4 years ago and has thyroid studies done annually. Last year, her thyroid panel was within normal limits. She is currently at 15 weeks' gestation, and has had a thyroid panel drawn today. Which of the following changes is likely to have occurred today as compared to last year's result?

   A. Elevation of serum TSH levels
   B. Elevation of serum total thyroxine levels
   C. Decrease in serum thyroid-binding globulin levels
   D. Decrease in serum-free T_4 levels
   E. No effect on TSH or total thyroxine levels

21.2 A 25-year-old G1P0 woman at 16 weeks' gestation complains of some intermittent palpitations, and feeling very warm despite the air conditioning. Which of the following is the best screening test for hyperthyroidism?

   A. Serum TSH levels
   B. Serum thyroid-binding globulin levels
   C. Serum antithyroid antibody levels
   D. Serum total thyroxine levels
   E. Serum transferrin levels

21.3 A 24-year-old woman delivered vaginally at term about 2 months previously. She was in good health until 1 week ago, when she began to complain of nervousness, tremulousness, and feeling palpitations. The TSH is 0.01 mIU/L (normal: 0.5–5). Which of the following is the most likely abnormality?

   A. Immunoglobulin G (IgG) antibodies stimulating the TSH receptor
   B. Antimicrosomal antibodies
   C. Dominant nodule of the thyroid gland
   D. Positive urine drug screen
   E. Urine catecholamines

21.4 A 23-year-old G1P0 woman at 16 weeks' gestation is suspected of hypothyroidism. Which of the following is most consistent with hypothyroidism in pregnancy?

	TSH	Free Thyroxine	Thyroid-Binding Globulin	Total Thyroxine
A.	Unchanged	Elevated	Decreased	Unchanged
B.	Decreased	Elevated	Unchanged	Decreased
C.	Increased	Decreased	Elevated	Unchanged
D.	Unchanged	Decreased	Decreased	Elevated
E.	Unchanged	Unchanged	Unchanged	Decreased

ANSWERS

21.1 **B.** The high estrogen levels during pregnancy lead to **increased levels of thyroid-binding globulin and total T_4, but the active or free T4 and TSH levels remain unchanged.** In general, pregnancy is a euthyroid state.

21.2 **A.** A **TSH level is considered the best screening test for hyperthyroidism.** A low level suggests hyperthyroidism; an elevated level suggests hypothyroidism. The diagnosis of hyperthyroidism is confirmed by the presence of an elevated free T_4 level. Maternal hyperthyroidism may result in either fetal hyperthyroidism or hypothyroidism. Failure to identify fetal thyrotoxicosis can result in nonimmune hydrops and fetal demise. For this reason, it is important to screen women in their prenatal screen for TSH levels. If the TSH is borderline or a more definitive diagnosis is sought, then free T_4 is a good follow-up test.

21.3 **B.** Overall, the most common cause of hyperthyroidism in the United States is Graves disease. However, in the postpartum period, women with hyperthyroidism are more likely to have destructive lymphocytic thyroiditis. This is because the high corticosteroid levels in pregnancy suppress the autoimmune antibodies, and a flare occurs postpartum when the corticosteroid levels fall after the placenta delivers. Often, **antimicrosomal and antiperoxidase antibodies are present.** Thus, the postpartum patient is unique in that the cause of hyperthyroidism is usually lymphocytic thyroiditis rather than Graves disease.

21.4 **C.** With **hypothyroidism, the TSH level is elevated** and the free T_4 is decreased. With hyperthyroidism, the TSH is decreased and the free T_4 is increased. Normally, with pregnancy, the only physiologic change is increased total T_4. With early or mild hypothyroidism, one may occasionally find the TSH level as normal (upper limits of normal) and free T_4 as low; however, the findings **most** consistent with hypothyroidism would be elevated TSH and low T_4.

CLINICAL PEARLS

▶ Graves disease is the most common cause of hyperthyroidism in pregnancy. Thyroid storm should be considered when central nervous system dysfunction and autonomic instability are present. The treatments for thyroid storm in pregnancy include MMI or PTU, steroids, and β-blockers.

▶ Maternal Graves disease may lead to fetal hyperthyroidism due to IgG antibodies crossing the placenta.

▶ Pregnancy (or use of estrogens) causes total thyroxine to be increased, free T_4 to be unchanged, TSH to be unchanged, and thyroid-binding globulin to be increased.

▶ Postpartum thyroiditis often occurs 1 to 4 months postpartum and is associated with antimicrosomal antibodies. After several months, hypothyroidism may result.

▶ After the first trimester, methimazole is the preferred agent due to the possibility of liver toxicity with PTU.

▶ Maternal hypothyroidism that is untreated can lead to neonatal and childhood neurodevelopmental delays.

▶ Hyperparathyroidism in pregnancy presents as kidney stones, lethargy, or pain. Surgery is the treatment of choice in the second trimester.

REFERENCES

American College of Obstetricians and Gynecologists. Thyroid disease in pregnancy. *ACOG Practice Bulletin 148*. Washington, DC; 2015.

American College of Obstetricians and Gynecologists. Subclinical hypothyroidism in pregnancy. *ACOG Committee Opinion 381*. Washington, DC; 2007.

Castro LC, Ognyemi D. Common medical and surgical conditions complicating pregnancy. In: Hacker NF, Gambone JC, Hobel CJ, eds. *Essentials of Obstetrics and Gynecology*. 5th ed. Philadelphia, PA: Saunders; 2009:191-218.

Cunningham FG, Leveno KJ, Bloom SL, Hauth JC, Dwight JR, Spong CY. Thyroid and other endocrine disorders. In: Cunningham FG, Leveno KJ, Bloom SL, Hauth JC, Gilstrap LC III, Wenstrom KD, eds. *Williams Obstetrics*. 24th ed. New York, NY: McGraw-Hill; 2014:1126-1144.

CASE 22

A 32-year-old primigravida is seen in your office at 33 weeks' gestation for a routine prenatal visit. Her gestational age (GA) was calculated by her last normal menstrual period, which was consistent with an ultrasound performed at 8 weeks' gestation. Her pregnancy has been uneventful to date, although she has continued to smoke one pack or more of cigarettes daily. She states that she has been feeling normal fetal movement and no uterine contractions. On examination, her height is 5 ft 6 in., her weight is 118 lb (53.5 kg), and her blood pressure (BP) is 90/60 mm Hg. Her fundal height is 26 cm. On ultrasound, you note a single pregnancy with an estimated fetal weight of 900 g, which is at the third percentile for gestational age.

▶ What is the most likely diagnosis?
▶ What other important items should be noted on the ultrasound?
▶ What is the next step in the management of this patient?
▶ What are potential complications of the patient's disorder?

ANSWERS TO CASE 22:
Intrauterine Growth Restriction

Summary: This is a 32-year-old woman at 33 weeks' gestation, who continues to smoke cigarettes during pregnancy, showing a growth-restricted fetus by ultrasound.

- **Most likely diagnosis:** Intrauterine growth restriction (IUGR), likely due to cigarette smoking.
- **Other ultrasound items:** (a) Determine whether this is symmetric or asymmetric IUGR, and (b) assess the amniotic fluid.
- **Next step:** Evaluate fetal well-being.
- **Potential complications:** Preterm birth, fetal stress, intrauterine demise.

ANALYSIS
Objectives

1. Describe the definition and risk factors for IUGR.
2. Understand signs in pregnancy that may indicate a growth-restricted fetus.
3. Be able to evaluate a patient with suspected IUGR.
4. Develop a plan of management for a patient whose fetus is growth restricted.

Considerations

This gravida's main risk for IUGR is that she is a smoker. Although there is overlap, once IUGR is diagnosed, the fetal ultrasound parameters are broadly categorized as symmetric (head affected) or asymmetric (head spared) IUGR. By comparing the relative measurements of the head circumference (HC) as compared to the abdominal circumference (AC) and femur length (FL), this determination can be made. In general, factors that affect the head growth include chromosomal abnormalities, and severe and early intrauterine infections (such as TORCH [TOxoplasmosis, Rubella, Cytomegalovirus, Herpes] infections). In situations of relative hypoxia or a decrease in nutrients provided to the fetus, the fetus will tend to preserve blood flow to the brain and heart, preserving HC, while losing growth on the AC and FL. The most common cause of asymmetric IUGR is a maternal vascular disorder such as hypertensive disease, smoking, or illicit drug use. The most common cause of symmetric "IUGR" is a constitutionally small baby with no adverse problems. However, estimated weight of less than 5th percentile, or 3rd percentile, is more likely a true growth restriction. After an attempt is made to determine symmetric versus asymmetric IUGR, fetal assessment should be undertaken to assess risk of fetal death. Biophysical profile, assessment of amniotic fluid volume, and Doppler flow studies of the umbilical artery are helpful. In the case of this patient, if the ultrasound parameters suggest asymmetric IUGR (eg, HC: 33 weeks, AC: 26 weeks, FL: 27 weeks), then cigarette smoking can be assumed to be the

Table 22-1 • SELECTED LIST OF RISK FACTORS FOR IUGR

Maternal factors:
- Hypertensive disease (chronic hypertension or preeclampsia)
- Renal disease
- Cardiac and respiratory diseases
- Underweight and/or poor pregnancy weight gain
- Significant anemia
- Substances: cocaine, tobacco

Uterine/placental factors:
- Abruptio placenta
- Placenta previa
- Infection

Fetal factors:
- Multiple gestation
- Aneuploidy
- Congenital syndromes
- Structural fetal malformations
- Infection

culprit provided there are no other risk factors (see Table 22–1). The decision for delivery depends on gestational age, severity of the IUGR, possibility of reversible causes, and findings on the fetal assessment (risk of fetal death). If the fetal testing for this patient is reasonably reassuring (eg, BPP shows 10/10 with normal amniotic fluid), then a careful observation with once or twice weekly fetal testing may be adopted. Repeat ultrasound for fetal growth in 3 weeks can help to evaluate the severity of the process. In other words, no growth at all after 3 weeks indicates a profound IUGR, whereas normal interval growth may indicate a constitutionally small baby or an underlying process that is not as severe.

APPROACH TO: IUGR

DEFINITIONS

IUGR: The most commonly used definition is a **birthweight less than the 10th percentile** for GA.

ASSYMETRIC IUGR: Preservation of the HC while the AC and FL lag behind.

SYMMETRIC IUGR: All parameters including the HC are small.

BIOPHYSICAL PROFILE: Combination of ultrasound criteria and NST to assess for fetal well-being conducted over 30 minutes. Fetal breathing, movement, tone, and amniotic fluid are assessed.

DOPPLER FLOW STUDIES: Using ultrasound to assess for flow through vessels. With IUGR, Doppler flow in the umbilical artery is helpful.

END-DIASTOLIC FLOW: The flow through the umbilical artery measured by Doppler ultrasound. Reverse end-diastolic flow is associated with a high stillbirth rate within 48 hours. Absent end-diastolic flow has a moderately high stillbirth risk, and in some settings can be closely observed.

CLINICAL APPROACH

Diagnosis

By definition, 10% of infants in a population will have a birthweight less than the 10th percentile. This designation notes that while defining a pathologic condition using a 10th-percentile cutoff makes statistical sense, it may not be clinically relevant. The clinical challenge of greatest relevance: distinguishing the small-but-healthy fetus from the one who is compromised. Bernstein and Gabbe elegantly **define the IUGR fetus as one who suffers morbidity and/or mortality associated with the failure to reach growth potential.** This is in contrast to a fetus that is constitutionally small. When a patient has had an early ultrasound establishing the gestational age, then a "dating error" is not a consideration. In those patients who present with late prenatal care, the possibility of wrong dates is likely (eg, menstrual history suggests 36 weeks but ultrasound measures 30 weeks). A repeat ultrasound in 2 to 3 weeks showing adequate interval growth is highly suggestive of a dating error, whereas lagging growth suggests IUGR.

Symmetric or Asymmetric

Early insults to fetal growth are thought to more commonly manifest as symmetric IUGR. Symmetric IUGR may be caused by aneuploidy or early transplacental infection. On the other hand, asymmetric IUGR describes a pattern with a relatively smaller abdominal circumference in comparison to the fetal head circumference, and it is thought to reflect a more recent insult to fetal growth. An example of this type of situation occurs in association with hypertension developing late in the pregnancy. The patterns may ultimately merge in the setting of long-standing complications, such as preexisting hypertension.

The excess morbidity and mortality in the setting of IUGR are significant. An early study of infants born between 38 and 42 weeks with a birthweight between 1500 and 2500 g found that **perinatal morbidity and mortality were up to 30 times greater than that seen in infants born between the 10th and the 90th percentile.** Expert commentary on this study offered the following perspective: "An infant with a weight of 1250 g at 38 to 42 weeks' gestation has a greater perinatal mortality risk than one born with similar weight at 32 weeks."

Some of the neonatal morbidities associated with IUGR include increased meconium aspiration, necrotizing enterocolitis, hypoglycemia, respiratory distress, hypothermia, and thrombocytopenia.

It has been suggested that IUGR has long-term consequences, beyond those seen in the immediate postnatal period. The Barker hypothesis states that undernutrition during fetal life—a time of great developmental plasticity—increases the risk of adult-onset coronary artery disease, type II diabetes, stroke, and hypertension (HTN). This increased morbidity is thought to be secondary to the allocation of energy to one trait (such as brain growth) at the expense of allocation to traits such as tissue repair processes.

Risk Factors and Etiology

There are many risk factors for IUGR, which may be divided into three broad categories: maternal, uterine/placental, and fetal (see Table 22–1).

Maternal factors include HTN, cardiac disease, respiratory diseases, renal disease, anemia, toxic habits, and malnutrition. HTN—whether antecedent to pregnancy or first appearing during pregnancy—places the fetus at risk for IUGR. Cardiac and respiratory diseases may impact oxygenation, and maternal oxygenation, in turn, is associated with IUGR. Gravidas with severe anemia are at increased risk of having a fetus with IUGR. Toxic habits, such as drug and tobacco use, are potentially the most modifiable risk factors for IUGR. Evidence suggests that advanced maternal age is a risk for IUGR.

Uterine/placental factors include abruptio, placenta previa, and infection. Abruptio is more common in women with HTN, as well as in those who smoke. Cocaine use is a risk factor for abruption. Toxoplasmosis, herpes, and parvovirus have all been associated with IUGR. Early-onset IUGR (<20 weeks) is associated with cytomegalovirus.

Fetal factors include multiple pregnancy, aneuploidy, structural malformations, and infection. Multiple gestations are at increased risk of IUGR. Aneuploid fetuses—trisomy 13, trisomy 18, and trisomy 21—are typically smaller than their euploid siblings. Many syndromes are associated with IUGR, including Russel–Silver syndrome, Bloom syndrome, and cretinism (hypothyroidism). Fetal structural malformations, such as gastroschisis or omphalocele, place the fetus at risk for IUGR. As noted above, infection is also associated with IUGR.

Diagnostic Strategy

Once a diagnosis of IUGR is suspected, the clinical challenge is to distinguish the small and sick (IUGR) fetus from the one who is small but healthy. Several tools help make this distinction: clinical history and risk factors, fetal assessment tools such as the BPP, the amniotic fluid assessment, and Doppler studies (see Table 22–2).

A detailed history and physical should unearth any factors that would increase the risk of a pathologically small fetus. In the sample patient, for

Table 22–2 • EVALUATION OF IUGR

- Detailed history and physical
- Close attention to current blood pressure and blood pressure trend
- Detailed fetal anatomic ultrasound survey
- If indicated, consider amniocentesis
  - Karyotype: Increased risk of aneuploidy in the setting of IUGR
  - Infectious workup (such as cytomegalovirus assessment)
  - Fetal lung maturity studies depending upon the GA at presentation
- Modified or complete BPP
- Umbilical artery Doppler studies
- Antenatal corticosteroids if less than 34 weeks' GA

example, the low body mass index, poor weight gain, and smoking all point toward a pathologically—rather than constitutionally—small fetus.

First- or second-trimester screening results are important, as aneuploidy is associated with IUGR. **Amniocentesis is often indicated**, although this will depend on the GA at presentation. While infection is associated with IUGR, the yield of an infectious workup after mid-gestation is low.

Decreased AFI is associated with IUGR, and may be the earliest pathological sign detected on ultrasound. Decreased perfusion of fetal kidneys and decreased urine output explain the low AFI. **In general, pregnancies with the most severe oligohydramnios have the highest perinatal mortality rate, incidence of anomalies, and incidence of IUGR.** At the other extreme, polyhydramnios and IUGR have been dubbed an "ominous combination." This combination is associated with a high rate of structural and chromosomal anomalies.

Doppler studies have proven to be a powerful tool in the evaluation of a suspected IUGR fetus. Increased resistance in the placental circulation manifests as increased Doppler blood flow indices in the umbilical arteries. This finding has been demonstrated by many investigators in both animal and human models.

By signaling an underlying pathology, the utilization of umbilical artery Doppler flow measurements improves clinical outcomes. Numerous trials confirm that **the use of Doppler flow measurements can significantly reduce both perinatal death and unnecessary induction of labor** (iatrogenic preterm birth of the small-but-healthy fetus). Absence or reversal of end-diastolic flow in the umbilical artery is suggestive of poor fetal condition. Conversely, normal flow is rarely associated with significant morbidity.

Management

Treatment of the fetus with suspected IUGR will depend upon the clinical circumstances, particularly the gestational age. In general, pregnancies of <34 weeks' GA should **receive a course of antenatal corticosteroids to enhance lung maturation since preterm delivery is commonly encountered.** In fact, the use of antenatal corticosteroids is associated with a 50% reduction in neonatal death, a 50% reduction in RDS, and a 33% reduction in intraventricular hemorrhage; its use is the single most important intervention to improve neonatal outcome. Doppler studies are very useful. Antenatal testing with BPP or modified BPP—along with a repeat growth scan in 2 to 4 weeks—is suggested (see Table 22–3).

Emerging Concepts

There are ongoing trials to assess whether the use of low-dose aspirin with or without dipyridamole can improve or reduce the risk of IUGR; the speculated mechanism is to alter the thromboxane-to-prostacyclin ratio. To date, the results are inconclusive.

CASE CORRELATION

- See also Case 19 (Parvovirus Infection in Pregnancy) to see how Doppler is used to assess for fetal anemia (middle cerebral artery) versus growth restriction (umbilical artery).

Table 22-3 • SUGGESTED GUIDELINES FOR TIMING OF DELIVERY IUGR	
Gestational Age	**Circumstances for Delivery**
Term (37+ weeks): (risk of prematurity low)	Deliver since risks of prematurity are low
32-36 weeks (prematurity risks intermediate)	• Severe hypertension despite therapy • Absence of growth over 2-4 weeks • Nonreassuring fetal testing • Absent or reversal of end-diastolic flow on Doppler studies
<32 weeks (prematurity risks high)	• Reverse end-diastolic flow • Persistent nonreassuring fetal testing despite measures to optimize placental perfusion • Significant or ominous fetal testing results

COMPREHENSION QUESTIONS

22.1 A 21-year-old G1P0 woman is seen for her first prenatal visit at the obstetrician's office. Based on the LMP, the patient is 36 weeks' gestation. On ultrasound, the measurements indicate 32 weeks for all parameters including the HC, AC, and FL. Which of the following is the best management for this patient?

A. Antenatal steroids for probably IUGR

B. Recommend amniocentesis for karyotype

C. Delivery in 1 week (at term)

D. Continued monitoring and repeat ultrasound

22.2 A 27-year-old G2P1 woman is at 37 weeks' gestation supported by LMP and a 10-week ultrasound. The estimated fetal weight is 2000 g, which is less than the 3rd percentile for gestational age. The Doppler studies indicate the presence of forward end-diastolic flow. You recommend delivery for this patient. Which of the following is the best reason for your recommendation?

A. A fetal weight of 2000 g correlates with a high survival in the nursery

B. IUGR carries a significant risk of fetal death

C. The Doppler studies indicate a concern for continuing the pregnancy

D. With delivery, further diagnostic studies such as karyotype and viral studies can be conducted

22.3 An 18-year-old G1P0 woman at 38 weeks' gestation confirmed by a 12-week ultrasound has a fundal height of 34 cm. The patient has gained 20 lbs during the pregnancy. She denies smoking or alcohol or illicit substance use. Her BP is 110/70 mm Hg. Which of the following is the best management of this patient?

A. Perform a basic ultrasound study
B. Schedule for delivery since the patient has reached a term gestational age
C. Schedule biophysical profile and Doppler studies for this patient
D. Send her urine for a drug screen and consider ordering serum TORCH titers

ANSWERS

22.1 **D.** This patient presents for her first prenatal visit at 36 weeks' gestation. Although the baby measures small on ultrasound, there is a strong likelihood of wrong dates. Thus, rather than presume IUGR, this patient should be monitored with fetal surveillance such as BPP each week and a repeat ultrasound in 3 weeks to assess for interval growth. Normal growth would confirm wrong dates. In contrast, lack of growth would suggest IUGR.

22.2 **B.** Doppler flow showing forward diastolic flow is normal. Ominous signs would be reverse end-diastolic flow or absent end-distolic flow. The most concerning complication of IUGR is fetal death. The reason for delivery at term is to avoid stillbirth or other complications.

22.3 **A.** The first step in evaluating size less than dates is to perform an ultrasound for fetal weight. Sometimes due to the fetal position, or fetal head descending into the maternal pelvis, the fundal height may be decreased. If the ultrasound demonstrates fetal weight less than the 10th percentile, then further management may be contemplated.

CLINICAL PEARLS

- In general, the diagnosis of IUGR is made by the estimated fetal weight of less than the 10th percentile for gestational age.
- It is often helpful to categorize the IUGR as asymmetric (head sparing) or symmetric (head affected).
- Causes of symmetric IUGR include fetal chromosomal abnormalities, congenital syndromes, or severe fetal infections.
- Causes of asymmetric IUGR include maternal vascular disorders such as hypertensive disease.
- Antenatal corticosteroid use prior to delivery of an infant of <34 weeks' gestation is associated with dramatically improved outcome.
- Delivery is typically indicated when IUGR is coupled with oligohydramnios due to the greatly increased risk of fetal death.
- Umbilical artery Doppler is a useful tool in distinguishing the constitutionally small fetus from the pathologically small fetus. The use of Doppler has been shown to significantly reduce perinatal death and unnecessary preterm delivery.
- Timing of delivery is based on the clinical circumstances. Hypertension, the absence of growth over a 2- to 4-week period, and nonreassuring testing typically trigger delivery.
- When the Doppler flow reveals **reverse** end-diastolic umbilical artery flow, there is a high perinatal death within 48 hours, and usually delivery is performed.
- Absent end-diastolic flow is also worrisome although the risk for fetal death is not as ominous.

REFERENCES

American College of Obstetricians and Gynecologists. Fetal growth restriction. *Practice Bulletin* 124, May 2013.

Chamberlain PF, Manning FA, Morrison I, Harman CR, Lange IR. Ultrasound evaluation of amniotic fluid volume. The relationship of marginal and decreased amniotic fluid volumes to perinatal outcome. *Am J Obstet Gynecol.* 1984;150(3):245-249.

Miller J, Turan S, Baschat AA. Fetal growth restriction. *SeminPerinatol.* 2008;32(4):274-280.

Ott WJ. Diagnosis of IUGR: comparison of ultrasound parameters. *Am J Perinatol.* 2002;19(3):133-137.

CASE 23

A 20-year-old G1P0 woman at 29 weeks' gestation is hospitalized for acute pyelonephritis. She has no history of pyelonephritis in the past. She has been receiving intravenous (IV) ampicillin and gentamicin for 48 hours. She complains of acute shortness of breath. On examination, her temperature is 99°F, heart rate is 100 beats per minute (bpm), respiratory rate (RR) is 24 bpm and labored, and blood pressure (BP) is 120/70 mm Hg. Right costovertebral angle tenderness is elicited. The fetal heart tones are in the range of 140 to 150 bpm. The urine culture reveals *Escherichia coli* sensitive to ampicillin.

- What is the most likely diagnosis?
- What is the most likely mechanism for this patient's condition?

ANSWER TO CASE 23:
Pyelonephritis, Unresponsive

Summary: A 20-year-old G1P0 woman at 29 weeks' gestation is undergoing treatment of pyelonephritis with an appropriate antibiotic regimen and now complains of shortness of breath.

- **Most likely diagnosis:** Acute respiratory distress syndrome (ARDS).
- **Mechanism:** Endotoxin-mediated pulmonary injury.

ANALYSIS
Objectives

1. Understand the clinical presentation of pyelonephritis.
2. Know that the primary treatment of pyelonephritis is intravenous antibiotic therapy.
3. Understand that endotoxins can cause pulmonary damage, leading to ARDS.

Considerations

The patient is a 20-year-old woman at 29 weeks' gestation, who presented with pyelonephritis. She was started on intravenous ampicillin and gentamicin. Urine culture confirmed the diagnosis of infection with *E. coli*. The patient now complains of dyspnea and tachypnea. The most likely etiology for her respiratory symptoms is ARDS, with pulmonary injury secondary to endotoxin release. This typically occurs after antibiotics have begun to lyse the bacteria, leading to endotoxemia. Endotoxins can damage a variety of organs including lung, heart, liver, and kidney. The pathophysiology of ARDS is leaky capillaries, which allow fluid from the intravascular space to permeate into the alveolar areas. Chest x-ray may reveal patchy infiltrates; however, if the disease process is early, the chest radiograph may be normal. Treatment includes oxygen supplementation, careful monitoring of fluid status, and supportive measures. Occasionally, a patient may require intubation, but typically, the condition stabilizes and improves with time.

APPROACH TO:
Pyelonephritis in Pregnancy

DEFINITIONS

PYELONEPHRITIS: Kidney parenchymal infection, most commonly caused by gram-negative aerobic bacteria, such as *E. coli*.

ENDOTOXIN: A lipopolysaccharide that is released upon lysis of the cell wall of bacteria, especially gram-negative bacteria.

ACUTE RESPIRATORY DISTRESS SYNDROME: Alveolar and endothelial injury leading to leaky pulmonary capillaries, clinically causing hypoxemia, markedly increased alveolar–arterial gradient, and loss of lung volume.

CLINICAL APPROACH

Pyelonephritis in pregnancy can be a very serious medical condition, with an incidence of 1% to 2% of all pregnancies. It is the most common cause of sepsis in pregnant women. Studies show an increase risk of pyelonephritis in pregnant women who are young, Hispanic or Black, less educated, who smoke and have late entry to prenatal care. Pyelonephritis can lead to preterm labor, preterm delivery, and ARDS. The patient generally presents with complaints of dysuria and abrupt onset of flank tenderness, fever, chills, and, possibly, nausea and vomiting. Urinalysis typically shows pyuria and bacteriuria; a urine culture revealing >100 000 colony-forming units/mL of a single uropathogen is diagnostic. About 15% to 20% of women may also have bacteremia. The most common organism is *E. coli*, seen in about 80% of cases. *Klebsiella pneumoniae*, *Staphylococcus aureus*, *Enterobacter*, and *Proteus mirabilis* may also be isolated.

Pregnant women with acute pyelonephritis should be hospitalized and given intravenous antibiotics. Cephalosporins, such as cefotetan or ceftriaxone, or the combination of ampicillin and gentamicin are usually effective. IV antibiotics should be continued until fever and flank tenderness have substantially improved, and then the patient may be switched to oral antimicrobial therapy. Suppressive therapy should be prescribed for the remainder of the pregnancy as recurrent infection may develop in 30% to 40% of women after treatment of pyelonephritis. This can be achieved using nitrofurantoin 100 mg orally on a daily basis. A repeat urine culture should be obtained to ensure eradication of the infection. **If clinical improvement has not occurred after 48 to 72 hours of appropriate antibiotic therapy, urinary tract obstruction (ie, ureterolithiasis) or perinephric abscess should be suspected.** Ultrasound and/or computed tomography imaging may be helpful in this situation to assess for hydronephrosis, stone, or abscess.

Approximately 2% to 5% of pregnant women with pyelonephritis will develop ARDS, defined as pulmonary injury due to sepsis, usually mediated by endotoxins. The endotoxins derived from the gram-negative bacterial cell wall enter the blood stream, especially after antibiotic therapy is initiated, and may induce transient elevation of the serum creatinine as well as liver enzymes. Also, the endotoxemia may cause uterine contractions and result in preterm labor. Diffuse bilateral or interstitial infiltrates are typically seen in chest radiograph (Figure 23–1).

The treatment of ARDS is supportive care, with priorities on oxygenation and careful fluid management. In severe cases, mechanical ventilation may be required to maintain adequate oxygen levels.

Prevention

Normal physiologic changes in the urinary tract system occur in pregnancy that may increase the risk of infections. Progesterone induces relaxation of the smooth muscle that makes up part of the renal calyces and ureters. Some vesicoureteral reflux also occurs during pregnancy which can add to the increased risk of upper

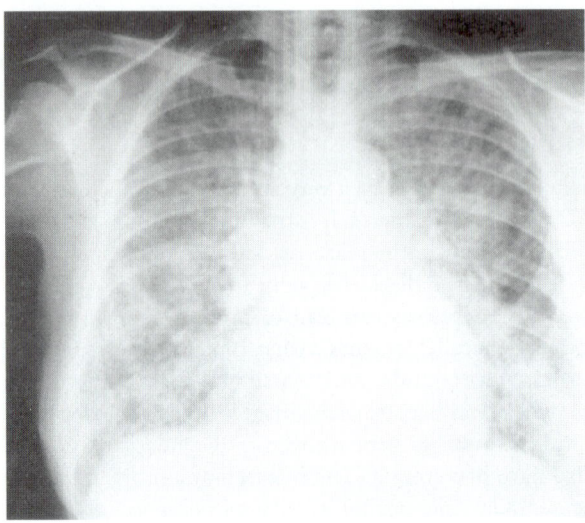

Figure 23–1. Acute respiratory distress syndrome. Chest radiograph depicts acute respiratory distress syndrome with diffuse pulmonary infiltrates. (*Reproduced with permission from Kasper DL, et al. Harrison's Principles of Internal Medicine. 16th ed. New York, NY: McGraw-Hill; 2005:1593.*)

tract infection. Up to 8% of pregnant women will have asymptomatic bacteriuria, persistent, actively multiplying bacteria within the urinary tract. When untreated, about 25% of women will develop pyelonephritis in the pregnancy. In contrast, when asymptomatic bacteriuria is identified and treated in the first trimester, the risk of pyelonephritis is reduced to 1% to 4%. For this reason, a urine culture should be performed in the first trimester, or entry into prenatal care, and follow-up cultures performed to ensure eradication of the urinary tract infection. The recurrence rate for asymptomatic bacteriuria (ASB) is about 30%; therefore, periodic surveillance is necessary after treatment to prevent recurrent infections.

CASE CORRELATON

- See also Case 15 (Pulmonary Embolism in Pregnancy), Case 16 (Preeclampsia), and Case 17 (Preterm Labor) to see other mechanisms of dyspnea and hypoxemia in pregnancy. The mechanisms are different:
- **Pulmonary embolism:** Intrapulmonary shunt with deoxygenated blood
- **Preeclampsia–pulmonary edema:** Leaky capillaries and iatrogenic fluid overload
- **Preterm labor with tocolytic agent:** Pulmonary edema due to tocolytic agent especially beta-mimetics
- **Pyelonephritis:** Endotoxin-mediated pulmonary injury (ARDS)

COMPREHENSION QUESTIONS

23.1 A 36-year-old G1P0 woman at 27 weeks' gestation is noted to have fever, right flank tenderness, and pyuria. She is diagnosed with pyelonephritis. A urine culture is performed. Which of the following is the most commonly isolated etiologic agent causing pyelonephritis in pregnancy?

   A. *Proteus* species
   B. *Candida* species
   C. *Escherichia coli*
   D. *Klebsiella* species

23.2 A 21-year-old G1P0 woman at 15 weeks' gestation is noted to have fever of 101°F (38.3°C), BP of 80/40 mm Hg, and decreased urine output. Which of the following is the most common cause of septic shock in pregnancy?

   A. Pelvic inflammatory disease
   B. Pyelonephritis
   C. Wound infection
   D. Mastitis

23.3 When a pregnant woman with pyelonephritis does not improve on adequate antibiotic therapy for 48 hours and experiences continued severe flank tenderness and fever, which of the following should be next considered?

   A. Obstruction of the urinary tract
   B. Anaerobic organisms
   C. Hemolytic uremic syndrome
   D. Factitious fever

23.4 Asymptomatic bacteriuria is best identified by which of the following?

   A. Careful questioning for dysuria or urinary frequency
   B. Urine culture on the first prenatal visit
   C. Urine culture at 35 weeks' gestation
   D. Urinalysis for any patient with family history of urinary tract infection (UTI)

ANSWERS

23.1 **C.** *Escherichia coli* is the most commonly isolated bacteria in pyelonephritis. *Proteus* and *Klebsiella* may also be found, but they are not the most common. Pregnant women with acute pyelonephritis should be hospitalized and given IV hydration and antibiotics. Cephalosporins, or the combination of ampicillin and gentamicin, are usually effective. The patient should be treated with IV medicines until the fever and flank pain resolve, and then switched to oral medication for the remainder of the pregnancy. *Candida* species are more often associated with vaginitis and not an infection associated with the urinary tract or kidneys.

23.2 **B.** Pyelonephritis is the most common cause of septic shock in pregnancy. Endotoxins derived from the gram-negative bacterial cell wall enter the bloodstream, especially after antibiotic therapy, and may induce transient elevation of serum creatinine as well as liver enzyme levels. The endotoxemia may cause uterine contractions and place a patient into preterm labor. Another complication that may arise is the development of ARDS, pulmonary injury due to sepsis. Mastitis typically occurs postpartum and, though rare, if left untreated can lead to abscess formation or sepsis. The agent most commonly responsible for mastitis is *S. aureus*, typically acquired from the back of the baby's throat during breastfeeding. An unattended wound infection can lead to postpartum sepsis as well; especially, after cesarean delivery. Pelvic inflammatory disease typically does not lead to sepsis; however, if a tubo-ovarian abscess forms and then ruptures, the patient is likely to go into septic shock. This is a surgical emergency that could be fatal.

23.3 **A.** Urinary obstruction, such as with a stone, should be considered with continued fever and flank tenderness after a 48- to 72-hour course of appropriate antibiotic therapy. Pyelonephritis is typically caused by **aerobic** bacteria such as *E. coli, Klebsiella, Proteus,* and *S. aureus*. Hemolytic uremic syndrome (HUS) is a disease characterized by hemolytic anemia, acute renal failure (uremia), and thrombocytopenia, but is not associated with pyelonephritis; however, like pyelonephritis, its etiology is usually due to *E. coli* (in HUS, a strain of *E. coli* that expresses a Shiga-like toxin). Patients typically present with bloody diarrhea rather than fever and flank pain. Factitious fever is also not associated with pyelonephritis, since the fever associated with this infection is legitimate.

23.4 **B.** Urine culture for every patient at the first prenatal visit helps to identify asymptomatic bacteriuria. Treatment prevents sequelae such as preterm labor and pyelonephritis during pregnancy. Careful questioning would not be of much use since the bacteriuria is asymptomatic. A urine culture at 35 weeks would not be helpful either; by this point, the asymptomatic bacteria may have already led to unfavorable consequences such as preterm labor or pyelonephritis. It is cost-effective and a good practice of preventative medicine for patients to get a urinalysis at every prenatal visit, regardless of family history which does not affect the likelihood of having bacteriuria.

CLINICAL PEARLS

▶ The most common cause of septic shock in pregnancy is pyelonephritis.

▶ When dyspnea occurs in a pregnant woman who is being treated for pyelonephritis, ARDS should be considered.

▶ When pyelonephritis is unresponsive after 48 to 72 hours of antibiotics, resistant organisms, obstructed urinary tract (stone), or perinephric abscess should be considered.

▶ Endotoxin release from gram-negative bacteria is the cause of acute respiratory distress syndrome associated with pyelonephritis.

REFERENCES

Cunningham FG, Leveno KJ, Bloom SL, Hauth JC, Rouse DJ, Spong CY. Renal and urinary tract disorders. In: *Williams Obstetrics*. 24th ed. New York, NY: McGraw-Hill; 2014:1033-1038.

Cunningham FG, Leveno KJ, Bloom SL, Hauth JC, Rouse DJ, Spong CY. Renal and urinary tract disorders. In: *Williams Obstetrics*. 24th ed. New York, NY: McGraw-Hill; 2014:1051-1068.

Wing DA, Fasset MJ, Getahun D. Acute pyelonephritis in pregnancy: an 18-year retrospective analysis. *Am J ObstetGynecol*. 2014;210:219.e1-6.

Hooton, TM. Urinary tract infections and asymptomatic bacteriuria in pregnancy. *UpToDate Inc*. Update December 19, 2011; Accessed 5.02.2012.

CASE 24

A 28-year-old woman who underwent a cesarean delivery 1 week ago is brought into the emergency room with a blood pressure of 60/40 mm Hg. The patient's husband states that she had 2 days of nausea and vomiting, fever up to 102°F (38.8°C), and myalgias. The reason for the cesarean was arrest of active phase, with cervical dilation at 5 cm for 3 hours despite strong uterine contractions. She was discharged home on postoperative day 3 in good condition. On examination, the patient appears lethargic and has mental confusion. Auscultation of her heart reveals tachycardia. The lung examination demonstrates slight crackles at the lung bases. The abdomen is tender throughout, and the fundus of the uterus is slightly tender. The skin incision is tender, red, and indurated. Upon opening the incision, purulent material is expressed. The underlying tissue is palpated and has a brawny texture with crepitance noted. The laboratory evaluation reveals a hemoglobin level of 15 g/dL and a serum creatinine of 2.1 mg/dL.

▶ What is the most likely diagnosis?
▶ What is the next step in therapy?

ANSWERS TO CASE 24:
Necrotizing Fasciitis

Summary: A 28-year-old woman who underwent an uncomplicated cesarean 1 week ago has fever up to 102°F (38.8°C), myalgias, vomiting, hypotension, confusion, and a skin incision that is infected with underlying tissue revealing a brawny texture and crepitance. She has evidence of hemoconcentration and renal insufficiency.

- **Most likely diagnosis:** Necrotizing fasciitis.

- **Next step in therapy:** Isotonic intravenous (IV) fluids, broad-spectrum antibiotics, and immediate surgical debridement.

ANALYSIS
Objectives

1. Recognize the manifestations of shock.

2. Understand that necrotizing fasciitis is a rare but potentially fatal infection that can affect patients.

3. Understand that aggressive fluid resuscitation, broad-spectrum antibiotics, and immediate surgical debridement are fundamental in the treatment of necrotizing fasciitis.

Considerations

This patient presents with multiple life-threatening issues. First, the hypotension must be recognized, since her blood pressure is 60/40 mm Hg. Her mean arterial pressure is 47 mm Hg, which is insufficient to maintain cerebral perfusion. Regardless of the etiology, the blood pressure needs to be supported immediately. Because the patient has a fever of 102°F (38.8°C) with hypotension and no history of hemorrhage or postpartum bleeding, septic shock is the most likely diagnosis. **The first step in resuscitation should be to support the blood pressure when low**, with aggressive use of intravenous isotonic fluids. A Foley catheter can help to assess urine output and indirectly kidney perfusion, particularly since the patient has an elevated serum creatinine level. The goal is to keep the mean arterial blood pressure at least 65 mm Hg to perfuse her vital organs. Ideally, this patient would have a urine output of at least 25 to 30 mL/h (depending on the degree of renal insufficiency). Furthermore, this woman most likely has **necrotizing fasciitis** since the underlying infected tissue has an abnormal consistency upon palpation. The crepitance is due to gas in the soft tissue, most likely due to anaerobic bacteria. Her myalgias, fever, nausea, and vomiting indicate the systemic nature of the infection.

APPROACH TO:
Necrotizing Fasciitis

DEFINITIONS

NECROTIZING FASCIITIS: A serious infection of the muscle and fascia usually caused by multiple organisms or anaerobes. It can involve surgical infections, traumatic injury, or rarely Group A Streptococci (flesh-eating bacteria).

GROUP A STREPTOCOCCAL TOXIC SHOCK SYNDROME: Rapidly progressing infection of the episiotomy or cesarean delivery incision ("flesh-eating bacteria" syndrome).

SHOCK: Condition of circulatory insufficiency where tissue perfusion needs are not met.

SEPTIC SHOCK: Circulatory insufficiency due to infection or the body's response to infection, commonly caused by gram-negative endotoxins.

$$\text{Mean arterial pressure (MAP)} = [(2 \times \text{Diastolic blood pressure}) + (1 \times \text{Systolic blood pressure})]/3$$

CLINICAL APPROACH

The management of septic shock includes copious intravenous fluids with close monitoring of urine output and blood pressure. At times, invasive hemodynamic monitoring with a central venous catheter or Swan–Ganz line is needed. Intravenous antibiotics should be broad spectrum to include penicillin, gentamicin, and metronidazole or other anaerobic agent, and dopamine or dobutamine is sometimes required when fluids alone are insufficient to maintain the blood pressure. Addressing the underlying etiology of the septic shock is important. When dealing with an aggressive wound infection, immediate surgical debridement, sometimes very radical or wide excisional procedures, is warranted. Necrotic and infected tissue must be removed, and sometimes, it requires multiple surgeries. Methicillin-resistant *Staphylococcus aureus* sometimes complicates wound infections; this is associated with a worse prognosis.

Monitoring of blood pressure, heart rate, oxygen saturation, urine output, and neurological status is important. Once the patient is stabilized, treating the underlying cause typically leads to resolution. Septic shock initially presents as decreased urine output and if untreated, proceeds to ischemia of vital organs and death.

COMPREHENSION QUESTIONS

24.1 A 35-year-old woman is noted to have a blood pressure of 80/40 mm Hg, fever, and abdominal pain. Which of the following is the likely mechanism of the patient's hypotension?
A. Cardiac contractility dysfunction
B. Cardiac bradycardia
C. Third spacing of fluid
D. Vasodilation

24.2 A 45-year-old woman is noted to have a surgical incision site that is suspicious for necrotizing fasciitis. Which of the following is most consistent with necrotizing fasciitis?
A. Redness of the surgical incision
B. Induration and edema of the surgical incision
C. Gas in the surgical tissue
D. Gram-negative rods growing from blood culture

24.3 A 30-year-old woman is brought into the emergency department with fever and a blood pressure of 70/40 mm Hg. She is presumed to be in septic shock. Which of the following is a fundamental principle for the treatment?
A. Intravenous normal saline
B. Plasmapheresis
C. Oral fluid resuscitation
D. Await blood culture results prior to initiation of antibiotic therapy

ANSWERS

24.1 **D.** The pathophysiology of septic shock is vasodilation usually due to endotoxins, although at times, such as with *S. aureus* (toxic shock syndrome), exotoxins can be causative. The vasodilation leads to hypotension, and is treated with IV fluids. If the IV fluids are insufficient to produce a correction in hypotension, then vasoconstrictors are indicated, such as dopamine. Late in the course of septic shock, cardiac dysfunction can occur; however, at this stage, the patient is typically in a near terminal condition.

24.2 **C.** Gas in the muscle or fascia is indicative of necrotizing fasciitis, likely due to a clostridial species. Induration and redness of the surgical wound are suggestive of a superficial wound infection, in which the skin and subcutaneous tissue are infected. This is a superficial surgical site infection, and needs to be opened. The superficial wound infection is not as lifethreatening as when a deep surgical site infection occurs.

24.3 **A.** Intravenous isotonic fluids are the initial treatment of choice for septic shock. The cornerstones of therapy include removing the nidus of infection, antibiotic therapy, and support of the blood pressure. Plasmapheresis is not a major part of the treatment of septic shock.

CLINICAL PEARLS

▶ The cornerstones of treatment of septic shock include aggressive intravenous fluids, source control, antibiotic therapy, and monitoring perfusion and organ function.

▶ Source control in septic shock means removing the etiology of the infection.

▶ The sunburn-like rash and/or desquamation are typical for *S. aureus* infections.

▶ The initial antibiotic therapy for serious *S. aureus* infections is generally intravenous nafcillin or methicillin unless methicillin resistance is suspected, in which case vancomycin is used.

▶ Hypotension that persists despite intravenous isotonic fluid replacement generally requires pressor support such as with intravenous infusion of dopamine.

REFERENCES

Cunningham FG, Leveno KJ, Bloom SL, Hauth JC, Gilstrap LC III, Wenstrom KD. Puerperal infection. In: *Williams Obstetrics*. 24th ed. New York, NY: McGraw-Hill; 2014:671-688.

Gambone JC. Gynecologic procedures. In: Hacker NF, Gambone JC, Hobel CJ, eds. *Essentials of Obstetrics and Gynecology*. 5th ed. Philadelphia, PA: Saunders; 2009:332-344.

Katz VL. Postoperative counseling and management. In: Katz VL, Lentz GM, Lobo RA, Gersenson DM, eds. *Comprehensive Gynecology*. 6th ed. St. Louis, MO: Mosby-Year Book; 2012:661-710.

CASE 25

A 24-year-old G1P1 woman underwent a low-transverse cesarean section 2 days ago for arrest of active phase of labor. She required oxytocin and an internal uterine pressure catheter. She reached and persisted at 6-cm dilation for 3 hours despite adequate uterine contractions as judged by 240 Montevideo units. Her baby weighed 8 lb 9 oz. The past medical and surgical histories were unremarkable. She denies a cough or dysuria. On examination, the temperature is 102°F (38.8°C), heart rate is 80 beats per minute, blood pressure is 120/70 mm Hg, and respiratory rate is 12 breaths per minute. The breasts are nontender. The lungs are clear to auscultation. There is no costovertebral angle tenderness. The abdomen reveals that the skin incision is without erythema or tenderness. The uterine fundus is firm, at the level of the umbilicus, and somewhat tender. No lower extremity cords are palpated.

- ▶ What is the most likely diagnosis?
- ▶ What is the most likely etiology of the condition?
- ▶ What is the best therapy for the condition?

ANSWERS TO CASE 25:
Postpartum Endomyometritis

Summary: A 24-year-old G1P1 woman, who underwent a cesarean delivery 2 days previously for arrest of labor, has a fever of 102°F (38.8°C). She denies cough or dysuria. There are no abnormalities of the breasts, lungs, costovertebral region, or skin incision. The uterine fundus is somewhat tender.

- **Most likely diagnosis:** Endomyometritis.
- **Most likely etiology of the condition:** Ascending infection of vaginal organisms (anaerobic predominance but also Gram-negative rods).
- **Best therapy for the condition:** Intravenous antibiotics with anaerobic coverage (eg, gentamicin and clindamycin).

ANALYSIS
Objectives

1. Know that the most common cause of fever for a woman who has undergone cesarean delivery is endomyometritis.
2. Know the mechanism of the endomyometritis, that is, ascending infection of "polymicrobial" vaginal organisms.
3. Know that the differential diagnosis of fever in the woman who has undergone cesarean delivery includes mastitis, wound infection, atelectasis (if general anesthesia), and pyelonephritis.

Considerations

This 24-year-old woman underwent cesarean delivery for arrest of dilation with adequate uterine contractions (see Case 1 for criteria). She presumably had a long labor, an intrauterine pressure catheter, and numerous vaginal examinations. These are all risk factors for the development of postpartum endomyometritis. Other risk factors include low socioeconomic status, multiple gestations, young maternal age, Group B Step infection, chlamydia and manual extraction of the placenta. On examination, she has a fever up to 102°F (38.8°C). The scenario reveals that there are no abnormalities of the breasts, which rules out mastitis. The lungs are normal to auscultation, which speaks against atelectasis; in the obstetric patient, atelectasis is an uncommon cause of postoperative fever since the majority of cesarean deliveries are performed under regional anesthesia. This patient's wound appears normal. There is no costovertebral angle tenderness, so the likelihood of pyelonephritis is low. Urinary tract infections involving only the bladder do not usually cause fever. The uterus is only somewhat tender, which does not overtly point to endomyometritis. However, when the remainder of the examination does not reveal a focus, the majority of women who have fever after cesarean delivery have endomyometritis.

APPROACH TO:
Fever after Cesarean Delivery

DEFINITIONS

FEBRILE MORBIDITY: Temperature after cesarean delivery equal to or >100.4°F (38°C) taken on two occasions at least 6 hours apart, exclusive of the first 24 hours.

ENDOMYOMETRITIS: Infection of the decidua, myometrium, and, sometimes, the parametrial tissues.

SEPTIC PELVIC THROMBOPHLEBITIS (SPT): Bacterial infection of pelvic venous thrombi, usually involving the ovarian vein.

CLINICAL APPROACH

A woman who has febrile morbidity after cesarean delivery most likely has endomyometritis. The use of perioperative antibiotics has decreased postoperative infection rate more than any other intervention but infections can still occur. The mechanism of infection is ascension of bacteria, a mixture of organisms from the normal vaginal flora. In other words, postcesarean delivery infection is almost always "polymicrobial," with a mix of both aerobic and anaerobic bacteria. The uterine incision site, being devitalized and containing foreign material (ie, suture), is commonly the site for infection. Typically, the fever occurs on postoperative day 2. When intra-amniotic infection occurs during labor, the fever usually continues postpartum. The patient may complain of abdominal tenderness or a foul-smelling lochia. Uterine tenderness is common. **Broad-spectrum antimicrobial therapy** especially with **anaerobic coverage** is important. Intravenous gentamicin and clindamycin is a well-studied regimen and effective in 90% of cases. Other choices include extended penicillins or cephalosporins. In contrast to postcesarean infection, endometritis after vaginal delivery does not necessarily require anaerobic antimicrobial coverage, and ampicillin and gentamicin are usually sufficient. Regardless of route of delivery, the fever usually improves significantly after 48 hours of antimicrobial therapy. Enterococcal infection may be one reason for nonresponse; ampicillin is the treatment for this organism and often is added if fever persists after 48 hours of therapy. If fever persists despite triple antibiotic therapy for 48 to 72 hours, a computed tomography (CT) scan of the abdomen and pelvis may reveal an abscess, infected hematoma, or pelvic thrombophlebitis.

Another cause of fever after cesarean delivery is wound infection. Prophylactic antibiotics are given prior to surgery to decrease the incidence of infection. Thus, women who are scheduled to have cesarean, whether elective or in labor, should have a single-dose antibiotic prophylaxis prior to skin incision; this practice reduces the infection risk by about 75%. When a patient fails to respond to antibiotic therapy, wound infection is the most likely etiology. The fever usually occurs on postoperative day 4. Erythema or drainage may be present in the wound site. The organisms are often the same as those involved with endomyometritis. The treatment includes surgical opening of the wound (and dressing changes) and

Table 25–1 • APPROACH TO POSTPARTUM FEVER
Evaluate for pulmonary etiology: Cough? Atelectasis?
Evaluate for pyelonephritis: Costovertebral angle tenderness? Dysuria? Pyuria?
Evaluate for breast engorgement: Are breasts engorged, tender, red?
Evaluate for wound infection: Is the wound indurated, erythematous? Is there drainage?
Evaluate for endometritis: Is the uterus tender? Foul-smelling lochia?
If endometritis, begin intravenous gentamicin and clindamycin if cesarean, and can be ampicillin and gentamicin for vaginal delivery.
If no response in 48 h, reevaluate and if endometritis is still considered, add ampicillin for enterococcus coverage.
If no response after 48 h of triple antibiotics, reevaluate (especially look for wound infection). Consider CT imaging to assess for abscess, hematoma, or septic pelvic thrombophlebitis.

antimicrobial agents. The fascia must be inspected for integrity. Necrotizing fasciitis is a serious life-threatening infection that can affect the cesarean wound. Infections in the first 24 hours postoperatively can implicate group A streptococcus, the so-called "flesh-eating bacteria." Immediate and extensive surgical debridement is indicated. Community-acquired methicillin-resistant *Staphylococcus aureus* has also been isolated with increasing frequency, affecting the skin incision.

Septic pelvic thrombophlebitis is a rare bacterial infection affecting thrombosed pelvic veins, usually the ovarian vessels. The bacterial infection at the placental implantation site spreads to the ovarian venous plexuses or to the common iliac veins, sometimes extending to the inferior vena cava. Women with SPT typically have recurrent high fevers and sometimes have a palpable pelvic mass. The diagnosis may be confirmed by a CT scan or magnetic resonance imaging. Treatment includes antimicrobial therapy and some practitioners will also use heparin therapy.

Other considerations in a febrile, woman should include pyelonephritis (fever, flank tenderness, leukocytes in the urine), pelvic abscess or infected pelvic hematoma, and breast engorgement (Table 25–1).

CASE CORRELATON

- See also Case 24 (Necrotizing Fasciitis)

COMPREHENSION QUESTIONS

25.1 A 30-year-old G1P1 who underwent a cesarean section 3 days previously has a fever of 101°F (38.3°C). The skin incision is indurated, tender, and erythematous. Which of the following is the best management?

   A. Initiation of intravenous ampicillin
   B. Initiation of intravenous heparin
   C. Placement of a warm compress on the wound
   D. Opening of the wound

25.2 A 29-year-old woman is diagnosed with postpartum endometritis based on fever, abdominal pain, fundal tenderness, and elimination of other etiologies. Which of the following is the most significant risk factor for postpartum endomyometritis?
  A. Numerous vaginal examinations
  B. Bacterial vaginosis
  C. Cesarean delivery
  D. Internal uterine pressure monitors
  E. Prolonged rupture of membranes

25.3 A 27-year-old G1P0 woman at 39 weeks' gestation is noted to be in labor. She underwent artificial rupture of membranes, and experiences fetal bradycardia. Palpation of the vagina reveals a rope-like structure prolapsing through the cervix. She is diagnosed with a cord prolapse and underwent stat cesarean delivery. On postoperative day 2, the patient has a temperature of 102°F (38.8°C), and is diagnosed with endometritis. The patient who works in the microbiology laboratory asks which of the following is the most commonly isolated bacteria in her infection?
  A. Peptostreptococcus species
  B. *Staphylococcus aureus*
  C. Group B Streptococcus
  D. *Escherichia coli*

25.4 A 22-year-old woman who underwent cesarean delivery has persistent fever of 102°F (38.8°C), despite the use of triple antibiotic therapy (ampicillin, gentamicin, and clindamycin). The urinalysis, wound, breasts, and uterine fundus are normal on examination. A CT scan of the pelvis is suggestive of septic pelvic thrombophlebitis. Which of the following is the best therapy for this condition?
  A. Hysterectomy
  B. Discontinue antibiotic therapy and initiate intravenous heparin
  C. Continue antibiotic therapy and begin intravenous heparin
  D. Surgical embolectomy
  E. Streptokinase therapy

ANSWERS

25.1 **D.** The best treatment of a wound infection is **opening of the wound**. Prophylactic antibiotics given during surgery decrease the likelihood of becoming infected. In addition to opening the wound, the patient should undergo dressing changes and be started on antimicrobial agents. The fascia must be inspected for integrity. In cesarean wound infections, there are two distinct populations of organisms that may be involved: skin organisms versus vaginal organisms. A Gram stain of the wound may direct toward the correct antibiotic regimen that would be effective for the possible bacteria.

25.2 **C. Cesarean delivery greatly increases the risk of endometritis** due to the fact that the patient most likely had prolonged rupture of membranes, numerous vaginal examinations, and an intrauterine pressure monitor due, for example, to an arrest of labor. Endometritis after vaginal delivery may occur as well, though less frequent, but does not necessarily require anaerobic antimicrobial coverage; therefore, ampicillin and gentamicin are usually sufficient.

25.3 **A. Anaerobic bacteria** are the most commonly isolated organisms in endomyometritis in patients who have undergone cesarean delivery. Peptostreptococcus and peptococcus are the most likely pathogens 45% of the time and bacteriodes 9%. The other organisms listed are aerobes.

25.4 **C. Continue antibiotic therapy and begin intravenous heparin.** Although there is no universal agreement, the best treatment for septic pelvic thrombophlebitis seems to be the combination of antibiotics and heparin. There are some practitioners who believe that antibiotics alone are sufficient to treat SPT. Heparin alone is not effective. Hysterectomy is not indicated.

CLINICAL PEARLS

▶ The most common cause of fever after cesarean delivery is endomyometritis.

▶ The major organisms responsible for postcesarean endomyometritis are anaerobic bacteria with the most commonly isolated organisms include peptostreptococcus, peptococcus, and *Bacteroides* species.

▶ Atelectasis is rare in obstetric patients due to the large number of women who have regional anesthesia.

▶ When fever in a cesarean patient persists on triple antibiotic therapy, CT imaging should be performed.

▶ Antibiotic therapy and heparin are an accepted treatment for septic pelvic thrombophlebitis.

REFERENCES

Aronoff DM, Mulla ZD. Postpartum invasive group A Streptococcal disease in the modern era. *Infect Dis Obstet Gynecol.* 2008;796-892.

Costantine MM, Rahman M, Ghulmiyah L, et al. Timing of perioperative antibiotics for cesarean delivery: a metaanalysis. *Am J Obstet Gynecol.* 2008;199(3):301.e1.

Cunningham FG, Leveno KJ, Bloom SL, Hauth JC, Gilstrap LC III, Wenstrom KD. Puerperal infection. In: *Williams Obstetrics.* 24th ed. New York, NY: McGraw-Hill; 2014:711-724, 661-668.

Henderson K, Fuller K, Morosky C. ACOG: Green Journal Manual Exploration of the Uterus as a Risk Factor for Postpartum Endometritis. *Obstetrics & Gynecology.* 2015;124:81S.

Kim M, Hyashi RH, Gambone JC. Obstetrical hemorrhage and puerperal sepsis. In: Hacker NF, Gambone JC, Hobel CJ, eds. *Essentials of Obstetrics and Gynecology.* 5th ed. Philadelphia, PA: Saunders; 2009:128-138.

CASE 26

A 20-year-old parous woman complains of right breast pain and fever. She states that 3 weeks previously, she underwent a normal spontaneous vaginal delivery. She had been breastfeeding without difficulty until 2 days ago, when she noted progressive pain, induration, and redness to the right breast. On examination, her temperature is 102°F (38.8°C), blood pressure is 100/70 mm Hg, and heart rate is 110 beats per minute. Her neck is supple. Her right breast has induration on the upper outer region with redness and tenderness. There is also significant fluctuance noted in the breast tissue. The abdomen is nontender and there is no costovertebral angle tenderness. The pelvic examination is unremarkable.

- ▶ What is the most likely diagnosis?
- ▶ What is your next step in therapy?
- ▶ What is the etiology of the condition?

ANSWERS TO CASE 26:
Breast Abscess and Mastitis

Summary: A 20-year-old breast-feeding woman who is 3 weeks' postpartum complains of right breast pain and fever of 2 days' duration. She notes progressive pain, induration, and redness in the right breast. Her temperature is 102°F (38.8°C). There is also significant fluctuance noted in the right breast.

- **Most likely diagnosis:** Abscess of the right breast.
- **Next step in therapy:** Incision and drainage of the abscess and antibiotic therapy.
- **Etiology of the condition:** *Staphylococcus aureus*.

ANALYSIS
Objectives

1. Know the clinical presentation of postpartum mastitis.
2. Know that *S. aureus* is the most common etiology in postpartum mastitis.
3. Understand that the presence of fluctuance in the breast probably represents an abscess that needs incision and drainage.

Considerations

This woman is 3 weeks' postpartum with breast pain and fever. This is a typical presentation of a breast infection, since mastitis usually presents in the third or fourth postpartum week. Induration and redness of the breast accompanied by fever and chills are also consistent. The treatment for this condition is an antistaphylococcal agent such as dicloxacillin. Provided that the offending agent is not methicillin resistant, improvement should be rapid. Affected women are instructed to continue to breast feed or drain the breast by pump. This patient has fluctuance of the breast that speaks for an abscess, which usually requires surgical drainage and will not generally improve with antibiotics alone. If there is uncertainty about the diagnosis, ultrasound examination may be helpful in identifying a fluid collection.

APPROACH TO:
Breast Infections

DEFINITIONS
MASTITIS: Infection of the breast parenchyma typically caused by *S aureus*.

BREAST ABSCESS: The presence of a collection of purulent material in the breast, which requires drainage.

GALACTOCELE: A noninfected collection of milk due to a blocked mammary duct leading to a palpable mass and symptoms of breast pressure and pain.

CLINICAL APPROACH

Postpartum breast disorders and infections are common. They include cracked nipples, breast engorgement, mastitis, breast abscesses, and galactoceles. Cracked nipples usually arise from dryness, and may be exacerbated by harsh soap or water-soluble lotions. Treatment includes air drying the nipples, washing with mild soap and water, the use of a nipple shield, and the application of a lanolin-based lotion.

Breast engorgement is usually noted during the first-week postpartum and is due to vascular congestion and milk accumulation. The patient will generally complain of breast pain and induration, and may have a low-grade fever. Infant feedings around-the-clock usually help to alleviate this condition. Fever seldom persists for more than 12 to 24 hours. Treatment consists of a breast binder, ice packs, and analgesics.

Postpartum mastitis is an infection of the breast parenchyma, affecting about 2% of lactating women. These infections usually occur between the second and fourth week after delivery. Other signs and symptoms include malaise, fever, chills, tachycardia, and a red, tender, swollen breast. Importantly, there should be no fluctuance of the breast, which would indicate abscess formation. The most commonly isolated organism is *S. aureus*, usually arising from the infant's nose and throat. The treatment for mastitis should be prompt to prevent abscess formation, consisting of an antistaphylococcal agent such as dicloxacillin. If the patient has a penicillin allergy, then clarithromycin orally for 10 to 14 days has been effective. For MRSA, clindamycin or trimethoprim/sulfa orally for 10 to 14 days has been used as empiric therapy pending cultures. Breastfeeding or pumping should be continued to prevent the development of abscess. A culture of the breast milk sent prior to initiating treatment is useful for determining bacterial sensitivities and nosocomial surveillance.

About 1 in 10 cases of mastitis is complicated by **abscess**, which should be suspected with persistent fever after 48 hours of antibiotic therapy or the presence of a fluctuant mass. Ultrasound examination may be performed to confirm the diagnosis. The purulent collection is best treated by surgical drainage, or alternatively by ultrasound-guided aspiration; antistaphylococcal antibiotics should also be used.

The **galactocele** or milk-retention cyst is caused by blockage of a milk duct. The milk accumulates in one or more breast lobes, leading to a nonerythematous fluctuant mass. They usually resolve spontaneously, but may need aspiration.

Breastfeeding has many benefits (Table 26–1). Breast milk contains nearly all of the nutrients required with the exception of several vitamins (K and D), and is more easily tolerated than formula. The infant has a strong suckling reflex in its first hour of life. For this reason, the American College of Obstetricians and Gynecologists and the American Academy of Pediatrics (AAP) recommend that that a healthy baby have a skin-to-skin contact with the mother immediately after delivery with an encouragement for breastfeeding.

Table 26–1 • BENEFITS OF BREASTFEEDING
Neonatal   Decreased incidence of: GI: diarrhea, NEC   Infectious: lower respiratory infections, otitis media, bacteremia, UTI   Other possible benefits: protective against SIDS, allergies, and type 1 DM; slightly higher performance on standardized tests
Maternal   Decreased weight retention   Decreased risk of breast cancer   Decreased risk of ovarian and endometrial cancer   Decreased risk of diabetes   Decreased risk of osteoporosis

COMPREHENSION QUESTIONS

26.1 A 32-year-old woman has just delivered a 40-week baby vaginally. Her physician recommends that she should not breastfeed because of a medical condition. Which of the following conditions is most likely to be present?

A. Ampicillin therapy for cystitis

B. Maternal Dilantin therapy for seizure disorder

C. Maternal human immunodeficiency virus (HIV) infection

D. Maternal inverted nipples

26.2 A 22-year-old nulliparous woman is noted to have a tender, red, right breast and enlarged, tender axillary lymph nodes that have persisted despite antibiotics for 3 weeks. She denies manipulation of her breasts and is not lactating. Which of the following is the most appropriate next step?

A. Course of oral antibiotic therapy

B. Sonographic examination of the breasts

C. Mammographic examination of the breasts

D. Check the serum prolactin level

E. Biopsy of the breast

26.3 A 28-year-old G1P1 woman has delivered vaginally 3 weeks ago. She is breastfeeding and notes that the baby prefers to breastfeed from the right breast. On the left breast, she notes a 3-day history of a tender mass on the upper outer quadrant. On examination, she is afebrile. The left breast has a fluctuant mass of 4 × 8 cm of the upper outer quadrant without redness. It is somewhat tender. Which of the following is the best treatment for this condition?

A. Oral antibiotic therapy

B. Oral antifungal therapy

C. Bromocriptine therapy

D. Aspiration

E. Mastectomy

26.4 A 29-year-old G1P1 woman desires to breastfeed her infant, which is 1 day old. The infant received an injection of vitamin K. You counsel the patient on positive health consequences of breastfeeding, including immunological, bonding, neurodevelopmental, and gastrointestinal (GI) effects. Which of the following requires supplementation in the first 6 months as it is not present in breast milk?

A. Iron
B. Vitamin D
C. Vitamin E
D. Vitamin K

ANSWERS

26.1 **C. Maternal HIV infection is a contraindication for breastfeeding** because the neonate may contract the infection from infected breast milk. Dilantin and ampicillin are safe to take during pregnancy. Though challenging, women with inverted nipples are still able to breastfeed. There are very few **contraindications** to breastfeeding: infants with classic galactosemia (galactose 1-phosphate uridyltransferase deficiency), mothers who have active untreated tuberculosis disease or HIV infection, mothers who are receiving diagnostic or therapeutic radioactive isotopes or have had exposure to radioactive materials, mothers who are receiving antimetabolites or chemotherapeutic agents or a small number of other medications until they clear the milk, mothers who are using drugs of abuse ("street drugs"), and mothers who have herpes simplex lesions on a breast.

26.2 **E.** This woman has had persistent tenderness and redness of the breast despite not lactating and not having trauma to the breast; these symptoms have worsened despite antibiotic therapy. There is a concern about inflammatory breast carcinoma (see Case 47), and she should undergo biopsy. Inflammatory breast cancer presents with redness, tenderness, and warmth and can mimic mastitis. It is an aggressive type of malignancy with cancer cells located in the skin lymphatics.

26.3 **D.** This patient has a galactocele. It is not an abscess since there is no fever or redness, although untreated, this could become an abscess. The best treatment of a **galactocele** (milk-retention cyst) is aspiration if it does not resolve spontaneously. This is done to prevent a breast abscess. A galactocele forms when a milk duct is blocked and the milk accumulates in one or more breast lobes, leading to a nonerythematous fluctuant mass. It is not an infection, therefore antibiotics and antifungals are unnecessary; it is also not cancerous, so a mastectomy is not indicated. **Bromocriptine** is an ergot alkaloid that blocks the release of prolactin from the pituitary (typically in the setting of a prolactinoma), mostly as an attempt to allow a woman to be able to have normal menstrual cycles.

26.4 **B.** Vitamin D should be supplemented at 2 months of age. The American Academy of Pediatrics recommends that unless contraindicated, each infant be breastfed exclusively for the first 6 months of life because of the health benefits to the baby. Breast-fed babies have less infections including meningitis, urinary tract infections, and sepsis thought to be due to immunoglobulin and leukocytes in the breast milk. They have slightly better neurodevelopmental outcomes, and there is evidence of less risk of diabetes and childhood obesity in later life. Breast milk consists of two proteins, whey and casein, and has lower casein proportion than formula milk, allowing for easier digestion. Lactoferrin (inhibits certain iron-dependent bacteria of the GI tract), secretory IgA, and lysozyme (enzyme which protects against *Escherichia coli* and other bacteria) are also found in breast milk, along with fats and carbohydrates (lactose). All the vitamins are found in breast milk provided the mother's nutrition is sufficient, with the exception of vitamin D. The AAP recommends supplementation of vitamin D drops at 2 months of age for infants exclusively breastfed.

CLINICAL PEARLS

▶ The best treatment for postpartum mastitis is an oral antistaphylococcal antibiotic, such as dicloxacillin, and continued breastfeeding or pumping.

▶ The presence of fluctuance in a red, tender, indurated breast suggests abscess, which needs surgical drainage.

▶ The best treatment of cracked nipples is air drying and the avoidance of using a harsh soap.

▶ Breast engorgement rarely causes high fever persisting more than 24 hours.

REFERENCES

American College of Obstetricians and Gynecologists. Breast-feeding: maternal and infant aspects. *ACOG Committee Opinion 361*. 2007. (Reaffirmed 2013.)

Cunningham FG, Leveno KJ, Bloom SL, Hauth JC, Rouse DJ, Spong CY. The puerperium. In: *Williams Obstetrics*. 24th ed. New York, NY: McGraw-Hill; 2014:652-654.

Hobel CJ, Zakowski M. Normal labor, delivery, and postpartum care: anatomic considerations, obstetric and analgesia, and resuscitation of the newborn. In: Hacker NF, Gambone JC, Hobel CJ, eds. *Essentials of Obstetrics and Gynecology*. 5th ed. Philadelphia, PA: Saunders; 2009:91-118.

CASE 27

A 27-year-old G3P0020 who is at 32 weeks' gestation presents to the Obstetrical Unit for fatigue and lethargy. The patient has a history of type 1 diabetes for 12 years. She denies hypertension, retinopathy, and renal disease. Her obstetric history is significant for two first trimester pregnancy losses occurring 1 and 3 years previously. Her medications include twice-daily subcutaneous insulin. On examination, her blood pressure (BP) is 84/44 mm Hg, heart rate (HR) is 120 bpm, and respiratory rate (RR) is 32 breaths per minute. She appears sleepy and confused. The mucous membranes are dry. The urine on dipstick shows a specific gravity of 1.030, 4+ glucose, and 3+ ketones. The fingerstick glucose is 280 mg/dL. The fetal heart tones' rate tracing is noted below (Figure 27–1).

▶ What is the most likely diagnosis?
▶ What is the next step in therapy for this patient?
▶ What does the fetal heart rate (FHR) tracing indicate?
▶ What is the best management for the pregnancy?

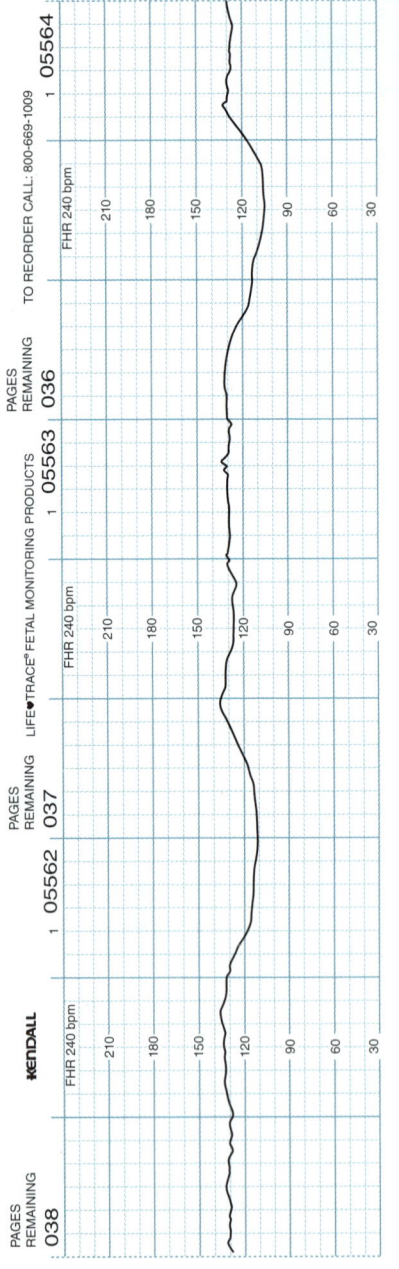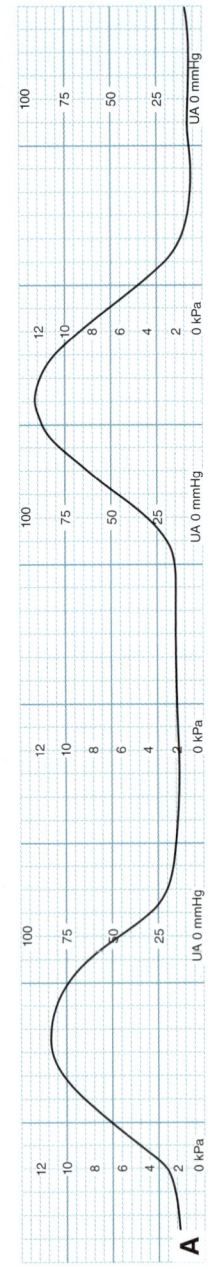

Figure 27–1. (A) and (B) FHR tracing. (Reproduced with permission from Eugene C. Toy, MD.)

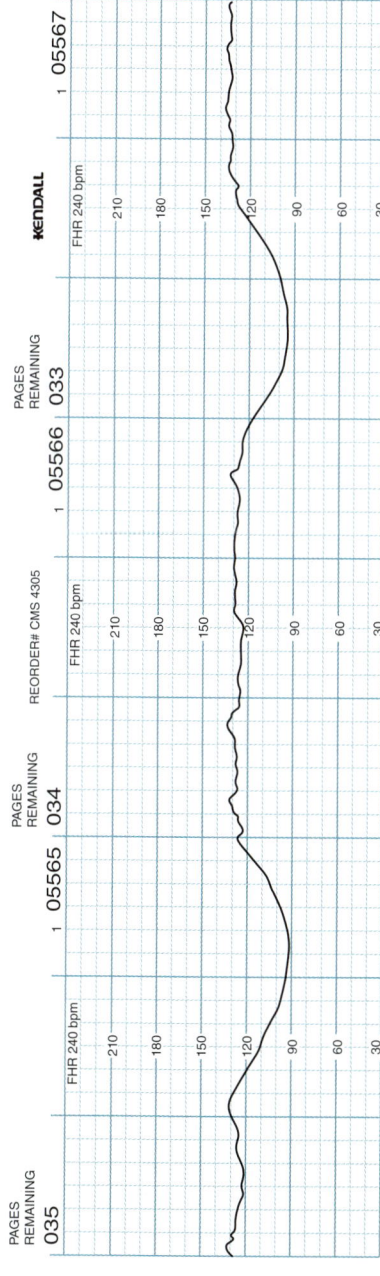
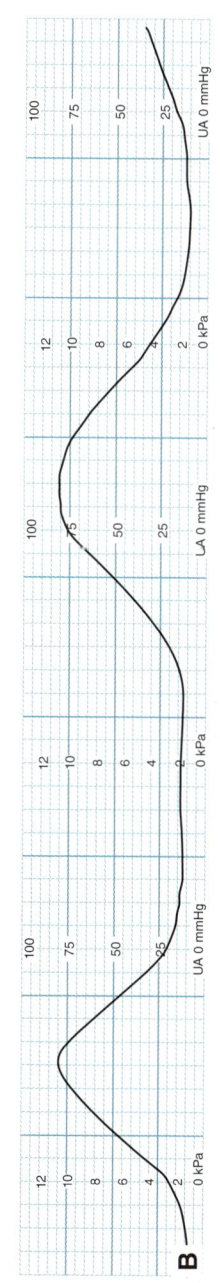

Figure 27–1. *(Continued)*

ANSWERS TO CASE 27:
Diabetes in Pregnancy

Summary: A 27-year-old G3P0020 type 1 insulin-requiring diabetic with multiple miscarriages is at 32 weeks' gestation. She is presenting with fatigue and lethargy. She denies hypertension, retinopathy, and renal disease. Her blood pressure (BP) is 84/44 mm Hg, heart rate (HR) is 120 bpm, and respiratory rate (RR) is 32 breaths per minute. She appears sleepy and confused, and her mucous membranes are dry. The urinalysis shows a specific gravity of 1.030, 4+ glucose, and 3+ ketones. The fingerstick glucose is 280 mg/dL. The fetal heart tones' rate tracing demonstrates late decelerations and decreased variability.

- **Most likely diagnosis:** Diabetic ketoacidosis (DKA). This should be confirmed with a STAT arterial blood gas, blood sugar, electrolytes with anion gap (AG), and serum ketones.

- **Next step in therapy for this patient:** Aggressive isotonic fluid hydration begins intravenous (IV) insulin infusion to lower the glucose, remedy any electrolyte abnormalities, and treat the trigger of the DKA (such as infection).

- **Fetal heart rate tracing:** Baseline of 140 bpm with decreased variability and recurrent late decelerations, indicative of severe hypoxia or acidosis.

- **Best management for the pregnancy:** Treat the DKA and observe the FHR tracing carefully.

ANALYSIS:

Objectives

1. Describe the maternal and fetal complications associated with **pregestational** diabetes.
2. Describe the maternal and fetal complications associated with **gestational** diabetes.
3. Be aware that DKA can occur with lower blood sugars and more rapidly in pregnancy.
4. List the differences in the pathophysiology and clinical manifestations of pregestational versus gestational diabetes.

Considerations

This pregnant woman at 32 weeks' gestation presents with lethargy, hypotension, tachycardia, dry mucous membranes, hyperglycemia, and ketonuria. She has a 12-year history of type 1 diabetes. **This is most likely diabetic ketoacidosis, which is a medical emergency. DKA can be difficult to diagnose during pregnancy.** Note that this patient's blood sugar is only 280 mg/dL; **pregnant diabetics can develop DKA with lower blood sugars and more rapidly than nonpregnant patients.** The priority in this patient should be IV fluid infusion with two large bore IVs using an isotonic solution such as NS, since these individuals may have up to a 5-L deficit. This is the most important initial management. Arterial pH will confirm acidosis. Serum electrolytes should also be obtained especially to assess the potassium level and the anion gap. The management of DKA is similar to that of the nonpregnant patient: (a) IV fluid hydration, (b) correction of acidosis, (c) insulin to correct glucose (usually takes 6-10 hours), (d) correction of electrolyte and other metabolic abnormalities, and (e) treatment of the underlying etiology. The fetal pH is dependent on the maternal pH to clear excessive acids; the fetal pH is generally 0.1 units less than the maternal pH. Thus, maternal acidosis will cause fetal acidosis, which accounts for the late decelerations on the FHR tracing. The FHR pattern of late decelerations is a reflection of the maternal acidosis. Generally, correction of the maternal DKA will correct the FHR pattern as the fetal pH is normalized. Usually, it is an error to take the DKA patient for an emergency cesarean due to the late decelerations, since the acidosis is correctable, and these individuals are unstable. In this case, the baby is also preterm. The patient could suffer significant complications if rushed for an emergency surgery. Thus, as uncomfortable as it is, careful observation in the face of persistent late decelerations and quickly treating the maternal DKA is the best treatment course.

APPROACH TO:
Diabetes in Pregnancy

DEFINITIONS

ANION GAP: Defined as $Na-(Cl+HCO3)$. An abnormal AG > 12 mEq/L. Possible causes include DKA, uremia, lactic acidosis, ethylene glycol or methanol ingestion, and salicylates.

DIABETIC KETOACIDOSIS: Life-threatening complication of diabetes in pregnancy associated with hyperglycemia and ketoacidosis that requires emergency treatment with insulin and intravenous fluids.

DKA IN PREGNANCY: Serious medical emergency with hyperglycemia, anion gap acidosis, and increased serum ketones. Lab values differ from a nonpregnant patient since the baseline acid base values are different (Table 27–1).

GESTATIONAL DIABETES: Condition of hyperglycemia caused by insulin resistance that occurs during the pregnancy. There are two principal diagnostic criteria for this condition and no consensus about the best approach.

PREGESTATIONAL DIABETES: Condition of hyperglycemia which existed prior to pregnancy, and can be associated with type 1 or type 2 diabetes.

TYPE 1 DIABETES: Condition of absolute insulin deficiency leading to hyperglycemia, usually having its onset in the childhood or teen years.

Table 27–1 • DIAGNOSTIC CRITERIA FOR DKA IN PREGNANCY
pH < 7.35
Blood sugar of 200 mg/dL or greater (rarely can be less)
Serum ketones >5 mEq/L
Often also serum bicarbonate level <18 mEq/L and ketonuria

TYPE 2 DIABETES: Condition of relative insulin deficiency due to insulin resistance leading to hyperglycemia. The absolute insulin levels are often normal or even increased.

WHITE CLASSIFICATION: System of characterizing diabetes in pregnancy using letters (A, B, C, D, F, H, etc) based on duration of disease and presence of end-organ dysfunction.

CLINICAL APPROACH

Diabetes affects approximately eight million women annually and complicates approximately 1% of all pregnancies. Pregestational diabetes accounts for about 10% of cases, and gestational diabetes accounts for 90%. Because pregestational diabetes may cause high blood sugars at conception and during embryo organogenesis, **pregestational diabetes is associated with miscarriage and congenital anomalies.** In contrast, gestational diabetes is due to insulin resistance as a process of the pregnancy, and typically elevated glucose levels are not seen until the second trimester. Thus, gestational diabetics are **not** at risk for congenital anomalies or miscarriage. Additionally, pregestational diabetics are at risk for vascular and renal disease, whereas gestational diabetics do not have the same risk. Pregestational diabetics may be classified as type 1, which is an insulin deficiency (prone to DKA) and type 2 which is an insulin resistant.

Physiologic changes of pregnancy cause insulin resistance resulting in a need to adjust insulin dosing as the pregnancy progresses. (See Table 27–2 for maternal and neonatal complications associated with diabetes in pregnancy.) Additionally,

Table 27–2 • MATERNAL AND NEONATAL COMPLICATIONS OF DIABETES IN PREGNANCY		
	Neonatal	Maternal
All diabetics (gestational and pregestational)	Birth injury NICU admission Hypoglycemia Hyperbilirubinemia Macrosomia Hydramnios Long-term: childhood obesity	Increased risk for cesarean Increased maternal lacerations and injury Preeclampsia Long-term: metabolic syndrome, overt diabetes
Pregestational diabetics	Congenital anomalies Growth restriction Miscarriage Prematurity	Worsening proliferative retinopathy Worsening nephropathy (if moderate/severe preexisting)

DKA is seen more often in the second and third trimesters. There are physiologic mechanisms to ensure the availability of glucose, the primary fuel source for the fetus; these mechanisms also decrease maternal utilization of glucose. The placenta produces **diabetogenic hormones such as growth hormone, corticotrophin-releasing hormone, human placental lactogen (hPL), and progesterone** which create an insulin-resistant state.

PREGESTATIONAL DIABETES

The White classification has been used in the past based on duration of disease and presence of end-organ dysfunction to predict maternal and fetal outcome. Today, this classification has proven to be less useful than categorizing the disease as type 1 (insulin deficiency) and type 2 (insulin resistance), and presence or absence of end-organ disease.

Fetal Risks

Diabetics with suboptimal glycemic control have higher rates of pregnancy loss, birth defects, preterm delivery, disturbances in fetal growth, and stillbirth. **Long-standing diabetes, presence of vascular, hypertensive, or renal disease are particular risk factors for growth restriction.** Fetal monitoring and intermittent ultrasound examinations for fetal growth are warranted. Fetal macrosomia can also be seen with maternal hyperglycemia. The incidence of fetal anomalies is a function of glucose control at conception and organogenesis (up to 8 weeks' gestational age), correlating to the **HbA_{1c} level.**

Maternal Risks

Women with pregestational diabetes often experience hyperglycemia during pregnancy. They are also at increased risk of **chronic hypertension, preeclampsia, diabetic retinopathy, and cesarean delivery.**

Diabetic retinopathy is the leading cause of blindness in reproductive age women. Diabetic retinopathy is often accelerated during pregnancy. Rapid changes in glucose control are associated with worsening retinopathy; for this reason, it is preferred that control be achieved **prior** to pregnancy in a gradual manner. Laser photocoagulation during pregnancy may be necessary.

Renal damage, with minimal preexisting disease, does not appear to be worsened by pregnancy. However, women with **moderate-to-severe preexisting renal damage**, such as creatinine levels exceeding 1.4 mg/dL, microalbuminuria or proteinuria, often will experience a worsening of renal pathology and also develop hypertensive disorders.

Hypertensive disorders, both chronic hypertension and preeclampsia, are major complications of pregnant pregestational diabetics. Frequently, it is the severity of the hypertension that leads to morbidity and subsequent iatrogenic preterm delivery. In other words, the usual scenario necessitating preterm scheduled delivery involves markedly elevated blood pressures, or significant proteinuria. The incidence of preeclampsia increases with the number of risk factors of renal disease and/or retinopathy.

Management

Frequent physician visits are vital to monitor glycemic control. **Fasting targets should be <105 mg/dL and 1-hour postprandial targets <140 mg/dL (or 2-hour postprandial sugars <120 mg/dL).** Those diabetics that are "brittle" and prone to dramatic swings from hyperglycemia to hypoglycemia may benefit from a less strict insulin regimen to avoid life-threatening hypoglycemia. Other monitoring usually includes:

- Ophthalmologic evaluations every trimester and during the postpartum period.
- Detailed anatomy ultrasound and potentially a fetal echocardiogram during the second trimester.
- Fetal surveillance with antenatal testing and serial growth ultrasounds.
- If glycemic control is optimal, in the absence of comorbidities, delivery should occur between 38 and 39 weeks' gestation.
- Women with suboptimal control should be delivered prior to 39 weeks after fetal lung maturity is confirmed.
- Route of delivery should be based on the estimated fetal weight (EFW) by ultrasound and most would agree that **elective cesarean delivery should be considered in diabetics with EFW of >4500 g** due to the potential for shoulder dystocia.

Glycemic control is critically important during labor and delivery. Maternal hyperglycemia can lead to neonatal hypoglycemia after birth. Infants born with neonatal hypoglycemia are more likely to have neurodevelopmental delay. Insulin therapy should be titrated to achieve and maintain glucose levels between 80 and 110 mg/dL.

Preconception Counseling

Preconception counseling can optimize pregnancy outcome as well as maternal well-being. A detailed history and physical examination including baseline laboratory testing should be completed to assess the disease severity. Effective contraception should be offered to delay conception until diabetic control is optimized. A glycosylated hemoglobin level (HbA_{1c}) <7% correlates to neonatal morbidity and mortality rates similar to the general population. In contrast, **those with HbA_{1c} levels >10% experience rates of congenital anomalies (typically cardiac, skeletal dysplasias, and neural tube defects) as high as 20% to 25%. Folate supplementation is extremely important to decrease the risk of NTDs.** Other important tests include: thyroid and renal function, 24-hour urine for protein, and an ophthalmological examination for retinopathy. **ACE inhibitors should be discontinued** prior to conception, since they are associated with teratogenicity.

Diabetic Ketoacidosis (DKA)

DKA is a serious medical emergency associated with a fetal loss rate of up to 25% and maternal mortality rate of about 1%. The **diagnostic criteria are different from that of nonpregnant patients** (see Table 27–1), and the diagnosis is more difficult to reach in pregnant women. Although its prevalence is higher in patients with type 1 diabetes, ketoacidosis may also occur in patients with type 2 diabetes or even with gestational diabetes. DKA occurs more in the second and third trimesters since serum hPL levels are higher. It can occur with **blood glucose levels as low as 200 mg, and should be suspected with an arterial pH of <7.35.**

DKA usually develops as a consequence of absolute or relative insulin deficiency that is accompanied by an increase in counterregulatory hormones (ie, glucagon, cortisol, growth hormone, epinephrine). This type of hormonal imbalance enhances hepatic gluconeogenesis, glycogenolysis, and lipolysis. In pregnancy, several physiological factors predispose to DKA:

- Increased counterregulatory hormones including hPL, progesterone, and cortisol which cause insulin resistance.

- Decreased serum bicarbonate levels to compensate for the primary respiratory alkalosis, which reduces the buffering capacity.

- Increased tendency for ketosis with increased lipolysis and free fatty acids and ketones.

Precipitating factors include emesis, infection, noncompliance or unrecognized new onset of diabetes, and maternal steroid use. Signs and symptoms are similar to those in the nonpregnancy state; however, they also may mimic normal symptoms of pregnancy (Table 27–3). Because of the high risk of morbidity and mortality, and subtle findings, **every diabetic pregnant woman who has vague complaints should be assessed for DKA by checking blood sugar and urine for ketones.**

Aggressive and early resuscitation is the key to effective management of DKA. Fluid replacement should begin with 1 to 2 L of isotonic saline during the first hour followed by 300 to 500 mL/h of normal saline. As glucose levels approach 250 mg/dL, 5% dextrose may be added. Insulin therapy should also be initiated as soon as the diagnosis is made. An appropriate loading dose of regular insulin is 0.2 to 0.4 U/kg regular insulin followed by continuous insulin infusion of 6 to 10 U/h. When glucose levels approach 200 to 250 mg/dL, the insulin infusion rate may be decreased to 1 to 2 U/h.

Electrolyte replacement should be provided as needed. Inevitably, the total body potassium is depleted, even though the serum potassium may be normal or even elevated due to the shifting of potassium extracellularly as the excess hydrogen ions move intracellularly. If serum potassium is elevated, potassium replacement should be provided at 20 mEq/h after urine output is established. If serum potassium is below normal, replacement should be initiated immediately at the above rate. Serum magnesium and phosphorus levels should be evaluated and provided as needed.

Table 27–3 • SYMPTOMS AND SIGNS OF DKA IN PREGNANCY

General: Malaise, weight loss
CNS: Headache, confusion, or lethargy
Volume: Dehydration, excessive thirst, dry mouth
GI: Abdominal pain, nausea, and vomiting
Renal: Polyuria/polydipsia, oliguria
Metabolic: Shortness of breath

The fetal heart rate pattern will often exhibit loss of variability and late decelerations due to the maternal acidosis. This will almost always correct with resolution of the DKA. **Delivery of the fetus for heart rate abnormalities should not be performed unless the abnormalities are persistent even after maternal stabilization.**

GESTATIONAL DIABETES

Diagnosis

There has been much debate about whether diabetic screening should be selective or universal, and which screening test to use. Selective screening based on risk factors would reduce the number of women requiring screening by 10% to 15%, however, it would fail to identify one-third to one-half of affected individuals. For this reason, the American College of Obstetrics and Gynecology (ACOG) supports universal screening in all persons except those deemed to be at low risk. Many practitioners perform early screening at 16 weeks' gestation for those at high risk for diabetes, and repeated at 26 weeks. **Routine screening is usually performed at 26 to 28 weeks' gestation.**

Traditional diagnostic strategy (two steps): A two-step approach has been recommended in order to identify women with GDM. The first step involves a 50-g 1-hour screening test, and the second step utilizes a 100-g 3-hour diagnostic test for those women identified via the initial screening test. The threshold for an abnormal 1-hour test varies from 130 to 140 mg/dL depending on the practice's philosophy of false positive and false negatives. The diagnosis of gestational diabetes depends on noting two abnormal values on the 100-g 3-hour test with variations on the cutoffs. Common thresholds are as follows:

- Fasting: 95 to 105 mg/dL
- 1 hour: 180 to 190 mg/dL
- 2 hours: 155 to 165 mg/dL
- 3 hours: 140 to 145 mg/dL

IADPSG diagnostic strategy (one step): The new International Association of Diabetes in Pregnancy Study Group (IADPSG) supports the use of a **2-hour 75-g** diagnostic test utilizing values concurrent with fasting, 1- and 2-hour values. A positive result requires at least two abnormal values (Table 27–4). The American

Table 27–4 • DIAGNOSTIC CRITERIA FOR GESTATIONAL DIABETES		
	Traditional 3-h 100-g GTT (mg/dL)	International Association of Diabetes in Pregnancy Study Groups (IADPSG) 2-h 75-g GTT (mg/dL)
Fasting	95-105	92
1 h	180-190	180
2 h	155-165	153
3 h	140-145	

Diabetes Association recognizes this as an acceptable option although at this time, the 100-g test is generally used in the United States. In 2008, the **hyperglycemia and adverse pregnancy outcome (HAPO)** trial published its findings of maternal and fetal implications of maternal hyperglycemia less than that which is diagnostic for diabetes. The HAPO trial utilized a one-step diagnostic process with a 75-g 2-hour test. They found a linear relationship between maternal glucose levels and adverse outcomes, even at glucose concentrations below those that are usually diagnostic of GDM. The results of this study are likely to alter not only classification criteria for GDM but are also likely to modify treatment modalities.

Those who have not adopted the IADPSG diagnostic strategy claim that up to 13% to 15% of pregnant women would be diagnosed with diabetes using the 2-hour 75-g test, and that there are not yet **prospective** randomly controlled trials to show that using this new criterion leads to improved outcomes.

Risk factors for GDM for developing gestational diabetes including age >25 years, belonging to an ethnic group with an increased risk for the development of type 2 diabetes, obesity, and prior macrosomic infant.

Treatment options: Diet is the first line of therapy for GDM. For those patients who fail dietary treatment, insulin is the gold standard for diabetes therapy, although the use of glyburide, an oral hypoglycemic agent, has been found to be effective in select patients. Targets for glucose control include fasting glucose of 90 to 105 mg/dL and 1-hour postprandial glucose of <140 mg/dL. Potential maternal and fetal complications are summarized in Table 27–2.

Postpartum management: All women diagnosed with GDM should be screened for overt diabetes mellitus using a **75-g oral glucose tolerance test at 6 weeks' postpartum**. Fasting glucose levels >126 mg/dL or 2-hour values >200 mg/dL are diagnostic for diabetes mellitus. Contraception options are very important to consider in this population as we know that recurrent pregnancies in a woman with GDM increases her risk for overt diabetes mellitus (see Case 44).

Breast-feeding should be encouraged for both infant and maternal benefits. Breast-feeding is associated with a greater decrease in maternal weight, which may reduce their risk of developing type 2 diabetes. It may also decrease the risk of childhood obesity and the development of diabetes mellitus compared to formula-fed infants.

Controversies

- Oral hypoglycemic medications in pregnancy are being used with some success. More research needs to be performed to understand its exact role.
- Patients in whom the estimated fetal weight exceeds 4500 g should be offered cesarean delivery in order to decrease risk of traumatic delivery.
- Carpenter and Coustan diagnostic criteria for the 3-hour 100-g OGTT are recommended by the Fourth and Fifth International Workshop-Conference of GDM and endorsed by ACOG; however, these expert bodies recognize that the 2-hour 75-g diagnostic criteria tests are acceptable.
- Further data in pregnancy are needed before the use of metformin for the treatment of GDM can be recommended.

CASE CORRELATION

- See also Case 4 (Shoulder Dystocia) to review the two main risk factors for shoulder dystocia (macrosomia and diabetes), Case 19 (Parvovirus Infection in Pregnancy) since diabetes and parvovirus are two causes of hydramnios, and Case 22 (IUGR) (pregestational diabetes is a cause for IUGR).

COMPREHENSION QUESTIONS

27.1 A 36-year-old G2P1001 woman presents for her initial prenatal visit at 6 weeks' gestation. She has a 9-year history of type 2 diabetes mellitus which is managed with oral hypoglycemic medications. Which of the following is the best indicator for fetal outcome of the pregnancy?

A. Blood sugar value in the office
B. Hemoglobin A_{1c} value
C. Nuchal translucency on ultrasound
D. Umbilical artery Doppler studies at 18 weeks' gestation

27.2 A 32-year-old G3P2002 female presents for her postpartum visit. Her obstetrical history is significant for GDM with her last pregnancy only ending in a term delivery of a 7 lb (3 kg) infant, 8 weeks ago. Her body mass index (BMI) is 24 kg/m². Besides the routine examination and Pap smear, what is your next step regarding this patient?

A. Recommend fasting glucose and HbA_{1c} every 3 years
B. Recommend 3-hour 100-g GTT if she has a first-degree relative with DM
C. Recommend 2-hour 75-g GTT at this time
D. No intervention due to her optimal BMI

27.3 A 21-year-old G1P0 woman at 11 weeks' gestation is seen in the emergency center complaining of nausea, vomiting, abdominal pain, and fatigue. The patient is a known diabetic since age 12 years and has been in good control. On examination, her BP is 90/60 mm Hg, HR 120 beats per minute, and RR 28 per minute. The arterial blood gas reveals a pH of 7.28, pO_2 of 100 mm Hg, pCO_2 of 22 mm Hg, and bicarbonate level of 12 mEq/L. Which of the following is the best management of this patient?

A. Administer 2 L of normal saline intravenously
B. Infuse two ampules of bicarbonate IV
C. Obtain a spiral computed tomography scan to assess for pulmonary embolism
D. Obtain an ultrasound for a possible concealed abruption

27.4 A 31-year-old woman is diagnosed with gestational diabetes based on two abnormal values on a 3-hour 100-g GTT. She is at 28 weeks' gestation. The patient is concerned about the risks of congenital anomalies after she has read about the adverse effects of diabetes on the Internet. What is your response to this patient?
   A. Your risk of fetal congenital anomalies is essentially the same as the general population since this is GDM.
   B. We can draw an HbA_{1c} test at this time, and your risk of fetal anomalies depends on the HbA_{1c} result.
   C. Tight glucose control from this point onward and during labor and delivery will determine the risk of congenital anomalies.
   D. The majority of GDMs had normal glucose levels at conception and no increased risk of fetal anomalies.

ANSWERS

27.1 **B.** The hemoglobin A_{1c} value correlates with the risk of fetal anomalies and fetal morbidity. An optimal HbA_{1c} is <7% and the fetal risks approach the general population with this value. In contrast, an HbA_{1c} of 11% corresponds to a risk of fetal anomalies as high as 25%. Nuchal translucency is one factor used to identify an increased risk of Down syndrome. Umbilical Dopplers are used in the evaluation of IUGR and fetal anemia.

27.2 **C.** All women with gestational DM should have a screening test at 6 weeks' postpartum for overt diabetes. The 2-hour 75-g GTT test is probably the optimal test for these individuals.

27.3 **A.** This patient likely has diabetic ketoacidosis. Pregnancy will often cause diabetes to become more difficult to control. The pH is acidotic, whereas the normal pH in pregnancy is slightly alkalotic. Together with the low bicarbonate level, this is consistent with an anion gap metabolic acidosis. The patient's oxygenation is good, and thus, a pulmonary embolus is not suspected. The pCO_2 is lower than the normal 28 mm Hg seen in pregnancy, which is indicative of partial respiratory compensation. The blood sugar is likely to be elevated. The cornerstones of management of DKA include IV fluid hydration, insulin intravenous drip to control the blood sugars and correct the acidosis, correction of metabolic abnormalities such as hypokalemia, hypophosphatemia, or hypomagnesemia, and addressing the etiological factor.

27.4 **D.** The vast majority of those patients with gestational diabetes are true **gestational** diabetics, and their glucose levels at conception and at organogenesis were normal; this means the risk of congenital anomalies were the same as the general population. However, a small fraction of the "so-called GDM" were type 2 pregestational diabetics who were not detected. In this setting, there could have been hyperglycemia at conception.

CLINICAL PEARLS

▶ Diabetic retinopathy or nephropathy may worsen during pregnancy and regular monitoring is warranted.

▶ Preeclampsia rates may be as high as 50% in some diabetic gravidas.

▶ HbA_{1c} levels <7% prior to conception is associated with neonatal morbidity and congenital anomaly rates are comparable to the general population.

▶ HbA_{1c} levels >10% prior to conception are associated with neonatal morbidity rates as high as 25%.

▶ The most common congenital anomalies associated with pregestational diabetes are cardiac and neural tube defects.

▶ DKA occurs more rapidly and at lower serum glucose levels during pregnancy compared to outside of pregnancy. Different DKA diagnostic criteria are used for pregnant women.

▶ Neonatal hypoglycemia can occur especially with maternal hyperglycemia during labor and delivery. Thus, tight control of maternal glucose during labor is crucial.

▶ Risks factors for GDM include maternal obesity, family history, polycystic ovarian syndrome, previous gestational diabetes, fetal macrosomia or unexplained fetal or neonatal demise.

▶ There is debate about the best diagnostic criteria for diagnosing GDM.

▶ All women with GDM should be screened for overt diabetes at 6 weeks' postpartum.

▶ Glyburide is considered a safe alternative to insulin for treatment of GDM.

▶ Most patients with GDM can be managed with diet alone, and when diet is inadequate, then insulin or oral therapy is used.

REFERENCES

ACOG Practice Bulletin. Gestational diabetes: clinical management guidelines for obstetrician-gynecologists. Number 137; 2013 (level III).

ACOG Practice Bulletin. Clinical management guidelines for obstetrician-gynecologists. Number 60, March 2005. Pregestational diabetes mellitus. *Obstet Gynecol.* 2005;105:675-685. (Reaffirmed 2014.)

Coustan DR. Pharmacological management of gestational diabetes: an overview. *Diabetes Care.* 2007;30(Suppl 2):S206-S208 (level III).

Diagnosis and classification of diabetes mellitus. *Diabetes Care.* 2006;29(Suppl 1):S43-S48.

Hollander MH, Paarlberg KM, Huisjes AJ. Gestational diabetes: a review of the current literature and guidelines. *Obstet Gynecol Surv.* 2007;62(2):125-136 (level III).

Kinsley B. Achieving better outcomes in pregnancies complicated by type 1 and type 2 diabetes mellitus. *Clin Ther*. 2007;29(Suppl D):S153-S160.

Langer O, Conway DL, Berkus MD, Xenakis EM, Gonzales O. A comparison of glyburide and insulin in women with gestational diabetes mellitus. *N Engl J Med*. 2000;343:1134-1138.

McFarland MB, Langer O, Conway DL, Berkus MD. Dietary therapy for gestational diabetes: how long is enough? *Obstet Gynecol*. 1999;93(6):978-982 (level II-2).

Metzger BE, Buchanan TA, Coustan DR, de Leiva A, et al. Summary and recommendations of the Fifth International Workshop-Conference on Gestational Diabetes Mellitus. *Diabetes Care*. 2007;30(Suppl 2):S251-S260 (level III).

Metzger BE, Lowe LP, Dyer AR, et al. Hyperglycemia and adverse pregnancy outcomes. *N Engl J Med*. 2008;358(19):1991-2002 (level I).

Moore TRCP. Diabetes in pregnancy. In: Creasy RK RR, Iams JD, Lockwood CJ, Moore TR, eds. *Creasy and Resnik's Maternal-Fetal Medicine, Principles and Practice*. Philadelphia, PA: Saunders Elsevier; 2009.

Nicholson W, Bolen S, Witkop CT, et al. Benefits and risks of oral diabetes agents compared with insulin in women with gestational diabetes: a systematic review. *Obstet Gynecol*. 2009;113(1):193-205 (level III).

Rosenn B, Miodovnik M, Kranias G, et al. Progression of diabetic retinopathy in pregnancy: association with hypertension in pregnancy. *Am J Obstet Gynecol*. 1992;166:1214-1218.

Rowan JA, Hague WM, Gao W, Battin MR, Moore MP. Metformin versus insulin for the treatment of gestational diabetes. *N Engl J Med*. 2008;358:2003-2015.

Wong SF, Lee-Tannock A, Amaraddio D, et al. Growth patterns in fetuses of women with pregestational diabetes mellitus. *Ultrasound Obstet Gynecol*. 2006;28:934-938.

CASE 28

A 35-year-old G2P1001 woman is seen for her first prenatal visit. Based on her last menstrual period, she is at 15 weeks' gestation. She has no complaints and has no significant medical history. She denies dysuria or urinary urgency. Her surgical history is remarkable only for "ear tubes" as a child. Her last delivery was a vaginal delivery and was uncomplicated. She has had Pap smears each year which to her memory "have been normal." On examination, she is a well-appearing white female in no distress. Her blood pressure is 100/65 mm Hg, heart rate is 90 beats per minute (bpm), respiratory rate is 12 breaths per minute, temperature is 98°F (36.6°C), and weight is 130 lb. Her general physical examination is normal. The breasts are nontender and without masses or skin changes. The heart reveals II/VI systolic ejection murmur. The lungs are clear. Her abdomen is nontender and her fundal height is at the level of the umbilicus. Fetal heart tones are 140 bpm. The pelvic examination reveals a normal external genitalia, normal-appearing vagina and cervix. The bimanual examination shows adequate pelvimetry, and nontender uterus without adnexal or other masses. The cervix is normal in consistency and without masses. Her extremities are without edema. Prenatal laboratories are obtained and reveal the following:

CBC: Hgb 10.0 g/dL, MCV 82 fLPlt, 150 000/mm^3, WBC 8000/mm^3

Rubella: nonimmune

Hepatitis B surface antigen: positive

Blood type: O, Rh-negative

Indirect Coombs (antibody screen): negative

HIV ELISA: negative

UC&S: 10 000 cfu/mL of group B streptococcus

RPR: negative

Pap smear: ASC-US

Gonorrhea assay: negative

Chlamydia assay: negative

▶ What items should be listed on the problem list?
▶ What is your next step for the problems listed?
▶ What other testing should be recommended to the patient?

ANSWERS TO CASE 28:
Prenatal Care

Summary: A 35-year-old G2P1001 white female at 15 weeks' gestation whose prior delivery was normal. Her fundal height is at the umbilicus. Fetal heart tones are 140 bpm. Prenatal laboratory results indicate a hemoglobin level of 10.0 g/dL with MCV 82 fL; hepatitis surface antigen positive; Rh-negative blood type, negative indirect Coombs; urine culture revealing 10 000 cfu/mL of group B streptococcus; and a Pap smear showing ASC-US.

- **Problem list:**

    1. Advanced maternal age (AMA)—age 35 or greater at estimated time of delivery.
    2. Size greater than dates (fundal height at umbilicus corresponds to 20 weeks).
    3. Mild microcytic anemia (Hgb < 10.5).
    4. Hepatitis B surface antigen (HBsAg) positive.
    5. Rh-negative blood type with negative indirect Coombs.
    6. Urine culture with GBS 10 000 cfu/mL, asymptomatic.
    7. Pap smear showing atypical squamous cells of undetermined significance (ASC-US).
    8. Rubella nonimmune.

- **Next steps:**

    1. AMA—genetic counseling and discuss invasive testing (amniocentesis) versus noninvasive prenatal testing.
    2. Size/dates—fetal ultrasound to assess gestational age, multiple gestation, or cell-free fetal DNA testing (see Case 7).
    3. Anemia—therapeutic trial of iron.
    4. HBsAg positive—check liver function tests and hepatitis B serology to assess for active hepatitis versus chronic carrier status.
    5. Rh-negative with indirect Coombs negative—RhoGAM at 28 weeks and at delivery if the baby proves to be Rh-positive.
    6. Urine culture with GBS—treat with ampicillin and reculture urine, penicillin IV prophylaxis in labor.
    7. Pap smear ASC-US—observe and repeat Pap smear postpartum.
    8. Rubella status—vaccinate postpartum.

- **Other testing:** Cystic fibrosis screening; consider early diabetic screen.

ANALYSIS

Objectives

1. Describe the routine prenatal care and the key screening strategies.
2. Be able to understand the principle of developing a problem list and its importance.
3. Be able to describe the "next steps" with any abnormal finding and know its significance.

Considerations

This is a 35-year-old woman who is seen for her first prenatal visit. Since pregnancy and delivery is a normal physiological process, the purpose of the prenatal care is to educate and build rapport with the patient and family, establish gestational age, screen for possible conditions that may impact maternal or fetal health, and monitor the progress of the pregnancy. During the first visit, a fairly extensive process is used to screen for at-risk conditions using a detailed history, general physical examination, and laboratory panel. This patient has a variety of conditions that need addressing. The best way to ensure that each issue is dealt with in a systematic manner and until resolution is to use a "problem list." Thus, numerous issues are written into the problem list, and investigation is performed until resolution of the problem. An understanding of the strategy and approach to addressing each issue is fundamental to the care of patients. Likewise, an understanding of the physiologic changes of pregnancy allows for interpretation of physical examination findings and impact of various diseases (see Table 28–1).

Table 28–1 • PHYSIOLOGICAL CHANGES IN PREGNANCY

	Parameter			Comment
Cardiovascular	Cardiac output and plasma volume increased 50%	Systemic vascular resistance decreased	Mean arterial pressure unchanged/slightly lower	Pregnancy increases intravascular volume
Respiratory	Respiratory rate unchanged	Tidal volume increased	Minute ventilation increased	Ventilation exceeds needs
Arterial blood gas	pH 7.45 (increased)	PCO_2 28 (decreased)	HCO_3 18 (decreased)	Primary respiratory alkalosis and partial metabolic compensation
Renal	GFR—increased 50%	Serum Cr decreased	Ureteral caliper dilated	GFR increased and creatinine clearance also increased
Hematologic	Hemoglobin decreased slightly	Platelet decreased slightly	Leukocyte count slightly increased	Physiologic anemia due to plasma volume increased more than red blood cell mass
Gastrointestinal	Delayed stomach emptying	Decreased lower esophageal sphincter tone	Decreased gut motility	

For instance, this 35-year-old patient has an early systolic ejection murmur, very common in pregnancy due to the increased cardiac output. A diastolic murmur, however, would be abnormal. Although the American College of Obstetricians and Gynecologists recommends counseling to every pregnant patient about cystic fibrosis screening; Caucasian patients are at particular risk with gene frequency being about 1 in 40. Also for women over the age of 30, some practitioners will perform a glucose screen for gestational diabetes early (eg, 18 weeks), and if negative, then again at the time of universal screening, 26 to 28 weeks' gestation.

APPROACH TO:
Prenatal Care

DEFINITIONS

ADVANCED MATERNAL AGE: Pregnant woman who will be 35 years or beyond at the estimated date of delivery.

ISOIMMUNIZATION: The development of specific antibodies as a result of antigenic stimulation by material from the red blood cells of another individual. For example, Rh isoimmunization means an Rh-negative woman who develops anti-D (Rh factor) antibodies in response to exposure to Rh (D) antigen.

ASYMPTOMATIC BACTERIURIA: Urine culture of 100 000 cfu/mL or more of a pure pathogen of a midstream-voided specimen.

GENETIC COUNSELING: An educational process provided by a health-care professional for individuals and families who have a genetic disease or who are at risk for such a disease. It is designed to provide patients and their families with information about their condition or potential condition and help them make informed decisions.

VERTICAL TRANSMISSION: The passage of infection from mother to fetus, whether in utero, during labor and delivery, or postpartum.

ANTENATAL TESTING: A procedure that attempts to identify whether the fetus is at risk for uteroplacental insufficiency and perinatal death. Some of these tests include nonstress test and biophysical profile.

BASIC OBSTETRICAL ULTRASOUND: Sonographic examination focused on fetal biometry (dating and fetal weight), number of fetuses, fetal presentation, placental location, amniotic fluid volume, and limited fetal anatomical survey.

COMPREHENSIVE (OR TARGETED) ULTRASOUND: Detailed anatomical evaluation to assess a suspected structural anomaly.

CLINICAL APPROACH

Physiological Changes

Pregnancy is associated with numerous physiological changes. An understanding of these changes is critical in the interpretation of laboratory tests, or a rational awareness of how disease processes may impact the pregnant patient. Some "seemingly abnormal" findings will be normal in pregnancy such as glycosuria due to the increased glomerular filtration rate delivering more glucose to the kidneys. Other findings in pregnancy will appear to be normal, but are "worrisome" in pregnancy; for instance, when the PCO_2 level is 40 mm Hg (normal for nonpregnant), it indicates significant CO_2 retention and possibly impending respiratory failure.

Dating

The priorities of prenatal care includes establishment of gestational age since all of the monitoring, assessments, and milestones are based on gestational age. History of the LMP, regularity of menses, medication use that may affect ovulation, physical examination, and early ultrasound help this determination. On examination, the fundal height in centimeters corresponds to the gestational age from 20 to 34 weeks. An ultrasound will be obtained when there is a discrepancy of 3 cm or more.

Prevention

Much of prenatal care involves educating the patient, screening for diseases or unsafe conditions (intimate partner violence), and preventive measures. Use of immunizations (influenza and RhoGAM), prenatal vitamin with folate, iron supplementation, and a balanced diet are recommended.

Screening for Conditions of Risk

Much of the time spent in caring for the pregnant patient is involved in trying to identify high-risk conditions and taking the proper steps to reduce the risk, or minimize complications (see Table 28–2).

Because both maternal and fetal health are being considered, any high-risk condition must be balanced from both perspectives. Many of the cases involve antepartum, intrapartum, or postpartum complications (see Table 28–3).

Table 28-2 • SUMMARY OF PRENATAL LABORATORIES, RAMIFICATIONS, AND EVALUATION

Lab Test	Finding	Ramifications	Next Step	Comments
Hemoglobin	<10.5 g/dL	Preterm delivery, low fetal iron stores, identify thalassemia	Mild therapeutic trial of iron, moderate ferritin and Hb electrophoresis	
Rubella	Negative	Nonimmune to rubella	Stay away from sick individuals, vaccinate postpartum	Live-attenuated vaccine
Blood type	Any type	May help pediatricians identify ABO incompatibility		
Rh factor	Negative	May be susceptible to Rh disease	If antibody screen negative, give RhoGAM at 28 wk, and if baby is Rh-positive, then also after delivery	
Antibody screen	Positive	May indicate isoimmunization	Need to identify the antibody, and then titer	Lewis lives, Kell kills, Duffy dies
HIV ELISA (or Fourth Generation Ag/Ab test)	Positive	May indicate infection with HIV	Western blot or PCR, if positive then place patient on anti-HIV medicines, offer elective cesarean, or IV ZDV in labor	Intervention reduces vertical transmission from 25% to 2%
RPR or VDRL	Positive	May indicate syphilis	Specific antibody such as MHA-TP, and if positive, then stage disease	Less than 1 yr, penicillin × 1; >1 year or unknown, penicillin IM each week × 3
Gonorrhea	Positive	May cause preterm labor, blindness	Ceftriaxone IM	
Chlamydia	Positive	May cause neonatal blindness, pneumonia	Azithromycin or amoxicillin orally	
Hepatitis B surface antigen	Positive	Patient is infectious	Check LFTs and hepatitis serology to determine if chronic carrier vs active hepatitis	Baby needs HBIG and hepatitis B vaccine

Urine culture	Positive	Asymptomatic bacteriuria may lead to pyelonephritis 25%	Treat with antibiotic and recheck urine culture	If GBS is organism, then give penicillin in labor
Pap smear	Positive	Only invasive cancer would alter management	ASC-US = re-Pap postpartum; LGSIL, HSIL = colposcopy	Reflexive HPV not recommended with ASC-US
Nuchal translucency (11-13 wk)	Positive	May indicate trisomy	Offer karyotype and follow-up ultrasounds	Increased NT means increased risk, not definitive diagnosis
Trisomy screen (16-20 wk)	Positive	At risk for trisomy or NTD	Basic ultrasound for dates; if dates confirmed, offer genetic amniocentesis	Most common reason for abnormal serum screening—wrong dates
1-h diabetic screen (26-28 wk)	Positive (elevated)	May indicate gestational diabetes	Go to 3-h GTT	About 15% of those screened will be positive
3-h glucose tolerance test	2 abnormal values	Gestational diabetes	Try ADA diet, monitor blood sugars, if elevated may need meds or insulin	About 15% of abnormal 1-h GCT will have gestational diabetes
GBS culture (35-37 wk)	Positive	GBS colonizing genital tract	Penicillin during labor	Helps to prevent early GBS sepsis of newborn

Table 28-3 • ANTENATAL, INTRAPARTUM, AND POSTPARTUM CASE CORRELATION

Pregnancy Phase	Condition	Diagnosis	Case Number
PRENATAL			
	Normal	Routine prenatal care	28
	Vaginal bleeding <20 wk gestation	Threatened and spontaneous abortion, ectopic pregnancy, septic abortion	42, 43, 45
	Vaginal bleeding >20 wk' gestation	Placenta previa, placenta abruption	10, 11
	Serum screening	Congenital anomalies	7
	Multiple gestations	Twin gestation	8
	Anemia in pregnancy	Thalassemia	2
	Abdominal pain in pregnancy	Torsion of ovary, ruptured corpus luteum	13
	Hypertensive disease	Preeclampsia	16
	Pruritus	Cholestasis of pregnancy	14
	Thromboembolism	DVT in pregnancy, pulmonary embolism	15
	Thyroid disease	Hyperthyroidism in pregnancy	21
	Infectious	Chlamydia and HIV in pregnancy, pyelonephritis, Parvovirus	20, 23, 19
INTRAPARTUM			
	Labor	Normal and abnormal	1
	Fetal heart rate	Fetal bradycardia	5
	Preterm birth	Preterm labor	17
	Infection	Intra-amniotic infection, HSV in labor	18, 9
DELIVERY			
	Complications of delivery	Shoulder dystocia	4
	Hemorrhage	Placenta accreta, postpartum hemorrhage (also under "postpartum")	12, 6
POSTPARTUM			
	Infection	Breast abscess, endometritis	26, 25
	Hemorrhage	Postpartum hemorrhage (also under delivery)	6

COMPREHENSION QUESTIONS

28.1 A 24-year-old woman G2P0010 had a pregnancy complicated by abruptio placentae leading to fetal death at 38 weeks' gestation. There was no etiology found after a diligent search. Which of the following statements is most accurate regarding this pregnancy?
   A. With no etiology found, the risk of abruption in this current pregnancy is the same as any other pregnant patient.
   B. Antenatal testing with biophysical profile should be considered starting at 34 to 35 weeks' gestation.
   C. Induction of labor should be considered at 37 to 38 weeks' gestation.
   D. Weekly ultrasound examinations screening for retroplacental hemorrhage should be considered starting at 32 weeks' gestation.

28.2 A 27-year-old G0P0 woman is contemplating becoming pregnant. In preparation, her obstetrician conducts a preconception counseling session, assesses rubella status, and prescribes supplemental folate. Which of the following is the best explanation of the purpose of the supplemental folate?
   A. Avoidance of megaloblastic anemia
   B. Decreasing fetal anomalies
   C. Enhancing absorption of iron
   D. Increasing maternal immune function

28.3 A 32-year-old G1P0 woman at 15 weeks' gestation is a physiologist, and is questioning the physician about the adaptations that occur in pregnancy. Which of the following statements is most accurate regarding the changes in pregnancy?
   A. Cardiac output is largely the same as the nonpregnant woman.
   B. The plasma volume is increased by about 50%.
   C. The systemic vascular resistance of a pregnant woman is slightly increased as compared to the nonpregnant woman.
   D. The pregnant woman typically has a short diastolic murmur which is physiologic.

28.4 A 29-year-old G1P0 woman at 18 weeks' gestation is noted to have a blood type of O, Rh-positive. Her antibody screen (indirect Coombs) is positive. Identification of the antibody is anti-Lewis. Which of the following is the most accurate statement regarding this patient?
   A. This fetus is at significant risk for fetal erythroblastosis if she/he is Lewis-positive.
   B. The father of the baby's Lewis antigen status should be evaluated.
   C. Ultrasound for fetal hydrops should be performed.
   D. Further testing is not indicated in this patient.

28.5 A 31-year-old G1P0 woman at 15 weeks' gestation is noted to have a positive hepatitis B surface antigen. Which of the following would most significantly increase the risk of vertical transmission?

A. Presence of positive hepatitis E antigen
B. Presence of positive antihepatitis B surface antibody
C. Presence of positive antihepatitis B core antibody
D. Presence of elevated liver function tests

28.6 A 31-year-old G2 P1001 woman is at 30 weeks' gestation and her obstetrician recommends that she receives the TdaP vaccine. The physician explains that this is to help prevent neonatal pertussis. The patient states that she received the vaccine after delivery of her first baby. Which of the following is the best next step?

A. If the patient received the TdaP vaccine within the last 5 years, no vaccine is needed.
B. If the patient received the TdaP vaccine at any time in her adult life, no vaccine is needed.
C. The vaccine should not be administered until postpartum.
D. The vaccine should be given regardless of whether has previously been given.

ANSWERS

28.1 **C.** A history of abruption that is unexplained confers an increased risk of abruption with subsequent pregnancies. Antenatal testing does not predict acute events such as abruption. Rather, fetal testing such as biophysical profile is designed to identify chronic uteroplacental insufficiency such as caused by chronic hypertension, renal insufficiency, or maternal lupus. Ultrasound has poor ability to identify retroplacental clots or abruption. Induction at or slightly before the time of abruption with the fetal loss, if at term, is a reasonable approach to avoid repeat abruption.

28.2 **B.** The main purpose of the supplemental folate prior to pregnancy is to help reduce fetal neural tube defects (NTDs). These conditions include anencephaly, a fatal anomaly where there are no cerebral hemispheres or fetal skull, or spina bifida which often leads to debilitation and inability to control bowel or bladder. Because the neural tube closes at 21 to 28 days embryonic age (5-6 weeks' gestational age), by the time the patient realizes she is pregnant, the "die is cast" regarding the neural tube. Folate supplementation reduces the risk of neural tube defects by 50%; thus, every woman in the reproductive age should take sufficient folate to reduce the risk of fetal NTDs.

28.3 **B.** In pregnancy, the plasma volume is increased by about 50%. The cardiac output likewise increases by 50%, as does the glomerular filtration rate. Both the stroke volume and heart rate increase to account for this elevated CO. The mean arterial pressure is unchanged to slightly decreased, meaning that the systemic vascular resistance is markedly decreased as compared to the nonpregnant patient. An early systolic ejection murmur is physiologic, whereas a diastolic murmur usually indicates a pathological etiology.

28.4 **D.** No further testing is indicated in this patient, because anti-Lewis antibodies do not cause hemolytic disease of the newborn. This is because Lewis antibodies are IgM and do not cross the placenta, whereas anti-D (Rh) are IgG. Other worrisome antibodies include anti-Kell and anti-Duffy. "Lewis lives, Kell kills, Duffy dies." This highlights the need to identify the antibody when the indirect Coombs (antibody screen) is positive. When a worrisome antibody is identified, the titer should be evaluated to assess the potential severity of the isoimmunization potential. In general, fetal risk is not great unless the titer is 1:8 or higher.

28.5 **A.** This patient has a positive hepatitis B surface antigen, meaning that the patient has been infected with hepatitis B virus and currently still infectious (virus actively replicating). Liver function tests would indicate whether this is a chronic carrier status (normal LFT) versus active hepatitis (elevated LFT). The hepatitis antibodies also will give a clue regarding acute versus chronic hepatitis. The presence of hepatitis Be antigen markedly increases the transmission. Regardless of whether E antigen is present, this baby when born should receive hepatitis B immune globulin to protect against immediate exposure, and then the active hepatitis B vaccine for lifelong immunity. Hepatitis B infections to the neonate often lead to cirrhosis and hepatocellular carcinoma.

28.6 **D.** The TdaP vaccine is a killed vaccine and is safe in pregnancy. It should be given between 28 and 36 weeks' gestation regardless of whether it has been given in prior pregnancies. The reason is so that the patient will augment an IgG antibody response, which will result in passive transmission to the fetus. This is the mechanism for reducing the risk of neonatal pertussis. Other adults who will be near the newborn such as spouses, grandparents, older siblings, or babysitters should also be vaccinated to reduce the risk of their acquisition of pertussis.

CLINICAL PEARLS

▶ Pregnancy and delivery is a normal physiological process. The objective of prenatal care is to educate the patient, prevent complications, and screen for significant conditions that can affect maternal or fetal health.

▶ Assessment of a pregnant woman depends on knowledge of the physiologic changes in pregnancy.

▶ Human immunodeficiency virus (HIV), hepatitis B, and syphilis are three infectious diseases in which intervention can dramatically impact neonatal well being.

▶ Identification and treatment of asymptomatic bacteriuria markedly decreases the risk of pyelonephritis in pregnancy.

▶ The main objective in assessing for cervical dysplasia/neoplasia is to identify invasive cervical cancer since that finding would change the management in pregnancy and treatment of other lesser findings would be deferred until after pregnancy.

▶ Advanced maternal age is defined as age of 35 or greater at the estimated date of delivery. These women are at increased risk for autosomal trisomies, and genetic counseling and genetic amniocentesis are usually offered.

▶ Screening for hypertension and proteinuria by semiquantitative urine dipstick at each prenatal visit is performed to screen for gestational hypertension or preeclampsia.

▶ Antepartum fetal testing is defined as a procedure that attempts to identify whether the fetus is at risk for uteroplacental insufficiency and perinatal death. Some of these tests include nonstress test and biophysical profile.

▶ Live-attenuated vaccines should be avoided in pregnancy, but killed vaccines are acceptable, and some, such as influenza vaccine, are indicated in pregnancy.

REFERENCES

Cunningham FG, Leveno KJ, Bloom SL, Hauth JC, Gilstrap LC III, Wenstrom KD. Prenatal care. In: *Williams Obstetrics*. 24th ed. New York, NY: McGraw-Hill; 2014:201-230.

Lu MC, Williams III, J, Hobel CJ. Antepartum care: preconception and prenatal care, genetic evaluation and teratology, and antenatal fetal assessment. In: Hacker NF, Gambone JC, Hobel CJ, eds. *Essentials of Obstetrics and Gynecology*. 5th ed. Philadelphia, PA: Saunders; 2009:71-90.

CASE 29

A 66-year-old woman comes in for a routine physical examination. Her menopause occurred at age 51 years, and she is currently taking an estrogen pill along with a progestin pill each day. The past medical history is unremarkable. Her family history includes one maternal cousin with ovarian cancer. On examination, she is found to have a blood pressure of 120/70 mm Hg, a heart rate of 70 beats per minute, and a temperature of 98°F (36.6°C). She weighs 140 lb and is 5 feet 4 in tall. The thyroid is normal to palpation. Examination of her breasts reveals no masses or discharge. The abdominal, cardiac, and lung evaluations are within normal limits. The pelvic examination shows a normal, multiparous cervix, a normal-sized uterus, and no adnexal masses. She had undergone mammography 3 months previously.

▶ What is your next step?
▶ What would be the most common cause of mortality for this patient?

ANSWERS TO CASE 29:
Health Maintenance, Age 66 Years

Summary: A 66-year-old woman comes for health maintenance. A mammogram has been performed 3 months previously.

- **Next step:** Each of the following should be performed: Calculate the body mass index, send stool for occult blood, colonoscopy, pneumococcal vaccine, influenza vaccine, tetanus and diphtheria vaccines (if not performed within the past 10 years), herpes zoster vaccine, lipid profile, fasting blood glucose, thyroid function tests, bone mineral density screening, and urinalysis.
- **Most common cause of mortality:** Cardiovascular disease.

ANALYSIS
Objectives

1. Understand which health maintenance studies should be performed for a 66-year-old woman.
2. Know the most common cause of mortality for a woman in this age group.
3. Understand that preventive maintenance consists of cancer screening, immunizations, and screening for common diseases.

Considerations

The approach to health maintenance includes three parts: (1) cancer screening, (2) immunizations, and (3) addressing common diseases for the particular patient group. For a 66-year-old woman, this includes annual mammography for breast cancer screening, colon cancer screening (annual stool test for occult blood and either intermittent colonoscopy or air contrast barium enema), tetanus, and diphtheria booster every 10 years, the pneumococcal vaccine, annual influenza immunization, and herpes zoster vaccine. She should undergo a lipid profile every 5 years up to the age of 75 years, thyroid function testing every 5 years, and fasting blood glucose levels every 3 years. Because urosepsis is common in geriatric patients, a urinalysis is also usually performed. Osteoporosis screening is indicated for women of age 65 and over. Finally, the most common cause of mortality in a woman in this age group is cardiovascular disease.

APPROACH TO:
Health Maintenance in Older Women

DEFINITIONS

SCREENING TEST: A study used to identify asymptomatic disease in the hope that early detection will lead to an improved outcome. An optimal screening test has high sensitivity and specificity, is inexpensive, and is easy to perform.

PRIMARY PREVENTION: Identifying and modifying risk factors in people who have never had the disease of concern.

SECONDARY PREVENTION: Actions taken to reduce morbidity or mortality once a disease has been diagnosed.

COST EFFECTIVENESS: A comparison of resources expended (dollars) in an intervention versus the benefit, which may be measured in life years or quality-adjusted life years.

CLINICAL APPROACH

In each age group, particular screening tests are recommended (Table 29–1).

Rationale

When the patient does not have any apparent disease or complaint, the goal of medical intervention is disease prevention. One method of targeting diseases is by using the patient's age. For example, the most common cause of death for a 16-year-old person is a motor vehicle accident; hence, the teenage patient would be well served by the physician encouraging him or her to wear seat belts and to avoid alcohol intoxication when driving. In contrast, a 56-year-old woman will most likely die of cardiovascular disease, so the physician should focus on exercise, weight loss, and screening for hyperlipidemia. In a woman beyond 65 years of age, if prior Pap smears have been normal, cervical cancer screening is not cost-effective. Patients who have had a total hysterectomy (removal of uterine corpus and cervix) do not require vaginal cytology (Pap smears) as long as the patient had no history of cervical dysplasia. (See Table 29–2 for cervical cytology screening guidelines).

Tobacco Cessation

The most important modifiable factor contributing to mortality is tobacco use. Thus, it is crucial that every patient be identified as to whether they are a smoker. Each patient who is a smoker should be approached on whether they are willing to stop, and if so, then one of the major effective interventions (bupropion, nicotine gum, nicotine inhaler, nicotine nasal spray, or nicotine patch) can be offered. Those unwilling to quit should be given a brief intervention based on the 5 R's:

- **Relevance**—indicate why quitting is personally relevant.
- **Risks**—help patient to identify negative consequences of smoking.

Table 29-1 · SCREENING BASED ON AGE

	13-18 Yr	19-39 Yr	40-64 Yr	65+ Yr
Cancer screening		• Pap smear: starting at *age 21*, q 3 yrs *Age 30*, then either pap alone q3yrs or co-testing (preferable) q 5 yrs	• Pap smear co-test q 5 yrs (preferable) or pap alone q 3 yrs, • Stool for occult blood, *age 50*, annual • Colonoscopy, *age 50*, q 10 yrs • Mammography[a]	• Pap smears not needed if hx negative • Stool for occult blood, annual • Colonoscopy q 10 yrs • Mammography[a]
Immunizations	• Tetanus + diphtheria booster once between *ages 11-18 yrs* • Hepatitis A • Hepatitis B • Human papillomavirus, *ages 9-26* • Meningococcus booster, *age 16* • Influenza, annual	• Tetanus + diphtheria q 10 yrs (substitute TdaP once) • Human papillomavirus, *ages 9-26* • Meningococcus[b], *ages 19-21* • Influenza, annual	• Tetanus + diphtheria q 10 yrs • Influenza, *age 50*, annual • Herpes zoster, *age 60*	• Tetanus + diphtheria q 10 yrs • Pneumococcal 23 valent vaccine • Influenza, annual • Herpes zoster
Other diseases	• Gonorrhea + Chlamydia, annual, if sexually active	• Gonorrhea + Chlamydia, annual, up to *age 25* • HIV, annual	• Lipid profile q 5 y at *age 45* • Fasting blood glucose q 3 y at *age 45* • TSH q 5 y at *age 50* • HIV, annual	• Lipid profile q 5 y • Fasting blood glucose q 3 y • Bone mineral density study at 65 *(earlier with risk factors)* • TSH q 5 y • Urinalysis
Most common causes of mortality	• Motor vehicle accidents • Cancer • Suicide	• Cancer • Accidents • Cardiovascular disease	• Cancer • Cardiovascular disease • Accidents	• Cardiovascular disease • Cancer • Cerebrovascular disease

[a]Some experts recommend mammography beginning at age 40 yr whereas others question its efficacy in decreasing mortality.
[b]Administer Meningococcus vaccine to students, ages 19-21, who are in first year of college or who live in residence halls.
(Data from ACOG Committee Opinion No. 534, 2012. Washington, DC: American College of Obstetricians and Gynecologists; 2012 [Reaffirmed 2014].)

Table 29–2 • SUMMARY OF CERVICAL CYTOLOGY SCREENING
• <21 years: No screening recommended • 21-29 years: Cytology (Pap smear) alone every 3 years • 30-65 years (two options): Cytology with HPV cotesting every 5 years (preferred) or cytology alone every 3 years (acceptable) • 65+ years: No screening recommended if adequate prior screening has been negative and high risk is not present

- **Rewards**—ask the patient to identify benefits of stopping tobacco use.
- **Roadblocks**—identify barriers to quitting.
- **Repetition**—motivational intervention should be repeated.

Screening in HIV-Positive Women

HIV-positive women have specific screening. There is a greater prevalence of abnormal pap smears and increased risk of progression to high grade disease or cancer, especially with a lower CD4 count. Pap smears twice in the first year after diagnosis or entry into care, and if normal, then annually; there does not seem to be a role for human papillomavirus (HPV) testing in this population. There is no data for when to discontinue (ie, perhaps continue cytology even after hysterectomy or after age 65). Although lung cancers occur more often in HIV-infected individuals, there is likely no utility for chest x-ray or sputum screening. There is a higher incidence of anal cancers in these individuals, and some experts recommend anal cytology, although there is no consensus. They should receive the usual immunizations except varicella zoster which is usually withheld. They should also receive the pneumococcal 13-valent vaccine, and if the vaccine is given when the CD4 count is below 200 cells/mm^3, it should be repeated.

Controversies

Recently, several clinical trials have refuted the clinical utility of the internal pelvic examination (bimanual examination) for low-risk and asymptomatic women. The American College of Physicians issued guidelines in 2014 recommending against performing screening speculum/bimanual pelvic examination in asymptomatic, nonpregnant adult women. There is poor sensitivity of the bimanual examination to detecting adnexal masses. The American College of Obstetricians and Gynecologists recommends annual pelvic examinations and advises that the physician should discuss the complete (internal speculum and/or bimanual) examination with the patient. Women with symptoms such as vaginal discharge, pelvic pain, urinary incontinence, or pelvic pressure should have a complete examination.

COMPREHENSION QUESTIONS

29.1 A 59-year-old woman is being seen for a health maintenance appointment. She has not seen a doctor for over 10 years. She had undergone a total hysterectomy for uterine fibroids 12 years ago. The patient takes supplemental calcium. The physician orders a fasting glucose level, lipid panel, mammogram, colonoscopy, and a Pap smear of the vaginal cuff. Which of the following statements is most accurate regarding the screening for this patient?

   A. The Pap smear of the vaginal cuff is unnecessary.
   B. In general, colon cancer screening should be initiated at age 50 but this patient has very sporadic care, therefore colonoscopy is reasonable.
   C. Because the patient takes supplemental calcium, a DEXA scan is not needed.
   D. Pneumococcal vaccination should be recommended.

29.2 A 63-year-old woman has had annual health maintenance appointments and has followed all the recommendations offered by her physician. The physician counsels her about varicella zoster vaccine. Which of the following is the most accurate statement about this vaccine?

   A. This vaccine is recommended for patients who are aged 50 and older.
   B. This vaccine is not recommended if a patient has already developed shingles.
   C. This vaccine is a live-attenuated immunization.
   D. This vaccine has some cross-reactivity with herpes simplex virus and offers some protection against HSV.

29.3 An 18-year-old adolescent female is being seen for a health maintenance appointment. She has not had a Pap smear previously. She currently takes oral contraceptive pills. She began sexual intercourse 1 year previously. Which of the following statements is most accurate regarding health maintenance for this individual?

   A. A Pap smear should not be performed in this patient at this time.
   B. The HPV vaccine should be administered only if she has a history of genital warts.
   C. The most common cause of mortality for this patient would be suicide.
   D. Hepatitis C vaccination should be offered to this patient.

29.4 A 39-year-old G1P1 woman who is HIV positive is being seen for a well woman examination. The CD4 count is 600 cells/mm^3. She had a mammogram and cervical cytology 1 year ago which were both negative. Which of the following is most appropriate at this time?

A. Chest x-ray
B. Colonoscopy
C. Mammography
D. Cervical cytology
E. Pelvic ultrasound for ovarian cancer screening

ANSWERS

29.1 **A.** Cervical cytology of the vaginal cuff is unnecessary when the hysterectomy was for benign indications (not cervical dysplasia or cervical cancer) and when there is no history of abnormal Pap smears. Colon cancer screening is generally started at age 50. DEXA scan for osteoporosis screening should be considered in any postmenopausal woman at risk, such as having an osteoporosis-related fracture, a family history, or being thin and Caucasian. Pneumococcal vaccine is generally given at age 65.

29.2 **C.** The varicella zoster vaccine is a live-attenuated vaccine, recommended for individuals aged 60 and above, and has been shown to greatly reduce the incidence of herpes zoster (shingles), and the severity and likelihood of postherpetic neuralgia. It has no efficacy in preventing HSV.

29.3 **A.** Cervical cytology should be deferred until age 21. Adolescents frequently clear the HPV infection and allow an abnormal Pap smear to return to normal. Smoking inhibits the ability to clear HPV. The delayed screening prevents unnecessary and costly diagnostic procedures. The HPV vaccine should be recommended to all females between the ages of 9 and 26 regardless of exposure. The most common cause of mortality for adolescent females is motor vehicle accidents. The hepatitis C vaccine is undergoing testing for safety and efficacy and is not currently available.

29.4 **D.** Annual cervical cytology is indicated for HIV-infected women, and usually without HPV cotesting, since the prevalence is so high that there is little differentiation on triaging based on the result. There is no definite end date (age) to cervical cancer screening in these patients. Mammography and colon cancer screening is the same as HIV-negative patients.

CLINICAL PEARLS

▶ The basic approach to health maintenance is threefold: (1) cancer screening, (2) age-appropriate immunizations, and (3) screening for common diseases.

▶ The most common cause of mortality in a woman younger than 20 years is motor vehicle accidents.

▶ The most common cause of mortality of a woman older than 39 years is cardiovascular disease.

▶ Major conditions in women aged 65 years and older include osteoporosis, heart disease, breast cancer, and depression.

▶ Cervical cytology screening does not appear to be cost-effective in women older than age 65 when prior Pap smears have been normal.

▶ Tobacco use is the single most important modifiable risk factor contributing to mortality.

REFERENCE

American College of Obstetricians and Gynecologists. Low bone mass (osteopenia) and fracture risk. *ACOG Committee Opinion 407*. Washington, DC; 2008.

American College of Obstetricians and Gynecologists. Well-women visit. *ACOG Committee Opinion 534*. Washington, DC; 2012. (Reaffirmed 2014.)

American College of Obstetricians and Gynecologists. Primary and preventive care: periodic assessments. *ACOG Committee Opinion 483*. Washington, DC; 2011.

Centers for Disease Control. Immunization schedule for adults, 2015. www.cdc.gov/vaccines/recs/schedules/adult-schedule.htm#everyone. Accessed 25.08.2015.

Centers for Disease Control. Immunization schedule for persons 7 through 18 yrs, 2015. www.cdc.gov/vaccines/recs/schedules/downloads/child/7-18 yrs-schedule-pr.pdf. Accessed 25.08.2015.

Qaseem A, Humphrey LL, Harris R, et al. Screening pelvic examination in adult women: a clinical practice guideline from the American College of Physicians. *Ann Intern Med*. 2014;161 (1):67-71.

CASE 30

A 49-year-old woman complains of irregular menses over the past 6 months, feelings of inadequacy, vaginal dryness, difficulty sleeping, and episodes of warmth and sweating at night. On examination, her blood pressure is 120/68 mm Hg, heart rate is 90 beats per minute, and temperature is 99°F (37.2°C). Her thyroid gland is normal to palpation. The cardiac and lung examinations are unremarkable. The breasts are symmetric, without masses or discharge. Pelvic examination is without any masses or other abnormalities.

▶ What is the most likely diagnosis?
▶ What is your next diagnostic step?

ANSWERS TO CASE 30:
Perimenopause

Summary: A 49-year-old woman complains of irregular menses, feelings of inadequacy, sleeplessness, and episodes of warmth and sweating.

- **Most likely diagnosis:** Climacteric (perimenopausal state).
- **Next diagnostic step:** Serum follicle-stimulating hormone (FSH), luteinizing hormone (LH), and thyroid-stimulating hormone (TSH) levels.

ANALYSIS
Objectives

1. Understand the normal clinical presentation of women in the perimenopausal state.
2. Understand that the diagnosis of perimenopause is a clinical diagnosis and may include elevated serum FSH and LH levels. It is a diagnosis of exclusion and requires an awareness of disease processes that could also cause her symptoms.
3. Know that estrogen-replacement therapy is usually effective in treating the hot flushes.
4. Know the risks of continuous estrogen–progestin therapy.

Considerations

This 49-year-old woman complains of irregular menses, feelings of inadequacy, and intermittent sensations of warmth and sweating. **This constellation of symptoms is consistent with the perimenopause, or climacteric state.** The average age of menopause in the United States is 51 years old but can be anywhere from age 40 to 58 age range. The majority of women begin to experience the perimenopause for several years before and after the actual menopause. The predominant symptom of hypoestrogenemia is the hot flush. **Hot flushes are a vasomotor reaction associated with skin temperature elevation and sweating lasting for 3 to 4 minutes.** The low estrogen concentration also has an effect on the vagina by decreasing the epithelial thickness, leading to atrophy and dryness, but she will complain of symptoms long before actual signs are evident on pelvic examination of decreased vaginal rugation and moisture. With these changing levels of estrogen and progestin during the perimenopausal years leading up to the actual menopause, the woman will usually experience altered menstrual cycles, with sometimes a skipped menses, a lighter one, or a prolonged one. Elevated serum FSH and LH levels may be helpful. However, these levels will fluctuate in the perimenopause leading up to actual menopause and cannot be relied upon until persistently elevated. The value is determined by the particular reference lab being used but in general is 30 mIU/mL or greater. Saliva testing of estrogen or other levels is not reliable and is expensive. Treatment for hot flushes may include clonidine, gabapentin, selective serotonin reuptake inhibitors (SSRIs) medications, or estrogen-replacement therapy with progestin, which is the most effective of the choices. When a woman still has her uterus, the addition of progestin to estrogen replacement is important in preventing endometrial cancer. When estrogen and progestin are used in combination, this is referred to as hormone-replacement therapy (HRT). For a woman who has had a hysterectomy, the estrogen alone is adequate, and is referred to as estrogen-replacement therapy. Until a woman reaches the menopause, treatment for the irregular menstrual cycle may include a progestin or a low-dose oral contraceptive (dependent on her risk factors). This also has the added benefit of providing a back-up method for contraception. The choice of therapy depends on a careful review of the patient's medical conditions and risk factors for thrombosis, cardiovascular disease, and breast cancer weighed against the severity of the hot flushes. Bioidentical hormones or pharmacy-compounded hormones are not recommended as they are not as closely regulated as FDA-approved medications, and there are no studies that prove their safety or efficacy above standard therapies.

Note: The selective estrogen receptor modulator (SERM), raloxifene, does not treat hot flushes.

APPROACH TO:
Menopause

DEFINITIONS

MENOPAUSE: The point in time in a woman's life when there is cessation of menses for 12 months due to follicular atresia occurring after age 40 years (mean age 51 years). It describes the final menstrual cycle, but is commonly used to describe the time in a woman's life after that point.

PERIMENOPAUSE (CLIMACTERIC): The transitional few, sometimes several years, spanning from before to 1 year after the menopause. It is characterized in the years leading up to the menopause by irregular menstrual cycles. If hot flushes occur, they usually increase in frequency as menopause is reached. The hot flushing may continue for several years after menopause.

HOT FLUSHES (FLASHES): Irregular unpredictable episodes of increased skin temperature and sweating lasting about 3 to 4 minutes caused by vasomotor changes. Women often complain of night sweats, another form of hot flushes, which must be differentiated from a disease process or other causes.

PREMATURE OVARIAN FAILURE: The cessation of ovarian function due to atresia of follicles prior to age 40 years. At ages younger than 30 years, autoimmune diseases or karyotypic abnormalities should be considered.

CLINICAL APPROACH

At about 47 years of age, most women experience perimenopausal symptoms due to the ovaries' impending failure. **This is a clinical diagnosis, although lab tests can help** somewhat. Symptoms include irregular menses due to anovulatory cycles, vasomotor symptoms such as hot flushes, and decreased estrogen and androgen levels. Because ovarian inhibin levels are decreased, FSH and LH levels rise even before estradiol levels fall. The decreased estradiol concentrations lead to vaginal atrophy, bone loss, and vasomotor symptoms. While most clinicians agree that hormone-replacement therapy is currently the best treatment for the vasomotor symptoms and to prevent osteoporosis, scientific data raises concerns about the risks of this therapy. The Women's Health Initiative Study of continuous estrogen–progestin treatment reported a small but significant increased risk of breast cancer, heart disease, pulmonary embolism, and stroke. The cardiovascular risk was not seen in the women who were in the 50 to 59 age group—those women who were most likely to benefit from beginning HRT in the early menopause years. Women on hormone-replacement therapy had fewer fractures and a lower incidence of colon cancer.

Short-term hormone-replacement therapy (5 years or less) is indicated for vasomotor symptoms, and should be used for as short a duration as possible in the smallest dose. It is the most effective therapy for relief of symptoms. For women who cannot or choose not to take estrogen, clonidine, or gabapentin may help with the vasomotor symptoms. Another class of pharmaceuticals that may be helpful to relieve the hot flushes is the selective serotonin reuptake inhibitors. A selective estrogen receptor modulator, such as raloxifene, is helpful in preventing bone loss, but does not alter the hot flushes. Weight-bearing exercise, calcium and vitamin D supplementation, and estrogen replacement are important cornerstones in maintaining bone mass. Because FSH responds to feedback by inhibin, the FSH level cannot be used to titrate the estrogen-replacement dose. In other words, the FSH concentration will still be elevated even though the estrogen replacement may be sufficient.

Other diseases that are important to consider in the perimenopausal woman include hypothyroidism, diabetes mellitus, hypertension, and breast cancer. Women in this stage of life may also experience depression, whether spontaneous in its onset or situational due to grief or midlife adjustments. The practitioner should advocate aerobic exercise at least three times a week, again, with weight-bearing exercise being advantageous for the prevention of osteoporosis. Bone mineral density (BMD) testing, such as by dual-energy X-ray absorptiometry (DEXA), is useful in the early identification of osteoporosis and osteopenia. BMD testing is indicated for all postmenopausal women aged 65 years or older and postmenopausal women at risk for osteoporosis and presenting with a bone fracture. Alcohol abuse may be seen in up to 10% of postmenopausal women, and requires clinical suspicion to establish the diagnosis.

EMERGING CONCEPTS

The Stages of Reproductive Aging Workshop (STRAW) research group published a system in 2012 that attempted to predict when women would go into menopause and also characterized the clinical and laboratory changes in the various reproductive stages from adolescence through menopausal transition and into menopause. The next step is to individualize patients based on stage and risk factors into the treatment of these women (Table 30–1). Anti-Mullerian hormone (AMH) is the

Table 30–1 • REPRODUCTIVE AGING

Early vs Late Menopause	Early	Early	Early ≥ Late	Late	Late
Menstrual cycle	Regular	Variable cycle length	Oligomenorrhea		
FSH	Low	Variable	Elevated/normal	Elevated	Elevated
AMH	Normal≥ Low	Low	Low	Low	Very Low
Inhibin B	Normal	Low/variable	Low	Very Low	Very Low
Antral follicle count	Normal	Low	Low	Very Low	Very Low
Vasomotor symptoms			Likely	Very Likely	
Vaginal/vulvar atrophy				Slight	Very likely

Data from STRAW+10 Workgroup; 2012.
Data from Fritz MA, Speroff L. *Clinical Gynecologic Endocrinology and Infertility*. 8th ed. Philadelphia, PA: Lippincott Williams & Wilkins; 2011:673-748.

earliest marker to indicate decreased ovarian reserve. Inhibin B is the next serum marker to decrease. Finally, estradiol falls.

> **CASE CORRELATION**
> - See also Case 29 for health maintenance of menopausal women since the case focuses on health maintenance in the older patient.

COMPREHENSION QUESTIONS

Which of the following single best direct mechanisms for amenorrhea (A-H) best matches the clinical situations described (30.1-30.6)?

    A. Gonadotropin receptor insensitivity
    B. Pituitary dysfunction
    C. Ovarian failure
    D. Ovarian cortical atrophy syndrome
    E. Peritoneal interference with ovulation
    F. Hypothalamic dysfunction
    G. Estrogen excess
    H. Immune downregulation of ovary

30.1 A 51-year-old woman with oligomenorrhea and hot flushes.

30.2 A 22-year-old nonpregnant woman with hyperprolactinemia due to psychotropic medication use.

30.3 A 25-year-old woman slightly obese, slightly hirsute, and with a long history of irregular menses.

30.4 An 18-year-old adolescent female with infantile breast development who has not started her menses. She has some webbing of the neck region.

30.5 A 19-year-old nonpregnant woman marathon runner with amenorrhea.

30.6 A 33-year-old woman who has not started her menses since a vaginal delivery 1 year previously complicated by postpartum hemorrhage. She was unable to breast-feed her baby.

30.7 A 25-year-old woman has a history of 1 year of amenorrhea due to hyperprolactinemia. She has bilateral galactorrhea due to a prolactin-secreting adenoma. Which of the following tests is also likely to reveal an abnormal finding?
A. DEXA scan of the spine
B. Endometrial biopsy
C. Mammography of the breasts
D. Thyroid-stimulating hormone level

ANSWERS

30.1 **C.** Ovarian failure due to follicular atresia is the reason for oligo-ovulation in the perimenopausal years. During perimenopause (or climacteric), follicular atresia occurs from *hypo*estrogenemia, as do the vasomotor changes that lead to hot flushes. There is nothing dysfunctional occurring in this scenario, as it is a common occurrence in a perimenopausal patient.

30.2 **F.** Both hypothyroidism and hyperprolactinemia may cause hypothalamic dysfunction, which inhibits gonadotropin-releasing hormone (GnRH) pulsations, which in turn inhibit pituitary FSH and LH release. The lack of gonadotropins, FSH and LH, leads to hypoestrogenic amenorrhea. A common cause of hyperprolactinemia in a girl of this age is a prolactinoma. This is not a pituitary problem, nor a receptor insensitivity issue. There is no pathology related to the ovaries; however, this patient will most likely be amenorrheic due to the lack of stimulation to the ovaries by the gonadotropins.

30.3 **G.** This patient most likely has polycystic ovarian syndrome (PCOS). Women with PCOS often are obese and hirsute, have anovulation and insulin resistance, but an estrogen excess. Because of this, they are often prescribed progesterone alone or combination oral contraceptive pills to induce vaginal bleeding and to prevent endometrial hyperplasia.

30.4 **C.** Ovarian failure is the most likely etiology in this woman with probable Turner syndrome (45,X). It would be reflected by elevated gonadotropin levels and streaked ovaries. She most likely has decreased estrogen levels as well, which predisposes her to complications such as osteoporosis later in life. This patient's symptoms result from a chromosomal abnormality and not a hypothalamic or pituitary dysfunction.

30.5 **F.** Excessive exercise may lead to hypothalamic dysfunction, but many times simple weight gain will lead to its restoration of function. This patient has amenorrhea, and therefore is in a hypoestrogenic state. This puts this patient at an increased risk of bone fractures. The "female athlete triad" of eating disorder, amenorrhea, and osteoporosis is associated with hypothalamic dysfunction and hypoestrogenemia. Many times these individuals are placed on oral contraceptive pills (OCPs) in order to maintain normal hypothalamic function. There is no pathology related to the ovaries or pituitary in this scenario.

30.6 **B.** Sheehan syndrome is when the anterior pituitary suffers from hemorrhagic necrosis associated with postpartum hemorrhage. She is unable to breast-feed due to her inability to release prolactin from the anterior pituitary. This patient's symptoms are unrelated to the ovaries and hypothalamus. This patient would be in a hypoestrogenic state due to the lack of gonadotropin stimulation. Treatment for this would be supplemental hormonal replacement.

30.7 **A.** Amenorrhea due to hyperprolactinemia causes a hypoestrogenic state due to decreased GnRH release, and decreased FSH and LH secretion. Ovarian estrogen levels are decreased, leading to decreased bone mineral density. Hence, the DEXA scan is most likely to be abnormal. The endometrial biopsy is likely to be normal, or perhaps show atrophic changes due to the hypoestrogenic state, and certainly not likely to show hyperplasia or cancer. The mammogram would not be affected. The thyroid gland is not affected by hyperprolactinemia; rather, hypothyroidism can lead to hyperprolactinemia, not vice versa.

CLINICAL PEARLS

▶ Hot flushes and irregular menses after the age of 45 years are most likely due to the climacteric state (or perimenopause). These symptoms usually respond to estrogen recommended to be given as a combination of estrogen and progestin (HRT).

▶ Significant vasomotor symptoms are the current indication for hormone-replacement therapy in the menopausal woman, and the lowest dose should be used for the shortest duration feasible.

▶ The most common location of an osteoporosis-associated fracture is the thoracic spine as a compression fracture.

▶ Weight-bearing exercise, calcium and vitamin D supplementation, and estrogen-replacement therapy are the important cornerstones in the prevention of osteoporosis.

▶ Progestin should be added to estrogen-replacement therapy when a woman has her uterus, to prevent endometrial cancer.

▶ Continuous estrogen–progestin therapy may be associated with a small but significant risk of cardiovascular disease and breast cancer.

▶ The sequence of biochemical markers in the life of the ovary is as follows: AMH falls first, inhibin B next, and then finally estradiol.

▶ Pregnancy should be ruled out in any patient who presents with amenorrhea.

REFERENCES

American College of Obstetricians and Gynecologists. Hormone therapy and heart disease. *ACOG Committee Opinion 420*. Washington, DC; 2008.

American College of Obstetricians and Gynecologists. Low bone mass (osteopenia) and fracture risk. *ACOG Committee Opinion 407*. Washington, DC; 2008.

Harlow SD, Glass M, Hall JE, et al. Executive summary of the stages of reproductive aging workshop +10: addressing the unfinished agenda of staging reproductive aging. *Fert Steril.* 2012;87(4):843-851.

Laufer LR, Gambone JC. Climacteric: menopause and peri and post-menopause. In: Hacker NF, Gambone JC, Hobel CJ, eds. *Essentials of Obstetrics and Gynecology.* 5th ed. Philadelphia, PA: Saunders; 2009:379-385.

Lobo RA. Menopause. In: Katz VL, Lentz GM, Lobo RA, Gersenson DM, eds. *Comprehensive Gynecology.* 5th ed. St. Louis, MO: Mosby-Year Book; 2007:1039-1072.

Writing Group for the Women's Health Initiative Investigators. Risks and benefits of estrogen plus progestin in healthy postmenopausal women. *JAMA.* 2002;288(3):321-333.

CASE 31

A 24-year-old G0P0 woman is brought into the emergency center by police due to a sexual assault. The preliminary information is that the woman was attacked by an unknown male assailant while she was jogging in a nearby park. She reported that she is not sexually active and uses no form of contraception. She experienced vaginal penetrated penile intercourse while being threatened with a knife. On examination, the patient appears anxious and tearful. Her blood pressure (BP) is 130/70 mmHg, heart rate (HR) is 90 beats per minute (bpm), and she is afebrile.

- ▶ What are the priorities in the management of this patient?
- ▶ What special approach must be undertaken in the examination?
- ▶ What infections are most likely to be acquired?
- ▶ What medications (if any) should be offered?

ANSWERS TO CASE 31:
Sexual Assault

Summary: A 24-year-old nulliparous woman is brought into the emergency center by police due to a sexual assault. She is not currently sexually active and does not use contraception. She experienced vaginal penetrated penile intercourse by an unknown male assailant, and was threatened with a knife. On examination, the patient appears anxious and tearful. Her vital signs are normal.

- **Priorities in management:** Treat acute and/or life-threatening medical issues, perform a careful history and physical examination, order appropriate lab and sexually transmitted infection (STI) testing, arrange for emergency contraception and STI prophylaxis, and provide psychosocial support and counseling.

- **Special approach in the examination:** Exercise patience and gentleness, gain informed consent, approach the exam with sensitivity, and collect samples appropriate for local regulation and ensuring the chain of custody for legal reasons.

- **Most common infections:** Trichomonas, Chlamydia, gonorrhea, and hepatitis B.

- **Medications offered:** Ceftriaxone intramuscular (IM), oral metronidazole, and oral azithromycin, and if not previously vaccinated, hepatitis B immune globulin (HBIG) and hepatitis B vaccine, as well as emergency contraception.

ANALYSIS
Objectives

1. Define sexual assault and the incidence and prevalence.
2. Describe the legal, emotional, social, and medical approach to the sexual assault victim.
3. Describe postexposure prophylaxis for the sexual assault victim.
4. Be aware of elder abuse and describe physical exam findings.
5. Be aware of domestic abuse, recognize the signs, and the interventions.

Considerations

This is a case of a 24-year-old nulliparous woman brought into the emergency center by police due to a sexual assault. She reports to have been raped at knifepoint by an unknown male assailant at a nearby park. The patient appears anxious and tearful. Sexual assault is a crime of violence, and can result in significant physical and emotional trauma and injury. A coordinated and multidisciplinary approach is optimal to minimize trauma and connect the patient to community resources. The exam should be victim-centered, meaning that the order of the exam may need to be modified depending on the patient's cultural or emotional needs. Informed consent is crucial, and should be gained through the process including medical care, pregnancy testing, testing and prophylaxis for STI, human immunodeficiency virus (HIV) prophylaxis, photographs, and permission to contact the patient for follow-up on test results. The first priority is to identify and treat any life threatening injury. As much as possible, the examination should be coordinated with evidence collection to minimize discomfort to the patient. Many emergency centers have Sexual Assault Forensic Examiners, who have special training, expertise, and knowledge of how to collect evidence to meet legal requirements. The patient should be counseled in a language that is most comfortable. Confidentiality is complex in these settings, and should be carefully discussed with the patient, so that the patient may be aware of what information may be part of the criminal justice record (information shared with law enforcement, justice system advocates, etc), and what evidence and lab results may become legal evidence and not privileged. Testing for sexually transmitted infections should be individualized. A pregnancy test should be performed. The most common infections identified after a sexual assault are trichomonas, gonorrhea, chlamydia and hepatitis B. Thus, the patient should be encouraged to accept STI prophylaxis. A common regimen is ceftriaxone 250 mg IM, metronidazole 2 g orally, and azithromycin 1 g orally. If the patient has not been vaccinated for hepatitis B, then HBIG as well as the full hepatitis B vaccine is recommended. HIV postexposure prophylaxis should be discussed with the patient, taking into account the risk factors for exposure. Pregnancy prevention should be discussed and emergency contraception should be offered. Finally, support to community resources, arrangements for follow-up, and referral for reporting to the legal authorities should be undertaken if not already done.

APPROACH TO:
Sexual Assault and Domestic Violence

DEFINITIONS

SEXUAL ASSAULT: Any sexual act, ranging from sexual coercion to contact abuse to rape including genital, oral, or anal penetration, performed by one person on another without consent.

ACQUAINTANCE RAPE: Sexual assault committed by someone known to the victim.

DATE RAPE: When the sexual assault occurs in the context of a dating relationship.

STATUTORY RAPE: Sexual intercourse with a person under an age specified by state law, in many states it is 16 to 18 years old.

CHILD SEXUAL ABUSE: Refers to an interaction between a child and an adult, when the child is being used for sexual stimulation of the adult.

INTIMATE PARTNER VIOLENCE: Control by one partner over another in a dating, marital, or live-in relationship. The control can include physical, sexual, emotional or economic abuse and/or threats, and isolation.

INCEST: A form of acquaintance rape, in which the assailant is a family member; includes parental figures who live in the home.

ELDERLY ABUSE: A single or repeated act, or lack of appropriate actions, which causes injury or distress to an individual 60 years older and occurs within a relationship where there is an assumption of trust, or when the act is directed toward an elder person due to their age or impairments. It can be physical, psychological, emotional, or sexual abuse, neglect, abandonment, or financial exploitation.

MARITAL RAPE: Forced coitus or related sexual acts within a marital relationship without consent of the partner.

SEXUAL COERCION: The use of nonphysical tactics to gain sexual contact with a nonconsenting partner, may include intentional use of drugs or alcohol to lower inhibitions.

POSTTRAUMATIC STRESS DISORDER: A disorder developing after a traumatic event that involves re-experiencing the trauma, avoidance of activities that may be associated with the trauma, and a state of hyperarousal.

CLINICAL APPROACH

Sexual assault is a term that encompasses rape, unwanted genital touching, and sexual coercion. It is a complex problem with many medical, psychological, and legal aspects. The lifetime prevalence of sexual assault is reported as approximately 20% but this is likely an underestimation due to reporting bias. The majority of reported assailants are known to the victim—either a current or former intimate partner, acquaintance, or family member. Fourteen percent of reported assailants are strangers. Those at increased risk for sexual assault include the physically or mentally disabled, homeless, and persons who are gay, lesbian, bisexual, or transgendered. Other populations at risk are college students, alcohol and drug users, and persons under age 25 years.

Sexual assault can lead to physical injury in approximately half of cases, and emotional trauma, fear, and embarrassment in the majority of cases. Many victims fear that they will not be heard or believed, or that details about their assault will be released to the public. They may also fear for their safety, or fear that their case will not be successfully prosecuted. Sexual assault victims may be hesitant to seek medical attention after the inciting event so it is important for healthcare providers to understand that the patient may be guarded in her verbal and nonverbal responses. Prior to examination, the patient must be instructed not to bathe, eat, drink, clean fingernails, smoke, urinate nor defecate. All of these actions may alter important legal data collection.

The initial role of the healthcare provider is to rule out any life-threatening injuries as with any patient triaged through a medical facility. Although most physical injuries are reported as minor, about 1% report major injuries needing hospitalization or operative repair, and 0.1% suffer fatality. After life-threatening injuries have been ruled out, the patient must be moved to a quiet, private room for the remainder of the exam and informed consent must be obtained (Figure 31–1). A thorough history and physical examination must be taken that includes: details of the event with

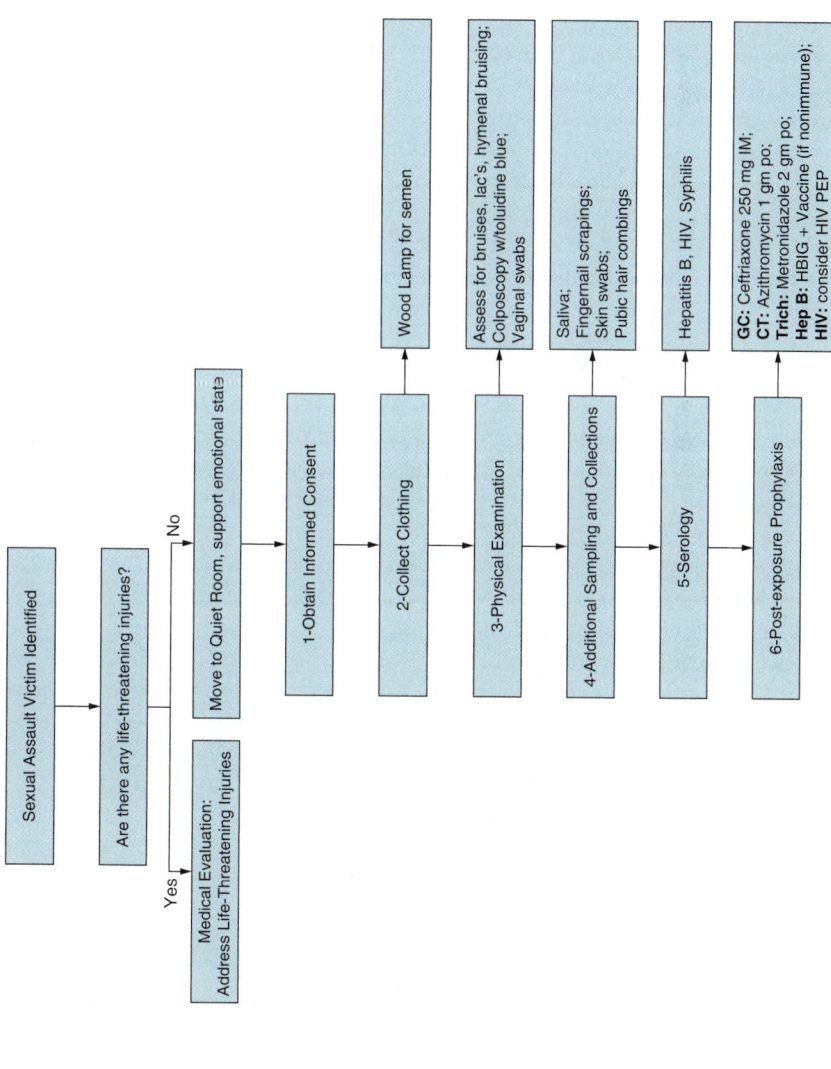

Figure 31–1. Examination of a sexual assault victim.

a description of her attacker, last menstrual period, and contraceptive use. Next, patient should be instructed to undress on a white sheet and the clothes collected for legal purposes. A head to toe examination needs to be performed, searching for bruises, lacerations, and bite marks, including a thorough documentation of the pelvic examination. Photographs may be placed in the medical record to aid in the documentation.

Vaginal swabs should be taken on speculum exam, which can be used to perform deoxyribonucleic acid (DNA) evaluation, noting the presence of motile sperm on microscopy, as well as cultures for *Neisseria gonorrhea*, *Chlamydia trachomatis*, and *Trichomonas vaginalis*. Pubic hair combings, fingernail scrapings, and skin washings need to be collected as well. A Wood's lamp can be used to assess clothing for semen. Colposcopic evaluation with toluidine blue can assess microscopic abrasions that may be missed on gross examination. **Serologic tests for hepatitis B virus, HIV, and Syphilis should also be performed.** Collection of these samples and thorough documentation play a pivotal role from a legal and medical perspective, and any healthcare provider that does not feel comfortable proceeding with the necessary steps, must seek assistance from experienced personnel (see Figure 31–1 for algorithm of the examination of a sexual assault victim).

The risk of pregnancy after sexual assault is estimated to be between 2% and 4%. Emergency contraceptives should be given within 72 hours of the assault, but may be effective if given within 120 hours. A serum pregnancy test must be documented in the chart prior to administering any method of contraception to rule out a pre-existing pregnancy. The **most effective form of emergency contraception is the copper intrauterine device** if inserted **within 120 hours postcoital** and patients may benefit from the long-term retention.

There are three main regimens for oral emergency contraception: progestin-only pills, combined oral contraceptives, and antiprogesterone pills (Table 31–1). See also case 44 (contraception) for more details.

Prophylactic antibiotics for sexually transmitted infections are indicated for chlamydial, gonococcal, and trichomonal infections. **Administering ceftriaxone 250mg intramuscularly in a single dose, metronidazole 2g orally in a single dose, as well as azithromycin 1g orally in a single dose or doxycycline 100mg twice daily orally for 7 days are the recommended treatment for these infections** (see Table 31–2).

Post exposure prophylaxis (PEP) is also recommended for hepatitis B virus and risk individualization for HIV. The regimen according to the 2015 CDC guidelines

Table 31–1 • EMERGENCY CONTRACEPTION	
Medication	**Regimen**
Combined OCPs (Yuzpe method)	Two doses (100mcg EE + 0.5mg P), 12 hours apart
Single-dose progestin only	Levonorgestrel 1.5mg
Two-dose progestin only	Levonorgestrel 0.75mg, 12-24 hours apart
Copper intrauterine device	Nonhormonal, <120 hours after coitus
Ulipristal acetate	One 30mg pill

EE, ethynyl estradiol; P, progestin (levonorgestrel).

Table 31–2 • POST-EXPOSURE PROPHYLAXIS	
Infection	Regimen
Chlamydia trachomatis	Azithromycin or doxycycline
Neisseria gonorrhea	Ceftriaxone IM
Trichomonas vaginalis	Metronidazole
Hepatitis B*	Hepatitis B vaccine, hepatitis B immune globulin
HIV**	Zidovudine
HPV*	HPV vaccine

*If victim unvaccinated.
**If substantial exposure risk.

include receiving both **hepatitis B immunoglobulin in addition to hepatitis B vaccine** if the assailant is hepatitis B positive and the victim unvaccinated. **HIV PEP is risk dependent;** however, the CDC recommends administering 28 days of zidovudine within 72 hours of assault, to higher risk patients outlined in the algorithm (Figure 31–2). Additionally, Human Papilloma Virus vaccine is recommended for female victims aged 9 to 26 years, and may be offered to the victim of sexual assault.

Sexual assault leads to a variety of acute emotional reactions ranging from severe distress to numbing of emotions, anger, and denial. There is no universal reaction. Medical providers should emphasize that the victim is not to blame. After the assault, a **rape-trauma syndrome** frequently occurs. This syndrome is characterized by an acute disorganized phase, then a delayed phase of organization. The acute phase lasts days to weeks and is characterized by physical reactions such as body aches, alterations of appetite and sleeping, and a variety of emotional reactions including anger, fear, anxiety, guilt, humiliation, embarrassment, self-blame, and mood swings. The later phase occurs in the weeks to months following and is characterized by flashbacks, nightmares, and phobias as well as somatic and gynecologic symptoms. Victims of sexual assault are at increased risk for post-traumatic stress disorder, major depression, and contemplation of suicide, or actual suicide attempt.

Rape survivors are also at increased risk for some chronic medical problems including chronic pelvic pain, fibromyalgia, and functional gastrointestinal disorders. It is important to consult with social workers and rape crisis counselors to provide immediate intervention, evaluate future emotional and safety needs, and to ensure proper follow-up. Rape crisis centers can provide ongoing support to victims and a list of these types of resources should be provided. In some centers, a sexual assault nurse examiner (SANE) who is extensively trained in this area is not only responsible for examining the victim and collecting evidence, but also can offer support and community referrals. Close follow-up is important not only for psychological support, but also to ensure that all vaccine schedules are followed, as well as to repeat STI testing at appropriate intervals.

Elder Abuse

Elder abuse is a widespread issue that impacts the well-being of approximately **1 in 10 adults over age 60,** with an estimated 4 million older affected per year in

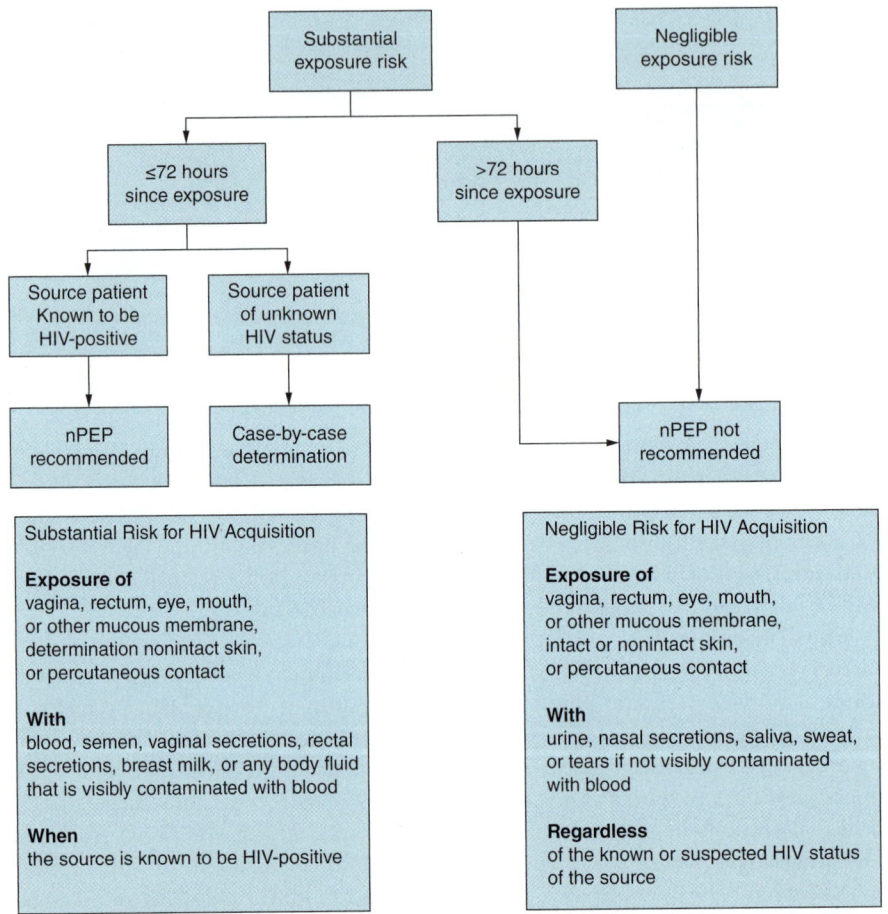

Figure 31–2. Algorithm for evaluation and treatment of possible nonoccupational HIV exposures (CDC 2015 STD Guideline Reference).

the United States. Elder abuse can be physical, emotional, psychological, or sexual abuse, or many be in the form of neglect, abandonment, or financial exploitation. Contrary to common assumptions, most incidents of elder abuse does not happen in nursing homes or other institutional settings but **usually take place at home and often the family, other household members, or paid caregivers** are usually the abusers. Risk factors for elder abuse include cognitive impairment, depression and anxiety. There is no pathognomonic sign of elder abuse as signs can vary and may be subtle, and the majority of cases go undetected. It is important to screen all elderly women in order to identify victims and provide assistance.

A detailed social history can evaluate family structure, stability of social supports, identify financial stressors, and substance abuse or mental health history. Patients reporting high levels of stress, depression, or anxiety, sleeping or eating difficulties may be the victims of abuse. Special attention should be paid to a **history** of multiple falls, frequent emergency room visits or hospitalizations, or difficulty controlling chronic medical problems as these may indicate an unstable social or family structure and possibly abuse. **Poor hygiene, weight loss, unkempt appearance, missing assistive devices, and inappropriate attire** may be some signs of neglect. Most states mandate that health care providers report confirmed cases to Adult Protective Services so it is important to educate yourself on the laws in your state. Elder abuse comes in many forms but the effects are the same. Abuse creates potentially harmful situations and feelings of worthlessness, and isolates the elder person from those who can help.

Intimate Partner Violence

Intimate partner violence occurs in every culture, country, and age group, and affects individuals in all socioeconomic and religious backgrounds. It takes place in same sex as well as heterosexual relationships. According to a 2007 CDC report, 22% of women are physically assaulted by a partner or date during their lifetime, and nearly 25% of women have been raped and/or physically assaulted by an intimate partner at some time. Between 4% and 8% of pregnant women experience physical assault; thus, the CDC and ACOG recommend universal screening each trimester and postpartum. Lifelong consequences exist including physical impairment, emotional trauma, chronic health problems, and even fatality. Alcohol and/or substance abuse is much more prevalent in women who are victims as well as men who commit violent acts.

Because of the high prevalence, the ob/gyn physician must be particularly attuned to this problem. Sensitive, confidential, but direct questioning is the best approach: "Are you being hurt or threatened by anyone?" or "Do you feel safe at home?" It is paramount to assess lethality such as threats of homicide or suicide, abuse involving severe violence, use or and/or access to weapons, pregnancy, or a recent separation. When homicide or child abuse is suspected, it is mandatory to notify the authorities.

It must be reinforced to a victim of domestic abuse that they are not responsible for the abuse, and should be empowered to learn about the resources and support services, needs to make their own decisions, and discussions held in confidentiality (to the limits of the law). A safety plan may be discussed including packing a bag in advance, having personal documents ready, having an extra set of car/house keys, establishing a code with friends/family, and having a plan of where to go. They may agree to speak to a social worker or someone at the National Domestic Violence Hotline (1-800-799-SAFE [7233]). Nevertheless, even if the patient denies intimate partner violence, it is beneficial to discuss the issues in a caring manner and offer educational material.

COMPREHENSION QUESTIONS

31.1 A 22-year-old female college student is sexually assaulted by an unknown male assailant. Penile-to-vaginal intercourse occurred and the patient states she does not believe a condom was used. The patient is not using any form of birth control and is not sexually active. Prior to prescribing emergency contraception, which of the following is most important to order?

A. Chlamydia assay
B. Pregnancy test
C. Serum alcohol level
D. HIV test
E. Liver function tests

31.2 An 82-year-old woman is being seen for her annual well woman examination. She is brought in by her middle-aged son via wheelchair. The patient has advanced dementia and cannot give a history, but her son says there have been no problems. On examination, you note that the patient is unkempt in appearance. Her BP is 140/85 mmHg and HR is 90 bpm. There are multiple bedsores on the sacral and back area. The patient has a diaper on. A red rash is noted on the introital region, and also some bruising on the vulvar and perineal area. Which of the following is the most likely diagnosis?

A. Behcet's disease
B. Chronic alcoholism
C. Elder abuse
D. Lichen sclerosis
E. Squamous cell carcinoma

31.3 A third year medical student is doing research into intimate partner violence in pregnancy. Which of the following statements is most accurate?

A. Although violence does occur against pregnant women, homicide is rare.
B. The CDC recommends screening of intimate partner violence once during the pregnancy, usually at the first prenatal visit.
C. Intimate partner violence can lead to preterm delivery and low birth weight.
D. Usually intimate partner violence lessens during pregnancy due to concern about hurting the fetus.

31.4 A 28-year-old G1P1 woman is the victim of sexual assault. She has recently immigrated to the country and has not been vaccinated against hepatitis B. The assailant is unknown and his hepatitis B status is unknown. Which of the following is best management of the patient?

A. Administer HBIG only
B. Administer the hepatitis B vaccine only
C. Administer both HBIG and the hepatitis B vaccine
D. Expectant management since the hepatitis B status is unknown

ANSWERS

31.1 **B.** Prior to emergency contraception (EC), it is vital to assess an immediate pregnancy test, even for those patients who state that they are not sexually active or have never been sexually active. Because the EC may have a deleterious effect on any current pregnancy, a pregnancy test is mandatory.

31.2 **C.** An elderly patient who has dementia is at risk for elder abuse, because they have high needs and also cannot report the abuse. This patient has signs of neglect such as bedsores and unkempt appearance, and likely prolonged soiling without diaper changes. The vulvar bruising is highly suggestive of sexual abuse. Notification of the authorities is mandatory in a situation such as this.

31.3 **C.** Intimate partner violence increases in pregnancy and can lead to preterm delivery, low birth weight, and placental abruption. Homicide, usually in the first trimester, is the second leading cause of injury-related deaths to pregnant women after motor vehicle accidents. ACOG and the CDC recommends universal screening at the first prenatal visit and also each trimester and also postpartum.

31.4 **C.** After a sexual assault, hepatitis B immune globulin (HBIG) and the vaccine should be given if the assailant is thought to be hepatitis B positive and the patient has not been vaccinated previously. In a situation when the status of the assailant is unknown, the usual practice is still HBIG for any acute exposure, and then hepatitis B vaccination for longer term immunity.

CLINICAL PEARLS

▶ The most common type of rape are date rape and acquaintance rape.

▶ It is important to screen for sexual assault at every visit.

▶ Sexual assault is a traumatic experience and allowing the patient to dictate the order of events at evaluation is important.

▶ Emergency contraception is most effective if given within the first 72 hours from the assault.

▶ Post-exposure prophylaxis is indicated to cover C. trachomatis, N. Gonorrhea, T. vaginalis, and hepatitis B.

▶ If not comfortable with the initial exam and specimen collection, contact a provider who is in order to ensure property evidence handling.

▶ Repetitive visits, falls, and poor control of medical conditions may be signs of elder abuse.

▶ Intimate partner violence (IPV) is common and is best screened by sensitive and direct questioning.

▶ Mandatory reporting is required in situations where impending homicide or child abuse is suspected.

REFERENCES

American College of Obstetricians and Gynecologists. Intimate partner violence. *ACOG Committee Opinion 518*, 2012.

American College of Obstetricians and Gynecologists. Emergency contraception. Practice Bulletin No. 112. *Obstet Gynecol.* 2010;115:1100-1109.

American College of Obstetricians and Gynecologists. Elder abuse and women's health. Committee Opinion No. 568. *Obstet Gynecol.* 2013;122:187-191.

American College of Obstetricians and Gynecologists. Reproductive and sexual coercion. Committee Opinion No. 554. *Obstet Gynecol.* 2013;121:411-415.

American College of Obstetricians and Gynecologists. Sexual assault. Committee Opinion No. 592. *Obstet Gynecol.* 2014;123:905-909.

Centers for Disease Control and Prevention. The National Intimate Partner and Sexual Violence Survey; 2013a. Available at: cdc.gov/violenceprevention/nisvs; Accessed 23.07.2015.

Federal Bureau of Investigation. Summary Reporting System (SRS) User Manual, version 1.0. Criminal Justice Information Services (CJIS) Division, Uniform Crime Reporting (UCR) Program. DC: FBI; 2013. Available at: http://www.fbi.gov/about-us/cjis/ucr/nibrs/summary-reporting-system-srs-user-manual; Accessed 30.07.2015.

Hoffman BL, Schorge JO, Schaffer JI, et al. Psychosocial issues and female sexuality. In: Hoffman BL, Schorge JO, Schaffer JI, eds. *Williams Gynecology*; New York: McGraw-Hill 2012, Chap. 13,2e.

Linden JA. Clinical practice. Care of the adult patient after sexual assault. *N Engl J Med.* 2011;365: 834-841.

Lu MC, Lu JS, Halfin VP. Domestic violence &sexual assault. In: DeCherney AH, Nathan L, Laufer N, Roman AS, eds. *Current Diagnosis & Treatment: Obstetrics & Gynecology*; 2013, Chap. 60, 11e.

Richardson AR, Maltz FN. Ulipristal acetate: review of the efficacy and safety of a newly approved agent for emergency contraception. *Clin Ther.* 2012;34:24-36.

CASE 32

A 45-year-old woman underwent a total laparoscopic hysterectomy for symptomatic endometriosis 2 days ago. Today, she complains of new onset right flank tenderness. On examination, her temperature is 102°F (38.8°C), heart rate (HR) is 100 beats per minute, and blood pressure (BP) is 130/90 mm Hg. Her heart and lung examinations are normal. The abdomen is slightly tender diffusely with normal bowel sounds. The small incisions appear within normal limits. Exquisite right costovertebral angle tenderness is noted.

▶ What would be your next diagnostic step?
▶ What is the most likely diagnosis?

ANSWERS TO CASE 32:
Ureteral Injury after Hysterectomy

Summary: A 45-year-old woman who underwent a total laparoscopic hysterectomy for symptomatic endometriosis 2 days previously has right flank tenderness, fever of 102°F (38.8°C), and exquisite costovertebral angle tenderness. The small incisions appear normal.

- **Next step:** Intravenous pyelogram (IVP) or computed tomography (CT) scan of the abdomen with intravenous contrast.
- **Most likely diagnosis:** Right ureteral obstruction or injury.

ANALYSIS
Objectives

1. Understand that the urinary tract is sometimes injured in pelvic surgery.
2. Know the common presentations of ureteral and bladder injuries after gynecologic surgery.
3. Know some of the conditions that predispose patients to urinary tract injury.

Considerations

This patient has a clinical picture identical to pyelonephritis; however, because she has recently undergone a hysterectomy, injury to or obstruction of the ureter is of paramount concern. Endometriosis tends to obliterate tissue planes, making ureteral injury more likely. Either an intravenous pyelogram (IVP) or a CT scan of the abdomen and pelvis with intravenous contrast would also be diagnostic. In the past, IVP would have been the preferred imaging study, but more recently, CT imaging has emerged as the examination of choice due to its availability and ease of performance. If the same clinical picture were present without the recent surgery, then the most likely diagnosis would be pyelonephritis and the next step would be intravenous antibiotics and urine culture. Finally, the wound incisions are normal, which argues against a wound infection causing the postoperative fever. Laparoscopic hysterectomies can cause injury to the ureter by mechanical ligation, for instance, if a stapling device were used. Thermal injury can also cause ureteral injury either directly to the ureter, or thermal spread. Thermal spread injury occurs when the ureter is not directly in contact with the electrocautery device but close enough so that the injury evolves over time. Typically, it is a delayed presentation such as 7 to 10 days following surgery. At this time, the tissue becomes devitalized and the injury presents clinically.

SECTION II: CASES   319

APPROACH TO:
Ureteral Injuries

DEFINITIONS

CARDINAL LIGAMENT: The attachments of the uterine cervix to the pelvic side walls through which the uterine arteries traverse.

CYSTOSCOPY: A procedure in which a scope is introduced through the urethra to examine the bladder lumen and its ureteral orifices. Various procedures, such as placement of stents into the ureters, can be performed.

INTRAVENOUS PYELOGRAM: Radiologic study in which intravenous dye is injected and radiographs are taken of the kidneys, ureters, and bladder.

HYDRONEPHROSIS: Dilation of the renal collecting system, which gives evidence of urinary obstruction.

PERCUTANEOUS NEPHROSTOMY: Placement of a stent into the renal pelvis through the skin under radiologic guidance to relieve a urinary obstruction.

CLINICAL APPROACH

Rates for ureteral injury for total laparoscopic hysterectomies are 17 per 1000 procedures. Cancer, extensive adhesions, endometriosis, tubo-ovarian abscess, residual ovaries, and interligamentous leiomyomata are risk factors. Any gynecologic procedure, including laparoscopy or vaginal hysterectomy, may result in ureteral injury; however, the majority of the injuries are associated with abdominal hysterectomy. The **most common location for ureteral injury is at the cardinal ligament**, where the ureter is only 2- to 3-cm lateral to the cervix. The ureter is just under the uterine artery, "water under the bridge" (Figure 32–1). Other locations of ureteral injuries

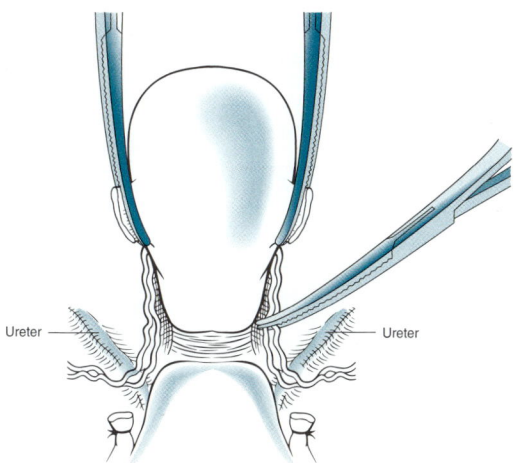

Figure 32–1. Location of ureters during hysterectomy. The ureters are within 2- to 3-cm lateral to the internal cervical os and can be injured upon clamping of the uterine arteries.

include the pelvic brim, at which injury occurs during the ligation of the ovarian vessels (infundibular pelvic ligament), and at the uterovesicular junction, the point at which the ureter enters the bladder (anterior to the vagina, when the vaginal cuff is ligated at the end of the hysterectomy). Ureteral injuries include suture ligation, trans-section, crushing with clamps, ischemia-induced damage from stripping the blood supply, and laparoscopic injury.

If the IVP shows possible obstruction with hydronephrosis and/or hydroureter (Figure 32–2), the next steps include antibiotic administration and cystoscopy to attempt retrograde stent passage. This procedure is performed in the hope that the ureter is kinked but not occluded. Relief of the obstruction is critically important in preventing renal damage. The decision for immediate ureteral repair versus initial percutaneous nephrostomy with later ureteral repair should be individualized.

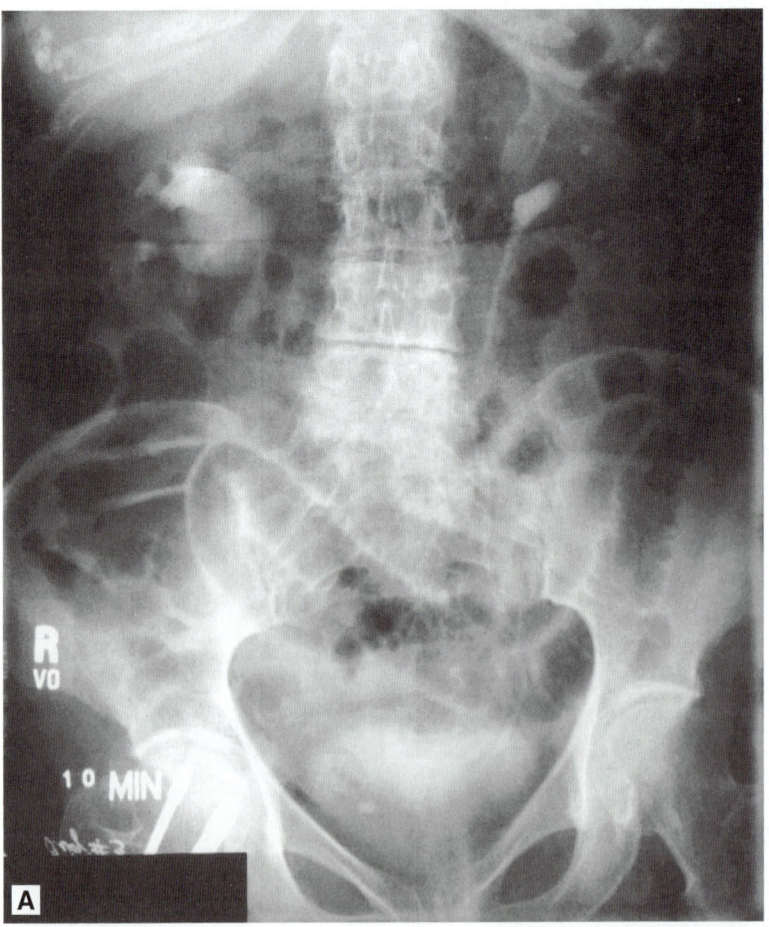

Figure 32–2. Intravenous pyelogram. Right hydronephrosis is reflected by dilation of the renal collecting system and hydroureter, whereas the left collecting system is normal (**A**). Delayed film of the same patient shows the right hydroureter more prominently (**B**). (Courtesy of Dr John E. Bertini.)

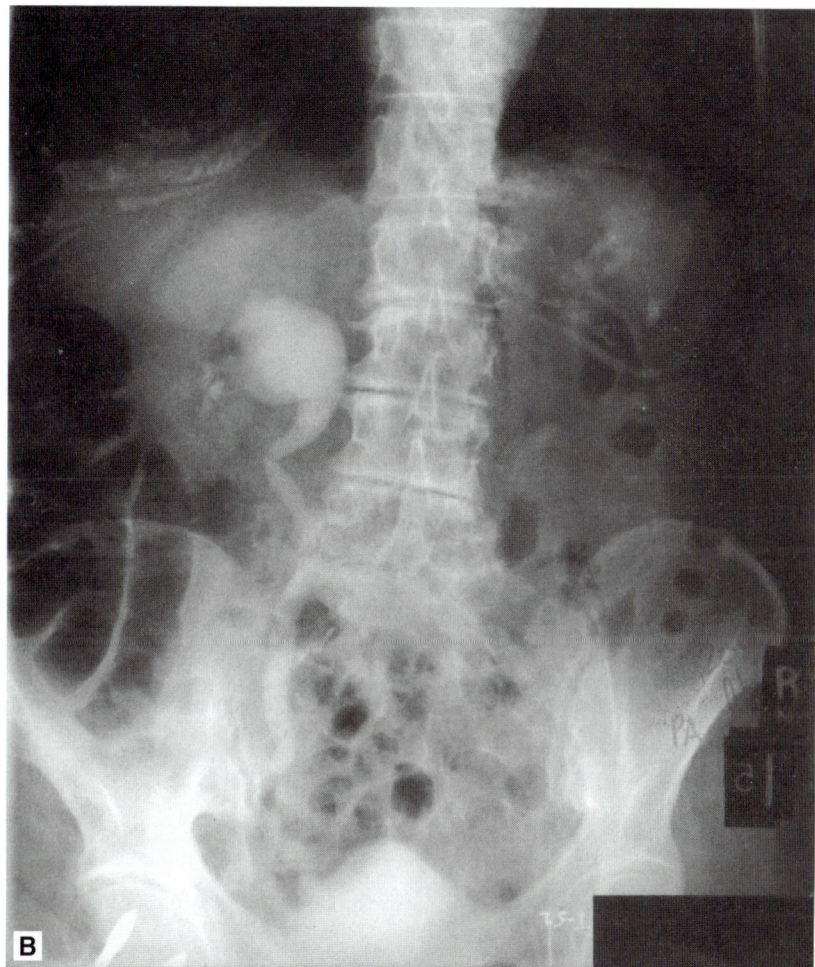

Figure 32–2. (Continued)

In general, bladder lacerations on the dome (top) of the bladder can be sutured at the time of surgery; however, injury in the trigone area (lower) may need ureteral stent placement to prevent ureteral stricture.

Ureteral injury is not a common cause of postoperative fever but must be considered after hysterectomy. Table 32–1 shows more common etiologies (5W's) of postoperative fever.

Prevention of Complications

The most important intervention in preventing surgical site infections after hysterectomy is the use of preoperative antibiotics, typically a first generation cephalosporin agent 15 to 60 minutes prior to incision time (see Case 33). Another important complication is venous thromboembolism prevention. Table 32–2 shows how to grade VTE risk and the prophylactic measures recommended.

Table 32-1 • COMMON CAUSES OF POSTOPERATIVE FEVER

5 W's	Disease Process	Postoperative Day
Wind	Atelectasis, pneumonia	1
Water	Urinary tract infection	3
Walking	DVT or PE	5
Wound	Wound infection	7
Wonder drugs	Drug-induced fever	>7

NOTE: Table 32-1 was 31-1 in 4e.

Table 32-2 • VTE PROPHYLAXIS

Risk Level	Examples	Prophylaxis
Low risk	Minor surgery in patients aged <40 with no additional risk factors	None needed, early and "aggressive" ambulation
Moderate risk	Minor surgery in patients with additional risk factors; surgery in patients aged 40-60 with no additional risk factors	Low molecular weight heparin or intermittent pneumatic compression
High risk	surgery in patients aged >60, or aged 40-60 with additional risk factors (prior VTE, cancer, molecular hypercoagulability)	Low molecular weight heparin or intermittent pneumatic compression
Highest risk	Cancer, prior VTE, hypercoagulable state	Combined LMWH and intermittent pneumatic compression

COMPREHENSION QUESTIONS

Match the following processes (A-E) to the most likely clinical situations (32.1-32.4).

- A. Vesicovaginal fistula
- B. Ureteral ligation
- C. Ureteral ischemia leading to injury
- D. Ureteral thermal injury
- E. Bladder perforation injury

32.1 A 55-year-old woman undergoes a total laparoscopic hysterectomy and develops fever and flank tenderness.

32.2 A 33-year-old woman undergoes pelvic lymphadenectomy for cervical cancer. During the procedure, the right ureter is meticulously and cleanly dissected free and a Penrose drain is placed around it to ensure its safety. She is asymptomatic until postoperative day 9, when she develops profuse nausea and vomiting, and is noted to have ascites on ultrasound.

32.3 A 55-year-old woman, who underwent a vaginal hysterectomy for third-degree vaginal prolapse 1 month ago, complains of constant leakage of fluid per vagina of 7 days duration.

32.4 A 44-year-old woman undergoes a right salpingo-oophorectomy laparoscopically. Bipolar cautery is used to ligate the infundibular pelvic ligament. The next day, she complains of fever and flank tenderness.

ANSWERS

32.1 **B.** There are many risk factors associated with ureteral injury; however, the majority are associated with laparoscopic hysterectomies. Other risk factors include: cancer, extensive adhesions, endometriosis, tubo-ovarian abscess, residual ovaries, interligamentous leiomyomata, and most gynecological procedures. Also, the presentation of fever and flank tenderness after surgery makes the diagnosis of ureteral ligation most likely in comparison to the other options. When the ureter is ligated, the patient is at an increased risk of hydronephrosis and/or hydroureter. Antibiotic treatment and relief of the obstruction should be administered promptly to avoid the situation in this scenario of pyelonephritis. Patients with a bladder perforation injury typically present with gross hematuria, pain, or tenderness in the suprapubic region and difficulty in voiding. Ureters are not typically "dissected out" during a hysterectomy; therefore, it would be unlikely for ischemia to occur in this situation.

32.2 **C.** Over dissection of the ureter may lead to devascularization injury because the ureter receives its blood supply from various arteries along its course and flows along its adventitial sheath. Urine is leaked into the abdominal cavity and causes irritation to the intestines and induces nausea and emesis. With a vesicovaginal fistula, urine is continuously leaking out the vagina, but not into the abdominal cavity. Nausea and vomiting are not associated with any of the other answer choices except for bladder perforation. In bladder perforation injuries, patients present with pain in the suprapubic region.

32.3 **A.** Constant urinary leakage after pelvic surgery is a typical history for vesicovaginal fistula (see Case 34—Urinary Incontinence). In other words, there is a constant connection between the bladder and vagina. Any type of pelvic surgery predisposes to fistula formation. Surgery is necessary to remove the fistula.

32.4 **D.** Thermal injury can spread from cauterized tissue to surrounding structures. As with the patient diagnosed with a ureteral ligation, this patient presents with fever and flank tenderness. The fact that the procedure in this scenario was performed using bipolar cautery, the likelihood that the symptoms deal with thermal injury versus ligation is much higher.

CLINICAL PEARLS

▶ Ureteral injury should be suspected when a patient develops flank tenderness and fever after a hysterectomy or oophorectomy.

▶ Meticulous ureteral dissection can lead to devascularization injury to the ureter since the vascular channels run along the adventitia of the ureter.

▶ A fistula should be considered when there is constant leakage or drainage from the vagina after surgery or radiation therapy.

▶ An intravenous pyelogram (IVP) is the imaging test of choice to assess a postoperative patient with a suspected ureteral injury.

REFERENCES

American College of Obstetricians and Gynecologists. The role of cystourethroscopy in the generalist obstetrician–gynecologist practice. *ACOG Committee Opinion 372*. Washington, DC; 2007.

Gambone JC. Gynecologic procedures. In: Hacker NF, Gambone JC, Hobel CJ, eds. *Essentials of Obstetrics and Gynecology*. 5th ed. Philadelphia, PA: Saunders; 2009:332-344.

Underwood P. Operative injuries to the ureter: prevention, recognition, and management. In: Rock JA, Jones III HW, eds. *TeLinde's Operative Gynecology*. 10th ed. Philadelphia, PA: Lippincott; 2008: 960-971.

CASE 33

A 55-year-old G3P3 woman complains of a 1-month history of pelvic pressure and feeling as though there is "something falling out of my vagina." She underwent a total abdominal hysterectomy 10 years ago for symptomatic uterine fibroids. She had three vaginal deliveries. She denies other medical problems. She has no urinary incontinence or dysuria. On examination, her blood pressure (BP) is 120/70 mm Hg, heart rate (HR) is 90 beats per minute (bpm), respiratory rate (RR) is 12 breaths per minute, temperature is 98°F (36.6°C), height is 5 ft 1 in, and weight is 160 lb. Her breasts are nontender and without masses. Her heart and lung examinations are normal. On pelvic examination, her external genitalia are somewhat atrophic but without lesions. At the introitus, a mucosal bulging is seen, which increases in size with the patient bearing down. This mass is reducible upon digital pelvic examination. Upon inspection with one blade of the speculum, both the anterior vaginal wall and posterior vaginal wall show no evidence of bulging. There are no adnexal masses. The physician places a cotton tip applicator into the urethra, but there is no movement of the applicator with Valsalva. On rectal examination, there is normal sphincter tone.

▶ What is the most likely diagnosis?
▶ What is the underlying etiology?
▶ What are the options for therapy?

ANSWERS TO CASE 33:
Pelvic Organ Prolapse

Summary: This 55-year-old G3P3 woman, who underwent a total abdominal hysterectomy previously, has a 1-month history of pelvic pressure and a sensation of "something falling out of her vagina." On examination, there is vulvar atrophy. There is a mucosal bulging through the introitus. The remainder of the pelvic examination including the rectal examination and Q-tip test is normal.

- **Most likely diagnosis:** Vaginal vault prolapse.

- **Underlying etiology:** Enterocele with small bowel in hernia sac behind the vaginal cuff.

- **Options for therapy:** Pessary device or surgical fixation of the vagina to a sturdy structure such as the sacrospinous ligament, the uterosacral ligaments, or the sacrum.

ANALYSIS
Objectives

1. Understand the anatomical support of the pelvic organs provided by the pelvic diaphragm and endopelvic fascia.

2. Describe the types of pelvic organ prolapse (POP) based on location: cystocele (anterior), enterocele (central), rectocele (posterior), paravaginal (lateral).

3. Describe the symptoms of the various types of POP defects and treatment options.

Considerations

This 55-year-old patient has a sensation of something falling out of the vagina. She has had three vaginal deliveries and a total abdominal hysterectomy in the past, both of which are risk factors for developing POP. On examination, the vaginal cuff is noted at the introitus. Examination of the anterior compartment (bladder) is normal in support, including Q-tip test. If the urethra were not well supported, the finding of urethral hypermobility might be present causing the urethral Q-tip to rotate through a large angle on Valsava. The posterior compartment is also well supported (rectum). There is no mention of the lateral support. Almost inevitably, an enterocele is present associated with vaginal vault prolapse. It is unlikely that conservative measures, such as pelvic muscle strengthening exercises, will alleviate this patient's symptoms. This patient is overweight at 160 lb. Some studies suggest that a 10% decrease in weight may significantly decrease prolapse symptoms. Thus, this patient should be counseled regarding weight loss, which may alleviate symptoms, or at the least, reduce surgical risks and make the procedure technically easier to accomplish. Therefore, the best treatments include either pessary, which is a synthetic device used to act as a "hammock" to suspend the pelvic organs, or surgery.

Surgical repair includes dissection and ligation of the hernia sac associated with the enterocele. Fixation of the vagina is then achieved to a sturdy structure such as the sacrospinous ligament or the uterosacral ligaments (vaginal approach), or abdominal sacrocolpopexy (fixing the vaginal cuff to the sacrum using a synthetic mesh).

APPROACH TO:
Pelvic Organ Prolapse

DEFINITIONS

CYSTOCELE: Defect of the pelvic muscular support of the anterior vagina allowing the bladder to descend into the vagina. Often the urethra is hypermobile. This is an anterior POP defect.

ENTEROCELE: Defect of the pelvic muscular support of the uterus and cervix (if still in situ) or the vaginal cuff (if hysterectomy). The small bowel and/or omentum descend into the vagina. This is a central POP defect.

RECTOCELE: Defect of the pelvic muscular support of the rectum, allowing the rectum to impinge into the vagina. The patient may have constipation or difficulty evacuating stool. This is a posterior POP defect.

PARAVAGINAL DEFECT: Defect in the levatorani attachment to the lateral pelvic side wall leading to lack of support of the vagina, known as a lateral pelvic defect.

CLINICAL APPROACH

Pelvic organ prolapse has a prevalence of 30% to 50% in parous women with 4% to 8% becoming symptomatic, particularly those over the age of 40 years, and with greater incidence after menopause. The symptoms vary and can include a heaviness or pressure sensation in the pelvis, a bulging mass (central), difficulty voiding or incomplete bladder emptying, urinary incontinence (anterior), constipation or having to use one's fingers to apply pressure on the vagina as a splint to achieve a bowel movement (posterior), sexual dysfunction or pain with intercourse (see Figure 33–1).

The pelvic diaphragm, a muscular and ligamentous network, which attaches from the pubic bone to the sacrum to the lateral pelvic side walls acts to support the pelvic organs. The **pelvic diaphragm** consists of multiple muscles such as the **pubococcygeus, puborectalis,** and **levatorani**. The bladder sits on the pelvic diaphragm and defects will lead to its descent from the normal location. Known risk factors for POP include multiple vaginal births, aging, prior pelvic surgery, hysterectomy, constipation, irritable bowel syndrome, genetic predisposition, lack of estrogen, and obesity. Potential, but still debated, risk factors include episiotomy, high birth weight infants, chronic cough, exercise, heavy lifting, and lower education.

Physical examination can be revealing and indicate what type of defect is present. The examination should be conducted with the patient in the lithotomy as well as standing positions. The bladder should be examined for support, with a

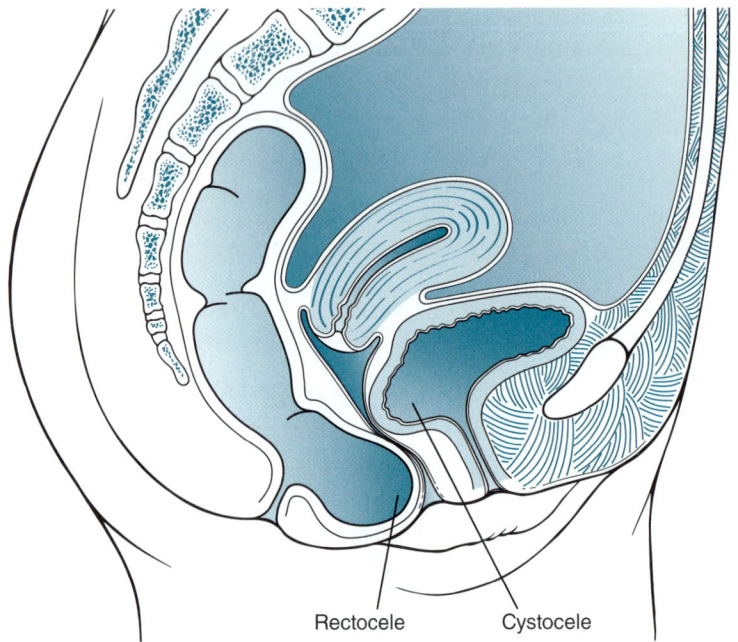

Figure 33–1. Note the types of anatomic pelvic organ prolapse such as cystocele and rectocele.

cystocele noted if it is bulging into the vagina. When the patient bears down, it should be noted whether the bladder moves further downward. Additionally, a cotton applicator tip may be placed into the urethra and the angle of excursion of the Q-tip should be observed at rest and with Valsalva. Hypermobility includes a resting urethral angle >30° or a maximal angle strain during Valsava >30°. The rectum should likewise be examined both vaginally and with a rectal examination. The perineal body is often attenuated and weakened with a posterior defect. If the patient has her uterus and cervix, then its position should be noted in relationship to the hymenal ring. With bearing down, the cervix may descend. Various systems are used to grade the degree of uterine prolapse; one such system is to delineate mild (above the hymen), moderate (at the hymen), complete (beyond the hymen). Sometimes the entire uterus is prolapsed out of the patient's introitus, the so-called procidentia. Women who have had a hysterectomy previously are at risk for vaginal cuff prolapse due to failure to fix the vagina to supporting cardinal or uterosacral ligaments. A paravaginal defect is assessed by palpating the lateral aspects of the vagina for its support and mobility.

Once the extent and type of POP is discerned, the patient can be counseled about therapy. In general, mild POP defects can be treated with pelvic floor strengthening exercises and observation. More significant defects may be treated by pessary devices, which act as a hammock to support the pelvic structures. Different pessary devices are made for different types of defects (see Figure 33–2, pessary). Surgical approaches to vaginal vault prolapse from an enterocele include resection of redundant tissue, identification of hernia sac and resection if applicable, and

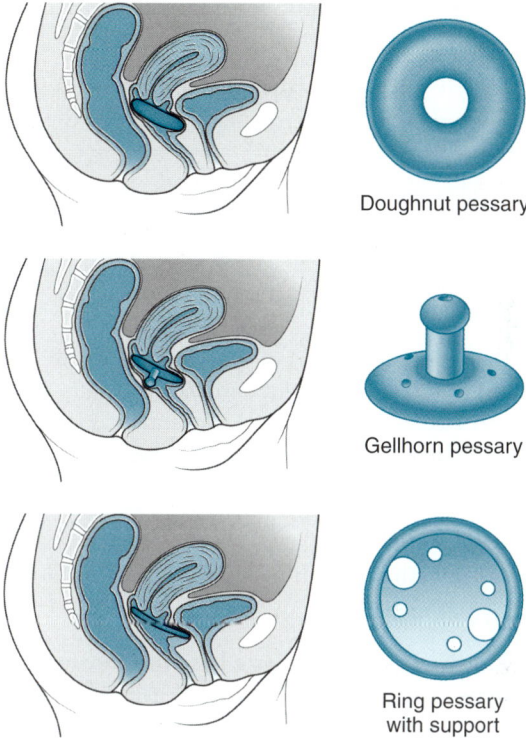

Figure 33–2. Pessary devices.

then support of the pelvic muscular defect either with suture to a ligamentous support, or using synthetic mesh. Fixation of the vaginal cuff to the sacrospinous ligament for instance is called a sacrospinous ligament fixation procedure. The use of vaginal mesh has been controversial recently, and its use is generally reserved for large defects with thorough informed consent. Using a synthetic material to fix the vaginal cuff to the sacral bone is called a sacrocolpopexy. Recently, the FDA has issued warnings that synthetic meshes in the vagina may lead to erosion and other complications.

CASE CORRELATION
- See also Case 35 (Urinary Incontinence).

COMPREHENSION QUESTIONS

33.1 A 48-year-old G3P3 woman has leakage of urine with coughing and sneezing. She denies dysuria or urinary urgency. Which of the following is likely to be present on physical examination?

A. Hypermobile urethra
B. Rectocele
C. Hypertrophic bladder
D. Paravaginal defect

33.2 A 62-year-old woman complains of constipation and difficulty having bowel movements. She states that she often needs to use her fingers to push her vagina backward to achieve a bowel movement. Her history is otherwise unremarkable. Which of the following is the best treatment for this patient?

A. Hysterectomy
B. Anterior colporrhaphy
C. Posterior colporrhaphy
D. Resection and repair of enterocele

33.3 A 35-year-old woman is undergoing a hysterectomy for uterine fibroids that have been symptomatic and failed medical therapy. The surgeon is attempting to ensure that the patient does not have subsequent vaginal vault prolapse. One step that is taken is to use suture to fix the vaginal vault to the uterosacral ligaments. The patient is also noted to have a spacious cul-de-sac area. Which of the following techniques may be used to further decrease the likelihood of vaginal vault prolapse?

A. Obliteration of the vaginal cavity
B. Fixation of the vagina to the anterior abdominal wall
C. Obliteration of the cul-de-sac
D. Prophylactic pessary

ANSWERS

33.1 **A.** This patient has symptoms consistent with pure stress urinary incontinence, typically due to the bladder falling out of its normal intra-abdominal position. When she bears down (Valsalva), the pressure to the bladder causes loss of urine. Another component of the urinary incontinence is loss of the vesicourethral angle and hypermobile urethra. The common denominator is probably childbirth, leading to damage of the pelvic support.

33.2 **C.** This woman has symptoms of a rectocele, which is a posterior vaginal defect. Because the support structure to the rectum is defective, the rectum is impinging into the vagina. When the patient bears down to have a bowel movement, the stool gathers in the pouch toward the vagina, instead of out the anal opening. When the patient splints against the rectum with her fingers, she acts as to alleviate the damaged muscular "endopelvic fascia," and simultaneous with Valsalva, the stool can be directed toward the anal opening. The surgical repair in this instance is a posterior colporrhaphy consisting of incision of the vaginal mucosa posteriorly, identification of the edges of the endopelvic fascia, and surgical repair of these edges that have separated.

33.3 **C.** One important risk factor for subsequent vaginal vault prolapse is a very spacious and deep cul-de-sac. A surgical technique of obliterating the cul-de-sac region is called culdoplasty. For instance, a circumferential sequence of purse-string sutures can be used to suture the cul-de-sac area closed. This procedure reduces the opportunity for the small bowel to push into the vaginal vault and enterocele formation. Caution must be taken to avoid injury to the rectum and the ureter.

CLINICAL PEARLS

▶ Pelvic organ prolapse is very common and is associated with multiparous women over the age of 40 years.

▶ Treatment of POP can entail pessary devices or surgical repair.

▶ Anterior defects lead to cystoceles and possibly urinary incontinence. If conservative treatment fails, surgical treatment includes anterior colporrhaphy, often in conjunction with a midurethral sling for stress urinary incontinence.

▶ Central defects lead to enteroceles and vaginal vault prolapse or uterine prolapse. The treatment is resection of the enterocele hernia sac and fixation of the vagina to secure ligamentous tissue.

▶ Posterior defects may lead to rectoceles and constipation or difficulty having bowel movements. Treatment is surgical repair (posterior colporrhaphy).

▶ Lateral defects lead to lack of lateral vaginal support. Repair is a paravaginal repair, reattachment of the levatorani muscle to its tendinous insertion site of the pelvic side wall.

REFERENCES

American College of Obstetricians and Gynecologists. Pelvic organ prolapse. *ACOG Practice Bulletin* 85. Washington, DC; 2007. (Reaffirmed 2013.)

Lentz GM. Anatomical defects of the abdominal wall and pelvic floor. In: Katz VL, Lentz GM, Lobo RA, Gersenson DM, eds. *Comprehensive Gynecology*. 6th ed. Philadelphia, PA: Mosby; 2012: 453-474.

Tarnay CM. Urinary incontinence & pelvic floor disorders. In: DeCherney AH, Nathan L, Laufer N, Roman AS, eds. *Current Diagnosis & Treatment: Obstetrics & Gynecology*. 11th ed. New York, NY: McGraw-Hill; 2013, Chap. 42, 671-700.

Tarnay CM, Bhatia NN. Genitourinary dysfunction, pelvic organ prolapse, urinary incontinence, and infections. In: Hacker NF, Gambone JC, Hobel CJ, eds. *Essentials of Obstetrics and Gynecology*. 5th ed. Philadelphia, PA: Saunders; 2009:276-289.

CASE 34

A 55-year-old woman complains of profuse serosanguineous drainage from her abdominal incision site that has persisted over 4 hours and has soaked several large towels. The patient states that the incision had been somewhat red and tender for several days. She underwent a staging laparotomy for ovarian cancer 7 days previously. She states that her vaginal bleeding was scant, and she denies the passage of blood clots or foul smelling lochia. Her past medical history is significant for type 2 diabetes mellitus, and her surgical history is unremarkable. On examination, her weight is 270 lb, blood pressure (BP) is 100/70 mm Hg, heart rate (HR) is 80 beats per minute, respiratory rate (RR) is 12 breaths per minute, and she is afebrile. The thyroid is normal to palpation. The heart and lung examinations are normal. The remainder of the physical examination is unremarkable except for the abdominal incision.

▶ What is the most likely diagnosis?
▶ What is the most appropriate therapy?

ANSWERS TO CASE 34:
Fascial Disruption

Summary: A 55-year-old obese woman complains of a 4-hour history of profuse serosanguineous drainage from her abdominal incision site. She had undergone staging surgery for ovarian cancer 7 days previously.

- **Most likely diagnosis:** Surgical site infection (deep incisional) with fascial disruption.

- **Most appropriate therapy:** Immediate surgical closure and broad-spectrum antibiotic therapy.

ANALYSIS
Objectives

1. Know the classic presentation of surgical site infection (SSI) with fascial disruption.
2. Understand that both fascial disruption and fascial evisceration are surgical emergencies.
3. Know the risk factors for wound disruptions.
4. Describe measures to prevent SSIs.

Considerations

This 55-year-old diabetic woman underwent ovarian cancer staging surgery 7 days previously. She now complains of 4 hours of profuse and continuous serosanguineous drainage from her abdominal incision. This is the typical presentation for fascial disruption. Because the rectus fascia is interrupted, the peritoneal fluid escapes through the wound. If this were only a superficial fascial separation, caused by a seroma or other small fluid collection in the subcutaneous fat tissue, then the patient would have only complained of a limited amount of drainage. The patient does not have intestines or omentum penetrating through the incision; thus, an evisceration is not suspected. Nevertheless, deep SSI with fascial disruption is a surgical emergency requiring immediate surgical repair. Broad-spectrum antibiotic therapy is usually administered. This patient has numerous risk factors for fascial dehiscence including obesity, diabetes, cancer, and a probable vertical incision. The time frame from the surgery is fairly typical, which is usually 7 to 10 days following surgery.

APPROACH TO:
Wound Complications

DEFINITIONS

WOUND DEHISCENCE: A separation of part of the surgical incision, but with an intact peritoneum.

FASCIAL DISRUPTION: Separation of the fascial layer, usually leading to a communication of the peritoneal cavity with the skin.

SEROSANGUINEOUS: Blood-tinged drainage.

EVISCERATION: A disruption of all layers of the incision with omentum or bowel protruding through the incision.

SURGICAL SITE INFECTION (SSI): Infection related to the operative procedure that occurs at or near the surgical incision within 30 days of an operation. **Deep SSI** involves (involves) the deep soft tissue such as fascia or muscle.

CLINICAL APPROACH

Wound Disorders

Wound complications include superficial separation, dehiscence, and evisceration. Separations of the subcutaneous tissue anterior to the fascia are usually associated with infection or hematoma. They affect about 3% to 5% of abdominal hysterectomy incisions. The affected patient usually presents with a red, tender, indurated incision and fever 4 to 10 days postoperatively. The treatment is opening the wound and draining the purulence. A broad-spectrum antimicrobial agent is recommended, with wet-to-dry dressing changes. The wound may be allowed to close secondarily, or be approximated after several days.

Fascial disruption, separation of the fascia but not the peritoneum, occurs in about 1% of all abdominal surgeries, and about 0.5% of abdominal incisions. It is more common with vertical incisions, obesity, intra-abdominal distension, diabetes, exposure to radiation, corticosteroid use, infection, coughing, and malnutrition. This condition often presents as profuse drainage from the incision 5 to 14 days after surgery. SSI with fascial disruption requires repair as soon as possible with the initiation of broad-spectrum antibiotics.

Evisceration is defined as protrusion of bowel or omentum through the incision, which connotes complete separation of all layers of the wound. This condition carries a significant mortality due to sepsis, and is considered a surgical emergency. When encountered, a sterile sponge wet with saline should be placed over the bowel, and the patient taken to the operating room. Antibiotics should be immediately started. The presentation is similar to that of wound dehiscence.

Prevention

Antibiotic prophylaxis is the single most important factor in preventing a SSI. Typically, it is a single dose of first generation cephalosporin such as cefazolin 1g given IV about 15 to 60 minutes prior to surgical incision. An additional dose is given for prolonged open abdominal cases (>4 hours) or if the estimated blood loss exceeds 1500 mL. Doubling of the dose is recommended for obese patients (>35 BMI [body mass index]). For penicillin allergic individuals, a combination of clindamycin and gentamicin is a reasonable choice. **Antibiotics should be given for clean-contaminated surgeries such as hysterectomies** (because of entry into the vaginal area); however, antibiotic prophylaxis is not given for clean uncomplicated cases (no entry into vaginal or uterus) such as laparoscopic oophorectomy. Antibiotics are not recommended for hysteroscopy, missed or incomplete abortion, or IUD insertion; it is recommended for pelvic organ prolapse surgery and/or stress urinary incontinence surgery and for induced (therapeutic abortion). Hair on the skin should not be routinely removed, and if required, then electric clippers rather than razors should be used immediately before the incision.

CASE CORRELATION
- See also Case 24 (Necrotizing Fasciitis).

COMPREHENSION QUESTIONS

34.1 Which of the following is a risk for wound dehiscence?
A. Diabetes mellitus
B. Use of monofilament suture
C. Horizontal incision
D. Addison disease

34.2 Which of the following is the most common reason for fascial disruption?
A. Suture becomes untied
B. Suture breakage
C. Suture tears through fascia
D. Defective suture material
E. Suture hydrolytic process

34.3 A 59-year-old woman who had staging surgery for ovarian cancer is noted to have clear serous drainage from her incision. The surgeon is concerned that it may represent lymphatic drainage versus a fistula from the urinary tract. Which of the following studies of the fluid would most likely help to differentiate between these two entities?
A. Creatinine level
B. Leukocyte count
C. pH
D. Hemoglobin level
E. CA-125 level

34.4 A 38-year-old woman had an abdominal hysterectomy for symptomatic uterine fibroids, namely menorrhagia that had failed to respond to medical therapy. One week later, she complains of low-grade fever and lower abdominal pain. On examination, she is noted to have a temperature of 100.8°F (38.22°C) and the Pfannenstiel (low transverse) incision is red, indurated, and tender. Which of the following is the best therapy for this condition?

A. Oral antibiotic therapy and follow up in 1 week
B. Observation
C. Opening the incision and draining the infection
D. Antibiotic ointment to the affected area
E. Interferon therapy

34.5 A 40-year-old woman is undergoing a laparoscopic salpingectomy. Which of the following is accurate regarding antibiotic prophylaxis?

A. Cefazolin 1 g IV should be given
B. Erythromycin IV should be given if penicillin allergic
C. An additional dose should be given if the patient is obese
D. No antibiotics are required

ANSWERS

34.1 **A.** Diabetes is associated with an increased risk for fascial separation because it is more difficult for wounds to heal in patients with this disease. The integrity of blood vessels is disrupted in a wound; this, along with the fact that diabetics typically have poor blood circulation, makes it more difficult to adequately perfuse the wounded area (blood contains the necessary clotting factors and immunoglobulins required to heal a wound and prevent infection). As a result, diabetics are also at a greater risk for a serious infection. A vertical incision as opposed to a transverse incision is associated with a greater risk of fascial disruption. Addison disease is a state of hypocortisolism, whereas Cushing disease is a state of hypercortisolism. Since increased cortisol levels are associated with immunosuppression, wound dehiscence would be more likely to occur in Cushing disease, not Addison disease.

34.2 **C.** Fascial breakdown (disruption) is not usually due to suture breakage or knot slippage, but rather due to the suture tearing through the fascia. It is more common with vertical incisions, obesity, intra-abdominal distension, diabetes, exposure to radiation, corticosteroid use, infection, coughing, and malnutrition. This condition requires immediate repair and broad-spectrum antibiotics. Fascial disruption and evisceration typically occur between 5 and 14 days postoperatively.

34.3 **A.** Fluid may appear to be serous and can be clinically indistinguishable between urine and peritoneal fluid. A creatinine level may distinguish between urine and lymphatic fluid. The creatinine level would be significantly more elevated in urine.

34.4 **C.** This patient has a superficial wound infection. The best treatment is to open the wound and drain the purulence. A broad-spectrum antimicrobial agent is recommended, with wet-to-dry dressing changes. The wound can be allowed to close secondarily or be approximated after several days. Observation in the face of infection would not be the best management and may lead to septicemia. Ointments and oral antibiotic therapy are not sufficient treatment options until the drainage is removed.

34.5 **D.** Because the uterus and vagina are not entered, and there is no overt infection, no prophylactic antibiotics are required. If the patient were penicillin allergic, then clindamycin and gentamicin should be given. For obese patients with BMI exceeding 35 kg/m^2, then a doubling of the cephalosporin dose should be considered.

CLINICAL PEARLS

▶ Fascial disruption is a concern when copious amounts of serosanguineous fluid are draining from an abdominal incision.

▶ An SSI with fascial disruption or evisceration should be immediately repaired.

▶ The most common time period in which fascial disruption or evisceration occurs is 5 to 14 days postoperatively.

▶ A superficial wound separation usually occurs due to infection or hematoma, and is treated by opening the wound and using wet-to-dry dressing changes.

▶ Obesity, malnutrition, and chronic cough are risk factors for fascial disruption.

REFERENCES

Centers for Disease Control and Prevention. Definitions of healthcare associated infections; August 2015. www.cdc.gov; Accessed 08.10.2015.

Hoffman BL. Surgeries for benign gynecologic conditions. In: Hoffman B, Schorge J, Schaffer J, Halvorson L, Bradshaw K, Cunningham F, eds. In: *Williams Gynecology*. 2nd ed. New York, NY: McGraw-Hill; 2012.

Katz VL. Preoperative counseling and management. In: Lentz GM, Lobo RA, Gersenson DM, Katz VL, eds. *Comprehensive Gynecology*. 5th ed. St. Louis, MO: Mosby-Year Book; 2012.

CASE 35

A 48-year-old G3P3 woman complains of a 2-year history of loss of urine four to five times each day, typically occurring with coughing, sneezing, or lifting; she denies dysuria or the urge to void during these episodes. These events cause her embarrassment and interfere with her daily activities. The patient is otherwise in good health. A urine culture performed 1 month previously was negative. On examination, she is slightly obese. Her blood pressure is 130/80 mm Hg, her heart rate is 80 beats per minute, and her temperature is 99°F (37.2°C). The breast examination is normal without masses. Her heart has a regular rate and rhythm without murmurs. The abdominal examination reveals no masses or tenderness. A midstream voided urinalysis is unremarkable.

- What is the most likely diagnosis?
- What physical examination finding is most likely to be present?
- What is the best initial treatment?

ANSWERS TO CASE 35:
Urinary Incontinence

Summary: A 48-year-old multiparous woman complains of urinary incontinence, which is related to stress activities. There is no urge component, and no delay from the Valsalva maneuver to the loss of urine.

- **Most likely diagnosis:** Genuine stress incontinence.
- **Physical examination finding:** Hypermobile urethra, cystocele, loss of urethrovesical angle, or positive cough stress test.
- **Best initial treatment:** Lifestyle modifications, Kegel exercises, and bladder training.

ANALYSIS
Objectives

1. Discern between the typical history of genuine stress urinary incontinence (GSUI) versus urge urinary incontinence (UUI).
2. Know that the cystometric examination can be used to distinguish between the two etiologies.
3. Know the treatments for both entities (GSUI and UUI).

Considerations
This patient's history is very typical for genuine stress incontinence. She has loss of urine concurrent with coughing, sneezing, or lifting. There is no urge component or a delay from cough, as these findings would be consistent with urge incontinence. There is no evidence of diabetes or a neuropathy, making overflow incontinence unlikely. The pelvic examination likely reveals a cystocele (bladder bulging into the anterior vagina) or a loss of the normal bladder–urethral angle (hypermobile urethra); both of these findings of pelvic relaxation may be associated with the anatomic problem of GSUI, the bladder neck being below the abdominal cavity. In patients with urge incontinence, or mixed symptoms (loss of urine with Valsalva and urge to void), cystometric examination can be helpful to differentiate between genuine stress and urge incontinence. An accurate diagnosis is important, since the therapies for these two conditions are very different, and surgical therapy may actually worsen urge incontinence.

With genuine stress urinary incontinence, initial treatment usually entails pelvic floor strengthening exercises, called Kegel exercises. If these are unsuccessful, then options for treatment include pessaries or surgical management. Pessaries support the pelvic structures, and some compress the urethra. Surgical management focuses on restoring urethral support through various methods (suburethral slings, retropubic colposuspension). Suburethral slings include bladder neck slings and midurethral slings. A bladder neck sling is placed at the level of the proximal urethra and bladder. A midurethral sling is placed at the level of the midurethra. Retropubic colposuspension (Burch procedure) involves suspending the vaginal wall adjacent to the proximal urethra and bladder neck to a ligament (Cooper's ligament) next to the pubic bone. Today, the midurethral sling procedures are the most popular methods to address this issue.

If a patient is a poor surgical candidate and does not desire pessary management, then urethral bulking agents that aim to approximate urethral mucosa may be used. This is generally used in patients with low leak point pressure.

APPROACH TO:
Urinary Incontinence

DEFINITIONS

URINARY INCONTINENCE: The involuntary loss of urine that is objectively demonstrable and creates social or hygienic concern.

GENUINE STRESS INCONTINENCE: Incontinence through the urethra due to sudden increase in intra-abdominal pressure, in the absence of bladder muscle spasm. See Table 35-1.

URGE INCONTINENCE: Loss of urine due to an uninhibited and sudden bladder detrusor muscle contraction.

Table 35-1 • DIFFERENTIAL DIAGNOSIS OF URINARY INCONTINENCE

	Mechanism	History	Diagnostic Test	Treatment
Genuine Stress urinary incontinence	Bladder neck has fallen out of its normal intra-abdominal position	Painless loss of urine concurrent with Valsalva; no urge to void	Physical examination: loss of bladder angle; cystocele; hypermobile urethra; cystometric examination	Urethropexy (urethral sling or urethropexy) to return proximal urethra back to intra-abdominal position
Urge incontinence	Detrusor muscle is overactive and contracts unpredictably	Urge component, "I have to go to the bathroom and can not make it there in time."	Cystometric examination shows uninhibited contractions	Anticholinergic medication to relax detrusor muscle(surgery may worsen)
Overflow incontinence	Over distended bladder due to hypotonic bladder	Loss of urine with Valsalva; dribbling; diabetes or spinal cord injury	Postvoid residual (catheterization) shows large amount of urine	Intermittent self-catheterization
Fistula	Communication between bladder or ureter and vagina	Constant leakage after surgery or prolonged labor	Dye into bladder shows vaginal discoloration	Surgical repair of fistulous tract

OVERFLOW INCONTINENCE: Loss of urine associated with an overdistended, hypotonic bladder in the absence of detrusor contractions. This is often associated with diabetes mellitus, spinal cord injuries, or lower motor neuropathies. It may also be caused by urethral edema after pelvic surgery.

CYSTOMETRIC EVALUATION (URODYNAMICS): Investigation of pressure and volume changes in the bladder with the filling of known volumes. It is often used to discern between GSUI and UUI.

PESSARY: A device that is inserted into the vagina to treat pelvic support problems and urinary incontinence. Pessaries support the pelvic structures, and some compress the urethra. They come in all shapes and sizes. They are useful for women who do not want or cannot have surgery to correct their incontinence.

MIDURETHRAL SLING PROCEDURES: Procedure that relieves the symptoms of GSUI by supporting the mid urethra with a hammock-like effect, with procedures such as tension-free vaginal tape (TVT), or transobturator tape (TOT).

TRANSVAGINAL TAPE PROCEDURE: A minimally invasive procedure used to fix the midurethra through the retropubic space via a blind technique using a special hook-like instrument to place a synthetic tape under the urethra, which is the most commonly used procedure for stress incontinence.

TRANSOBTURATOR TAPE (TOT) PROCEDURE: A minimally invasive procedure similar to the TVT but originating laterally to try to avoid the bladder or bowel injuries that have been reported with the TVT procedures. The Trial of Midurethral Slings (TOMUS) study found that both procedures were comparable, but with TVTs having a slightly higher efficacy at the cost of greater rates of bladder perforation, bowel injury, and postoperative voiding dysfunction.

LEAK POINT PRESSURE: The intravesical pressure at which urine leakage occurs due to increased abdominal pressure (Valsalva or cough) in the absence of a detrusor contraction.

CLINICAL APPROACH

Normal Physiology

Urinary continence is maintained when the urethral pressure exceeds the intravesicular (bladder) pressure. The bladder and proximal urethra are normally intra-abdominal in position, that is, above the pelvic diaphragm. In this situation, a Valsalva maneuver transmits pressure to both the bladder and proximal urethra so that continence is maintained. In the normal anatomic situation, the urethral pressure exceeds the bladder pressure, and also the pelvic diaphragm supports the bladder and urethra.

Mechanisms of Incontinence

Genuine Stress Incontinence: Following trauma and/or other causes of weakness of the pelvic diaphragm (such as childbearing), the proximal urethra may fall below the pelvic diaphragm. When the patient coughs, intra-abdominal pressure is exerted to the bladder, but not to the proximal urethra. When the bladder pressure equals or exceeds the maximal urethral pressure, urinary flow occurs. Because this is a mechanical problem, the patient feels no urge to void, and the loss of urine occurs simultaneously with coughing. There is no delay from cough to incontinence. Urethropexy replaces the proximal urethra and urethrovesical junction back to its intra-abdominal position (Figure 35–1). More recently, narrow strips

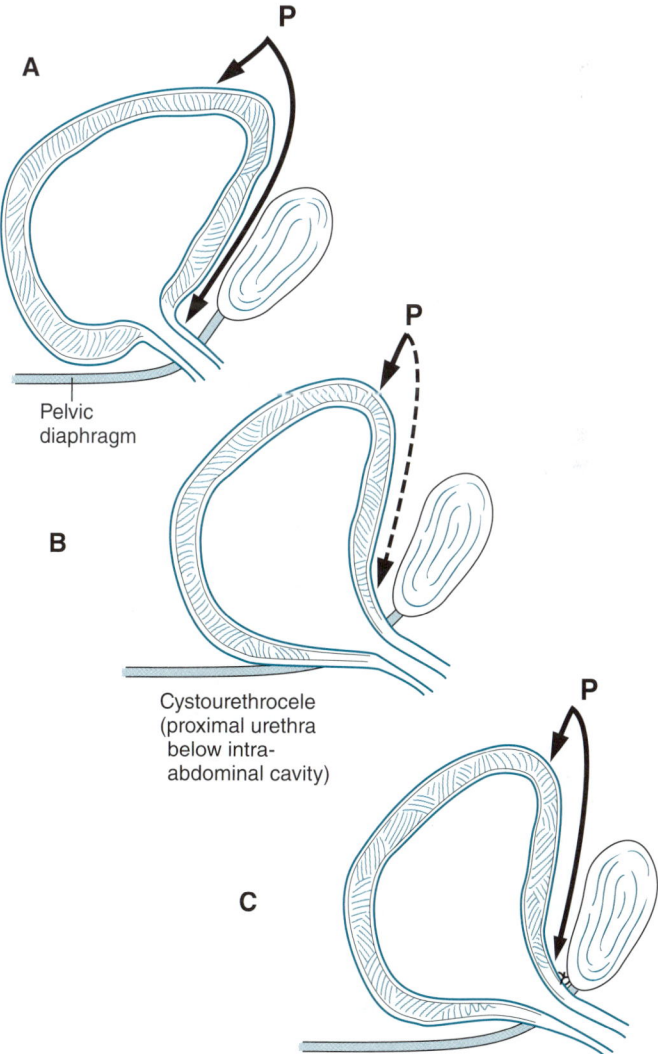

Figure 35–1. Bladder position: normal, genuine stress urinary incontinence, and after urethropexy. Normally, a Valsalva maneuver causes the increased intra-abdominal pressure (P) to be transmitted equally to the bladder and urethra (**A**). With genuine stress urinary incontinence, the proximal urethra has fallen outside the abdominal cavity (**B**) so that the intra-abdominal pressure no longer is transferred to the proximal urethra, leading to incontinence. After urethropexy (**C**), pressure is again transmitted to the urethra.

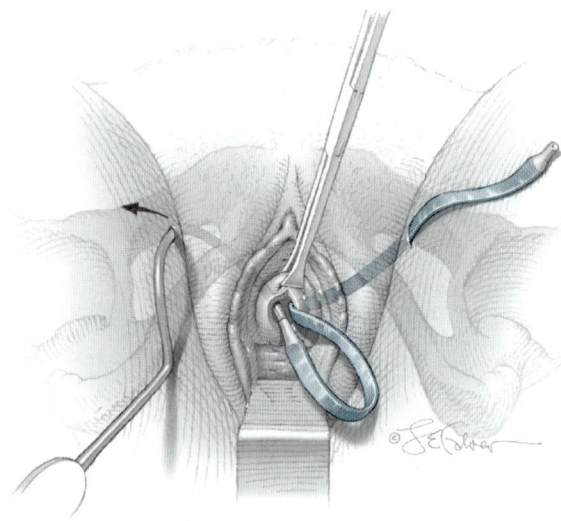

Figure 35–2. Placement of transobturator tape sling. Note that the hooked applicator instrument is used to pass through the obturator foramen, and then tension is adjusted. (*Reproduced, with permission, from Schorge JO, Schaffer Ji, Halvorson LM, et al. Williams Gynecology. www.accessmedicine.com, Figures 42–4.3.*)

of polypropylene mesh have been used to suspend the mid urethra due to the theory that urinary incontinence occurs due to pubourethral ligament insufficiency. These procedures act as a hammock to support the urethra, and also act to compress the urethra somewhat. These include various tension-free vaginal or obturator tape procedures, and outcomes are favorable as compared to urethropexy (Figure 35–2). Because of the minimally invasive nature of these procedures and shorter operating times, they have gained popularity. Nevertheless, there is concern about erosion of the synthetic material into the bladder or vagina prompting an FDA warning in 2008, which was reaffirmed in 2011. Although the FDA excluded the bladder sling procedures, some patients have been reluctant to opt for the mesh slings. A large NIH-funded study was published in 2007, which demonstrated that the sling procedure using autologous fascia was superior to the Burch colposuspension to treat GSUI.

Urge Incontinence: With uninhibited spasms of the detrusor muscle, the bladder pressure overcomes the urethral pressure. Dysuria and/or the urge to void are prominent symptoms, reflecting the bladder spasms. Sometimes, coughing or sneezing can provoke a bladder spasm, so that a delay of several seconds is noted before urine loss.

Overflow Incontinence: With an over distended bladder, coughing will increase the bladder pressure and eventually lead to dribbling or small loss of urine.

Work-Up

The history, physical examination, urinalysis, and postvoid residual are part of the initial evaluation of urinary incontinence.

Lifestyle modifications, bladder training (including timed voiding), and pelvic musculature strengthening, seem to have a role and generally should be the first line of treatment. Lifestyle modifications include weight loss, dietary changes (less caffeine/alcohol), avoiding constipation, and smoking cessation.

> **CASE CORRELATION**
>
> - See also Case 33 (Pelvic Organ Prolapse) since a cystocele is often associated with genuine stress urinary incontinence.

Note: A combined stress and mixed incontinence is probably the most common type of incontinence encountered; these patients will have symptoms of both stress and urge.

COMPREHENSION QUESTIONS

35.1 A 55-year-old woman notes constant wetness from her vagina following a total vaginal hysterectomy procedure, which she had undergone 2 months previously. She denies dysuria or urgency to void. The urine analysis is normal. Which of the following is the best method to diagnose the etiology of urinary incontinence?

   A. Cystometric examination
   B. Dye instillation into bladder
   C. Postvoid catheterization of the bladder
   D. Neurological profile of the sacral nerves

Match the following *single* best therapy (A-G) that will most likely help in the clinical situation described (35.2-35.4):

   A. Suburethral sling procedure (with or without preceding Pessary trial)
   B. Oxybutynin (Ditropan, an anticholinergic medication)
   C. Placement of ureteral stents
   D. Surgical repair of the fistulous tract
   E. Propranolol (Inderal)
   F. Placement of an artificial urethral sphincter
   G. Intermittent self-catheterization

35.2 A 42-year-old woman with long-standing diabetes mellitus complains of small amounts of constant dribbling of urine loss with coughing or lifting.

35.3 A 39-year-old woman wets her underpants two to three times each day. She feels as though she needs to void, but cannot make it to the restroom in time.

35.4 A 35-year-old woman has undergone four vaginal deliveries. She notes urinary loss six to seven times a day concurrently with coughing or sneezing. She denies dysuria or an urge to void. Her urine culture is negative.

35.5 A 43-year-old woman has undergone a TVT procedure for genuine stress incontinence approximately 4 hours previously. She tolerated the procedure well. Postoperatively, the patient is noted to be voiding but "feels like the bladder is still full." A postvoid residual is performed with 400 cc found in the bladder. Which of the following is the best management of this patient?

A. Discharge the patient home
B. Immediate surgery to remove the TVT sling
C. Perform a second voiding trial. Place a Foley catheter and discharge the patient with catheter if second voiding trial fails.
D. Order CT imaging to assess for hematoma or bowel injury

35.6 A 69-year-old woman is brought into your office with urinary incontinence. She has severe coronary artery disease, COPD, and renal insufficiency. On examination, she has a large cystocele and moderate uterine prolapse. What is the best treatment for this patient?

A. Artificial sphincter
B. Intermittent self-catherization
C. Midurethral sling procedure
D. Oxybutinin
E. Pessary device

ANSWERS

35.1 **B.** This patient likely has a vesicovaginal (between bladder and vagina) fistula from the surgery. A dye instilled into the bladder would be seen leaking into the vagina. If the leakage is slow, sometimes a tampon is placed into the vagina and removed after 30 to 60 minutes. Constant wetness after a pelvic operation suggests a fistula, such as vesicovaginal fistula, which is best treated with surgical repair, since it is an anatomic problem. Medications would not be helpful in this situation. The operation would include excision of the fistulous tract which usually may be infected or weakened, and then closure of the opening. Other common fistulae that may occur after pelvic surgery include ureterovaginal (between ureter and vagina) and rectovaginal fistulas (between rectum and vagina).

35.2 **G.** This patient has long-standing diabetes mellitus, which is a risk factor for a neurogenic bladder, leading to overflow incontinence. Other causes include spinal cord injury or multiple sclerosis. These patients generally do not feel the urge to void and accumulate large amounts of urine in their bladders. The best therapy for overflow incontinence (neurogenic bladder) is intermittent self-catheterization. Neither surgery (indicated for fistula repair), nor Burch urethropexy (indicated for genuine stress incontinence) would be appropriate for this scenario because it is not an anatomic problem. The medications listed would also not be indicated for neurogenic bladder; however, Bethanechol is a commonly prescribed drug to help stimulate bladder contractions by selectively acting on muscarinic receptors in the bladder muscles in individuals with overflow incontinence.

35.3 **B.** This woman's prominent urge component makes urge incontinence the most likely diagnosis, best treated with anticholinergic medications. Anticholinergics relax the overactive detrusor muscle. Surgery would not be indicated in this situation, and in fact, may worsen the situation by further damaging nerves and muscles of the bladder. An artificial urethral sphincter would not improve the patient's symptoms because the problem has to do with the detrusor muscle, and not the urethral sphincter. The patient is not having a problem with overflow, so self-catheterization would not be helpful either.

35.4 **A.** This clinical presentation is consistent with GSUI and is best treated by a pessary or sling procedure. Pessaries have been shown to have a ~40% to 60% patient satisfaction rate. However, patients can choose to have surgery without trying a pessary. There is some evidence that vaginal deliveries may increase the incidence of GSUI due to trauma to the pelvic diaphragm. The medications listed would not be indicated for this patient because her symptoms are due to a weakening of the pelvic diaphragm versus a problem with the bladder itself, or muscles of the bladder, as with urge incontinence. Unlike urge incontinence, the patient feels no urge to void, and there is no delay noted before urine loss after a cough or sneeze. A cystometric or urodynamic evaluation helps to differentiate between urge and genuine stress incontinence.

35.5 **C.** The patient should undergo a second voiding trial prior to discharge. If the voiding trial fails, the patient should be discharged with a urethral catheter in place. A normal post void residual is less than 100 cc or one-third of the instilled volume (if <300 mL is instilled into bladder for voiding trial). This patient's PVR of 400 cc is clearly abnormal. Bladder retention is a known outcome of suburethral sling procedures. This patient's bladder retention is mild since she is able to void somewhat, and usually will improve with time. She should be seen in the office in several days. If the patient was unable to void at all, the sling could be too tight, and the patient could benefit from loosening the sling prior to hospital discharge.

35.6 **E.** A pessary device would be the best initial treatment in this patient who likely has genuine stress incontinence based on the uterine prolapse, and due to her numerous and significant medical complications. A ring pessary with a knob may be able to support the urethra and bladder and address the urinary incontinence.

CLINICAL PEARLS

▶ In a woman who presents with urinary incontinence, a urinary tract infection should be ruled out. A voiding diary should also be collected.

▶ The definitive treatment of genuine stress incontinence is surgical, whereas the best treatment of urge incontinence is medical.

▶ Midurethral sling procedures have emerged as the most commonly performed procedures to treat GSUI because they have been demonstrated to have at least equal efficacy, shorter hospitalizations, shorter surgeries, and less pain as compared to the Burch urethropexy.

▶ The tension-free vaginal tape (TVT) procedure has the most long-term outcome data but has slightly increased risk of bleeding and bowel injury.

▶ Because of the concern for mesh erosion, even though the FDA warning excluded concern about urethral sling procedures, some patients will opt for the traditional urethropexy.

▶ Cystometric or urodynamic evaluation helps to differentiate genuine from urge incontinence.

▶ A postvoid catheterization showing a large residual volume suggests overflow incontinence.

▶ Loss of urine occurs when the intravesicular pressure equals (or exceeds) the sphincter pressure.

REFERENCES

Albo ME, Richter HE, Brubaker L. Burch colposuspension versus fascial sling to reduce urinary incontinence. *N Engl J Med*. 2007;356:2143-2155.

American College of Obstetricians and Gynecologists. Evaluation of uncomplicated stress urinary incontinence in women before surgical treatment. In: *ACOG Committee Opinion 603*. Washington, DC; 2014.

American College of Obstetricians and Gynecologists. Pelvic organ prolapse. *ACOG Practice Bulletin 85*. Washington, DC; 2007.

American College of Obstetricians and Gynecologists. Urinary incontinence in women. In: *ACOG Practice Bulletin 63*. Washington, DC; 2005. (Reaffirmed in 2011.)

Lentz GM. Urogynecology. In: Katz VL, Lentz GM, Lobo RA, Gersenson DM, eds. *Comprehensive Gynecology*. 5th ed. St. Louis, MO: Mosby-Year Book; 2007:537-568.

Rahn, D.D. Urinary Incontinence. *Williams Gynecology*. New York: McGraw-Hill Medical;2008:620-621.

Richter, HE. A trial of continence pessary vs behavioral therapy vs combined therapy for stress incontinence. *Obstet Gynecol*. 2010;115(3):609-617.

Richter, HE. Retropubic versus transobturator midurethal slings for stress incontinence. *N Engl J Med*. 2010 Jun 3;362(22):2066-2076.

Tarnay CM, Bhatia NN. Genitourinary dysfunction, pelvic organ prolapse, urinary incontinence, and infections. In: Hacker NF, Gambone JC, Hobel CJ, eds. *Essentials of Obstetrics and Gynecology*. 5th ed. Philadelphia, PA: Saunders; 2009:276-289.

CASE 36

A 23-year-old G0P0 woman complains of lower abdominal tenderness and subjective fever. She states that her last menstrual period started 5 days previously and was heavier than usual. She also complains of dyspareunia of recent onset. She denies vaginal discharge or prior sexually transmitted diseases. Her appetite has been somewhat diminished. She has urinary urgency or frequency. On examination, her temperature is 100.8°F (38.2°C), blood pressure (BP) is 90/70 mm Hg, and heart rate (HR) is 90 beats per minute (bpm). Her heart and lung examinations are normal. The abdomen has slight lower abdominal tenderness. There is no rebound tenderness and no masses. No costovertebral angle tenderness is noted. On pelvic examination, the external genitalia are normal. The cervix is somewhat hyperemic, and the uterus as well as adnexa are bilaterally exquisitely tender. The pregnancy test is negative.

▶ What is the most likely diagnosis?
▶ What are long-term complications that can occur with this condition?

ANSWERS TO CASE 36:
Salpingitis, Acute

Summary: A 23-year-old G0P0 nonpregnant woman complains of lower abdominal tenderness, subjective fever, heavier menses than usual, and dyspareunia. Her temperature is 100.8°F (38.2°C). The cervix is hyperemic, and the uterus and adnexa are bilaterally exquisitely tender.

- **Most likely diagnosis:** Pelvic inflammatory disease (PID).
- **Long-term complications that can occur with this condition:** Infertility or ectopic pregnancy.

ANALYSIS
Objectives

1. Know the clinical presentation, complications, and treatment of gonococcal cervicitis.
2. Understand the clinical diagnostic criteria of salpingitis.
3. Understand that the long-term complications of salpingitis are infertility, ectopic pregnancy, and chronic pelvic pain.
4. Know that one of the outpatient treatment regimens of salpingitis is intramuscular ceftriaxone and oral doxycycline.

Considerations

This nulliparous woman has lower abdominal pain, adnexal tenderness, and cervical motion tenderness. The presence of cervical motion tenderness is indirect, based on the dyspareunia and hyperemic cervix. The patient also has fever. These are the clinical criteria for pelvic inflammatory disease or salpingitis (infection of the fallopian tubes). Salpingitis is most commonly caused by pathogenic bacteria of the endocervix that ascend to the tubes. In the tubes, the rule is multiple organisms such as Gram-negative rods, gonorrhea or *Chlamydia*, and anaerobes. The fallopian tubes can become damaged by the infection, leading to tubal occlusion and infertility or ectopic pregnancy. The pain occurs around the time of menses, and ascending infection often occurs at the time of menses, during endometrial breakdown. This patient has lower abdominal tenderness, which indicates peritoneal irritation of the pelvis; generalized peritonitis such as involving the entire peritoneal cavity may indicate a more extensive process, such as purulent material throughout the abdominal cavity, or another process. The differential diagnosis of salpingitis includes pyelonephritis, appendicitis, cholecystitis, diverticulitis, pancreatitis, ovarian torsion, and gastroenteritis. A tubo-ovarian abscess is difficult to diagnose on physical examination and can present without fever; thus, a pelvic ultrasound is typically performed on patients with suspected PID to assess for TOA.

APPROACH TO:
Cervicitis and Salpingitis

DEFINITIONS

FITZ-HUGH–CURTIS: Perihepatitis caused by purulent tubal discharge which ascends to the right upper quadrant area. The patient will complain of right upper quadrant pain.

MUCOPURULENT CERVICITIS: Yellow exudative discharge arising from the endocervix with 10 or more polymorphonucleocytes per high-power field on microscopy.

LOWER GENITAL TRACT: The vulva, vagina, and cervix.

UPPER GENITAL TRACT: The uterine corpus, fallopian tubes, and ovaries.

PELVIC INFLAMMATORY DISEASE: Synonymous with salpingitis, or infection of the fallopian tubes.

CERVICAL MOTION TENDERNESS: Extreme tenderness when the uterine cervix is manipulated digitally, which suggests salpingitis.

ASCENDING INFECTION: Mechanism of upper genital tract infection whereby the offending microorganisms arise from the lower genital tract.

TUBO-OVARIAN ABSCESS (TOA): Collection of purulent material around the distal tube and ovary, which unlike the typical abscess, is often treatable by antibiotic therapy rather than requiring surgical drainage.

CLINICAL APPROACH

Lower Genital Tract Infections

An infection of the cervix is analogous to an infection of the urethra in the male. Thus, sexually transmitted pathogens, such as *Chlamydia trachomatis*, *N. gonorrhoeae*, or herpes simplex virus, may infect the cervix. Gonococcal and chlamydial organisms have a propensity for the columnar cells of the endocervix. Often, erythema of the endocervix is noted, leading to friability; these patients may complain of postcoital spotting. Mucopurulent cervical discharge is a common complaint, again analogous to the exudative urethral discharge of the male. The most common organism implicated in mucopurulent cervical discharge is *C. trachomatis*, although gonorrhea may also be a pathogen.

When a patient presents with purulent vaginal discharge, a speculum examination should be performed to discern the source of the discharge: to determine whether the source is vaginal versus cervical. Cervicitis will typically be mucopurulent discharge in the endocervix, and the cervix will be friable and bleed easily when touched. A primary vaginitis reveals frothy or green vaginal discharge, or erythematous vaginal mucosa. *Trichomonas* or HSV-2 can also cause a cervicitis. The patient should have a wet mount examination for Trichomonads, and assays for gonorrhea or chlamydial organisms. Treatment is based on the clinical impression, since microbiological confirmation may take several days.

When a patient presents with this type of cervical discharge, Gram stain may be helpful if available; if evidence of gonorrhea is present, that is, intracellular Gram-negative diplococci, then treatment should be directed toward gonococcal disease (ceftriaxone 125 to 250 mg IM). Because of the frequency of coexisting chlamydial infection, azithromycin 1 g orally or doxycycline 100 mg orally bid for 7 to 10 days is also often given. If the Gram stain of the cervical discharge is negative, then antimicrobial therapy directed at *Chlamydia* is warranted. Nevertheless, assays for both organisms should be performed. If the symptoms resolve, no follow-up tests need to be done (see Figure 36–1 for one suggested management scheme). Additionally, it is important that the partner receives treatment in order to prevent reinfection. Many states have expedited partner therapy enabling the patient's physician to provide medication for partners. Finally, the patient and partner should be counseled and offered testing for other sexually transmitted organisms such as HIV, syphilis, and hepatitis B and C.

Recently, urine nucleic acid amplification tests (NAAT) have been approved for confirmation of gonococcal or chlamydial cervicitis. For those patients who refuse

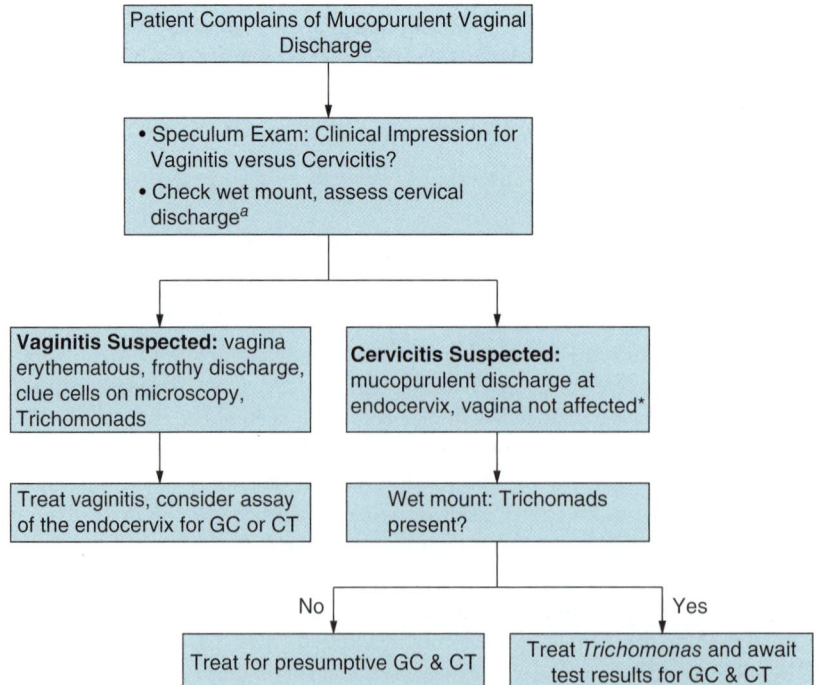

*a*If gram stain available, cervical/vaginal discharge Gram stain showing gram-negative intracellular diplococcic highly suggestive of GC; this should be treated for both GC and CT.

Figure 36–1. Example of algorithm to assess vaginal discharge.

a speculum examination, this test is helpful, with sensitivities and specificities slightly lower than that of directly sampling the endocervix.

Gonococcal cervicitis may lead to more serious complications. The organism may ascend and infect the fallopian tubes, causing salpingitis. The term pelvic inflammatory disease is usually synonymous with acute salpingitis. The tubal infection in turn predisposes the patient to infertility and ectopic pregnancies due to tubal occlusion and/or adhesions. If the infection is associated with profuse tubal discharge, the pus can ascend to the right upper quadrant region and cause a perihepatitis. These patients have right upper quadrant pain.

Gonococcal infections may lead to an infectious arthritis, usually involving the large joints, and classically is migratory. In fact, in the United States, gonorrhea is the most common cause of septic arthritis in young women. Disseminated gonorrhea can occur also; affected individuals will usually have eruptions of painful pustules with an erythematous base on the skin. The diagnosis is made by Gram stain and culture of the pustules.

Upper Genital Tract Infections

Pelvic inflammatory disease, or salpingitis, usually involves *Chlamydia*, gonorrhea, and other vaginal organisms, such as anaerobic bacteria. The mechanism is usually by ascending infection. A common presentation would be a young, nulliparous female complaining of lower abdominal or pelvic pain and vaginal discharge. The patient may also have fever, and nausea and vomiting if the upper abdomen is involved. The cervix is inflamed and, therefore, the patient often complains of dyspareunia.

The diagnosis of acute salpingitis is made clinically by abdominal tenderness, cervical motion tenderness, and/or adnexal tenderness (Table 36–1). Most episodes are asymptomatic or have mild symptoms; previously, all three criteria were thought to be required before a diagnosis and treatment was initiated, which likely led to insufficient treatment and tubal damage. Consideration of purulent vaginal discharge and the patient's risk for STDs also play a role. Confirmatory tests may include a positive *Neisseria gonorrhea* or *Chlamydia* culture, or an ultrasound suggesting a tubo-ovarian abscess. Other diseases that must be considered are acute appendicitis, especially if the patient has right-sided abdominal pain and ovarian torsion, which usually presents as colicky pain and is associated with an ovarian cyst on ultrasound. Renal disorders, such as pyelonephritis or nephrolithiasis, must also be considered. Right upper quadrant pain may be seen with salpingitis when perihepatic adhesions are present, the so-called Fitz-Hugh and Curtis syndrome.

Table 36–1 • SIGNS AND SYMPTOMS OF ACUTE SALPINGITIS

Abdominal tenderness
Cervical motion tenderness
Adnexal tenderness
Vaginal discharge
Fever
Pelvic mass on physical examination or ultrasound

Table 36–2 • CRITERIA FOR HOSPITALIZATION FOR PID
Surgical emergencies cannot be ruled out (such as appendicitis)
Pregnancy
Unresponsive to outpatient therapy after 48 hours
Unable to tolerate oral therapy (nausea/vomiting)
Severe illness, upper peritoneal signs, fever >102°F
Tubo-ovarian abscess

Findings highly suggestive of PID include endometrial biopsy showing endometritis, or transvaginal ultrasound or magnetic resonance imaging (MRI) showing thickened or fluid-filled tubes. However, its absence does not rule out PID. When the diagnosis is in doubt, the best method for confirmation is laparoscopy. The surgeon would look for purulent discharge exuding from the fimbria of the tubes.

The treatment of acute salpingitis depends on whether the patient is a candidate for inpatient versus outpatient therapy (see Table 36–2). Criteria for outpatient management include low-grade fever, tolerance of oral medication, and the absence of peritoneal signs. The woman must also be compliant. Single agent quinolone therapy had gained popularity previously, but recent evidence has shown increasing bacterial resistance. It is paramount to re-evaluate the patient in 48 hours for improvement. If the patient fails outpatient therapy, or is pregnant, or at the extremes of age, or cannot tolerate oral medication, she would be a candidate for inpatient therapy.

- One outpatient regimen: IM **ceftriaxone 250 mg, as a single injection, and oral doxycycline 100 mg twice a day for 14 days, with or without metronidazole twice a day for 14 days.**

- One inpatient regimen: Intravenous cefotetan 2 g IV every 12 hours and oral or IV doxycycline 100 mg twice daily to continue 24 hours after clinical improvement, then discharge on doxycycline 100 mg twice daily for 14 days.

Again, if the patient does not improve within 48 to 72 hours, the clinician should consider laparoscopy to assess the disease.

One important sequelae of salpingitis is **tubo-ovarian abscess.** This disorder generally has anaerobic predominance and necessitates the corresponding antibiotic coverage (clindamycin or metronidazole). The physical examination may suggest an adnexal mass, or the ultrasound may reveal a complex ovarian mass. A devastating complication of TOA is rupture, which is a surgical emergency and one that leads to mortality if unattended. In contrast to most abscesses, TOAs can often be treated with antibiotic therapy without surgical drainage; radiological percutaneous drainage may sometimes be used to hasten resolution.

Long-term complications of salpingitis include chronic pelvic pain, involuntary infertility, and ectopic pregnancy. The risk of infertility due to tubal damage is directly related to the number of episodes of PID. The intrauterine contraceptive device (IUD) places the patient at greater risk for PID, whereas oral contraceptive agents (progestin thickens the cervical mucus) decrease the risk of PID.

CASE CORRELATION

- See also Case 20 (Chlamydial Cervicitis in Pregnancy). The majority of chlamydial infection is asymptomatic. *Gonococcal cervicitis* can also be asymptomatic but more often produces mucopurulent discharge.

COMPREHENSION QUESTIONS

36.1 An 18-year-old adolescent female undergoes laparoscopy for an acute abdomen. Erythematous fallopian tubes are noted and a diagnosis of PID is made. Cultures of the purulent drainage would most likely reveal which of the following?

A. Multiple organisms
B. *Neisseria gonorrhoeae*
C. *Chlamydia trachomatis*
D. *Peptostreptococcus species*
E. *Treponema pallidum*

36.2 An 18-year-old adolescent female presents to the emergency department with a 36-hour history of abdominal pain and nausea. Her temperature is 100.5°F (38.05°C). Her abdominal examination reveals tenderness in the right lower quadrant with some mild rebound tenderness. Pelvic examination shows some cervical motion tenderness and adnexal tenderness, and also some right-sided abdominal tenderness. The pregnancy test is negative. In considering the differential diagnosis of appendicitis versus PID, which of the following is the most accurate method of making the diagnosis?

A. Following serial abdominal examinations
B. Sonography of the pelvis and abdomen
C. Serum leukocyte count and cell differential
D. Laparoscopy

36.3 A 24-year-old G0P0 woman is seen at the local sexually transmitted disease (STD) clinic. *Chlamydia* is discovered colonizing the endocervix. The patient is given oral azithromycin therapy and warned about the dangers of upper genital tract infection, such as PID. The physician notes that the patient is at risk for PID. Which of the following is a risk factor for developing PID?

A. Nulliparity
B. *Candida vaginitis*
C. Oral contraceptive agents
D. Depot medroxyprogesterone acetate

36.4 A 33-year-old woman with an intrauterine contraceptive device develops symptoms of acute salpingitis. On laparoscopy, sulfur granules appear at the fimbria of the tubes. Which of the following is the most likely organism?
   A. *C. trachomatis*
   B. *Nocardia* species
   C. *N. gonorrhoeae*
   D. *T. pallidum*
   E. *Actinomyces* species

36.5 A 28-year-old woman complains of lower abdominal pain for the last 6 months. The pain is worsened with menses. Which of the following descriptions for the pelvic pain is most accurate?
   A. An elevated inhibin level corresponds to endometriosis
   B. The presence of trigger points corresponds to fibromyalgia
   C. The presence of microscopic hematuria corresponds to interstitial cystitis
   D. Cyclic pain is consistent with the chronic pelvic pain of PID

36.6 An 18-year-old adolescent female has a yellowish vaginal discharge. On examination, the cervix is erythematous and the discharge reveals numerous leukocytes. The wet mount does not reveal trichomonads. Which of the following is the most likely etiology?
   A. *Neisseria gonorrhea*
   B. *Chlamydia trachomatis*
   C. *Ureaplasma* species
   D. *Bacterial vaginosis*

36.7 A 21-year-old college student has a sexually transmitted pharyngitis. Which of the following most likely corresponds to the etiology?
   A. *Neisseria gonorrhea*
   B. *Chlamydia trachomatis*
   C. Human papillomavirus
   D. HIV pharyngitis

ANSWERS

36.1 **A.** Multiple organisms are most likely encountered in acute salpingitis. *N. gonorrhoeae* and *C. trachomatis* are the two most common organisms involved. Other vaginal organisms, such as anaerobic bacteria, are also usually involved in the mix. Peptostreptococci are anaerobic, Gram-negative bacteria that are a natural part of human flora along the gastrointestinal (GI) and urinary tracts. They are not involved in salpingitis. Syphilis is not a common cause of salpingitis, although it is an STD like *Chlamydia* and gonorrhea. In the first stage of syphilis, chancres may appear on the external genitalia or along the vaginal wall, but not in the endocervix as with *Chlamydia* and gonorrhea.

36.2 **D.** Laparoscopy is considered the "gold standard" for diagnosing salpingitis. The surgeon has direct visualization of the tubes with this method, and looks for purulent discharge exuding from the fimbria of the tubes. Clinical criteria and sonography are not specific enough for this diagnosis, although findings of hydrosalpinx or TOA would be highly suggestive. The clinical criteria that may support this diagnosis include: abdominal tenderness, cervical motion tenderness, adnexal tenderness, vaginal discharge, fever, and pelvic mass on physical examination or ultrasound. A pelvic mass, such as a tubo-ovarian abscess, may be visualized using sonography; however, it would still not specify the origin of the mass. Of the imaging tests, CT scan is most helpful when appendicitis is suspected.

36.3 **A.** Nulliparity is associated with an increased risk of PID. IUD use increases the risk of PID. The most typical way this occurs is during the placement of the IUD, since it breaks the endocervical barrier as it enters the uterus and can spread infection from the endocervix into the tubes. Oral contraceptive agents, including depot medroxyprogesterone acetate, decrease the risk of PID by virtue of the progestin thickening the cervical mucus and thinning the endometrium. *Candida vaginitis* is a fungal infection, commonly called a yeast infection, that manifests due to an overgrowth of naturally occurring vaginal flora; fungal infections are typically not involved in the development of PID, and patients typically present with a chief complaint of severe itching and burning of the vagina with curd-like vaginal discharge.

36.4 **E.** Sulfur granules are classic for *Actinomyces*, which occurs more often in the presence of an IUD. *Actinomycesisraelii* is a Gram-positive anaerobe, which is generally sensitive to penicillin. *Chlamydia* and gonorrhea are the only other answer choices typically involved in the development of acute salpingitis; however, neither one of them are associated with sulfur granules.

36.5 **B.** Trigger points suggest a diagnosis of fibromyalgia. Chronic pelvic pain is defined as lower abdominal pain for 6 months. The differential diagnosis is lengthy. A careful history and physical exam is required. Central location of the pain and exacerbation with menses are more suggestive of a gynecologic etiology. Endometriosis is associated with a moderately elevated CA-125 level; irritable bowel syndrome should be suspected with bowel symptoms; pelvic adhesive disease from infection or adhesions is typically constant in nature; psychiatric disorders are common including depressive disorder; interstitial cystitis is diagnosed by cystoscopy. If a gynecologic etiology is suspected, then pelvic sonography is performed, and NSAID and/or oral contraceptive agents are usually used, and if ineffective, then laparoscopy can be considered.

36.6 **B.** *Chlamydial cervicitis* is the most common cause of mucopurulent cervical discharge. Although gonorrhea is also associated with a mucopurulent discharge, it is less common than *Chlamydia*. The mucus in the mucopurulent discharge is due to involvement of the columnar (mucin-containing) glandular cells of the endocervix.

36.7 **A.** The diagnosis of gonococcal pharyngitis is made by swabbing the throat. The infection is typically located on the tonsils and back of the throat. Patients who engage in oral sex are at increased risk of acquiring gonococcal pharyngitis. Typically, no symptoms are noted by the patient unless the disease disseminates. *Chlamydia* is not a common cause of pharyngitis most likely because, unlike *Neisseria gonorrhoeae*, it lacks the pili that allow the gonococcal bacteria to adhere to the surface of the columnar epithelium at the back of the throat.

CLINICAL PEARLS

▶ The two most common etiologies of mucopurulent cervical discharge are chlamydial infection and gonorrhea (of which chlamydial infection is more common).

▶ Purulent vaginal discharge should be evaluated for originating from the cervix or vagina. *Trichomonas* is a common "imitator" of cervicitis.

▶ Gram-negative intracellular diplococci are highly suggestive of *N. gonorrhoeae*.

▶ *Chlamydia* often coexists with gonococcal cervicitis.

▶ Ceftriaxone treats gonorrhea, whereas doxycycline or azithromycin treat chlamydial infections.

▶ The organisms responsible for salpingitis are polymicrobial including *N. gonorrhea*, *Chlamydia*, anaerobes, and Gram-negative rods. Therefore, the antibiotic therapy must be broad spectrum.

▶ The classic clinical triad of PID is lower abdominal tenderness, cervical motion tenderness, and adnexal tenderness; however, the patient may present with only one finding.

▶ Laparoscopy is the "gold standard" in the diagnosis of acute salpingitis, by the operator visualizing purulent drainage from the fallopian tubes.

▶ Long-term sequelae of acute salpingitis include chronic pelvic pain, ectopic pregnancy, and involuntary infertility.

▶ A tubo-ovarian abscess (TOA) should be suspected when there is an adnexal mass with clinical PID. Patients may present with subtle findings and sonography is usually required for diagnosis.

▶ TOAs are often treated medically with IV antibiotics especially with anaerobic coverage.

REFERENCES

Centers for Disease Control and Prevention (CDC). *Sexually-Transmitted Diseases Treatment Guidelines;* 2015. http://www.cdc.gov/std/tg2015/; Accessed 18.10.2015.

McGregor JA, Lench JB. Vulvovaginitis, sexually transmitted infections, and pelvic inflammatory disease. In: Hacker NF, Gambone JC, Hobel CJ, eds. *Essentials of Obstetrics and Gynecology.* 5th ed. Philadelphia, PA: Saunders; 2009:265-275.

Eckert LO, Lentz GM. Infections of the lower and upper genital tract. In: Lentz GM, Lobo RA, Gershenson DM, Katz VL, eds. *Comprehensive Gynecology,* 6e. Philadelphia, PA: Mosby; 2012:519-561.

CASE 37

A 42-year-old G2P2 woman complains of severe lower abdominal pain over the past 3 years, which is worsening. She states that the pain is worse with menses. She denied pain with intercourse. She had no medical problems. On examination, her blood pressure (BP) is 100/60 mm Hg, heart rate (HR) is 78 beats per minute (bpm), and temperature is 99°F (37.2°C). The heart and lung examinations are normal. Her abdomen is nontender and without masses. Her pelvic examination shows no tenderness or trigger points. Her pregnancy test is negative.

▶ What is the most likely diagnosis?
▶ What is the differential diagnosis?
▶ What is the next step?

ANSWERS TO CASE 37:
Chronic Pelvic Pain

Summary: A 42-year-old parous woman complains of a 3-year history of progressive lower abdominal and pelvic pain which worsened with menses.

- **Most likely diagnosis:** Chronic pelvic pain.
- **Differential diagnosis:** The differential diagnosis is broad and complex, and consists of gynecologic conditions such as endometriosis or adenomyosis, urinary conditions such as chronic urinary tract infections, GI conditions such as irritable bowel syndrome, neurologic conditions such as nerve entrapment, psychiatric conditions such as depression or sexual abuse, and rheumatologic conditions such as fibromyalgia.
- **Next step:** Careful history and physical examination to try to discern what general category the pain seems to belong, and if nongynecologic, refer to the appropriate consultant.

ANALYSIS
Objectives

1. Know the definition of chronic pelvic pain.
2. Describe the categories of conditions in the differential diagnosis of chronic pelvic pain (CPP).
3. List the evaluation of CPP.
4. Describe the treatment of CPP.

Considerations

This is a 42-year-old G2P2 woman with worsening lower abdominal/pelvic pain of 3 years' duration. The pain seems to be worse with menses. The physical examination appears to be normal. We are not given further information about the nature of the pain, but this is critically important to try to reach a presumptive diagnosis. For instance, pain that is associated with bloating, diarrhea/constipation may be gastrointestinal (GI) in nature; urinary urgency or frequency suggests urinary etiology; a patient with a history of depression or sexual abuse may suggest a psychological disorder; pain that is burning or radiating may be neurologic. Finally, excessive vaginal bleeding associated with CPP may be adenomyosis or uterine fibroids, and dyspareunia or dyschezia may be endometriosis. A history of PID may be chronic pelvic inflammatory disease and adhesions. Pregnancy should be ruled out. If the pregnancy test is negative, then typically the baseline work-up would include chlamydia and gonorrhea assays, urinalysis and urine culture and sensitivity, complete blood count, and then pelvic ultrasound. After a diligent search, nonsteroidal anti-inflammatory drugs such as ibuprofen and/or an oral contraceptive agent are usually initiated for a 3-month trial. If there is no response, an additional careful history and physical examination should be repeated. If there is no nongynecologic etiology noted, then a diagnostic laparoscopy is reasonable to assess for endometriosis.

APPROACH TO: Chronic Pelvic Pain

DEFINITIONS

ACUTE PELVIC PAIN: Pain in the lower abdomen and/or pelvis region for less than 2 weeks' duration.

SUBACUTE PELVIC PAIN: Pain in the lower abdomen and/or pelvis between 2 weeks' and 6 months' duration.

CHRONIC PELVIC PAIN: Persistent pain in the lower abdomen or pelvis for at least 6 months' duration, typically not related to pregnancy that has a significant effect on daily function and quality of life.

CHRONIC PELVIC PAIN SYNDROME: CPP without any obvious etiology or infection after diligent search, often associated with sexual or emotional consequences.

DYSPAREUNIA: Pain in the pelvis associated with penetrative sexual intercourse.

DYSMENORRHEA: Pain in the lower abdomen, pelvis, and/or back that is associated with menses.

CLINICAL APPROACH

Background

CPP is a common complaint. Up to 20% of women between the age of 18 and 49 years have CPP that lasts more than 1 year. CPP comprises 20% to 30% of gynecologic visits and accounts for 15% of hysterectomies in the United States. Up to one-third of laparoscopies are performed for this complaint. Even after diligent investigation, up to one-third of women with CPP will have no underlying etiology. One-third of these patients will have endometriosis. Approximately 20% will have pelvic adhesions or chronic PID. The remaining 10% to 15% will have a variety of other causes such as genitourinary, gastrointestinal, neuromuscular, musculoskeletal, and psychological. Gynecologic causes are in Table 37–1, and non-gynecologic causes in Table 37–2.

History and Physical Exam

The approach to chronic pelvic pain begins with a careful history and physical examination. The physician should be patient, respectful, sensitive, and meticulous. Women often have been dismissed as histrionic or exaggerating, or "hormonal"; thus, the physician should be encouraging and validate the patient's perception of the pain. The character of the pain, duration, frequency, severity, exaggerating and

Table 37-1 • GYNECOLOGIC CAUSES OF CHRONIC PELVIC PAIN
Endometriosis
Adhesions
Chronic PID
Ovarian remnant syndrome
Leiomyomata (degenerating)
Adenomyosis
Pelvic floor and hip muscle pain

relieving factors, onset, and associated factors are important. The evolution of the pain over time and response to various treatments is likewise very important.

Pain that varies markedly over the menstrual cycle is likely due to a hormonal process such as endometriosis or adenomyosis. Pain that is constant in nature following a gynecologic surgery or pelvic infection (PID or ruptured appendicitis) may be caused by dense vascular adhesions. Cyclic pain in a patient who had undergone a bilateral oophorectomy may be due to residual ovarian syndrome, in which small amounts of ovarian tissue are trapped in the retroperitoneum. Suppression of ovulation can be confirmatory, and treatment with surgical excision is curative.

Gastrointestinal etiologies can include inflammatory bowel disease or irritable bowel syndrome. Associated symptoms of abdominal bloating are as follows.

Psychosocial Inquiries

In approaching possible psychological or psychosocial reasons, the physician must be very judicious in when and how these questions are asked. Affected patients may misperceive the line of query as "You think I'm crazy like the rest of the doctors". Sometimes, these topics are reserved for the second visit, or put in the review of system. Because traumatic events such as sexual abuse or assault are very difficult

Table 37-2 • NONGYNECOLOGIC CAUSES OF CHRONIC PELVIC PAIN

Genitourinary
  Urethral syndrome
  Interstitial cystitis

Gastrointestinal
  Irritable bowel syndrome
  Partial bowel obstruction
  Inflammatory bowel disease
  Diverticulitis
  Hernia

Neuromuscular
  Nerve entrapment syndrome
  Myofascial pain syndrome
  Fibromyalgia

Psychological
  Depression
  Post-traumatic stress disorder
  Anxiety disorder

to talk about, the manner of discussion is also important. A history of depression (or symptoms), anxiety, counseling are important.

Examination

The patient's mood and posture are important to observe—flat affect or anxiety or in pain. She should be observed for mobility and flexibility. The extremities and joints are important to assess for arthritis or arthalgias. The back should be examined particularly, the paraspinous muscles and SI joints. The abdomen should be observed carefully for distension, surgical scars, and discoloration. Bowel sounds should be auscultated carefully. The abdomen should be mapped carefully for location, radiation, and severity; the abdominal wall should be palpated with and without abdominal wall flexion to try to discern musculoskeletal condition. There should be an evaluation of trigger points, which are tender points that cause the patient to "jump." The legs should be raised to assess for sciatica or a herniated disc.

The vulva and vaginal area should be carefully palpated for tenderness, such as with a cotton-tipped applicator to assess for vulvodynia or vestibulitis, conditions of severe tenderness. Cervical motion tenderness should be sought, which may indicate PID. The adnexa and uterosacral ligaments should be palpated for endometriosis. The pelvic musculature such as the levator muscles, obturators, and periformis muscles should be carefully palpated. The examination should begin with the nontender regions initially and then moving toward the more painful areas. A painful, enlarged boggy uterus may indicate adenomyosis. Tender nodules of the uterosacral ligaments or a fixed retroverted uterus may suggest endometriosis.

Laboratories and Imaging

A reasonable panel of blood tests include a CBC, urinalysis, urine pregnancy test, and gonorrhea/chlamydia assay. A pelvic transvaginal ultrasound examination is important to assess for uterine masses, adnexal masses, and peritoneal fluid.

Consultation

The patient should be referred to the appropriate consultant if the history, physical, laboratory, or imaging suggests a nongynecologic etiology. For instance, if the patient has abdominal bloating, nausea, or diarrhea, then a gastrointestinal consultation is indicated. If the patient has a history of depression, sexual abuse, or trauma, then a psychiatric consultation is important. If there is no definite organ system identified, then an empiric trial of 3 months of NSAID such as ibuprofen or naproxen, and/or a low dose oral contraceptive course can be helpful. If a gynecologic etiology is suspected, then laparoscopy can be useful to establish a diagnosis: principally endometriosis or pelvic adhesions. If after a 3- to 6- month trial of medications there is no relief, and careful search does not reveal nongynecologic conditions, then a diagnostic laparoscopy is reasonable.

Pain Persisting Without Identifiable Cause

A significant portion of patients with CPP will have persistent pain and no discernible etiology. In these instances, it is often helpful to have a multidisciplinary team, such as a gynecologist, physical therapist, psychologist, sex therapist, pain specialist, and anesthesiologist. Sometimes acupuncture can be helpful. A trial of nonnarcotic analgesics, SSRIs, tricyclic antidepressants, and perhaps ovulation suppression such as oral contraceptives or depolupron can be helpful. Excisional surgical procedures such as hysterectomy, oophorectomy, or salpingectomy should be used judiciously, since pelvic pain may persist or even worsen if there is no clear indication for these operations. Ablation of endometrioic implants and/or hysterectomy and BSO is helpful for endometriosis. Acupuncture, nerve blocks and trigger point injections can alleviate pain.

CASE CORRELATION
- See also Cases 31 (Domestic/Sexual Abuse) and 36 (PID).

COMPREHENSION QUESTIONS

37.1 A 17-year-old G0P0 female complains of severe pain with menses for 3 years, which seems to be worsening. She has tried oral contraceptives and NSAIDs for 2 years without relief. Her pregnancy test is negative. Which of the following is the best next step?
   A. GnRH agonist therapy
   B. Opiate medical therapy
   C. Psychiatric evaluation
   D. Laparoscopy
   E. Trigger point injection

37.2 A-42-year old G2P2 woman complains of a 3-year history of chronic pelvic pain. By history, it seemed as though it would be neuropathic pain. Which of the following is the best therapy?
   A. Vitamin B6 supplementation
   B. H2 antihistamine therapy
   C. Tricyclic antidepressant therapy
   D. Oral hypoglycemic therapy

37.3 A-16-year-old G0P0 female complains of severe pain with menses which began within her first year of menses. The physical examination is normal. The pregnancy test is negative. Which of the following is the most likely mechanism?
   A. Pelvic adhesions
   B. High prostaglandin levels
   C. Tubal inflammation
   D. Endometriosis

ANSWERS

37.1 **D.** Even in an adolescent, when there is severe dysmenorrhea that persists despite oral contraceptive and NSAID use, a likely etiology is endometriosis and laparoscopy is an important next step. GnRH agonist therapy should not be used without a diagnosis, and particularly not in an adolescent, since this will induce a hypoestrogenic state and predispose to osteoporosis. Opiate medications should be used with extreme caution since addiction is common. Psychiatric evaluation should be obtained when there is a reason, such as depression or a history of abuse. Trigger point injection is efficacious with fibromyalgia.

37.2 **C.** In cases of neuropathic pain, tricyclic antidepressant therapy can be helpful. Additionally, acupuncture has been shown to have efficacy in clinical trials.

37.3 **B.** This 16-year-old nulliparous female has primary dysmenorrhea, which is a condition with pain usually starting within 6 months of menarche. The mechanism is elevated prostaglandin F2 alpha levels, leading to intense uterine contractions, causing the pain with menses. The best treatment is NSAIDs, prostaglandin synthetase inhibitors which reduces the endogenous prostaglandin levels.

CLINICAL PEARLS

▶ Chronic pelvic pain is defined as lower abdominal or pelvic pain of 6 months' duration or more and leading to a significant debilitation.

▶ In approximately one-third of CPP patients, no etiology is found.

▶ Nongynecologic causes include GI, GU, psychological, and neuromuscular disorders.

▶ A history of depression, sexual abuse or trauma is important to seek when treating a patient with CPP.

▶ Primary dysmenorrhea is due to elevated endometrial prostaglandin F compounds leading to strong uterine contractions with menses.

▶ CPP which markedly worsens during menses suggests a gynecologic etiology.

▶ After a trial of NSAIDs and oral contraceptive, it is reasonable to consider laparoscopy to assess for endometriosis or pelvic adhesive disease.

REFERENCES

APGO. *Chronic Pelvic Pain: An Integrated Approach*. APGO Educational Series on Women's Health Issues. Washington, DC: APGO; January 2000.

APGO Medical Student Educational Objectives. 9th ed. *Educational Topic 39*; 2009:82-83.

Beckmann CRB, Ling FW, Barzansky BM, Herbert WNP, Laube DW, Smith RP, eds. *Obstetrics and Gynecology*. 6th ed. 2010, Chap. 30, 279-282.

Hacker NF, Gambone JC, Hobel CJ. *Hacker and Moore's Essentials of Obstetrics and Gynecology*. 5th ed. 2009, Chap. 21, 259-264.

Katz V, Lentz G, Lobo R, Gershenson D. *Comprehensive Gynecology*. 5th ed. 2007, Chap. 8.

CASE 38

An 18-year-old nulliparous woman complains of a vaginal discharge with a fishy odor over the past 2 weeks. She states that the odor is especially prominent after intercourse. Her last menstrual period was 3 weeks ago. She denies being treated for vaginitis or sexually transmitted diseases. She is in good health and takes no medications other than an oral contraceptive agent. On examination, her blood pressure (BP) is 110/70 mm Hg, heart rate (HR) is 80 beats per minute, and temperature is afebrile. The thyroid is normal to palpation. The heart and lung examinations are normal. Her breasts are Tanner stage V as is the pubic and axillary hair. The external genitalia are normal; the speculum examination reveals a homogeneous, white vaginal discharge and a fishy odor. No erythema or lesions of the vagina are noted.

▶ What is the most likely diagnosis?
▶ What is the best treatment for this condition?

ANSWERS TO CASE 38:
Bacterial Vaginosis

Summary: An 18-year-old nulliparous woman complains of a fishy vaginal discharge, which is worse after intercourse. The speculum examination reveals a homogeneous, white vaginal discharge and a fishy odor. No erythema or lesions of the vagina are noted.

- **Most likely diagnosis:** Bacterial vaginosis (BV).
- **Best treatment for this condition:** Metronidazole orally or vaginally; clindamycin is an alternative.

ANALYSIS
Objectives

1. Know the three common infectious causes of vaginitis or vaginosis, which are BV, Trichomoniasis, and *Candida vulvovaginitis*.
2. Know the diagnostic criteria for bacterial vaginosis.
3. Know the treatments for the corresponding causes of vaginitis and vaginosis.

Considerations

This 18-year-old woman complains of a vaginal discharge that has a fishy odor, which is the most common symptom of bacterial vaginosis. The discharge associated with BV has a typical white, homogenous vaginal coating, described as "spilled milk over the tissue." The pH is not given in this scenario, but it is likely alkaline. Although a whiff test was not performed with potassium hydroxide (KOH) in this patient, the worsening of the discharge after intercourse is presumably due to the alkaline semen. The vaginal epithelium is not erythematous or inflamed, which also fits with bacterial vaginosis. Of the three most common causes of infectious vaginal discharge (*Candida, Trichomonas,* and BV), bacterial vaginosis is the only etiology that is not inflammatory (hence the suffix "-osis" and not "-itis.") BV is a result of a predominance of anaerobic bacteria rather than a true infection. Therefore, antibiotic therapy targeting anaerobes, such as metronidazole or clindamycin, is appropriate.

APPROACH TO:
Vaginal Infections

DEFINITIONS
BACTERIAL VAGINOSIS: Condition of excessive anaerobic bacteria in the vagina, leading to a discharge that is alkaline.

CANDIDA VULVOVAGINITIS: Vaginal and/or vulvar infection caused by *Candida* species, usually with heterogeneous discharge and inflammation.

TRICHOMONAS VAGINITIS: Infection of the vagina caused by the protozoa *Trichomonas vaginalis*, usually associated with a frothy green discharge and intense inflammatory response.

CLINICAL APPROACH

The **three most common types of vaginal infections** are **bacterial vaginosis, trichomonal vaginitis,** and **candidal vulvovaginitis** (Table 38–1).

Bacterial vaginosis is not a true infection, but rather an overgrowth of anaerobic bacteria, which replaces the normal lactobacilli of the vagina. Although it may be sexually transmitted, this is not always the case. The most common symptom is a fishy or "musty" odor, often exacerbated by menses or intercourse. Since both of these situations introduce an alkaline substance, the vaginal pH is elevated above normal. The addition of 10% potassium hydroxide solution leads to the release of amines, causing a fishy odor (whiff test). There is no inflammatory reaction; hence, the patient will not complain of swelling or irritation, and typically, the microscopic examination does not usually reveal leukocytes. Microscopy of the discharge in normal saline (wet mount) typically shows clue cells (Figure 38–1), which are coccoid bacteria adherent to the external surfaces of epithelial cells. Three out of four Amsel's criteria are indicative of BV: (1) homogenous, gray–white discharge, (2) vaginal pH > 4.5, (3) positive whiff test, and (4) clue cells on wet mount. The Gram stain is considered the gold standard for diagnosing BV but is rarely performed clinically.

Bacterial vaginosis is associated with genital tract infections such as endometritis, pelvic inflammatory disease, and pregnancy complications such as preterm delivery and preterm premature rupture of membranes. Treatment includes oral or vaginal metronidazole. Patients should be instructed to avoid alcohol while taking metronidazole to avoid a disulfiram reaction. Clindamycin is another effective treatment.

Table 38–1 • CHARACTERISTICS OF VARIOUS VAGINAL INFECTIONS			
	Bacterial Vaginosis	**Trichomonal Vaginitis**	**Candidal Vulvovaginitis**
Appearance	Homogeneous, white discharge	Frothy, yellow to green	Curdy, lumpy
Vaginal pH	>4.5	>4.5	<4.5
Whiff test (fishy odor with KOH)	+	+	None
Microscopy	Clue cells (>20% of the cells seen)	Trichomonads	Pseudohyphae
Treatment	Metronidazole	Metronidazole	Oral fluconazole or imidazole cream

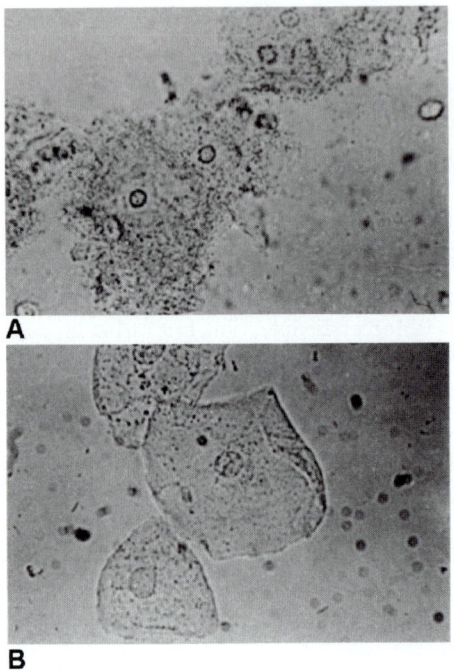

Figure 38–1. Vaginal epithelial "clue cells." Clue cells (**A**) with a granular appearance in contrast to normal cells (**B**). (Reproduced with permission from Kasper DL, et al. *Harrison's Principles of Internal Medicine*. 16th ed. New York, NY: McGraw-Hill; 2005:767.)

Trichomonas vaginalis is a single-cell anaerobic flagellated protozoan that induces an intense inflammatory reaction. It is a common sexually transmitted disease. *Trichomonas vaginalis* can survive for up to 6 hours on a wet surface. Aside from causing infection of the vagina, this organism can also inhabit the urethra or Skene's glands. The most common symptom associated with trichomoniasis is a profuse "frothy" yellow–green to gray vaginal discharge or vaginal irritation. Intense inflammation of the vagina or cervix may be noted, with the classic punctate lesions of the cervix (strawberry cervix). A fishy odor is also common with this disorder, which is somewhat exacerbated with KOH. Microscopy in saline will often display mobile, flagellated organisms. If the wet mount is cold or there are excess leukocytes present, the movement of the trichomonads may be inhibited. Nucleic acid amplification testing is more sensitive than wet mount microscopy. Optimal treatment consists of a fairly high dose of metronidazole (2 g orally) as a one-time dose, with the partner treated as well. Resistant cases may require the same dose every day for 7 days. A newer antiprotozoal agent, Tinidazole, has a similar dosing, side-effect profile, and contraindication for concurrent alcohol; due to its expense, its main role is for metronidazole-resistant cases. **Treatment usually does not include vaginal metronidazole because of low therapeutic levels in the urethra or Skene's glands where trichomonads may reside.**

Candidal vaginitis is usually caused by the fungus, *Candida albicans*, although other species may be causative. The lactobacilli in the vagina inhibit fungal growth;

thus, antibiotic therapy may decrease the lactobacilli concentration, leading to *Candida* overgrowth. Diabetes mellitus, which suppresses immune function, may also predispose patients to these infections. Candidiasis is usually not a sexually transmitted disease. The patient usually presents with intense vulvar or vaginal burning, irritation, and swelling. Dyspareunia (pain with intercourse) may also be a prominent complaint. The discharge usually appears curdy or like cottage cheese, in contrast to the homogenous discharge of bacterial vaginosis. Also, unlike the alkaline pH of BV and *Trichomonas* infection, the vaginal pH in candidiasis is typically normal (<4.5). The microscopic diagnosis is confirmed by identification of the hyphae or pseudohyphae after the discharge is mixed with potassium hydroxide. The KOH solution lyses the leukocytes and erythrocytes, making identification of the candidal organisms easier. Treatment includes oral fluconazole (Diflucan) or topical imidazoles, such as terconazole (Terazol), miconazole (Monistat), and clotrimazole (Lotrimin).

CASE CORRELATION

- See also Case 36 (Gonococcal Cervicitis) to understand the diagnostic approach of abnormal vaginal discharge and trying to discern a cervical versus a vaginal etiology.

COMPREHENSION QUESTIONS

38.1 An 18-year-old G0P0 adolescent female is being seen at the physician's office for vaginal discharge. A presumptive diagnosis of bacterial vaginosis is made. Which of the following is a finding consistent with BV?

A. pH less than 4.5
B. Frothy vaginal discharge
C. Predominance of anaerobes
D. Flagellated organisms

38.2 A 26-year-old woman completed a course of oral antibiotics for cystitis 1 week ago. She complains of a 1-day history of itching, burning, and a yellowish vaginal discharge. Which of the following is the best therapy?

A. Metronidazole
B. Erythromycin
C. Fluconazole
D. Hydrocortisone
E. Clindamycin

38.3 Which of the following organisms may be isolated from a wet surface 6 hours after inoculation?

A. *Candida albicans*
B. *Trichomonas vaginalis*
C. *Gardnerella* species
D. Peptostreptococci

38.4 A 27-year-old woman complains of a fishy odor and a vaginal discharge. The speculum examination reveals an erythematous vagina and punctuations of the cervix. Which of the following is the most likely treatment for this patient?

A. Oral fluconazole
B. Metronidazole gel applied vaginally
C. Metronidazole taken orally in a single dose
D. Intramuscular ceftriaxone and oral doxycycline

38.5 A 29-year-old woman has been treated for bacterial vaginosis and after 3 days of metronidazole, she notes abdominal discomfort, bloating, and diarrhea. Which of the following is most likely explanation?

A. Alcohol use
B. Clostridium difficile colitis
C. Medication side effect
D. Undiagnosed salpingitis

ANSWERS

38.1 **C.** There is a predominance of **anaerobes** in **bacterial vaginosis**. The vaginal pH in BV is usually >4.5, and the discharge is homogenous. The most common symptom is a **fishy or "musty" odor** when introduced to an alkaline substance (ie, 10% KOH, semen, or menses). **Clue cells** are found on microscopy. BV is associated with genital tract infection, such as endometritis, pelvic inflammatory disease, and pregnancy complications, such as preterm delivery and PPROM. Frothy discharge, normal to acidic pH, and flagellated organisms are more typical of trichomoniasis.

38.2 **C.** After **antibiotic therapy, candidal organisms** often **proliferate** and may induce an overt infection. The mechanism is likely that the lactobacilli are eliminated by the antibiotic, allowing overgrowth of yeast. Treatment of candidal vulvovaginitis is oral **fluconazole** or imidazole cream. **Metronidazole** is used to treat BV and *T. vaginalis*. Patients should be instructed to avoid alcohol while taking metronidazole to avoid a *disulfiram reaction*. **Erythromycin** may be used in the treatment of syphilis in nonpregnant women allergic to penicillin. **Clindamycin** is typically used in conjunction with gentamicin in the treatment of infections requiring broad-spectrum antibiotics, necessitating anaerobic coverage (ie, postpartum endomyometritis). Hydrocortisone is most commonly indicated for severe allergic reactions.

38.3 **B.** *Trichomonas vaginalis* is a hardy organism and may be isolated from a wet surface up to 6 hours after inoculation. The organism's difficulty to eradicate is the reason that therapy requires high tissue levels, metronidazole 2 g orally all at once, to be able to obtain sufficiently high tissue levels to be effective. Not uncommonly, a single course is not effective, and a 2- or 3-day course of metronidazole of high dose orally is needed.

38.4 **C.** The patient takes 2 g of metronidazole as a single dose to attain sufficient tissue levels to eradicate the trichomonads. Metronidazole gel is not as effective. Erythematous vagina and punctuations of the cervix (**strawberry cervix**) are classic findings of the inflammatory effects induced by trichomoniasis. Classic findings in candidal vaginitis include the curdy or cottage cheese appearance of the vaginal discharge with hyphae or pseudohyphae found on microscopy after discharge is mixed with KOH; this would be treated by fluconazole. HPV is associated with findings of cervical dysplasia. Ceftriaxone and doxycycline is the treatment for PID. Metronidazole gel would treat BV.

38.5 **C.** The most common side effects from metronidazole are gastrointestinal including nausea, abdominal discomfort, bloating or diarrhea. A disulfiram (Antabuse) effect that can be seen with metronidazole includes facial flushing, headache, hypotension, tachycardia, dizziness, and nausea and vomiting.

CLINICAL PEARLS

▶ The three most common types of vaginal infections are trichomoniasis, candidal vaginitis, and bacterial vaginosis.

▶ Both BV and trichomoniasis is associated with alkaline pH and positive whiff test.

▶ *Candidal vulvovaginitis* is a common infection in women who are pregnant, taking broad-spectrum antibiotics, diabetic, or immunocompromised.

▶ Bacterial vaginosis is associated with preterm delivery, postpartum endometritis, and pelvic inflammatory disease.

▶ *Trichomonal vaginitis* is associated with an intense inflammatory process and may induce punctuations of the cervix known as "strawberry cervix."

REFERENCES

American College of Obstetricians and Gynecologists. Vaginitis. *ACOG Practice Bulletin 72*. Washington, DC; 2006. (Reaffirmed 2015).

Amsel R, Totten PA, Spiegel CA, et al. Nonspecific vaginitis. Diagnostic criteria and microbial and epidemiologic associations. *Am J Med*. 1983;74:14-22.

Centers for Disease Control and Prevention (CDC). *Sexually-Transmitted Diseases Treatment Guidelines*; 2015. http://www.cdc.gov/std/tg2015/vaginal-discharge.htm; Accessed 30.06.15.

Eckert LO, Lentz GM. Infections of the lower and upper genital tracts. In: Lentz GM, Lobo RA, Gershenson DM, Katz VL, eds. *Comprehensive Gynecology*. 6th ed. Philadelphia, PA: Mosby; 2012: 531-539.

McGregor JA, Lench JB. Vulvovaginitis, sexually transmitted infections, and pelvic inflammatory disease. In: Hacker NF, Gambone JC, Hobel CJ, eds. *Essentials of Obstetrics and Gynecology*. 5th ed. Philadelphia, PA: Saunders; 2010:265-275.

Mohammadezadeh F, Dolatian M, Jorjani M, Alavi Majd H. Diagnostic value of Amsel's clinical criteria for diagnosis of bacterial vaginosis. *Global J Health Sci*. 2014;7(3):8-14.

CASE 39

A 31-year-old woman comes in for a well-woman examination. Her last menstrual period was 2 weeks ago. She has no significant past medical or surgical history. She denies having been treated for sexually transmitted diseases. On examination, her blood pressure (BP) is 130/70 mm Hg, heart rate (HR) is 70 beats per minute, and she is afebrile. Her thyroid is normal on palpation. Her heart and lung examinations are within normal limits. The abdomen is nontender and without masses. Examination of the external genitalia reveals a nontender, firm, ulcerated lesion approximately 1 cm in diameter, with raised borders and an indurated base located on the right labia majora. Bilateral inguinal lymph nodes are also noted that are nontender. Her pregnancy test is negative.

- What is the most likely diagnosis?
- What is your next step in diagnosis?
- What is the best therapy for this condition?

ANSWERS TO CASE 39:
Syphilitic Chancre

Summary: A 31-year-old woman who comes in for a well-woman examination is noted to have a nontender, firm, 1-cm ulcerated lesion of the vulva; it has raised borders and an indurated base. She also has bilateral, nontender inguinal lymphadenopathy.

- **Most likely diagnosis:** Syphilis (primary chancre).
- **Next step in diagnosis:** Syphilis serology (rapid plasma reagin [RPR] or Venereal Disease Research Laboratory [VDRL]) and, if negative, darkfield microscopy.
- **Best therapy for this condition:** Intramuscular penicillin.

ANALYSIS
Objectives

1. Know the classic appearance and presentation of the chancre lesion of primary syphilis.
2. Know that penicillin is the treatment of choice for syphilis.
3. Understand that the antibody tests (VDRL or RPR) may not yet turn positive with early syphilitic disease and that darkfield microscopy would then be the diagnostic test of choice.

Considerations

This 31-year-old woman came in for a well-woman examination. It was unexpected to find the lesion in the vulvar area. The patient denies any history of sexually transmitted diseases. Nevertheless, she has the classic lesion of primary syphilis, the painless chancre. It is typically a nontender reddish ulcer with clean-appearing edges, often accompanied by painless inguinal adenopathy. Painful ulcers are typically associated with herpes simplex virus (HSV). Because exam findings are variable, specific tests for evaluation of genital ulcers include (1) syphilis serology and darkfield examination, (2) culture for HSV orpolymerase chain reaction (PCR) testing for HSV, and (3) serologic testing for type-specific HSV antibody. Occasionally, the patient will have a negative nontreponemal test in the setting of primary syphilis. Primary syphilis usually manifests itself within 2 to 6 weeks after inoculation. The treatment for syphilis, that is less than 1-year duration, is one injection of long-acting penicillin. If this patient were older, for instance, in her postmenopausal years, squamous cell carcinoma of the vulva would be considered.

APPROACH TO:
Infectious Vulvar Ulcers

DEFINITIONS

NONTREPONEMAL TESTS: Nonspecific antitreponemal antibody tests, such as VDRL or RPR tests. These titers will fall with effective treatment.

SPECIFIC SEROLOGIC TESTS: Antibody tests that are directed against the treponemal organism such as the TP-PA (*Treponema pallidum* particle agglutination assay), MHA-TP (micro hemagglutinin antibody against *Treponema pallidum*) and FTA-ABS (fluorescent-labeled treponemal antibody absorption) tests. These tests will remain **positive for life** after infection.

CLINICAL APPROACH

The **two most common infectious causes of vulvar ulcers** in the United States are **herpes simplex virus and syphilis**, with chancroid being much less common. However, the differential diagnosis is complicated and can include trauma, other viral infections such as human immunodeficiency virus (HIV) or primary Epstein Barr virus (EBV) infection. Systemic diseases such as Behcet's disease, Candida infection, or vulvar neoplasms should also be considered. Biopsy of the lesion is often helpful. A careful history and physical queries about travel, contacts, prior STIs, drug use, possibly allergic reactions, and other systemic or autoimmune symptoms are important. If the clinical assessment is not revealing, then a reasonable diagnostic approach would be:

- Step 1: Assess for HSV (PCR or culture or lesion, and type-specific serology) and syphilis.
- Step 2: If negative, consider darkfield microscopy (biopsy may be needed).
- Step 3: If negative, assess for Candida, HIV, and EBV.
- Step 4: If negative, then reassess based on the wide differential diagnosis; biopsy may be helpful.

Herpes Simplex Virus

Genital herpes is a recurrent sexually transmitted infection (STI) for which there is no cure. It is the most prevalent STI in the United States. This organism is highly contagious, and it is thought that 20% of women in their child bearing years are infected. There are two types of herpes viruses, HSV type 1 and type 2. Approximately 50% of new genital infections, particularly in young women, are due to HSV-1. Recurrence is greater with HSV type 2. The primary episode is usually a systemic as well as local disease, with the woman often complaining of fever or general malaise. Local infection typically induces paresthesias before vesicles erupt on a red base. After the primary episode, the recurrent disease is local, with less severe symptoms. The recurrent herpes ulcers are small and superficial, and do not usually scar. The gold standard diagnostic test is viral culture, but polymerase chain reaction tests are increasingly used because they are more sensitive. Rarely, HSV infections may be severe enough to warrant hospitalization, such as those with encephalopathy or urinary retention. Oral acyclovir is effective in suppressing frequent recurrences.

Syphilis

Syphilis, caused by the bacteria *T. pallidum*, may induce a chronic infection. Infections occur rarely in the United States and tend to be concentrated in southern regions. The organism is extremely tightly wound, and too thin to be seen on light microscopy. The typical incubation period is 10 to 90 days. The disease can be divided into **primary, secondary, latent, and tertiary stages.** Primary syphilis classically presents as the **indurated, nontender chancre.** The ulcer usually arises 3 weeks after exposure and disappears spontaneously after 2 to 6 weeks without therapy. Nontreponemal tests (such as the RPR or VDRL) sometimes are not positive with the appearance of the chancre. **Darkfield** microscopy is an accepted diagnostic tool, but is limited in availability. **Secondary syphilis** is usually systemic, occurring about 9 weeks after the primary chancre. The classic macular papular rash may occur anywhere on the body, but usually on the palms and soles of the feet. Flat moist lesions called condylomatalata may be seen on the vulva (Figure 39–1), and have a high concentration of spirochetes. Treponemal and nontreponemal serologic tests are positive at this stage. Because nontreponemal tests can be falsely positive, a positive treponemal test is required to make a serologic diagnosis.

Latency of varying duration occurs after secondary disease; latency is subdivided into **early latent** (<1 year in duration), or **late latent** (>1 year). If untreated, about one-third of women may progress to tertiary syphilis, which may affect the cardiovascular system or central nervous system. Optic atrophy, tabes dorsalis, and aortic aneurysms are some of the manifestations. Penicillin G is the treatment of choice for all stages of syphilis. Because of the long replication time, prolonged therapy is required. **One injection** of long-acting benzathine penicillin G 2.4 million units intramuscularly is standard treatment for early disease (primary, secondary, and latent up to 1 year of duration). Patients with late-latent syphilis (>1 year) should be treated with a total of 7.2 million units intramuscularly divided as 2.4 million units every week for a total of three courses (Table 39–1). In pregnancy, penicillin is the only known effective treatment to prevent or treat congenital syphilis. The effectiveness of alternatives to penicillin in the treatment of early and latent syphilis has not been well documented. Treatment of nonpregnant penicillin-allergic women with doxycycline or tetracycline may be considered.

Neurosyphilis requires more intensive therapy, usually intravenous penicillin.

After therapy, clinical and serologic assessment should be performed at 6 and 12 months after treatment for early syphilis and additionally at 24 months after treating late latent or syphilis of unknown duration. An appropriate response is a four-fold fall in titers in 6 to 12 months, 12 to 24 months for late-latent syphilis. When the titer does not fall appropriately, one possible etiology is neurosyphilis, which may be diagnosed by lumbar puncture.

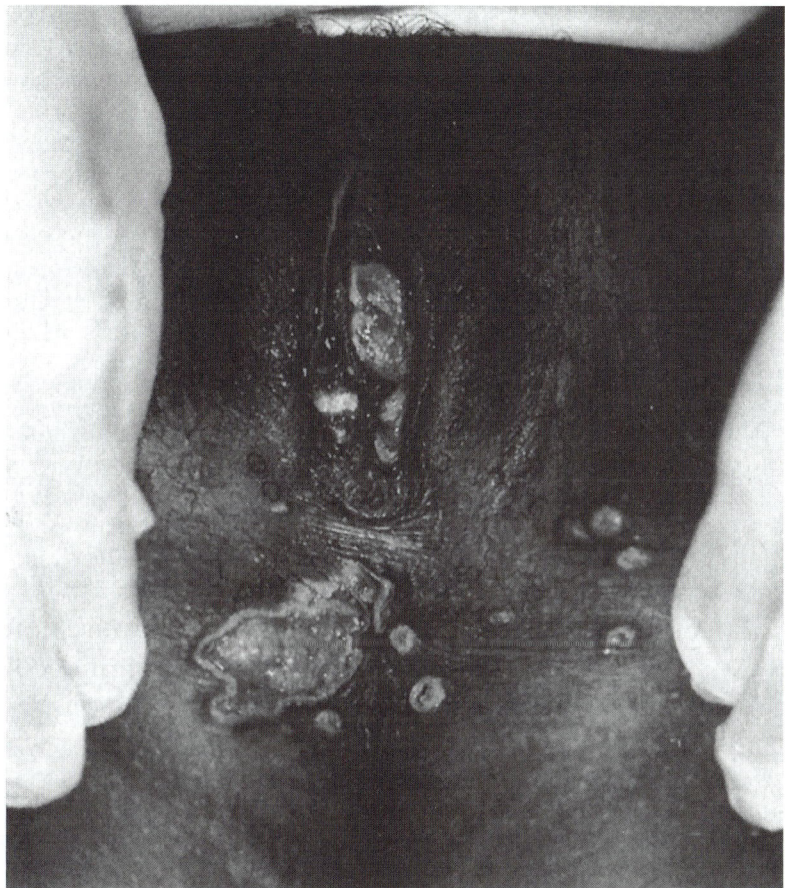

Figure 39–1. Genital condylomalata of secondary syphilis.(*Reproduced with permission from Cunningham FG, et al. Williams Obstetrics. 21st ed. New York, NY:McGraw-Hill; 2001:1487.*)

Chancroid

Chancroid is a sexually transmitted disease, usually manifesting a soft, painful ulcer of the vulva. Although common worldwide, it is very rare in the United States. It is more common in males than in females. The typical ulcer is tender, with ragged edges on a necrotic base. Tender lymphadenopathy may also coexist with these infections. The etiologic organism is *Haemophilusducreyi*, a small gram-negative

Table 39–1 • TREATMENT OF SYPHILIS	
Duration	Treatment
Primary, secondary, early latent	Benzathine penicillin G 2.4 million units IM
Late latent or unknown duration	Benzathine penicillin G 2.4 million units IM every week × 3 doses

rod. Gram stain usually reveals the classic "school of fish." After ruling out syphilis and herpes, chancroid should be suspected. Biopsy and/or culture help to establish the diagnosis. Treatment includes oral azithromycin or intramuscular ceftriaxone.

Lymphogranuloma Venereum

Lymphogranuloma Venereum (LGV) is caused by *Chlamydia trachomatis* subtypes L1, L2, or L3, and causes a painless papule or shallow ulceration/erosion (primary LGV). After 10 to 30 days following exposure, secondary LGV may lead to buboes (grossly enlarged tender nodes), and can lead to the "groove sign," separation of the lymph nodes by the inguinal ligament. The diagnosis is confirmed via culture although LGV titers can be helpful. The treatment is doxycycline.

Granuloma Inguinale (GI)

GI is a chronic bacterial infection characterized by intracellular inclusions in macrophages referred to as Donovan bodies. The organism is now called Klebsiellagranulomatis, a Gram-negative pleomorphic bacillus. Large painless ulcerative lesions of the mucus membranes is the typical presentation, usually without lymphadenopathy. The lesions are usually beefy red, and bleed easily. The diagnosis is confirmed with culture or smear for Donovan bodies.Treatment is by doxycycline or trimethroprim/sulfa.

COMPREHENSION QUESTIONS

39.1 A 19-year-old woman is noted to have an RPR titer of 1:16, and the confirmatory (TP-PA) test is positive. She had no history of syphilis. She is treated with benzathine penicillin G 2.4 million units intramuscularly. Six months after therapy, she is noted to have an RPR titer of 1:2. At 12 months, the titer is 1:1. Two months later, the repeat RPR is noted to be 1:32. Which of the following is the most likely diagnosis?

A. Resistant organism
B. Inadequately treated syphilis
C. Laboratory error
D. Reinfection
E. Systemic lupus erythematosus

39.2 Which of the following statements about *Tpallidum* is correct?

A. It is a protozoan.
B. Gram stain is a very sensitive method of diagnosis.
C. The spirochete does not cross the placenta during pregnancy.
D. Penicillin G is the recommended treatment for all stages of syphilis in nonpregnant women.

39.3 An 18-year-old G1P0 at 14 weeks' gestation is noted to have a positive RPR with a positive confirmatory MHA-TP test. The patient states that she is allergic to penicillin, with hives and swelling of the tongue and throat in the past. Which of the following is the most appropriate next step?

A. Desensitize and treat with penicillin
B. Oral erythromycin
C. Oral doxycycline
D. Pretreat with prednisone, then administer penicillin
E. Intramuscular ceftriaxone

39.4 A 29-year-old woman was diagnosed with syphilis. She is noted to have a persistently elevated RPR titer of 1:32, despite treatment with benzathine penicillin G 2.4 million units each week for a total of 3 weeks. She complains of slight dizziness and a clumsy gait of 6 months duration. Which of the following is the best test to diagnose neurosyphilis?

A. Plain x-ray films of the skull
B. Electroencephalograph (EEG)
C. CT scan of the head
D. Lumbar puncture
E. Psychiatric evaluation

39.5 A 35-year-old woman is seen for a "sore in the groin area" for an 8-day duration. On examination, she is noted to have a tender fluctuant mass which appears above and below the right inguinal ligament. Which of the following is the best treatment?

A. Acyclovir
B. Ceftriaxone
C. Doxycycline
D. Trimethroprim/sulfa
E. Penicillin

ANSWERS

39.1 **D.** When RPR titers fall in response to therapy and then suddenly rise, the most likely scenario is **reinfection**. It is not uncommon, for individuals with systemic lupus erythematosus to have a positive RPR, but they would not have a positive treponemal test without syphilis infection. Syphilis has not been noted to be resistant to penicillin.

39.2 **D.** Penicillin G is the recommended treatment for all stages of syphilis and data regarding effectiveness of alternatives to treatment for penicillin-allergic patients are limited. Syphilis is a bacteria and not a protozoan. It is very thin and tightly wound and therefore not visible on light microscopy. Transplacental infection during pregnancy is an important cause of congenital syphilis.

39.3 **A. Penicillin is the best treatment of syphilis in pregnancy.** When a pregnant woman with syphilis is allergic to penicillin, she should undergo desensitization and receive penicillin. Penicillin is the only known effective treatment for preventing congenital syphilis. Doxycycline use may lead to discoloration of the child's teeth, and erythromycin has not been shown to be an effective treatment in treating an infected fetus.

39.4 **D.** Typically, after a patient undergoes therapy for syphilis and their RPR titer does not fall appropriately, one possible etiology is **neurosyphilis**, which may be diagnosed by lumbar puncture. The classic examination of neurosyphilis is unsteady balance and Argyll Robertson pupils. Cerebrospinal fluid for RPR may point toward neurosyphilis, although there is no definitive test. Neurosyphilis requires more intensive therapy such as prolonged IV penicillin.

39.5 **C.** This is a description of the secondary stage of LGV, caused by Chlamydia trachomatis. The primary stage is a painless lesion (papule) which usually only appears for a few days, followed by unilateral painful inguinal adenopathy (secondary stage) usually occurring 30 to 60 days after infection. These can be fluctuant and even sometimes rupture. Because they grow cephalad and caudad to the inguinal ligament, there is the so called "groove sign" in which the inguinal ligament forms a groove in the lymphatic mass. The best treatment is doxycycline. Herpes is treated with acyclovir; gonorrhea is treated with ceftriaxone; and granuloma inguinale is treated with doxycycline or trimethroprim/sulfa.

CLINICAL PEARLS

► Syphilis of less than 1-year duration can be treated with a single intramuscular course of penicillin G; infection of greater than 1-year duration is treated by three courses of penicillin G at 1-week intervals.

► The nontender ulcer with indurated edges is typical of the chancre of primary syphilis. Darkfield examination and serologic testing is warranted.

► The best treatment for syphilis in pregnancy is penicillin.

► Pregnant women with syphilis and an allergy to penicillin should undergo penicillin desensitization and then receive penicillin.

► The most common infectious vulvar ulcers in the United States are herpes simplex virus and syphilis, and much less common is chancroid.

REFERENCES

Centers for Disease Control and Prevention. Sexually transmitted diseases treatment guidelines, 2010. *MMWR* 2010;59(RR-12):18-36.

Eckert LO, Lentz GM. Infections of the lower genital tract. In: Katz VL, Lentz GM, Lobo RA, Gersenson DM, eds. *Comprehensive Gynecology*. 5th ed. St. Louis, MO: Mosby-Year Book; 2007:569-606.

McGregor JA, Lench JB. Vulvovaginitis, sexually transmitted infections, and pelvic inflammatory disease sepsis. In: Hacker NF, Gambone JC, Hobel CJ, eds. *Essentials of Obstetrics and Gynecology*. 5th ed. Philadelphia, PA: Saunders; 2009:265-275.

CASE 40

A 29-year-old woman complains of a 2-day history of dysuria, urgency, and urinary frequency. She denies the use of medications and has no significant past medical history. On examination, her blood pressure (BP) is 100/70 mm Hg, heart rate (HR) is 90 beats per minute, and temperature is 98°F (36.6°C). The thyroid is normal on palpation. The heart and lung examinations are normal. She does not have back tenderness. The abdomen is nontender and without masses. The pelvic examination reveals normal female genitalia. There is no adnexal tenderness or masses.

- ▶ What is the most likely diagnosis?
- ▶ What is the next step in the diagnosis?
- ▶ What is the most likely etiology of the condition?

ANSWERS TO CASE 40:
Urinary Tract Infection (Cystitis)

Summary: A 29-year-old woman complains of a 2-day history of dysuria, urgency, and urinary frequency. Her temperature is 98°F (36.6°C). She does not have back tenderness. The abdomen is nontender and without masses. The pelvic examination is normal.

- **Most likely diagnosis:** Simple cystitis (bladder infection).
- **Next step in the diagnosis:** Urinalysis and/or urine culture.
- **Most likely etiology of the condition:** *Escherichia coli*.

ANALYSIS
Objectives

1. Recognize the symptoms of a urinary tract infection (cystitis).
2. Recall that the most common bacteria causing cystitis is *E. coli*.
3. Identify the evidence-based antibiotic therapies for cystitis.

Considerations

This 29-year-old woman has a 2-day history of urinary urgency, frequency, and dysuria, all of which are very typical symptoms of a lower urinary tract infection. Because she does not have fever or flank tenderness, she most likely has a bladder infection or simple cystitis. Other symptoms of cystitis may include hesitancy or hematuria (hemorrhagic cystitis). Urinalysis and/or urine culture and sensitivity (if antimicrobial resistance/complicated infection is suspected) would be the most appropriate test to confirm the diagnosis. Since *E. coli* is the most common etiologic agent, the empiric antibiotic treatment should be aimed at this organism. **Current evidence suggests a 3-day course of trimethoprim/sulfa (Bactrim) as the best agent for uncomplicated cystitis**, unless bacteriology patterns in the community point to resistance; in that case, a quinolone such as ciprofloxacin twice daily for 3 days is effective. If the urine culture demonstrates no growth of organisms and the patient still has symptoms, urethritis is a possibility (often caused by *Chlamydia trachomatis*). In this setting, urethral swabbing for chlamydial testing is advisable. Another possibility is candidalvulvovaginitis. Finally, some women with symptoms of bladder discomfort with persistently negative urine and urethral culture may have a chronic condition of urethral syndrome.

APPROACH TO:
Urinary Tract Infections

DEFINITIONS

CYSTITIS: Bacterial infection of the bladder defined as having greater than 100 000 colony-forming units of a single pathogenic organism on a midstream-voided specimen.

URETHRITIS: Infection of the urethra commonly caused by C. trachomatis.

URETHRAL SYNDROME: Recurrent episodes of urgency and dysuria caused by urethral inflammation of unknown etiology; urine cultures are persistently negative.

CLINICAL APPROACH

Urinary tract infections (UTI) may involve the kidneys (pyelonephritis), bladder (cystitis), and urethra (urethritis). More than one half of all women will acquire a UTI in their lifetime. The most commonly stated reason for the increased incidence of UTIs in women is the shorter length of the female urethra and its increased proximity to the rectum. Pregnancy further predisposes women to UTIs due to incomplete emptying of the bladder (urinary stasis), ureteral obstruction by the gravid uterus, and immune suppression. Causative bacteria include E. coli (isolated 80% of the time) followed by *Enterobacter, Klebsiella, Pseudomonas, Proteus,* group B streptococcus, *Staphylococcus saprophyticus,* and *Chlamydia.*

The most common symptoms of lower tract infection (cystitis) are dysuria, urgency, and urinary frequency. Occasionally, the infection may induce a hemorrhagic cystitis and the patient will have gross hematuria. Nevertheless, **gross hematuria should raise the suspicion of nephrolithiasis.** Fever is uncommon unless there is upper urinary tract/kidney involvement, which is usually reflected by flank tenderness. The diagnosis of cystitis hinges on identification of pathogenic bacteria in the urine; bacteriuria is defined as >100 000 colony-forming units per milliliter of a single uropathogen obtained from a midstream-voided clean catch urine culture. In symptomatic patients, as few as 1000 colony-forming units per milliliter may be significant. On a catheterized specimen, 10 000 colony-forming units per milliliter is considered bacteriuria. The presence of leukocytes in the urine (pyuria) is presumptive evidence of infection in a patient with symptoms.

Simple cystitis is the most common form of UTI and is diagnosed by the lower urinary tract symptoms in the absence of fever or flank tenderness. Oral antimicrobial therapy is effective, and varies from one dose to 3 days, to 7 days, or even 10 days. Trimethoprim/sulfa (Bactrim), nitrofurantoin, ciprofloxacin, norfloxacin, and fosfomycin are effective. Ampicillin and cephalosporins are generally *not* used as first-line agents due to the widespread resistance of common uropathogens. **However, current evidence points to a 3-day course of trimethorprim/sulfa as the treatment of choice for uncomplicated cystits.** The utility of urine cultures in the first episode of simple cystitis is unclear. Some practitioners will routinely obtain cultures, whereas others will reserve these studies for recurrences, persistent symptoms, or in pregnancy. In the pregnant woman, **asymptomatic bacteriuria (ASB) leads to acute infection in up to 25% of untreated women, and thus it should always be treated.**

A patient with *urethritis* has similar complaints to one with cystitis (ie, urgency, frequency, and dysuria). Sometimes, the urethra may be tender on palpation and purulent drainage expressed on examination. The most commonly isolated organisms are *Chlamydia, Gonococcus,* and *Trichomonas.* Urethritis should be suspected in a woman with typical symptoms of UTI, yet with no growth in culture (sterile pyuria) and no response to the standard antibiotics. Gram stain and cultures of the urethra for *Gonococcus* and *Chlamydia* should be performed, with reflex confirmatory nucleic acid amplification testing (NAAT). Treatment may be initiated empirically for *Chlamydia* with doxycycline; if *Neisseriagonorrhea* is suspected, intramuscular ceftriaxone with oral doxycycline is usually curative. Azithromycin should be substituted for doxycycline in pregnant women.

Women with *pyelonephritis* usually present with fever, chills, flank pain, nausea, and vomiting. Mild cases in the nonpregnant female may be treated with oral trimethoprim/sulfa or a fluoroquinolone for a 14-day course; these women should be re-examined within 48 to 72 hours. Sulfa agents are generally the most cost-effective. Those who do not begin clinically improving, are more toxic, unable to take oral medications, pregnant, or immunocompromised should be hospitalized and treated with intravenous antibiotics, such as ampicillin and gentamicin, 3rd gen cephalosporins such as ceftriaxone, intravenous fluroquinolones, a carbapenem, or piperacillin-tazobactam. Following resolution of fever and symptoms, pregnant women with acute pyelonephritis warrant suppressive antimicrobial therapy (such as nitrofurantoin macrocrystals 100 mg once daily) for the remainder of pregnancy.

CASE CORRELATION

- See also Case 23 (Pyelonephritis) to understand the different presentation of a lower urinary tract infection (frequency, urgency, dysuria) versus upper urinary tract process (flank tenderness, fever).

COMPREHENSION QUESTIONS

40.1 A 29-year-old G1P0 at 19 weeks' gestation is noted to have dysuria, urinary frequency, and urgency. A urine culture is performed, and growth is noted, which the microbiology laboratory notes as not *E. coli*. Which of the following is the most likely causative organism of cystitis?

A. *Chlamydia trachomatis*

B. *Klebsiella* species

C. *Peptostreptococcus*

D. *Bacteroides* species

40.2 A 19-year-old G2P1 woman at 13 weeks' gestation comes in for her first prenatal visit. Among other tests, a urine culture is performed showing 100 000 cfu/mL of *E. coli*. The patient has no symptoms, and has not had pyelonephritis, dysuria, or fever. Which of the following is best next step for this patient?

A. Observation, as no therapy is needed
B. No therapy needed unless the patient develops symptoms
C. Initiation of antibiotic therapy
D. No therapy needed at this time, but antibiotics should be given during labor

40.3 A 30-year-old G1P0 woman at 29 weeks' gestation is noted to have a urinary tract infection with 100 000 cfu/mL of *E. coli* growing on culture. Her obstetrician notes that an upper urinary tract infection leads to increased complications. Which of the following is a common manifestation of upper urinary tract infection rather than simple cystitis?

A. Fever
B. Urgency
C. Hesitancy
D. Dysuria

ANSWERS

40.1 **B.** The most common cause of UTIs in women is *E. coli*. Other causes include *Enterobacter*, *Klebsiella*, *Pseudomonas*, and *Proteus*. *Chlamydia trachomatis* is a common cause of urethritis along with *Gonococcus* and *Trichomonas*. *Peptostreptococcus* is a Gram-positive anaerobe that is a commensal organism with humans and usually does not cause pathology except in immunosuppressed individuals. Along with *Peptostreptococcus*, *Bacteroides* species live as gut flora in humans. *Bacteroides* is a Gram-negative anaerobe and, along with other anaerobes, rarely causes cystitis.

40.2 **C.** This patient has asymptomatic bacteriuria, which should be treated even without symptoms. If untreated, the patient has a 25% risk of developing pyelonephritis during the pregnancy. Asymptomatic bacteriuria (ASB) complicates approximately 8% to 10% of pregnant patients. Providing treatment of ASB at the first prenatal visit reduces the risk of pyelonephritis markedly.

40.3 **A.** Upper UTIs (including pyelonephritis) usually present with fever, costovertebral tenderness, chills, malaise, and often ill-appearing individual. They are at increased risk for septicemia, kidney dysfunction, or preterm labor. In severe cases, the patient should be hospitalized and started on intravenous antibiotics. Presenting symptoms of urgency, hesitancy, and dysuria are symptoms for a simple cystitis or urethritis. Urethritis can be differentiated from cystitis by a sterile culture and no response to antibiotics. Doxycycline (covers *Chlamydia*) with ceftriaxone (gonorrhea) is a good choice for suspected urethritis. Doxycycline should be avoided in pregnant women.

CLINICAL PEARLS

► The most common cause of uncomplicated cystitis is *E. coli*.

► For uncomplicated cystitis, a 3-day course of trimethoprim/sulfa is the treatment of choice.

► Complicated UTI's such as bladder retention, frequent infections, or indwelling catheters necessitate a longer course and perhaps a different antimicrobial agent.

► Bacteriuria caused by group B streptococcus in pregnancy necessitates the use of intravenous penicillin or ampicillin in labor to decrease the risk of neonatal GBS sepsis.

► Clinical features of pyelonephritis are flank tenderness and fever.

► Urethritis, commonly caused by *Chlamydia* or *N. gonorrhea*, should be suspected with negative urine cultures and symptoms of UTI.

► Asymptomatic bacteriuria has a high incidence in women with sickle cell trait.

REFERENCES

American College of Obstetricians and Gynecologists. Treatment of urinary tract infections in nonpregnant women. *ACOG Practice Bulletin 91*. Washington, DC; 2012.

Gupta, et al. International clinical practice guidelines for the treatment of acute uncomplicated cystitis and pyelonephritis in women. *Clin Infect Dis*. 2013;52(5):e103-e120.

CASE 41

A 40-year-old G5P5 woman complains of heavy vaginal bleeding with clots of 2-year duration. She denies bleeding or spotting between periods. She states that several years ago a doctor had told her that her uterus was enlarged. Her records indicate that 1 year ago she underwent a uterine dilation and curettage, with the tissue showing benign pathology. She denies fatigue, cold intolerance, or galactorrhea. She takes ibuprofen without relief of her vaginal bleeding. On examination, her blood pressure (BP) is 135/80 mm Hg, heart rate (HR) is 80 beats per minute (bpm), weight is 140 lb, and temperature is 98°F (36.6°C). The heart and lung examinations are normal. The abdomen reveals a lower abdominal midline irregular mass. On pelvic examination, the cervix is anteriorly displaced. An irregular midline mass approximately 18 weeks' size seems to move in conjunction with the cervix. No adnexal masses are palpated. Her pregnancy test is negative. Her hemoglobin level is 9.0 g/dL, leukocyte count is 6,000/mm^3, and platelet count is 160,000/mm^3.

▶ What is the most likely diagnosis?
▶ What is your next step?

ANSWERS TO CASE 41:
Uterine Leiomyomata

Summary: A 40-year-old G5P5 woman with a history of an enlarged uterus complains of menorrhagia and anemia despite ibuprofen. A prior uterine dilation and curettage showed benign pathology. Examination reveals an irregular midline mass approximately 18 weeks' size that is seemingly contiguous with the cervix, and there is an anteriorly displaced cervix.

- **Most likely diagnosis:** Symptomatic uterine leiomyomata.
- **Next step:** Offer the patient a hysterectomy.

ANALYSIS
Objectives

1. Understand that the most common reason for hysterectomy in the United States is symptomatic uterine fibroids.
2. Know that hysterectomy is generally reserved for women with symptomatic uterine fibroids that are refractory to an adequate trial of medical therapy.
3. Know that menorrhagia is the most common symptom of uterine leiomyomata.

Considerations

This 40-year-old woman complains of menorrhagia. The physical examination is consistent with uterine fibroids, because of the enlarged midline mass that is irregular and contiguous with the cervix. If the mass were lateral or moved apart from the cervix, another type of pelvic mass, such as ovarian, would be suspected. This patient complains of menorrhagia (excessive bleeding during menses), the most common symptom of uterine fibroids. If she had intermenstrual bleeding, the clinician would have to consider other diseases, such as endometrial hyperplasia, endometrial polyp, or uterine cancer, in addition to the uterine leiomyomata. Irregular cycles (menometrorrhagia) may suggest an anovulatory process. The patient has anemia despite medical therapy, constituting the indication for intervention, such as hysterectomy. If the uterus were smaller, consideration may be given toward another medical agent, such as medroxyprogesterone acetate (Provera). Also, a gonadotropin-releasing hormone (GnRH) agonist can be used to shrink the fibroids temporarily, to correct the anemia, or make the surgery easier. The maximum shrinkage of fibroids is usually seen after 3 months of GnRH agonist therapy. After the GnRH agonist is stopped, the fibroids would regrow.

APPROACH TO:
Suspected Uterine Leiomyomata

DEFINITIONS

LEIOMYOMATA: Benign, smooth muscle tumors, usually of the uterus.

LEIOMYOSARCOMA: Malignant, smooth muscle tumor, with numerous mitoses.

SUBMUCOSAL FIBROID: Leiomyomata that are primarily on the endometrial side of the uterus and protrude into the uterine cavity (Figure 41–1).

INTRAMURAL FIBROID: Leiomyomata that are primarily in the uterine muscle.

SUBSEROSAL FIBROID: Leiomyomata that are primarily on the outside of the uterus, on the serosal surface. Physical examination may reveal a "knobby" sensation.

PEDUNCULATED FIBROID: Leiomyoma that is on a stalk.

CARNEOUS DEGENERATION: Changes of the leiomyomata due to rapid growth; the center of the fibroid becomes red, causing pain. This is synonymous with red degeneration.

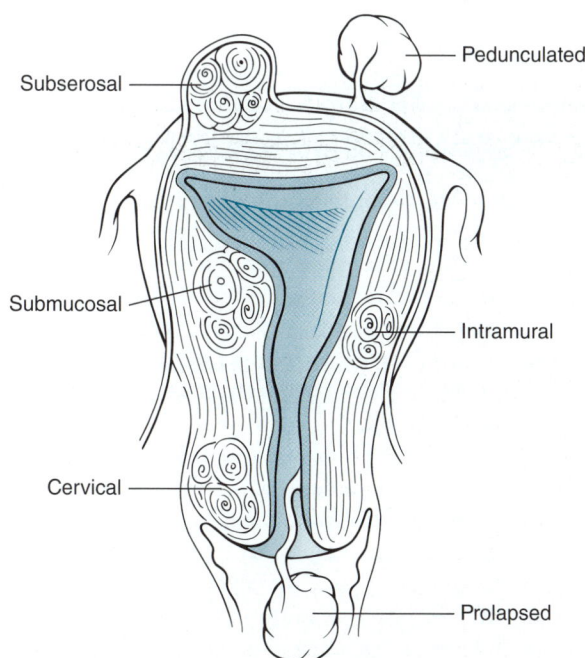

Figure 41–1. Uterine leiomyomata. Various uterine leiomyomata are depicted based on their location in the uterus.

CLINICAL APPROACH

Evaluation

Uterine leiomyomata are the most common tumors of the pelvis and the leading indication for hysterectomy in the United States. They occur in up to 25% of women, and have a variety of clinical presentations. The most common clinical manifestation is menorrhagia, or excessive bleeding during menses. The exact mechanism is unclear and may be due to an **increased endometrial surface area** or the **disruption of hemostatic mechanisms during menses** by the fibroids. Another speculated explanation is **ulceration** of the submucosal fibroid surfaces.

Many uterine fibroids are asymptomatic and only need to be monitored. Very rarely, uterine leiomyomata degenerate into leiomyosarcoma. Some signs of this process include rapid growth, such as an increase of more than 6 weeks' gestational size in 1 year. A history of radiation to the pelvis is a risk factor.

If the uterine leiomyomata are sufficiently large, patients may also complain of pressure to the pelvis, bladder, or rectum. Rarely, the uterine fibroid on a pedicle may twist, leading to necrosis and pain. Also, a submucous leiomyomata can prolapse through the cervix, leading to labor-like uterine contraction pain.

The physical examination typical of uterine leiomyomata is an irregular, midline, firm, nontender mass that moves contiguously with the cervix. This presentation is approximately 95% accurate. Most of the time, ultrasound examination is performed to confirm the diagnosis. Lateral, fixed, or fluctuant masses are not typical for fibroids. The differential diagnosis includes ovarian masses, tubo-ovarian masses, pelvic kidney, and endometrioma. Significant menorrhagia often leads to anemia.

Treatment

The initial treatment of uterine fibroids is pharmacological, such as with nonsteroidal anti-inflammatory agents or progestin therapy. Gonadotropin-releasing hormone agonists lead to a decrease in uterine fibroid size, reaching its maximal effect in 3 months. After the discontinuation of this agent, the leiomyomata usually regrow to the pretreatment size. Thus, GnRH agonist therapy is reserved for tumor shrinkage or correction of anemia prior to operative treatment. Other treatments include the levonorgestrel intrauterine device (IUD), selective progesterone receptor antagonists, or oral contraceptives. Notably, **the levonorgestrel IUD can be used for women with uterine fibroids without marked distortion of the uterine cavity.** With intracavitary (submucosal) uterine fibroids, hysteroscopic resection is the best conservative treatment option.

Hysterectomy is considered the proven treatment for symptomatic uterine fibroids when future pregnancy is undesired. The indication for surgery is persistent symptoms despite medical therapy. **Myomectomy** is still considered the procedure of choice for women with symptomatic uterine leiomyomata who desire pregnancy. One in four women who undergo myomectomy will require a hysterectomy in the following 20 years. Myomectomy can be accomplished through several approaches including hysteroscopic, open abdominal, laparoscopic and robotically. Advantages to robotic-assisted laparoscopic myomectomy include decreased intraoperative blood loss, shorter hospital stays; however, the technique incurs higher cost and greater intraoperative time. Myomectomy is not indicated in women who have uterine fibroids unless there have been pregnancy complications due to uterine fibroids in the past.

Uterine artery embolization is a technique performed by cannulizing the femoral artery and catheterizing both uterine arteries directly, and infusing embolization particles that preferentially float to the fibroid vessels. Fibroid infarction and subsequent hyalinization and fibrosis result. Short-term results appear promising; initial studies with follow-up over 5 years show symptom relief for approximately 75% of patients. This intervention should not be used in women who want to get pregnant in the future since there is an increased risk of placentation abnormalities. Very large uteri (>20 weeks size) or very large fibroids may not respond as well; also, submucosal fibroids may cause bleeding, pain, cramping, and expulsion which can be unpleasant for the patient. Pregnancy, a suspected gynecologic malignancy, history of PID, or renal failure are contraindications to the procedure.

Recent Advances

In 2014, the FDA issued a warning on the use of laparoscopic power morcellation during hysterectomy or myomectomy for women with suspected uterine fibroids due to the concerns of undiagnosed uterine leiomyosarcoma. This was due to concerns raised by the case of an unsuspected Boston anesthesiologist who underwent laparoscopic power morcellation for suspected fibroids. The risk calculated by the FDA was 1:350 cases, and that the power morcellation would spread the malignant cells in the peritoneal cavity and worsen the prognosis. Various hospitals and physicians have taken different approaches to this FDA warning; however, the use of laparoscopic power morcellation has been dramatically reduced.

COMPREHENSION QUESTIONS

41.1 A 29-year-old woman is noted to have three consecutive first-trimester spontaneous abortions. After an evaluation for the recurrent abortions including karyotype of the parents, hysterosalpingogram, vaginal sonogram, and testing for antiphospholipid syndrome, the obstetrician concludes the uterine fibroids are the etiology. Which of the following types of uterine fibroids would most likely lead to recurrent abortion?

  A. Submucosal
  B. Intramural
  C. Subserosal
  D. Parasitic
  E. Pedunculated

41.2 A 39-year-old woman is diagnosed as having probable uterine fibroids based on a pelvic examination revealing an enlarged irregular uterus. She is currently asymptomatic and expressed surprise that she had "growths" of the uterus. If she were to develop symptoms, which of the following would be the most common manifestation?

A. Infertility
B. Menorrhagia
C. Ureteral obstruction
D. Pelvic pain
E. Recurrent abortion

41.3 A 29-year-old G2P1 woman at 39 weeks' gestation had a myomectomy for infertility previously. While pushing during the second stage of labor, she is noted to have fetal bradycardia associated with some vaginal bleeding. The fetal head, which was previously at +2 station, is now noted to be at −3 station. Which of the following is the most likely diagnosis?

A. Submucosal myomata
B. Umbilical cord prolapse
C. Uterine rupture
D. Placental abruption
E. Fetal congenital heart block

41.4 A 65-year-old woman is noted to have suspected uterine fibroids on physical examination. Over the course of 1 year, she is noted to have enlargement of her uterus from approximately 12 weeks' size to 20 weeks' size. Which of the following is the best management?

A. Continued careful observation
B. Monitoring with ultrasound examinations
C. Exploratory laparotomy with hysterectomy
D. Gonadotropin-releasing hormone agonist
E. Progestin therapy

41.5 A 38-year-old woman is diagnosed with uterine fibroids of approximately 18 weeks' size and irregular in contour. She has significant menorrhagia with symptomatic anemia. The patient has finished her childbearing, but adamantly refuses surgical management for her fibroids. Which of the following is the best management for this patient?

A. Endometrial ablation procedure
B. Intramuscular GnRH agonist therapy
C. Levonorgestrel IUD
D. Oral contraceptive therapy
E. Uterine artery embolization

41.6. A 45-year-old G2P2 woman has significant heavy menstrual bleeding due to uterine fibroids. The pelvic ultrasound shows two large uterine fibroids—one in the anterior corpus and one in the uterine fundal region. The patient is considering uterine artery embolization. Which of the following is the best way to ensure that the uterine fibroids are not leiomyosarcoma?

A. Endometrial biopsy
B. Uterine dilatation and curettage
C. Percutaneous biopsy of the fibroid
D. Magnetic resonance imaging
E. Serum markers for CA125 and CEA

ANSWERS

41.1 **A.** Submucousal fibroids are the fibroids most likely to be associated with recurrent abortion because of their effect on the uterine cavity. The contours of the endometrium are altered and therefore, less favorable for implantation. There may be insufficient vasculature to provide adequate blood supply to the growing embryo if it were to implant along the side of the endometrium containing a submucosal fibroid. In the second trimester of pregnancy, the other answer choices are not associated with an increased risk of recurrent abortion because they do not alter the integrity of the endometrium.

41.2 **B.** Menorrhagia is the most common symptom of uterine fibroids, and severe menorrhagia often leads to anemia. Infertility and recurrent abortion may occur with submucosal fibroids due to the effects on the uterine cavity, whereas impingement on the ureters is most likely to occur with subserosal fibroids, but these are much less common than menorrhagia. Pelvic pain is not very common, and many uterine fibroids are asymptomatic and only require monitoring. If the uterine leiomyomata are large enough, patients may complain of pressure to the pelvis, bladder, or rectum. Though rare, a uterine fibroid on a pedicle may twist, leading to necrosis and severe pain.

41.3 **C.** Extensive myomectomies sometimes necessitate cesarean delivery because of the risk of uterine rupture. Most practitioners use the rule of thumb that if the endometrial cavity is entered during myomectomy, a cesarean delivery should be performed with pregnancy. As with uterine rupture, fetal bradycardia may also occur if the umbilical cord becomes prolapsed, but cord prolapse is not a risk factor from having a myomectomy. A submucosalmyomata is related to problems with fertility and implantation of the embryo, not problems during labor such as uterine rupture. Placental abruption is not associated with fetal bradycardia or as a risk after myomectomy. Myomectomies do not cause congenital anomalies or disease processes to occur in a developing fetus.

41.4 **C.** The rapid growth of the uterus suggests leiomyosarcoma; the diagnosis and treatment are surgical, especially in a woman of nonchildbearing age. Also, substantial growth of uterine fibroids in postmenopausal women is unusual due to the lower estrogen levels. In other words, uterine fibroids typically grow in response to estrogen. Once a fibroid degenerates into cancer, progestin therapy and gonadotropin-releasing hormone agonists have no more effect on the tumor and are no longer treatment options for shrinking the mass.

41.5 **E.** For a relatively large uterus due to fibroids, uterine artery embolization is the best alternative therapy to surgery. The majority of patients treated with this modality will have improvement. The IUD would likely not stay in place with an irregular uterine cavity; endometrial ablation is technically difficult if not impossible with a large irregular uterine cavity. GnRH agonist is useful in the short term (3-6 months) and is effective in shrinking the fibroids and slowing the bleeding; but its use is limited to 6 months due to the risk of osteoporosis.

41.6 **C.** Although rare, leiomyosarcoma does occur and can be very difficult if not impossible to distinguish from a uterine fibroid. MR imaging usually reveals a large heterogenous mass in the uterus with areas of both hyper- and hypoenhancement; however, there is considerable overlap between leiomyosarcoma and benign leiomyomata. Thus, percutaneous biopsy or even better surgical resection and pathological examination are the best ways to assess for leiomyosarcoma. Endometrial biopsy and uterine D&C are usually not helpful to evaluate for leiomyosarcoma.

CLINICAL PEARLS

▶ The most common reason for hysterectomy is symptomatic uterine fibroids.

▶ The most common symptom of uterine fibroids is menorrhagia, heavy bleeding **during** menses.

▶ The physical examination consistent with uterine leiomyomata is an irregular pelvic mass that is mobile, midline, and moves contiguously with the cervix.

▶ Leiomyosarcoma rarely arises from leiomyoma; rapid growth or a history of prior pelvic irradiation should raise the index of suspicion.

▶ Significant growth in suspected uterine fibroids in a postmenopausal woman is unusual and generally requires surgical evaluation.

▶ Asymptomatic uterine fibroids require surgical intervention in the presence of unexplained rapid growth, ureteral obstruction, or the inability to differentiate the fibroid from other types of pelvic masses.

REFERENCES

American College of Obstetricians and Gynecologists. Alternatives to hysterectomy in the management of leiomyomata. *ACOG Practice Bulletin 96.* Washington, DC; 2008. (Reaffirmed 2014.)

Barakat EE, Bedaiwy MA, Zimberg S, Nutter B, Nosseir M, Flacone T. Robotic-assisted, laparoscopic, and abdominal myomectomy: a comparison of surgical outcomes. *Obstet Gynecol.* 2011;117: 256-266.

FDA Safety Communication. FDA discourages use of laparoscopic power morcellation for removal of uterus or uterine fibroids. http://www.fda.gov/NewsEvents/Newsroom/PressAnnouncements/ucm393689.htm; Accessed 20.09.2015.

Katz VL. Benign gynecologic lesions. In: Lentz GM, Lobo RA, Gersenson DM, Katz VL, eds. *Comprehensive Gynecology.* 6th ed. St. Louis, MO: Mosby-Year Book; 2012:419-470.

Nelson AL, Gambone JC. Congenital anomalies and benign conditions of the uterine corpus and cervix. In: Hacker NF, Gambone JC, Hobel CJ, eds. *Essentials of Obstetrics and Gynecology.* 5th ed. Philadelphia, PA: Saunders; 2009:240-247.

Spies JB, Bruno J, Czeyda-Pommersheim F, Magee ST, Ascher SA, Jha RC. Long-term outcome of uterine artery embolization of leiomyomata. *Obstet Gynecol.* 2005;106:933.

Steward EA. Uterine fibroids. *New Engl J Med.* 2015;372:1646-1655.

CASE 42

Scenario 1: An 18-year-old G1P0 female, who is pregnant at 7 weeks' gestation by last menstrual period (LMP), complains of a 2-day history of vaginal spotting and lower abdominal pain. Her blood pressure (BP) is 130/60 mm Hg, heart rate (HR) is 70 beats per minute, and temperature is 99°F (37.2°C). The abdomen is nontender and without masses. On pelvic examination, the uterus is 4-week size and nontender, and there are no adnexal masses. The cervix is closed. The serum beta-human chorionic gonadotropin (β-hCG) level is 700 mIU/mL and a transvaginal ultrasound reveals an empty uterus and no adnexal masses.

▶ What is your next step in the management of this patient?

Scenario 2: A 35-year-old woman at 8 weeks' gestation complains of crampy lower abdominal pain and vaginal bleeding. She states that the pain was intense last night, and that something that looked like liver passed per vagina. After that, the pain subsided tremendously as did the vaginal bleeding. Her blood pressure (BP) is 130/80 mm Hg, heart rate (HR) is 90 beats per minute, and temperature is 98°F (36.6°C). Her abdominal examination is unremarkable. The pelvic examination reveals normal external female genitalia. The cervix is closed and nontender.

▶ What is the most likely diagnosis?
▶ What is your next step in management?

ANSWERS TO CASE 42:
Threatened Abortion and Spontaneous Abortion

Summary of Scenario 1: An 18-year-old adolescent female at 7 weeks' gestation by LMP complains of a 2-day history of vaginal spotting and lower abdominal pain. The physical examination reveals a 4-week-sized uterus and unremarkable adnexa. The β-hCG level is 700 mIU/mL and no intrauterine gestational sac is noted on endovaginal sonography.

- **Next step in management:** Follow-up β-hCG level in 48 hours.

Summary of Scenario 2: A 35-year-old woman at 8 weeks' gestational age had intense crampy lower abdominal pain and vaginal bleeding last night; after passing what looked like "liver," her pain and bleeding subsided tremendously. On examination, her cervix is closed.

- **Most likely diagnosis:** Completed abortion.
- **Next step in management:** Follow hCG levels to zero.

ANALYSIS
Objectives

1. Understand the concept of the hCG discriminatory zone or threshold, and its utility with transvaginal sonography.
2. Understand the principle of obtaining a follow-up hCG level when a patient is asymptomatic and has an hCG level that is below the discriminatory zone.
3. Know that a normal ultrasound examination does not rule out the presence of an ectopic pregnancy.
4. Know the typical characteristics of the different types of spontaneous abortions.
5. Understand the clinical presentations of and the treatments for the different types of abortions.

Considerations

In scenario 1, this 18-year-old patient complains of lower abdominal pain and vaginal spotting. Although there are numerous possible causes, the priority should be to assess for possible pregnancy and especially possible ectopic pregnancy. She does not have a history of sexually transmitted diseases, which if present would be a risk factor for an ectopic pregnancy. The physical examination is unremarkable and ultrasound does not show any adnexal masses. Of note, the hCG level is below the threshold whereby transvaginal sonography should reveal an intrauterine pregnancy (IUP; hCG threshold of 1500-2000 mIU/mL). Thus, the next step in management is to determine whether this pregnancy is a normal intrauterine gestation or an abnormal pregnancy. This may be accomplished by following serial hCG levels. In a normal intrauterine pregnancy, if the follow-up hCG level at 48 hours rises by at least 66%, then the patient most likely has a normal intrauterine pregnancy. If the follow-up hCG does not rise by 66% (particularly, if it rises by only 20%), then she most likely has an abnormal pregnancy. A subnormal rise in hCG does not indicate whether the abnormal pregnancy is in the uterus or the tube. The gestational age based on last menstrual period is not very reliable. Thus, the hCG levels and transvaginal ultrasound are generally the best tools for evaluating a possible ectopic pregnancy.

In scenario 2, the patient is pregnant at 8 weeks' gestation, which is in the first trimester. She noted intense cramping pain the night before and passed something that looked like liver to her. This may be tissue, although the gross appearance of presumed tissue can be misleading. The patient's pain and bleeding have subsided since the passage of the "liver." This is consistent with the complete expulsion of the pregnancy tissue. The clinical picture of passage of tissue, resolution of cramping and bleeding, and a closed cervical os are consistent with a completed abortion. To confirm that all of the pregnancy (trophoblastic) tissue has been expelled from the uterus, the clinician should follow serum quantitative hCG levels. It is expected that the hCG levels should halve every 48 to 72 hours. If the hCG levels plateau instead of falling, then the patient has residual pregnancy tissue (which may be either an incomplete abortion or an ectopic pregnancy). Notably, this patient is of advanced maternal age, and spontaneous abortions are more common in older patients. The most common cause identified with spontaneous abortion is a chromosomal abnormality of the embryo.

APPROACH TO:
Threatened Abortion and Spontaneous Abortion

DEFINITIONS

THREATENED ABORTION: Pregnancy with vaginal spotting during the first half of pregnancy. This does not delineate the viability of the pregnancy.

ECTOPIC PREGNANCY: Pregnancy outside of the normal uterine implantation site. Most of the time, this means a pregnancy in the fallopian tube.

HUMAN CHORIONIC GONADOTROPIN: "The pregnancy hormone," which is a glycoprotein that is secreted by the chorionic villi of a pregnancy. It is the hormone on which pregnancy tests are based. The normal pregnancy will have a logarithmic rise in early pregnancy.

hCG THRESHOLD: Level of serum hCG such that an intrauterine pregnancy should be seen on ultrasound. For endovaginal sonography, this level is 1500 to 2000 mIU/mL. When an intrauterine pregnancy is not seen on sonography and the hCG level exceeds the threshold, then it is highly probable that an ectopic pregnancy is present.

INEVITABLE ABORTION: A pregnancy <20 weeks' gestation associated with cramping, bleeding, and cervical dilation; there is no passage of tissue.

INCOMPLETE ABORTION: A pregnancy <20 weeks' gestation associated with cramping, vaginal bleeding, an open cervical os, and some passage of tissue per vagina, but also some retained tissue in utero. The cervix remains open due to the continued uterine contractions; the uterus continues to contract in an effort to expel the retained tissue.

COMPLETED ABORTION: A pregnancy <20 weeks' gestation in which all the products of conception have passed; the cervix is generally closed. Because all the tissue has passed, the uterus no longer contracts, and the cervix closes.

MISSED ABORTION: A pregnancy <20 weeks' gestation with embryonic or fetal demise but no symptoms such as bleeding or cramping.

CLINICAL APPROACH

Threatened Abortion

When a pregnant woman <20 weeks' gestation has vaginal bleeding, it is described as threatened abortion. The more difficult assessment is in the first 6 to 7 weeks of gestation when the status of the pregnancy and location of the pregnancy are uncertain. The gestational age based on LMP of patients with threatened abortion is unreliable due to the irregular bleeding. In general, patients with threatened abortion fall into three possible etiologies:

- Viable intrauterine pregnancy (about 50%)—bleeding will abate and pregnancy will continue
- Spontaneous abortion (nonviable IUP—about 35%)—the bleeding indicates a nonviable intrauterine pregnancy
- Ectopic pregnancy (nonviable pregnancy in tube; about 15%)

Of the three possibilities, ectopic pregnancy is the most dangerous; thus, the strategy in assessing threatened abortion or pregnant women with abdominal pain is to evaluate for possible ectopic pregnancy. It is of paramount importance to determine if the woman is hypotensive, volume depleted, or has severe abdominal or adnexal pain. These patients will most likely need laparoscopy or laparotomy since ectopic pregnancy is probable. For asymptomatic women, the quantitative human chorionic gonadotropin level is useful. When the hCG level is below the threshold for sonographic visualization of an intrauterine gestational sac, then repeat hCG level is generally performed in 48 hours to establish the viability of pregnancy. Another option would be a single progesterone level: levels >25 ng/mL almost always indicate a normal intrauterine gestation, whereas values <5 ng/mL usually correlate with a nonviable gestation. When a nonviable pregnancy is diagnosed either by an abnormal hCG rise or single progesterone assay (<5 ng/mL), it is still unclear whether the patient has a spontaneous abortion or an ectopic pregnancy. Many clinicians will perform a uterine curettage at this time to assess whether the patient has a miscarriage (histologic confirmation of chorionic villi) or an ectopic pregnancy (no villi from the curettage). Women with asymptomatic, small (<3.5 cm) ectopic pregnancies are ideal candidates for intramuscular methotrexate. A nonviable intrauterine pregnancy may be managed expectantly, surgically via dilation and curettage, or medically with vaginal misoprostol. Vaginal misoprostol has been reported to be effective in evacuating the pregnancy in about 80% of cases.

When the hCG level is greater than the ultrasound threshold, a transvaginal sonogram will dictate the next step. A patient in whom an intrauterine gestational sac is seen may be sent home with a diagnosis of threatened abortion and should have close follow-up. There is still a significant risk of miscarriage. When the hCG level is above the threshold, and there is no sonographic evidence of intrauterine pregnancy, the risk of ectopic pregnancy is high (about 85%), and thus laparoscopy is often undertaken to diagnose and treat the ectopic pregnancy. Because an intrauterine gestation is possible in this circumstance (about 15% of the time), methotrexate is usually not given; however, a high hCG level in the face of a sonographically empty uterus is almost always caused by an extrauterine gestation (see Figure 42–1 for one example of a management scheme). Finally, Rh-negative women with threatened abortion, spontaneous abortion, or ectopic pregnancy should receive RhoGAM to prevent isoimmunization.

Spontaneous Abortion

When the pregnancy is so early that a gestational sac is not able to be seen on ultrasound, then the status of the pregnancy is unsure. However, if the gestational sac or embryo is seen, or the patient presents with passage of tissue, then spontaneous abortion can be diagnosed. The history, physical examination, and/or sonography usually point to the category of spontaneous abortion (Table 42–1). Women with symptoms of spontaneous abortion should be instructed to bring in any passed tissue for histologic analysis.

Note: An inevitable abortion must be differentiated from an incompetent cervix. With an inevitable abortion, the uterine contractions (cramping) lead to the cervical dilation. With an insufficient cervix, the cervix opens spontaneously without uterine contractions and, therefore, affected women present with painless cervical dilation, usually in the second trimester. This disorder is treated with a surgical ligature at the level of the internal cervical os (cerclage). Hence, one of the main features used to distinguish between an insufficient cervix and an inevitable abortion is the presence or absence of uterine contractions.

The treatment of a **missed or incomplete abortion** includes expectant management for passage of tissue, medical management with mifepristone and misoprostol (misoprostol alone), and surgical management with dilatation and curettage of the uterus for immediate, definitive treatment. The primary complications of persistently retained tissue are bleeding and infection. A completed abortion is suspected by the history of having passed tissue and experiencing cramping abdominal pain, now resolved. The cervix is closed. Serum hCG levels are still followed to confirm that no further chorionic villi are contained in the uterus.

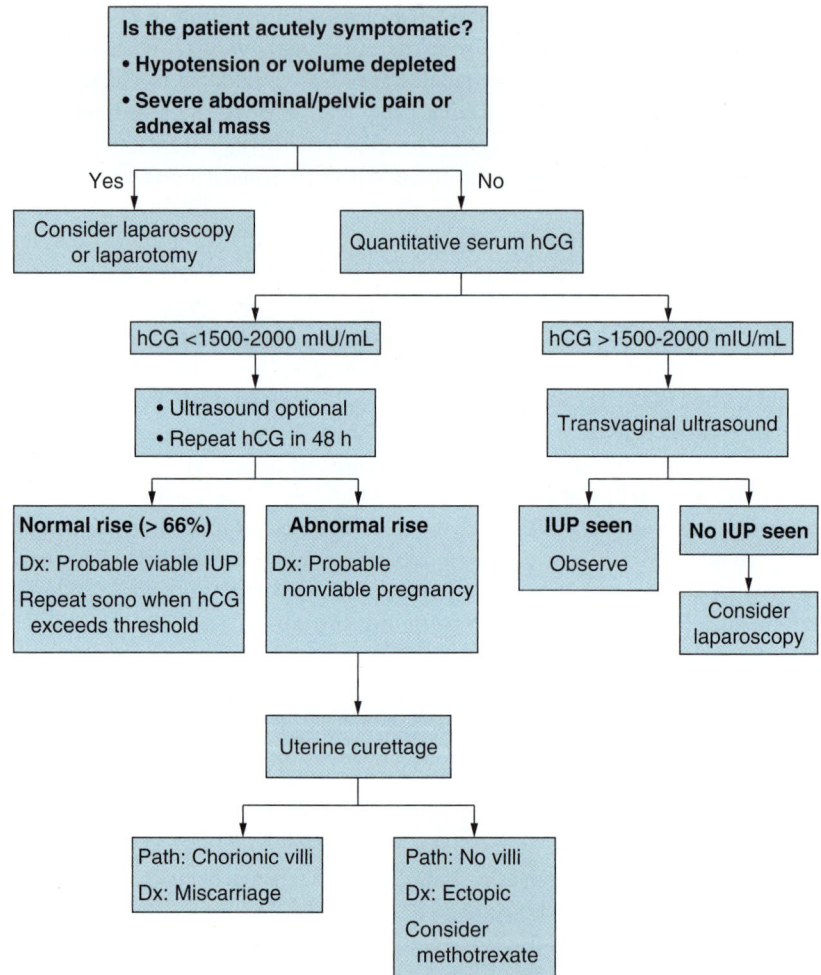

Figure 42–1. Algorithm for management of threatened abortion.

Differential Diagnosis

A pregnant patient who presents with abdominal pain and vaginal pain has a threatened abortion. The differential diagnosis includes: viable IUP, nonviable IUP, ectopic pregnancy, cervical or vaginal lesions/laceration, and more rarely molar pregnancy.

Molar Pregnancy

An unusual type of abnormal pregnancy is a **molar pregnancy (incidence 1:1200 pregnancies)**, which is trophoblastic tissue, or placenta-like tissue, usually without a fetus. The clinical presentation of molar pregnancy is vaginal spotting, absence of fetal heart tones, size greater than dates, and markedly elevated hCG levels. The diagnosis is by **ultrasound**, revealing a "snow storm"-like pattern in the

Table 42–1 • CLASSIFICATION OF SPONTANEOUS ABORTIONS					
Terminology	History	Passage of Tissue?	Cervical OS	Viability of Pregnancy?	Treatment
Threatened abortion	Vaginal bleeding	No	Closed	Uncertain; up to 50% will miscarry	Transvaginal ultrasound and hCG levels
Inevitable abortion	Cramping, bleeding	No	Open	Abortion is inevitable	D&C vs medical therapy vs expectant management
Incomplete abortion	Cramping, bleeding (still continuing)	Some but not all tissues passed	Open	Nonviable	D&C or medical therapy
Complete abortion	Cramping, bleeding previously but now subsided	All tissues passed	Closed	Nonviable	Follow hCG levels to negative
Missed abortion	No symptoms	No	Closed	Nonviable (diagnosed on ultrasound)	D&C vs medical therapy vs expectant management

uterus. Uterine suction curettage is the treatment. After curettage, patients are followed with weekly hCG levels because sometimes gestational trophoblastic disease persists after evacuation of the molar pregnancy. In these instances, chemotherapy is used.

CASE CORRELATION

- See also Case 43 (Ectopic Pregnancy). A patient with a threatened abortion may have a viable intrauterine pregnancy, a spontaneous abortion, or an ectopic pregnancy.

COMPREHENSION QUESTIONS

Match the single best treatment (A-E) with the clinical scenario (42.1-42.4).
  A. Laparoscopy
  B. Follow-up hCG level in 48 hours
  C. Cervical cerclage
  D. Dilation and curettage of uterus
  E. Expectant management

42.1 A 19-year-old G1P0 woman at 18 weeks' gestation, who had a prior cervical conization procedure, states that she has felt no abdominal cramping. She has a cervical dilation of 2 cm and effacement of 70%.

42.2 A 33-year-old woman at 10 weeks' gestation complains of vaginal bleeding and passage of a whitish substance along with something "meat-like." She continues to have cramping, and her cervix is 2 cm dilated.

42.3 A 20-year-old G2P1 woman at 12 weeks' gestation has had no problems with this pregnancy prior to today. She complains of some slight vaginal spotting. No fetal heart tones are heard on Doppler, and a transvaginal ultrasound reveals no uterine gestational sac and no adnexal masses. The hCG level is 700 mIU/mL.

42.4 A 28-year-old G3P2 woman at 22 weeks' gestation is noted to have vaginal spotting, and fetal heart tones are in the range of 140 to 145 bpm.

42.5 An 18-year-old adolescent female who is brought to the emergency room complains of vaginal spotting and lower abdominal pain. Her abdominal and pelvic examinations are normal. The hCG level is 700 mIU/mL and transvaginal sonogram shows no intrauterine gestational sac and no adnexal masses. Which of the following statements is most accurate regarding this patient's situation?

A. She has an unruptured ectopic pregnancy.

B. She has a viable intrauterine pregnancy that is too early to assess on ultrasound.

C. She has a nonviable intrauterine pregnancy.

D. There is insufficient information to draw a conclusion about the viability of this pregnancy.

E. A magnetic resonance imaging (MRI) scan would be useful in further assessing the possibility of an ectopic pregnancy.

42.6 A 22-year-old woman, who is pregnant at 5 weeks' gestation, complains of severe lower abdominal pain. On examination, she is noted to have a blood pressure of 86/44 mm Hg and heart rate of 120 bpm. Her abdomen is tender. The pelvic examination is difficult to perform due to guarding. The hCG level is 500 mIU/mL and the transvaginal sonogram reveals no intrauterine gestational sac and no adnexal masses. There is some free fluid in the cul-de-sac. Which of the following is the best management for this patient?

A. Repeat hCG level in 48 hours to assess for a rise of 66%

B. Check the serum progesterone level

C. Immediate surgery

D. Intramuscular methotrexate

E. Repeat sonography in 48 hours

ANSWERS

42.1 **C.** The hallmark of cervical insufficiency is painless dilation of the cervix. Cervical conization is a risk factor for an insufficient cervix. Other risk factors for incompetent cervix include: congenital manifestations (ie, short cervix or collagen disorder), trauma to the cervix, prolonged second stage of labor, and uterine overdistention as with a multiple gestation pregnancy. No contractions were felt by the patient in this scenario, so the diagnosis is less likely to be inevitable abortion. Cervical insufficiency may be treated with a surgical ligature known as a cerclage.

42.2 **D.** An open cervical os, a history of passing tissue, and continued cramping are all findings consistent with an incomplete abortion. If the cramping had stopped and the cervix closed, this would have been a complete abortion. The treatment of an incomplete abortion is dilation and curettage (D&C) of the uterus to prevent complications of retained tissue such as hemorrhage and infection. The products of conception obtained from the curettage are sent for pathology to confirm the diagnosis and to look for rare complications such as molar pregnancy.

42.3 **B.** This patient has a threatened abortion. Her hCG level is below the threshold when a gestational sac should be seen on transvaginal sonography (1500-2000 mIU/mL). Thus, it is unclear with the information at this time to discern whether she has a normal early intrauterine pregnancy, or an abnormal pregnancy (miscarriage or ectopic). Follow-up hCG level in 48 hours would be judicious; an appropriate rise in hCG of at least 66% is consistent with a normal intrauterine pregnancy, whereas a rise <66% is highly suggestive of an abnormal pregnancy.

42.4 **E.** This patient does not have an abortive process since she is at 22 weeks' gestation; she has antepartum bleeding. Abortions are described as <20 weeks' gestation. The two most common causes of antepartum bleeding are placenta previa and placental abruption. In abruption, the patient typically presents to triage with severe abdominal pain. The evaluation of this patient would include ultrasound to assess for placenta previa, and if this is ruled out, then speculum examination and assessment for abruption.

42.5 **D.** There is insufficient information in this scenario to establish viability of the pregnancy. A repeat hCG in 48 hours may be able to assess the state of the pregnancy. Since no conclusion may be drawn, it would be difficult to say whether this patient has an unruptured ectopic pregnancy, an intrauterine pregnancy that is too early to assess by ultrasound, or a nonviable intrauterine pregnancy. An MRI is not specific in evaluating for an ectopic versus viable intrauterine pregnancy; plus, it is costly and time-consuming.

42.6 **C.** Surgery is indicated because this patient is hypotensive and tachycardic due to a likely ruptured ectopic pregnancy. This patient is in shock, and immediate surgery is indicated to prevent end-organ damage that may immediately lead to or eventually result in death. Delaying treatment or relying on intramuscular (IM) methotrexate is not indicated for a patient in hemodynamic instability. Considering the patient's symptoms, methotrexate would be an ineffective treatment anyway since the ectopic pregnancy has most likely ruptured. A progesterone level would not be of use because tubal rupture in itself would indicate a nonviable gestation was present.

CLINICAL PEARLS

▶ Women with threatened abortion may have a viable IUP, a spontaneous abortion, or an ectopic pregnancy.

▶ When the hCG level is above the threshold and no intrauterine pregnancy is seen on transvaginal ultrasound, the patient most likely has an ectopic pregnancy.

▶ Early in the course of a normal intrauterine pregnancy, the β-hCG should rise by at least 66% over 48 hours.

▶ The presence of a true intrauterine gestational sac on ultrasound makes the risk of ectopic pregnancy very unlikely.

▶ Surgery is usually the best therapy in a patient with an early pregnancy who is hypotensive or has severe adnexal pain.

▶ When a pregnant woman has an open cervical os with uterine cramping and history of passage of tissue, she usually has an incomplete abortion, best treated by uterine curettage.

▶ The typical history of a completed abortion is resolution of cramping and vaginal bleeding following passage of tissue, and the finding of a small firm uterus and a closed cervical os.

▶ The most common cause of a first-trimester miscarriage is a fetal karyotypic abnormality.

▶ Cervical insufficiency, which is suspected with painless cervical dilation, is best treated with a cervical cerclage (ligature).

▶ A molar pregnancy is an unusual type of pregnancy characterized by vaginal spotting, absence of fetal heart tones, and size greater than dates. The diagnosis is made by sonography.

REFERENCES

American College of Obstetricians and Gynecologists. Medical management of ectopic pregnancy. *ACOG Practice Bulletin 94*. Washington, DC; 2008.

American College of Obstetricians and Gynecologists. Diagnosis and treatment of gestational trophoblastic disease. *ACOG Practice Bulletin 53*. Washington, DC; 2004.

American College of Obstetricians and Gynecologists. Medical management of abortion. *ACOG Practice Bulletin 67*. Washington, DC; 2005.

American College of Obstetricians and Gynecologists. Medical management of ectopic pregnancy. *ACOG Practice Bulletin 94*. Washington, DC; 2010.

Katz VL. Recurrent and spontaneous abortion. In: Katz VL, Lentz GM, Lobo RA, Gersenson DM, eds. *Comprehensive Gynecology*. 5th ed. St. Louis, MO: Mosby-Year Book; 2007:359-388.

Lobo RA. Ectopic pregnancy. In: Katz VL, Lentz GM, Lobo RA, Gersenson DM, eds. *Comprehensive Gynecology*. 5th ed. St. Louis, MO: Mosby-Year Book; 2007:389-410.

Lu MC, Williams III J, Hobel CJ. Antepartum care: preconception and prenatal care, genetic evaluation and teratology, and antenatal fetal assessment. In: Hacker NF, Gambone JC, Hobel CJ, eds. *Essentials of Obstetrics and Gynecology*. 5th ed. Philadelphia, PA: Saunders; 2009:71-90.

Shamonki M, Nelson AL, Gambone JC. Ectopic pregnancy. In: Hacker NF, Gambone JC, Hobel CJ, eds. *Essentials of Obstetrics and Gynecology*. 5th ed. Philadelphia, PA: Saunders; 2009:290-297.

Zhang J. A comparison of medical management with misoprostol and surgical management of early pregnancy failure. *N Eng J Med*. 2005;253(8):761-769.

CASE 43

A 19-year-old G2P0 Ab1 woman at 7 weeks' gestation by last menstrual period (LMP) complains of vaginal spotting. She denies the passage of tissue per vagina, any trauma, or recent intercourse. Her past medical history is significant for a pelvic infection approximately 3 years ago. She had used an oral contraceptive agent 1 year previously. Her appetite is normal. On examination, her blood pressure (BP) is 100/60 mm Hg, heart rate (HR) is 90 beats per minute (bpm), and temperature is afebrile. The abdomen is nontender with normoactive bowel sounds. On pelvic examination, the external genitalia are normal. The cervix is closed and nontender. The uterus is 4 weeks' size, and no adnexal tenderness is noted. The quantitative beta-human chorionic gonadotropin (β-hCG) is 2300 mIU/mL (Third International Standard). A transvaginal sonogram reveals an empty uterus and no adnexal masses.

▶ What is your next step?
▶ What is the most likely diagnosis?

ANSWERS TO CASE 43:
Ectopic Pregnancy

Summary: A 19-year-old G2Ab1 woman at 7 weeks' gestation by LMP has vaginal spotting. Her history is significant for a prior pelvic infection. Her BP is 100/60 mm Hg, HR is 90 bpm, and her abdomen is nontender. Pelvic examination shows a closed and nontender cervix, a uterus of 4 weeks' size, and no adnexal tenderness. The quantitative β-hCG is 2300 mIU/mL (Third International Standard). A transvaginal sonogram reveals an empty uterus and no adnexal masses.

- **Next step:** Laparoscopy.
- **Most likely diagnosis:** Ectopic pregnancy.

ANALYSIS
Objectives

1. Understand that any woman with amenorrhea and vaginal spotting or lower abdominal pain should have a pregnancy test to evaluate the possibility of ectopic pregnancy.
2. Understand the role of the hCG level and the threshold for transvaginal sonogram.
3. Know that the lack of clinical or ultrasound signs of ectopic pregnancy does not exclude the disease.

Considerations

The woman is at 7 weeks' gestation by last menstrual period and presents with vaginal spotting. Any woman with amenorrhea and vaginal spotting should have a pregnancy test. The physical examination is normal. Notably, the uterus is slightly enlarged at 4 weeks' gestational size. The enlarged uterus does not exclude the diagnosis of an ectopic pregnancy, due to the human chorionic gonadotropin effect on the uterus. The lack of adnexal mass or tenderness on physical examination likewise does not rule out an ectopic pregnancy. The hCG level and transvaginal ultrasound are key tests in the assessment of an extrauterine pregnancy. The ultrasound is primarily used to assess for the presence or absence of an intrauterine pregnancy (IUP), because a confirmed IUP would decrease the likelihood of an ectopic pregnancy significantly (risk 1:10,000 of both an intrauterine and ectopic pregnancy, that is, heterotopic pregnancy). Also, the presence of free fluid in the peritoneal cavity, or a complex adnexal mass, would make an extrauterine pregnancy more likely. This woman's hCG level of 2300 mIU/mL is greater than the threshold of 1500 to 2000 mIU/mL (transvaginal sonography); thus, the patient has a high likelihood of an ectopic pregnancy. Although the risk of an extrauterine pregnancy is high, it is not 100%. Therefore, laparoscopy is indicated, and not methotrexate, since the latter would destroy any intrauterine gestation.

SECTION II: CASES **417**

APPROACH TO:
Possible Ectopic Pregnancy

DEFINITIONS

ECTOPIC PREGNANCY: A gestation that exists outside of the normal endometrial implantation sites.

HUMAN CHORIONIC GONADOTROPIN: A glycoprotein produced by syncytiotrophoblasts, which is assayed in the standard pregnancy test.

THRESHOLD HCG LEVEL: The serum level of hCG where a pregnancy should be seen on ultrasound examination. When the hCG exceeds the threshold and no pregnancy is seen on ultrasound, there is a high likelihood of an ectopic pregnancy.

LAPAROSCOPY: Surgical technique to visualize the peritoneal cavity through a rigid telescopic instrument, known as a laparoscope.

CLINICAL APPROACH

See also Case 42 (Spontaneous Abortion).

The vast majority of ectopic pregnancies involve the fallopian tube (97%), but the cervix, or cornua (the portion of the tube that traverses the uterine muscle), abdominal cavity, and ovary have also been affected. In the United States, 2% of pregnancies are extrauterine. Hemorrhage from ectopic gestation is the most common reason for maternal mortality in the first 20 weeks of pregnancy. Risk factors for ectopic pregnancy are summarized in Table 43–1.

A woman with an ectopic pregnancy typically complains of abdominal pain, amenorrhea of 4 to 6 weeks' duration, and irregular vaginal spotting. In the case of a ruptured ectopic, the pain becomes acutely worse, and may lead to syncope. Shoulder pain can be a prominent complaint due to the blood irritating the diaphragm. An ectopic pregnancy can lead to tachycardia, hypotension, or orthostasis. Abdominal or adnexal tenderness is common. An adnexal mass is only palpable half the time; hence, the absence of a detectable mass does not exclude an ectopic pregnancy. The uterus may be normal in size, or slightly enlarged. A hemoperitoneum can be confirmed by the aspiration of nonclotting blood with a spinal needle piercing the posterior vaginal fornix into the cul-de-sac (culdocentesis).

Table 43–1 • RISK FACTORS FOR ECTOPIC PREGNANCY
Salpingitis, particularly with *Chlamydia trachomatis*
Tubal adhesive disease
Infertility
Progesterone-secreting IUD
Tubal surgery
Prior ectopic pregnancy
Ovulation induction
Congenital abnormalities of the tube
Assisted reproductive technology

Table 43–2 • DIFFERENTIAL DIAGNOSIS OF ECTOPIC PREGNANCY
Acute salpingitis
Abortion
Ruptured corpus luteum
Acute appendicitis
Dysfunctional uterine bleeding
Adnexal torsion
Degenerating leiomyomata
Endometriosis

The diagnosis of an ectopic pregnancy can be a clinical challenge. The differential diagnosis is noted in Table 43–2.

The usual strategy in ruling out an ectopic pregnancy is to try to prove whether an intrauterine pregnancy (IUP) exists. Because the likelihood of a coexisting intrauterine and extrauterine (heterotopic) gestation is so low, in the range of 1 in 10 000, if a definite IUP is demonstrated, the risk of ectopic pregnancy becomes very low. Transvaginal sonography is more sensitive than trans-abdominal sonography, and can detect pregnancies as early as 5.5 to 6 weeks' gestational age. Hence, the demonstration of a definite IUP by crown-rump length or yolk sac is reassuring. The "identification of a gestational sac" is sometimes misleading since an ectopic pregnancy can be associated with an irregularly shaped fluid collection in the midline of the uterine cavity, a so-called "pseudogestational sac." A normal gestational sac would be eccentrically located and have a decidual sign, which is an echogenic rim around the gestational sac that is absent in a pseudogestational sac. Other sonographic findings of an extrauterine gestation include an embryo seen outside the uterus, or a large amount of intra-abdominal free fluid, usually indicating blood.

Often, the quantitative human chorionic gonadotropin level is used in conjunction with transvaginal sonography. **When the hCG level equals or exceeds 1500 to 2000 mIU/mL, an intrauterine gestational sac is usually seen on transvaginal ultrasound; in fact, when the hCG level meets or exceeds this threshold and no gestational sac is seen, the patient has a high likelihood of an ectopic pregnancy.** (If there is a high suspicion of multiple gestation, where hCG levels can be higher than singletons at any comparable gestational age, this threshold may not apply.) Laparoscopy is usually performed in this situation. When the hCG level is less than the threshold, and the patient does not have severe abdominal pain, hypotension, or adnexal tenderness and/or mass, then a repeat hCG level in 48 hours is permissible. **A rise in the hCG of at least 53% above the initial level is good evidence of a normal pregnancy;** in contrast, a lack of an appropriate rise of the hCG is indicative of an abnormal pregnancy, although the abnormal change does not identify whether the pregnancy is in the uterus or the tube. Some practitioners will use a progesterone level instead of serial hCG levels to assess the health of the pregnancy. A progesterone level of greater than 25 ng/mL almost always correlates with a normal intrauterine pregnancy, whereas a level of <5 ng/mL almost always correlates with an abnormal pregnancy.

Treatment of an ectopic pregnancy may be surgical or medical. Salpingectomy (removal of the affected tube) is usually performed for those gestations too large

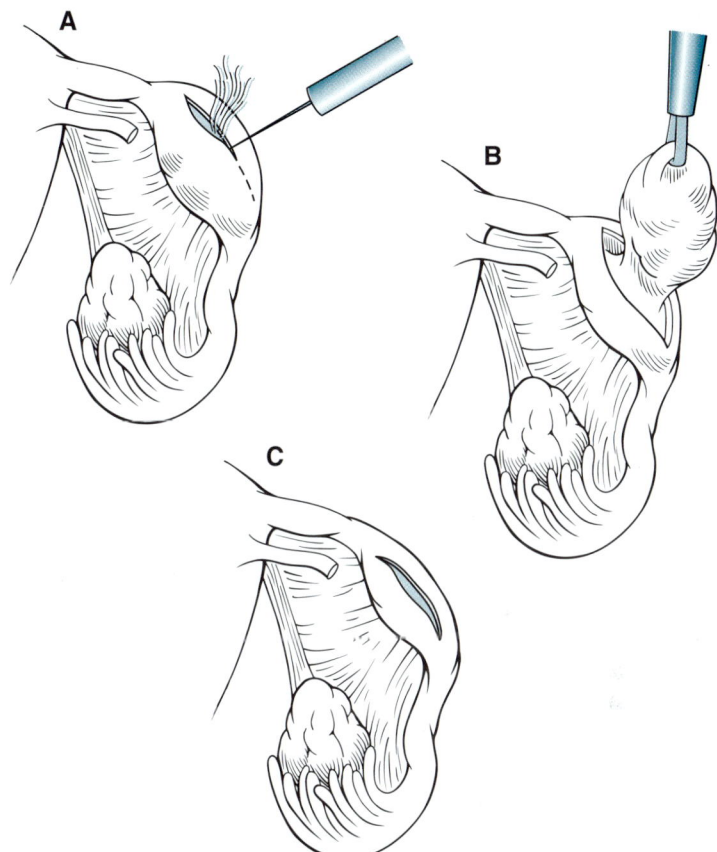

Figure 43–1. Salpingostomy. Needle-point cautery is used to incise over the ectopic pregnancy (**A**). The pregnancy tissue is extracted (**B**) and heals without closure of the incision (**C**).

for conservative therapy, when rupture has occurred, or for those women who do not want future fertility. For a woman who wants to preserve her fertility and has an unruptured tubal pregnancy, a salpingostomy can be performed (Figure 43–1).

An incision is carried out along the long axis of the tube, and the pregnancy tissue is removed. The incision on the tube is not re-approximated because suturing may lead to stricture formation. Conservative treatment of the tube is associated with a 10% to 15% chance of persistent ectopic pregnancy. Serial hCG levels are, therefore, required with conservative surgical therapy to identify this condition.

Methotrexate, a folic acid antagonist, is the principal form of medical therapy. It is usually given as a one-time, low-dose, intramuscular injection, reserved for ectopic pregnancies less than 3.5 cm in diameter, without fetal cardiac activity, and hCG levels <5000 mIU/mL. **Methotrexate is highly successful, leading to resolution of properly chosen ectopic pregnancies** in 85% to 90% of cases. Occasionally, a second dose is required because the hCG level does not fall. Between 3 and 7 days following therapy, a patient may complain of abdominal pain, which is usually due to tubal abortion and, less commonly, rupture. Most women may be observed; however, hypotension, worsening or persistent pain, or a falling hematocrit may indicate tubal rupture and necessitate surgery. About 10% of women treated with medical therapy will require surgical intervention.

Rare types of ectopic gestations such as cervical, ovarian, abdominal, or cornual (moved to above) pregnancies usually require surgical therapy.

> ### CASE CORRELATION
> - See also Case 13 (Abdominal Pain in Pregnancy), Case 41 (Threatened and Completed Abortion). A patient who presents with threatened abortion may have a normal IUP, an abnormal IUP (miscarriage), or an ectopic pregnancy.

COMPREHENSION QUESTIONS

43.1 A 22-year-old woman at 8 weeks' gestation has vaginal spotting. Her physical examination reveals no adnexal masses. The hCG level is 400 mIU/mL and the transvaginal ultrasound shows no pregnancy in the uterus and no adnexal masses. Which of the following is the next best step?

A. Laparoscopy

B. Methotrexate

C. Repeat the hCG level in 48 hours

D. Dilatation and curettage

43.2 A 26-year-old G2P1 woman at 7 weeks' gestation was seen 1 week ago with crampy lower abdominal pain and vaginal spotting. Her hCG level was 1000 mIU/mL at that time. Today, the woman does not have abdominal pain or passage of tissue per vagina. Her repeat hCG level is 1100 mIU/mL. A transvaginal ultrasound examination today shows no clear pregnancy in the uterus and no adnexal masses. Which of the following can be concluded based on the information presented?

A. The woman has a spontaneous abortion and needs a dilation and curettage.

B. The woman has an ectopic pregnancy.

C. No clear conclusion can be drawn from this information, and the hCG needs to be repeated in 48 hours.

D. The woman has a nonviable pregnancy, but its location is unclear.

43.3 A 17-year-old woman with lower abdominal pain and spotting comes into the emergency room. She is noted to have an hCG level of 1000 mIU/mL and a progesterone level of 26 ng/mL. Which of the following is the most likely diagnosis?
   A. This is most likely a normal intrauterine pregnancy.
   B. This is most likely an ectopic pregnancy.
   C. This is most likely a nonviable intrauterine pregnancy.
   D. No clear conclusion can be drawn from this information.

43.4 Which of the following statements describe the primary utility of the transvaginal ultrasound in the assessment of an ectopic pregnancy?
   A. Assessment of an intrauterine pregnancy
   B. Assessment of adnexal masses
   C. Assessment of fluid in the peritoneal cavity
   D. Color Doppler flow in the adnexal region

43.5 A 29-year-old woman complains of syncope. She is 6 weeks' pregnant and on examination has diffuse significant lower abdominal tenderness. The pelvic examination is difficult to accomplish due to guarding. Her hCG level is 400 mIU/mL and the transvaginal ultrasound shows no pregnancy in the uterus and no adnexal masses. Which of the following is the next best step?
   A. Follow-up hCG level in 48 hours
   B. Institution of methotrexate
   C. Observation in the hospital
   D. Surgical therapy

ANSWERS

43.1 **C.** When the hCG is *below the threshold* in an asymptomatic patient, the hCG level may be repeated in 48 hours to assess for viability. If the hCG level had been above the threshold in this patient, the chances that an extrauterine pregnancy exists would be even more likely (close to 100%), laparoscopy would be indicated to confirm suspicion. Since there is still a chance that this is a viable pregnancy, methotrexate should not be used since it could destroy any intrauterine gestation. Dilation and curettage would also destroy any viable intrauterine pregnancy, and would not be a good option for treatment of an ectopic pregnancy since they exist outside the uterus.

43.2 **D.** A plateau in hCG over 48 hours means it is a nonviable pregnancy; this finding does not identify the location of the pregnancy. Levels of hCG that plateau in the first 8 weeks of pregnancy indicate an abnormal pregnancy, which may be either a miscarriage or an ectopic pregnancy. It is unlikely that this patient had an incomplete or a completed abortion, given that she does not recall any passage of tissues.

43.3 **A.** A progesterone level greater than 25 ng/mL reflects a normal IUP. This patient's hCG level is below the threshold of being visible on ultrasound, so it is a very early pregnancy. Spotting and lower abdominal pain can be a normal occurrence in pregnancy, especially very early in the first trimester. Some patients have symptoms of lower abdominal pain, similar to menstrual cramps, and vaginal spotting during the first few weeks of pregnancy when the embryo implants into the wall of the uterus.

43.4 **A.** The best use of ultrasound for assessment of an ectopic pregnancy is to diagnose an IUP, as an IUP and coexisting ectopic pregnancy is very rare. Color Doppler flow in the adnexal region is typically used when there is suspicion of ovarian torsion and concern that the ovarian vessels are constricted and unable to perfuse the ovaries. Assessment of adnexal masses using transvaginal ultrasound is not very specific. A hemoperitoneum can be confirmed by culdocentesis, but not typically a transvaginal ultrasound (one could argue that with current ultrasound technology, clotted blood appears different from simple fluid and hemoperitoneum that is clotted can be diagnosed by ultrasound, especially if in pouch of Douglas).

43.5 **D.** Surgery is indicated. Although this woman has an hCG level lower than the threshold, she has an acute abdomen and this is most likely due to a ruptured ectopic pregnancy. If not addressed, the patient may exsanguinate. Methotrexate requires several days to weeks to act, and is appropriate in an asymptomatic patient with an ectopic pregnancy less than 3.5 cm in size.

CLINICAL PEARLS

▶ Levels of hCG that plateau in the first 8 weeks of pregnancy indicate an abnormal pregnancy, which may either be a miscarriage or an ectopic pregnancy.

▶ The classic triad of ectopic pregnancy is amenorrhea, vaginal spotting, and abdominal pain.

▶ When the quantitative hCG exceeds 1500 to 2000 mIU/mL and the transvaginal sonogram does not show an intrauterine gestational sac, then the risk of ectopic pregnancy is high.

REFERENCES

American College of Obstetricians and Gynecologists. Medical management of ectopic pregnancy. *ACOG Practice Bulletin 94*. Washington, DC; 2008. (Reaffirmed 2014.)

Lobo RA. Ectopic pregnancy. In: Lentz GM, Lobo RA, Gersenson DM, Katz VL, eds. *Comprehensive Gynecology*. 6th ed. Philadelphia, PA: Elsevier-Mosby; 2012:361-382.

Shamonki M, Nelson AL, Gambone JC. Ectopic pregnancy. In: Hacker NF, Gambone JC, Hobel CJ, eds. *Essentials of Obstetrics and Gynecology*. 6th ed. Philadelphia, PA: Saunders; 2015:290-297.

CASE 44

A 25-year-old G2P2002 desires contraception for the next 3 years. She reports that she had a deep venous thrombosis when she took the combination oral contraceptive pill 2 years ago. She cannot remember to take the pill every day and wants contraception that will allow her to be spontaneous. She does not take any medications and has no known allergies to medications. Menarche was age 13. Menstrual cycle is every 28 days, lasting for 7 days. She has quarter-size clots the first 3 days of her menstrual cycle. She has been married for 3 years and denies any sexually transmitted infections. Her blood pressure is 120/70 mm Hg, heart rate is 80 beats per minute (bpm), and temperature is 99°F (37.2°C). Heart and lung examinations are normal. The abdomen is nontender and without masses. Pelvic examination reveals a normal anteverted uterus and no adnexal masses.

▶ What would be the best contraceptive agent for this patient?
▶ What would be contraindications to the proposed contraceptive agent?

ANSWERS TO CASE 44:
Contraception

Summary: A 25-year-old multiparous woman, in a stable monogamous relationship, desires long-term contraception. She has had a deep venous thrombosis (DVT) while taking a combination oral contraceptive pill, is forgetful about taking pills every day, and wants contraception that will allow spontaneity. She reports heavy menses. Physical examination is within normal limits.

- **Best contraceptive agent for this patient**: The levonorgestrel-releasing intrauterine device (LNG-IUD).

- **Contraindications to the proposed contraceptive agent**: Contraindications include pregnancy, current or recent history of pelvic inflammatory disease, current sexually transmitted disease, current or recent puerperal or postabortion sepsis, purulent cervicitis, undiagnosed abnormal vaginal bleeding, malignancy of the genital tract, known uterine anomalies fibroids distorting the uterine cavity in a way incompatible with IUD insertion, or allergy to any component of the IUD.

ANALYSIS

Objectives

1. Know the various types of contraceptive agents including indications and contraindications, mechanisms of action, and efficacy.
2. Know benefits, risks, and contraindications for the combination oral contraceptive pill.
3. Know about intrauterine devices.
4. Know about emergency contraception.

Considerations

Each form of contraception has advantages and disadvantages, and the individual patient situation should be evaluated to find the best contraceptive choice. Factors that assist the physician in the counseling of the patient include agents requiring more patient action, such as remembering to take a pill each day, or putting on a barrier device (diaphragm or condom), duration of contraception desired, history of sexually transmitted infections, amount of vaginal bleeding, medical conditions, and contraception side effects. Because of the history of DVT, estrogen-containing contraception agents would be contraindicated. The desire for spontaneity would make barrier methods less desirable. Options for this patient would include depot medroxyprogesterone acetate (DMPA), nexplanon (progestin subdermal implant in the arm), or the levonorgestrel IUD. Because of the heavy menses, this 25-year-old would most benefit from a levonorgestrel-releasing intrauterine device or a progestin containing device (ie, Nexplanon), since the progestin would cause the endometrial lining to be thinner and decrease the amount of menstrual bleeding. LNG-IUD is a device placed inside the uterus by a provider during an office visit and can be left in place for up to 5 years. The progestin implant is inserted subdermally in the arm by a provider and can be left in place for up to 3 years. Both methods do not rely on the patient's memory for effectiveness. The progestin in these devices is released slowly over time and can decrease the amount and frequency of menses. The IUD does not protect against sexually transmitted infections. Also, this patient has had a DVT, which is a contraindication to any form of contraception that contains a combination of estrogen and progestin, like the combination oral contraceptive pill, patch, or ring. DMPA is not as effective as the LARCs (long acting reversible contraceptive options).

APPROACH TO:
Contraception

DEFINITIONS

INTRAUTERINE CONTRACEPTIVE DEVICES: Small T-shaped device, usually plastic with or without copper or a progestin, placed in the endometrial cavity as a method of long-term contraception.

TYPICAL USE EFFECTIVENESS: Overall efficacy in actual use, when forgetfulness and improper use occur.

PERFECT USE EFFECTIVENESS: Efficacy of a method when always used correctly, consistent, and reliably.

BARRIER CONTRACEPTIVE: Prevents sperm from entering upper female reproductive tract.

STEROID HORMONE CONTRACEPTION: Synthetic estrogen and/or progestin to provide contraception in various methods, including oral contraceptive pills, contraceptive patch, contraceptive ring, contraceptive injection, and implant.

YUZPE REGIMEN: Use of specific oral contraceptive regimen first reported by Dr Yuzpe, consisting of two tablets of 100 to 120 mcg of ethinyl estradiol, and 500-600 mcg of levonorgestrel at time zero and two tablets after 12 hours.

PLAN B (PROGESTIN ONLY): Levonorgestrel 0.75 mg taken orally at time zero and the same dose after 12 hours within 72 hours of unprotected intercourse.

PLAN B ONE-STEP: Enteric-coated levonorgestrel 1.5 mg taken as one pill.

ULIPRISTAL (ELLA): Selective progesterone receptor modulator taken as one dose.

CLINICAL APPROACH

Contraceptive agents have different effectiveness, which are characterized as theoretical (or perfect) and with typical use (see Table 44–1). The various agents

Table 44–1 • CONTRACEPTIVE FAILURE RATES COMPARING TYPICAL USE AND PERFECT USE

Method	% Failure Within First Year of Use	
	Perfect Use	Typical Use
No method	85	85
Periodic abstinence (calendar)	9	24
Diaphragm	6	12
Male condom	2	18
OC (combined and minipill)	0.3	9
Patch	0.3	9
Ring	0.3	9
Depo-Provera	0.3	6
Levonorgestrel implants (Nexplanon)	0.05	0.05
IUD (Levonorgestrel)	0.2	0.2
ParaGard (copper-T)	0.6	0.8
Female sterilization	0.5	0.5
Male sterilization	0.1	0.15

each have particular advantages and disadvantages and unique factors that may make one method better suited for a particular patient. Thus, the history and physical examination should focus on a patient's preference of method, factors such as the ability to remember to take a pill every day, and other medical conditions (see Table 44–2).

Barrier contraceptives prevent sperm from entering the upper female reproductive tract. Various forms include the male condom, female condom, vaginal diaphragm, cervical cap, and spermicides. The *male condom* is made of latex, polyurethane, or animal tissue. It is a sheath placed on an erect penis prior to intercourse and ejaculation. The latex condom is the most effective method of contraception to prevent transmission of sexually transmitted infections. It is the second most commonly used method of reversible contraception in the United States. The *female condom* is a sheath with two polyurethane rings. One ring is placed inside the vagina at the closed end of the sheath and provides an insertion mechanism and anchor. The second ring is at the outer edge of the device and is outside the vagina providing coverage for the labia and the base of the penis. The *vaginal diaphragm* must be fitted by a physician. It should be placed 1 to 2 hours before intercourse, should be used with a spermicide, and should be left in place for at least 8 hours after coitus. Drawbacks include higher rate of urinary tract infections and increased risk of ulceration to the vaginal epithelium with prolonged usage.

The *cervical cap* is also fitted by a physician. Compared to a diaphragm, the cap can be left in place for up to 48 hours and is more comfortable. It also carries a risk of ulceration and infection of the cervix if left in place for too long. However, the cap is only for use in women with normal cervical cytology due to concern of

Table 44–2 • CONTRACEPTION AGENTS COMPARED INCLUDING BEST-SUITED PATIENTS

Category	Agents	Mechanism	Best Suited For	Disadvantages and Contraindications
Barrier	Diaphragm Cervical caps Condoms (male and female)	Mechanical obstruction	Breast Feeding Not desiring hormones **Decrease sexually transmitted infections (male condom provides the best protection against STI)**	Patient discomfort with placing devices on genitals **Lack of spontaneity** Allergies to material Diaphragm may be associated with more UTIs and risk of toxic shock syndrome
Combined hormonal (estrogen and progestin)	Combined oral contraceptives Contraception patch Vaginal ring	Inhibit ovulation Thickens cervical mucous to inhibit sperm penetration Alters motility of uterus and fallopian tubes Thins endometrium	Iron-deficiency anemia Dysmenorrhea Ovarian cysts Endometriosis OCP—take pill each day PATCH—less to remember RING—less to remember, vaginal irritation, and discharge	Known thrombogenic mutations Prior thromboembolic event Cerebrovascular or coronary artery disease (current or remote) Cigarette smoking (>15 cigarettes/day) at or over the age of 35 Uncontrolled hypertension Diabetic retinopathy, nephropathy, peripheral vascular disease Known or suspected breast or endometrial cancer Undiagnosed vaginal bleeding Migraines with aura Benign or malignant liver tumors, active liver disease, liver failure Known or suspected pregnancy

(Continued)

Table 44-2 • CONTRACEPTION AGENTS COMPARED INCLUDING BEST-SUITED PATIENTS (CONTINUED)

Category	Agents	Mechanism	Best Suited For	Disadvantages and Contraindications
Progestin-only pill	Minipill	Thickens cervical mucous to inhibit sperm penetration Inhibit ovulation Alters motility of uterus and fallopian tubes Thins the endometrium	**Breastfeeding**	Very dependent on taking pill each day at same time Patient needs to remember to take pill
Injectables	Depot medroxy progesterone acetate	Inhibits ovulation Thins endometrium Alters cervical mucous to inhibit sperm penetration	Breastfeeding Iron-deficiency anemia **Sickle cell disease** **Epilepsy** Dysmenorrhea Ovarian cysts Endometriosis	Depression Osteopenia/osteoporosis Weight gain
Implants (subdermal in arm)	Etonorgestrel Implant (Nexplanon)	Inhibits ovulation Thins endometrium Thickens cervical mucous to inhibit sperm penetration	Breastfeeding Desires long-term contraception (lasts for 3 years) Iron-deficiency anemia Dysmenorrhea Ovarian cysts Endometriosis	Hepatic tumors (benign or malignant), active liver disease Undiagnosed abnormal vaginal bleeding Known or suspected carcinoma of the breast or personal history of breast cancer Hypersensitivity to any of the components of etonogestrel implant **May lead to irregular vaginal bleeding**

IUD	Levonorgestrel intrauterine device	Thickens cervical mucous to inhibit sperm penetration Thins endometrium	Breastfeeding Desires long-term, reversible contraception Stable, mutually monogamous relationship Menorrhagia Dysmenorrhea (NOTE: decreased bleeding and dysmenorrhea)	**Current STI or PID** Unexplained vaginal bleeding Malignant gestational trophoblastic disease Untreated cervical or endometrial cancer Current breast cancer Anatomical abnormalities distorting the uterine cavity Uterine fibroids distorting endometrial cavity
IUD	Copper-T	Inhibits sperm migration and viability Changes transport speed of ovum Damages ovum	Desires long-term reversible contraception (10 years) Stable, mutually monogamous relationship Contraindication to hormonal steroids	Current STI Current or PID within the past 3 months Unexplained vaginal bleeding Malignant gestational trophoblastic disease Untreated cervical or endometrial cancer Anatomical abnormalities distorting the uterine cavity Uterine fibroids distorting endometrial cavity **Wilson disease** **May cause more bleeding or dysmenorrhea**
Permanent sterilization	Bilateral tubal occlusion (can be postpartum, laparoscopic, or hysteroscopic)	Mechanical obstruction of tubes	Does not desire future fertility	Contraindications to surgery Risk of regret

traumatizing the cervix. *Spermicides* include gels, foams, suppositories, and jellies placed in the vagina. The active agent is nonoxynol-9 which disrupts the sperm cell membrane and provides a mechanical barrier. The contraceptive *sponge* is made of polyurethane impregnated with 1 mg of nonoxynol-9 and does not have to be inserted into the vagina before each act of intercourse. Because barrier methods are used only at time of coitus, the advantages include low cost, decreased transmission of certain sexually transmitted infections with condoms (not cervical cap or diaphragm), and no exposure to continuous hormones or ongoing IUD use. Disadvantages include relatively high failure rate (approximately 20%) due to required use with each act of intercourse.

Oral contraceptives were initially marketed in the United States in 1960. These quickly became the most-used method of reversible contraception among women. Oral steroid contraceptives come in combination pills at a fixed dose or a phased dose, or a progestin-only pill (minipill). The main effect of the progestin is to inhibit ovulation and cause cervical mucus thickening. The main effect of the estrogen is to maintain the endometrium, prevent unscheduled bleeding, and inhibit follicular development. The most common side effects are relatively mild and include nausea, breast tenderness, and fluid retention.

The **main risks of combined hormonal contraception** are due to the estrogen component and include **venous thromboembolism, strokes** in patients with migraines with aura, **myocardial infarction** in women who are heavy smokers (>15 cigarettes per day), and who are age 35 and older. There are many noncontraceptive benefits of hormonal oral contraceptives including decreasing the risk of developing ovarian, colon or endometrial cancer, shortening the duration of menses, decreasing blood loss during menses, improving pain from dysmenorrhea and endometriosis, decreasing abnormal uterine bleeding, and improving acne.

The **contraceptive patch** delivers norelgestromin and ethinyl estradiol transdermally. It is worn on the buttocks, upper outer arm, lower abdomen, or upper torso excluding the breast. It is changed weekly for 3 weeks followed by a week without a patch to allow for withdrawal bleed. In women weighing >90 kg, efficacy may be less. A recent FDA warning indicated the **risk of DVT was twice that of OCP**, although the data is conflicting. The **contraceptive ring** allows steroids to be absorbed through the vaginal epithelium into circulation. The ring is worn for 21 days and then removed for 7 days to allow for withdrawal bleed. The patch and ring have similar efficacy and side effects to combination oral contraceptives.

Only one **injectable contraceptive** is currently available in the United States, DMPA. It is administered subcutaneously every 3 months. Women receiving the injection have a relatively low pregnancy rate (but higher than that of LARCs). There is a significant disruption of the normal menstrual cycle that usually leads to amenorrhea.

A single subdermal **implant**, placed in a woman's upper arm, releases a steady amount of etonogestrel. The duration of action for this implant, named Nexplanon, is 3 years. Return to fertility is delayed about 2 weeks after cessation of pills, patches, or rings, but can take up to 9 to 10 months stopping contraceptive injection. Postpill amenorrhea may persist for up to 6 months.

An **intrauterine contraceptive device** is a small device, usually plastic with or without copper or a progestin, placed in the endometrial cavity as a method of contraception. Four IUDs are currently available in the United States: the copper T380A and three levonorgestrel-releasing intrauterine devices; the 5-year version (Mirena) and two 3-year versions, Skyla which is smaller and designed for younger women, and Liletta which is marketed for affordability. The copper T380A is **approved for use for 10 years** and has a 10-year cumulative pregnancy rate comparable to that of sterilization. Many mechanisms of action have been described for the copper-containing IUD, including inhibition of sperm migration and viability, change in transport speed of the ovum, and damage to or destruction of the ovum.

The **levonorgestrel-releasing intrauterine device** (Mirena) releases 20 µg of levonorgestrel daily and is **approved for use for 5 years; Skyla releases 14 µg/day and is approved for 3 years; and Liletta releases 18.6 µg/day and is approved for 3 years.** The main effect of the progestin is to cause thickening of the cervical mucus and decreasing fallopian tube motility, suppressing ovulation, and thinning the endometrium. The small amount of steroid causes minimal amounts of systemic side effects, and it also decreases menstrual bleeding due to the local effect on the endometrium. The levonorgestrel-releasing IUD also has noncontraceptive benefits and can be used to treat patients with menorrhagia, dysmenorrhea, and pain due to endometriosis and adenomyosis.

All IUDs have the advantage of requiring a single act of motivation for long-term use. The unintended pregnancy rate during the first year of use is 0.2% to 0.6%. They also have rapid return to fertility after removal of the device. Insertion has an infrequent association with uterine perforation (1:1000) and transiently increases the risk of upper genital infection (1:1000) due to endometrial contamination.

WHO contraindications to IUD insertion include current pregnancy, current sexually transmitted infection, current or pelvic inflammatory disease within the past 3 months, unexplained vaginal bleeding, malignant gestational trophoblastic disease, untreated cervical cancer, untreated endometrial cancer, uterine fibroids distorting the endometrial cavity, current breast cancer (for levonorgestrel-releasing IUD only), anatomical abnormalities distorting the uterine cavity, known pelvic tuberculosis, and allergy to component of IUD or Wilson disease (for copper-containing IUD).

Emergency contraception is the therapy for women who have had unprotected sexual intercourse, including victims of sexual assault. It is also known as the "morning after pill." The three most common regimens are progestin Plan B (two doses 12 hours apart), Plan B One-Step which is an enteric-coated levonorgestrel pill, and Ulipristal (ella) which is a progesterone agonist/antagonist. The copper IUD is another option (see Table 44-3). The combination oral contraceptive method, known as the Yuzpe method, which consists of two tablets of 100 to 120 mcg (total 200-240 mcg) of ethinyl estradiol, and 500-600 mcg (total of 1000-1200 mcg) of levonorgestrel in two doses, 12 hours apart, is only rarely used due to GI side effects. The efficacy of the pharmacologic methods is accepted to be about a 75% reduction in pregnancy rate, thus decreasing the risk of a midcycle coital pregnancy from 8 per 100 to about 2 per 100.

The mechanisms of action may include inhibition of ovulation, decreased tubal motility, and, possibly, interruption of implantation. There are no medical conditions where the risk of emergency contraception outweighs the benefits. Therefore, women with cardiovascular disease, migraines, liver disease, or who are breast feeding may use emergency contraception.

The major side effect of emergency contraception is nausea and/or emesis. Emergency contraception should not be used in patients with a suspected or

Table 44-3 · EMERGENCY CONTRACEPTION METHODS

Method	Dosing	Formulation	Efficacy	Number of Days after Intercourse	Comments
Plan B	Need 2 doses 12 hours apart	Levonorgestrel 750 mcg taken orally ASAP and also in 12 hours (available only by prescription to women below 17 yo, and available over the counter to women 17+ yo)	75% efficacy	72 hours	Well tolerated
Plan B: One-step	One dose	Levonorgestrel (1.5 mg or 1500 mcg) enteric-coated pill (available only by prescription to women below 17 yo, and available over the counter to women 17+ yo)	75% efficacy	72 hours	Well tolerated
Ulipristal (Ella)	One dose	Selective progesterone modulator, 30 mg tablet	75% efficacy	5 days (120 hours)	Frequent n&v
Copper IUD	One insertion		99% efficacy	Up to 5 days	
Combination estrogen and progestin (Preven)	Needs 2 doses 12 hours apart	Ethinyl Estradiol 200 mcg and Levonorgestrel 1 mg ASAP and in 12 hours	75% efficacy	72 hours	Rarely used; frequent n&v

known pregnancy, or those with abnormal vaginal bleeding. Those women who do not have onset of menses within 21 days following the emergency contraception should have a pregnancy test.

The copper IUD can be inserted up to 5 days after unprotected intercourse for emergency contraception. Women who receive the copper IUD under emergency conditions often choose to maintain the IUD for contraception. The levonorgestrel-releasing IUD is **not** effective for emergency contraception.

Emerging Concepts

At the time of this writing, postplacental IUD insertion was gaining interest in the United States. The insertion of an IUD immediate after delivery (within 10 minutes of placental expulsion) or at the time of hysterotomy closure during cesarean seems to be efficacious; however, there seems to be a higher expulsion rate.

> **CASE CORRELATION**
> - See also Case 31 (Sexual Assault).

COMPREHENSION QUESTIONS

44.1 A 17-year-old G0P0 woman desires a reversible form of contraception. After reviewing the various options, she chooses depot medroxyprogesterone acetate. Which of the following tests is most likely to be abnormal after 2 years of use?

   A. Dual energy x-ray absorptiometry (DEXA) scan
   B. Serum glucose level
   C. Serum creatinine level
   D. Ultrasound of the gallbladder

44.2 Which of the following patients can safely receive combination oral contraceptive pills?

   A. 35-year-old woman with diabetes with peripheral circulatory problems
   B. 37-year-old woman who smokes cigarettes, about 1 pack (20 cigarettes) per day
   C. 25-year-old woman with persistent tension headaches
   D. 30-year-old whose blood pressure is 160/90 mm Hg

44.3 A 28-year-old G1P1 woman has been prescribed an oral contraceptive agent. She was counseled about some risks, but also some benefits. Which of the following is a benefit of combination oral contraception?

   A. Decreased risk of breast cancer
   B. Decreased gallstone formation
   C. Decreased deep venous thrombosis risk
   D. Decreased benign breast masses

44.4 A 28-year-old woman experienced an episode of unprotected intercourse. Her last menstrual period was about 2 weeks previously. She receives a combination oral contraceptive agent for emergency contraception. Which of the following is the most common side effect of the Yuzpe regimen (combination OC)?

A. Vaginal spotting
B. Nausea and/or vomiting
C. Elevation of liver function enzymes
D. Glucose intolerance
E. Renal insufficiency

44.5 A 25-year-old nulliparous woman is being evaluated for possible IUD insertion. Which of the following characteristics is most acceptable for IUD use?

A. Current sexually transmitted disease
B. Nulliparity
C. Recent pelvic inflammatory disease
D. Enlarged uterus with an irregular cavity

44.6 A 29-year-old G1P1 woman requests emergency contraception for unprotected intercourse. She is given choices between the progestin-only (Plan B) regimen versus the Yuzpe (combination OC) regimen. Which of the following is the main effect of the progestin-only regimen as compared with the Yuzpe regimen in EC?

A. Higher ectopic pregnancy rate
B. Less effective prevention of pregnancy
C. Less nausea
D. More liver dysfunction

ANSWERS

44.1 **A.** Depot medroxyprogesterone acetate is associated with loss of bone mineral density particularly in adolescents. If it is the best type of contraception for the patient, then the loss in bone mineral density should not discourage the use of the agent, but it should be considered in the choice of the contraception agent.

44.2 **C.** Tension headaches are not a contraindication for oral contraceptive agents. Migraines with aura increase the risk of strokes in patient who take combination hormonal contraception. Other contraindications to combination hormonal contraception include diabetes with vascular disease, heavy smoker over the age of 35, and uncontrolled hypertension.

44.3 **D.** Oral contraceptives have many beneficial effects including decreasing the risk of endometrial and ovarian cancer, and decreasing the risk of benign breast disease; there may be a slight increase in risk of breast cancer and incidence of gallstones.

44.4 **B.** Because of the high dose of estrogens, nausea and vomiting are the most common side effects.

44.5 **B.** Nulliparity is not a contraindication to IUD insertion. Contraindications include pregnancy, current or recent history of pelvic inflammatory disease, current sexually transmitted disease, current or recent puerperal or postabortion sepsis, purulent cervicitis, undiagnosed abnormal vaginal bleeding, malignancy of the genital tract, known uterine anomalies or fibroids distorting the uterine cavity in a way incompatible with IUD insertion (*Note*: Small fibroid [3-4 cm] not impinging on the uterine cavity is not a contraindication), or allergy to any component of the IUD or Wilson disease.

44.6 **C.** As compared to the combination OC regimen, the progestin-only method has better efficacy and fewer side effects (nausea). Thus, it is the preferred method. Patients who are given the combination OC agents usually require an antiemetic agent.

CLINICAL PEARLS

- Emergency contraception is effective when initiated within 72 hours of intercourse.
- Emergency contraception consists of high-dose combination hormones, high-dose progestin, or insertion of an a copper IUD.
- The main side effects of combination hormonal emergency contraception therapy are nausea and vomiting.
- An advantage of copper IUD insertion for emergency contraception is that it can be retained for continuous long-term contraception.
- The levonorgestrel-releasing IUD can be used to improve bleeding profiles in patients with abnormal uterine bleeding.
- Nonuser-dependent methods (long acting reversible contraception) like the IUD and the subdermal implant, have the lowest failure rates.
- Oral contraceptives decrease the risk of ovarian and endometrial cancer; there may be a slightly increased risk of breast cancer.
- It decreases the duration of menses and the amount of blood loss per cycle.
- Smoking >15 cigarettes per day over the age of 35 years is an absolute contraindication for combination hormonal contraceptives.
- Sickle cell crisis and epilepsy occur less often with DMPA.
- The contraceptive patch may be associated with a greater risk of DVT.

REFERENCES

American College of Obstetricians and Gynecologists. Adolescents and long-acting reversible contraception: implants and intrauterine devices. *ACOG Committee Opinion 539.* Washington, DC; 2012.

American College of Obstetricians and Gynecologists. Contraception for adolescents. *Guidelines for Adolescent Health Care.* 2nd ed. Washington, DC; 2011:43-63.

American College of Obstetricians and Gynecologists. Depot medroxyprogesterone acetate and bone effects. *ACOG Committee Opinion 602.* Washington, DC; 2014.

American College of Obstetricians and Gynecologists. Emergency contraception. *ACOG Practice Bulletin 112.* Washington, DC; 2010. (Reaffirmed 2013.)

American College of Obstetricians and Gynecologists. Increasing use of contraceptive implants and intrauterine devices to reduce unintended pregnancy. *ACOG Committee Opinion 495.* Washington, DC; 2009. (Reaffirmed 2011.)

American College of Obstetricians and Gynecologists. Long-acting reversible contraception: implants and intrauterine devices. *ACOG Practice Bulletin 121.* Washington, DC; 2011. (Reaffirmed 2013.)

American College of Obstetricians and Gynecologists. Noncontraceptive uses of hormonal contraceptives. *ACOG Practice Bulletin 110.* Washington, DC; 2010. (Reaffirmed 2012.)

American College of Obstetricians and Gynecologists. Use of hormonal contraception in women with coexisting medical conditions. *ACOG Practice Bulletin 73.* Washington, DC; 2006. (Reaffirmed 2011.)

Centers for Disease Control and Prevention (CDC). U.S. medical eligibility criteria for contraceptive use, 2010. *MMWR Recomm Rep.* 2010;59(RR-4):1-86.

Centers for Disease Control and Prevention. U.S. selected practice recommendations for contraceptive use, 2013. *MMWR.* 2013;62:1-60.

Fine PM. Update on emergency contraception. *Adv Ther.* 2011;28(2):87-90.

Mishell DR Jr. Family planning. In: Katz VL, Lentz GM, Lobo RA, Gershenson DM, eds. *Comprehensive Gynecology.* 5th ed. Philadelphia, PA: Mosby Elsevier; 2007:275-325.

Nelson AL. Family planning: reversible contraception, sterilization, and abortion. In: Hacker NF, Gambone JC, Hobel CJ, eds. *Essentials of Obstetrics and Gynecology.* 5th ed. Philadelphia, PA: Saunders; 2009:304-314.

CASE 45

A 23-year-old woman underwent a dilation and curettage (D&C) for an incomplete abortion 3 days previously. She complains of continued vaginal bleeding and lower abdominal cramping. Over the last 24 hours, she notes significant fever and chills. On examination, her temperature is 102.5°F (39.2°C), blood pressure (BP) is 90/40 mm Hg, and heart rate (HR) is 120 beats per minute (bpm). The cardiac examination reveals tachycardia, and the lungs are clear. There is moderately severe lower abdominal tenderness. The pelvic examination shows the cervical os to be open to 1.5 cm, and there is uterine tenderness. The leukocyte count is 20,000/mm^3, and the hemoglobin level is 12 g/dL. The urinalysis shows 2 wbc/hpf.

▶ What is the most likely diagnosis?
▶ What is the next step in management?

ANSWERS TO CASE 45:
Abortion, Septic

Summary: A 23-year-old woman, who had undergone a dilatation and curettage procedure 3 days ago for an incomplete abortion, complains of continued vaginal bleeding, lower abdominal cramping, and fever and chills. Her temperature is 102.5°F (39.2°C), BP is 90/40 mm Hg, and HR is 120 bpm. The lungs are clear. There is moderately severe lower abdominal tenderness. The cervix is open, and there is uterine tenderness. The laboratory studies are significant for leukocytosis and a normal urinalysis.

- **Most likely diagnosis:** Septic abortion (with retained products of conception).
- **Next step in management:** Broad-spectrum antibiotics and fluid resuscitation followed by D&C of the uterus.

ANALYSIS
Objectives

1. Understand the clinical presentation of septic abortion.
2. Know that the treatment of septic abortion involves antibiotic therapy and fluid resuscitation with uterine curettage.

Considerations

This 23-year-old woman underwent a D&C procedure for an incomplete abortion 3 days previously and now presents with lower abdominal cramping, vaginal bleeding, fever, and chills. The open cervical os, lower abdominal cramping, and vaginal bleeding suggest retained products of conception (POC). The retained POC may lead to ongoing bleeding or infection. In this case, the fever, chills, and leukocytosis point toward infection. The retained tissue serves as a nidus for infection. The most common source of the bacteria is the vagina, via an ascending infection. The best treatment is broad-spectrum antibiotics with anaerobic coverage and a uterine curettage. Usually, surgery is delayed until antimicrobial agents are infused for up to 4 hours to allow for tissue levels to increase. Hemorrhage may occur with the curettage procedure, since risk of perforation is high in an infected uterus. Also, the patient should be monitored for septic shock.

APPROACH TO:
Septic Abortion

DEFINITIONS

SEPTIC ABORTION: Any type of abortion associated with a uterine infection.

SEPTIC SHOCK: The septic portion refers to the presence of an infection (usually bacterial), and the shock describes a process whereby the patient's cells, organs, and/or tissues are not being sufficiently supplied with nutrients and/or oxygen.

CLINICAL APPROACH

The two most common complications associated with spontaneous abortion are hemorrhage and infection. Septic abortion occurs in 1% to 2% of all spontaneous abortions and about 0.5% of induced abortions. This risk is increased if an abortion is performed with nonsterile instrumentation. This condition is potentially fatal in 0.4 to 0.6/100 000 spontaneous abortions.

Signs and symptoms of septic abortion are uterine bleeding and/or spotting in the first trimester with clinical signs of infection. The **infection ascends from the vagina or cervix** to the endometrium to myometrium to parametrium, and, eventually, the peritoneum. Affected women generally will have fever and leukocyte counts of >10 500 cells/μL. There is usually lower abdominal tenderness, cervical motion tenderness, and a foul-smelling vaginal discharge. The infection is almost always polymicrobial, involving anaerobic streptococci, bacteroidesspecies, *Escherichia coli* and other gram-negative rods, and group B β-hemolytic streptococci. Rarely, *Clostridium perfringens*, *Hemophilusinfluenzae*, and *Campylobacter jejuni* may be isolated.

When patients present with signs and symptoms of septic abortion, a CBC with differential, urinalysis, and blood chemistries including electrolytes should be obtained. A specimen of cervical discharge should be sent for Gram stain, as well as for culture and sensitivity. If the patient appears seriously ill or is hypotensive, blood cultures, a chest x-ray, and blood coagulability studies should be done. The blood pressure, oxygen saturation, heart rate, and urine output should be monitored.

The **treatment** has four general parts: (1) **maintain the blood pressure**; (2) **monitor** the blood pressure, oxygenation, and urine output; (3) start **antibiotic therapy**; and (4) perform a **uterine curettage**. Immediate therapeutic steps include intravenous isotonic fluid replacement, especially in the face of hypotension. Concurrently, intravenous broad-spectrum antibiotics with particular attention to anaerobic coverage should be infused. The combination of gentamicin and clindamycin has a favorable response 95% of the time. Alternatives include β-lactam antimicrobials (cephalosporins and extended-spectrum penicillins) or those with β-lactamase inhibitors. Another regimen includes metronidazole plus ampicillin and an aminoglycoside. Because retained POC are common in these situations, becoming a nidus for infection to develop, evacuation of the uterine contents is important. Uterine curettage is usually performed approximately 4 hours after antibiotics are begun, allowing serum levels to be achieved. If patient does not respond to curettage and antibiotic treatment, a hysterectomy can be the next step in controlling the source of infection. Currently, no evidence has shown that a full antibiotic course is required if the patient remains afebrile for 48 hours post-D&C.

Because oliguria is an early sign of septic shock, the urine output should be carefully observed. Also, for women in shock, a central venous pressure catheter may be warranted. Aggressive intravenous fluids are usually effective in maintaining the blood pressure; however, at times, vasopressor agents, such as a norepinephrine infusion, may be required. Other therapies include oxygen, digitalis, and steroids.

CASE CORRELATION

- See Case 42 (Spontaneous Abortion). Rarely, patients with spontaneous abortion with retained products of conception can develop a septic abortion.

COMPREHENSION QUESTIONS

45.1 A 34-year-old woman undergoes an elective termination of pregnancy at 12 weeks' gestation. She develops fever, uterine tenderness, and is diagnosed with a septic abortion. Which of the following is the most likely mechanism of her infection?

A. Instrumental contamination

B. Ascending infection

C. Skin organisms

D. Urinary tract penetration

E. Hematogenous infection

45.2 A 22-year-old woman is diagnosed with a septic abortion after an incomplete abortion, fever, and uterine tenderness. She is treated with triple IV antibiotics and D&C of the uterus. After 48 hours of antibiotic therapy, she still has a fever of 102°F (38.8°C), BP of 80/40 mm Hg, and HR of 105 bpm. A computed tomography (CT) scan of the abdomen and pelvis is performed revealing pockets of air within the muscle of the uterus. Which of the following is the best treatment for this patient?

A. Add extended anaerobic coverage to the antibiotic regimen

B. Add intravenous heparin to the regimen

C. Continue the present antibiotic therapy

D. Counsel the patient regarding need for hysterectomy

45.3 A 32-year-old G1P0 Hispanic female at 29 weeks' gestation presents to the obstetrical triage unit complaining of fever, chills, and nausea and vomiting of 3 days duration. She also has myalgias. She denies leakage of fluid per vagina and states that she has been in good health. She has not been out of the country for 2 years. Questions about dietary habits reveal that she does not eat raw or uncooked foods, does not eat raw shellfish, but she does eat a fair amount of soft goat cheese. Her temperature is 101°F (38.33°C), BP is 100/80 mm Hg, and HR is 110 bpm. Her abdominal examination reveals tenderness of the uterine fundus. The fetal heart rate is 170 bpm. An ultrasound reveals a single gestation that is viable consistent with 29 weeks' gestational age, and a normal amniotic fluid volume. An amniocentesis is performed revealing greenish dark fluid, and a Gram stain of the amniotic fluid shows gram-positive rods. Which of the following is the most likely diagnosis?

A. Group B streptococcus infection
B. Clostridial infection
C. *Listeria monocytogenes* infection
D. *Pasteurella multiforme* infection
E. Meconium-stained amniotic fluid with bacterial skin contaminant

ANSWERS

45.1 **B. Ascending infection** is the most likely mechanism of septic abortion. The bacteria involved are typically polymicrobial, particularly **anaerobes** that have ascended from the lower genital tract. Signs and symptoms include uterine bleeding and/or spotting in the first trimester with clinical signs of infection. There is usually lower abdominal tenderness, cervical motion tenderness, and a foul-smelling vaginal discharge. Also, careful attention should be given to the patient's **urine output** since oliguria is an early sign of septic shock.

45.2 **D.** This patient has a septic abortion which has been treated conventionally with IV antibiotics and D&C to remove the nidus of the infection. She is still febrile and hypotensive despite antibiotic therapy for 48 hours. Also, due to the pockets of gas noted on CT scan, she likely has a necrotizing metritis, with gas-forming bacteria such as *Clostridial* species. Hysterectomy should be performed urgently as she may suffer severe morbidity or mortality if the procedure is delayed.

45.3 **C.** Chorioamnionitis, also called intra-amniotic infection, almost always complicates pregnancies with rupture of membranes. One exception to this rule is the Gram-positive rod *Listeria monocytogenes*, which can be acquired through unpasteurized milk products such as soft goat cheese. The bacterial infection in the maternal gastrointestinal tract, which presents as a flu-like illness, then is spread hematogenously to the fetus, through the placenta. The diagnosis is largely from clinical suspicion and confirmed by amniocentesis. Often the amniotic fluid is meconium stained, and Gram-positive rods may be seen on Gram stain. The microbiology laboratory should be alerted not to dismiss this finding as skin (bacteroid) contaminants. Treatment is with IV ampicillin. Many times, the infection may be treated with antibiotic therapy and avoid delivery (again, an exception to the usual rule of needing to deliver the baby in chorioamnionitis). *Listeria* can also cause miscarriage and septic abortion.

> **CLINICAL PEARLS**
>
> ▶ The bacteria involved in septic abortion are usually polymicrobial, particularly anaerobes that have ascended from the lower genital tract.
>
> ▶ Hemorrhage, due to uterine perforation, can often complicate the curettage for septic abortion.
>
> ▶ Treatment of septic abortion consists of maintaining blood pressure; monitoring the blood pressure, oxygenation, and urine output; antibiotics; and uterine evacuation of infected tissue.

REFERENCES

Eschenbach, DA. Treating spontaneous and induced septic abortions. *Obstet Gynecol.* 2015;125: 1042-1048.

Euhus DM. First-trimester abortion. In: Hoffman B, Schorge J, Schaffer J, Halvorson L, Bradshaw K, Cunningham F, eds. *Williams Gynecology.* 2nd ed. New York, NY: McGraw-Hill; 2012.

Katz VL. Spontaneous and recurrent abortion. In: Katz VL, Lentz GM, Lobo RA, Gersenson DM, eds. *Comprehensive Gynecology.* 6th ed. St. Louis, MO: Mosby-Year Book; 2012:359-387.

CASE 46

A 22-year-old woman is seen by her physician for a routine physical examination. She seems to be up to date regarding her immunizations and has received the human papilloma virus (HPV) vaccine. She has no family history of breast cancer. She denies breast leakage or prior medical problems. On examination, her blood pressure (BP) is 100/60 mm Hg. Her physical examination is unremarkable except for 1-cm, right, nontender breast mass. Her neck is supple, and the heart and lung examinations are normal. Palpation of her right breast reveals a firm, mobile, nontender, rubbery 1-cm mass in the upper outer quadrant. There are no skin abnormalities noted. No adenopathy is noted. The left breast is normal to palpation.

▶ What is your next step?
▶ What is the most likely diagnosis?

ANSWERS TO CASE 46:
Fibroadenoma of the Breast

Summary: A 22-year-old woman is noted to have a 1-cm breast mass on routine physical examination. Palpation of her right breast reveals a firm, mobile, non-tender, rubbery 1-cm mass in the upper outer quadrant. No adenopathy is noted.

- **Next step:** Biopsy of the mass (fine-needle biopsy or core needle biopsy).
- **Most likely diagnosis:** Fibroadenoma of the breast.

ANALYSIS
Objectives

1. Understand that any three-dimensional (3D) dominant mass needs a biopsy.
2. Know the characteristic presentation of fibroadenomas of the breast.
3. Understand that the greater the risk of breast cancer, the more tissue that is needed for biopsy.

Considerations

This woman comes in for a health maintenance examination; the approach is generally immunizations, cancer screening, and assessment and prevention for common diseases. On the physical examination, she is found to have a dominant breast mass. The firm, nontender, rubbery description is classic for a fibroadenoma. Fibroadenomas, as opposed to fibrocystic changes, do not change with the menstrual cycle. Although the most likely etiology is a fibroadenoma, this diagnosis needs to be confirmed by biopsy. Ultrasound of the breast is probably the best imaging modality in a young patient, since mammography is hampered by the dense breast tissue. The three methods of biopsy are fine-needle aspiration (FNA), core needle stereotactic biopsy, and excisional biopsy. Both core needle and excisional biopsy remove more tissue but are more prone to bruising and pain; an excisional biopsy is a more extensive surgical procedure involving removal of the entire mass. In this case, FNA is acceptable since the patient is at low risk for breast cancer. She has no family history of breast cancer, is of a young age, and her examination does not contain any worrisome features of breast cancer. If the mass were fixed, or if there were nipple retraction or bloody nipple discharge, the better method of biopsy would be a core needle or excisional biopsy to remove more tissue for histologic analysis.

SECTION II: CASES 445

APPROACH TO:
Breast Masses

DEFINITIONS

CORE NEEDLE BIOPSY: A 14- to 16-gauge needle used to extract tissue from a breast mass, which preserves cellular architecture.

FINE-NEEDLE ASPIRATION: The use of a small-gauge needle with associated vacuum via a syringe to aspirate fluid or some cells from a breast mass and/or cyst. The histology from the FNA would be loose cells (cytology).

FIBROADENOMA: Benign, smooth muscle tumor of the breast, usually occurring in young women.

EXCISIONAL BIOPSY: Surgical procedure to remove the entire lesion.

CLINICAL APPROACH

Background

Breast masses can involve tissue that comprise the breast including ducts, lobules, connective tissue, and the overlying skin. Fibrocystic changes are the most common breast mass, and is found in up to 90% of females at autopsy. Fibroadenomas are the most common benign tumor, whereas infiltrating ductal carcinoma is the most common malignancy. Although fibroadenomas are the most common cause of a breast mass in a woman less than age 25, the atypical breast cancer must always be considered.

Evaluation

One of the key skills of any primary care physician is differentiating normal breast changes from abnormal ones, that is, identification of the **dominant breast mass. Fibrocystic changes,** the most common of the benign breast conditions, are described as **multiple, irregular, "lumpiness of the breast."** It is not a disease per se, but rather an exaggerated response to ovarian hormones. Fibrocystic changes are very common in premenopausal women, but rare following menopause. The clinical presentation is cyclic, painful, engorged breasts, more pronounced just before menstruation, and occasionally associated with serous or green breast discharge. Through careful physical examination, fibrocystic changes can usually be differentiated from the 3D-dominant mass suggestive of cancer, but occasionally, a fine-needle or core biopsy must be performed to establish the diagnosis. Treatment includes decreasing caffeine ingestion, and adding NSAIDs, a tight-fitting bra, oral contraceptives, or oral progestin therapy. With severe cases, danazol (a weak antiestrogen and androgenic compound) or even mastectomy are considered.

In a woman in the adolescent years or in her 20s, the most common cause of a dominant breast mass is a **fibroadenoma.** These tumors are **firm, rubbery, mobile, and solid in consistency.** They typically do not respond to ovarian hormones and do not vary during the menstrual cycle. Since any 3D-dominant mass necessitates histologic confirmation, a biopsy should be performed. In a woman less than age 35 years, an FNA or core needle biopsy is often chosen. The advantages of FNA are less expense, less pain, but higher nondiagnostic rate; advantages of core needle biopsy include higher sensitivity but higher cost.

The concept of the **triple assessment,** that is, clinical examination, imaging (ultrasound or mammography), and histology being concordant (all in agreement) has high reliability with either FNA or core needle biopsy. Nonconcordance usually indicates obtaining more tissue. If the histologic examination supports fibroadenoma (mature smooth muscle cells) and the mass is small and not growing, careful follow-up is possible. A rare tumor seen in adolescents and younger women, cystosarcoma phylloides, is diagnosed by biopsy. Nevertheless, many women choose to have excision of the mass. Most clinicians will excise any dominant 3D mass occurring in a woman over the age of 35 years, or in those with an increased likelihood of mammary cancer (family history).

BRCA Testing

Hereditary breast and ovarian cancer syndrome is most commonly related to mutations in BRCA 1 and BRCA 2 genes. Together, BRCA 1 and 2 account for 10% of ovarian cancer cases, and 3% to 5% of breast cancers. Women with BRCA-1 mutation have a 65% lifetime risk of breast cancer and 39% lifetime risk of ovarian cancer; those with BRCA-2 mutation have a 45% risk of breast and a 15% risk of ovarian cancer. These mutations are associated with an increased risk of fallopian tube, peritoneal, and pancreatic cancer. See Case 47 for more details.

COMPREHENSION QUESTIONS

Match the breast lesion (A-E) to the clinical presentation (46.1-46.4).

    A. Fibroadenoma

    B. Fibrocystic changes

    C. Intraductal papilloma

    D. Breast cancer

    E. Galactocele

46.1 A 34-year-old woman complains of unilateral serosanguineous nipple discharge from the breast, expressed from one duct. No mass is palpated.

46.2 A 27-year-old woman complains of breast pain, which increases with menses. The breast has a lumpy-bumpy sensation.

46.3 A 47-year-old woman has a 1.5-cm right breast mass with nipple retraction and skin dimpling over the mass.

46.4 An 18-year-old adolescent female has an asymptomatic, 1-cm, nontender, mobile right breast mass.

46.5 A 32-year-old G0P0 woman complains of a 1-week history of a red and tender breast. She denies trauma, insect bites, pustules, or other lesions. Her family history is negative for breast disease. She denies oral contraceptive use. On examination, her temperature is 98°F (36.6°C), heart rate (HR) is 80 beats per minute (bpm), and BP is 100/60 mm Hg. Her heart and lung examination is normal. The right breast reveals a 5 × 4 cm area of redness, induration, and tenderness. There is no breast discharge. Her right axillary lymph nodes are mildly tender and enlarged. Which of the following is the next best step for this patient?

A. Oral antibiotic therapy
B. Biopsy of the breast
C. Intravenous antibiotic therapy
D. Advise the use of a tight-fitting bra and avoid caffeine

46.6. A 25-year-old G0P0 woman states that her mother, who lives in another city, was diagnosed with breast cancer at age 45. There is also a history of ovarian cancer in a maternal aunt. Which of the following is the best next step?

A. Offer BRCA testing to the patient
B. Request that the patient's mother have BRCA testing
C. Offer the patient tamoxifen chemoprophylaxis
D. Offer the patient magnetic resonance imaging of bilateral breasts

ANSWERS

46.1 **C.** The most common cause of bloody (serosanguineous) nipple discharge when only one duct is involved and in the absence of a breast mass is intraductal papilloma. These are typically small, benign tumors that grow in the milk ducts. The highest incidence of this condition is in the 35 to 55 age group; causes and risk factors are unknown. The discharge is typically serosanguineous like the woman in this scenario. Because malignancy is also a common cause of bloody nipple discharge (second most common cause!), ductal exploration is required to rule out cancer.

46.2 **B.** A diffuse "lumpy-bumpy" examination suggests fibrocystic changes. They are very common in premenopausal women but rare following menopause. The classic clinical picture includes cyclic, painful, engorged breasts, more pronounced just before menstruation, and occasionally associated with breast discharge. Treatment includes decreasing caffeine intake and adding NSAIDs, a tight-fitting bra, oral contraceptives, or oral progestin therapy. With severe cases, danazol (a weak antiestrogen and androgenic compound) or even mastectomy is considered. A patient who presents with painful, engorged breasts may also have a galactocele; however, a galactocele does not have a "lumpy-bumpy" breast examination, nor is it associated with hormonal changes or the menstrual cycle. Galactoceles are mammary gland tumors that are cystic in nature and contain milk or milky fluid. They typically occur when there is any sort of obstruction of milk flow in the lactating breast.

46.3 **D.** Nipple retraction or skin dimpling over a mass is very suggestive of malignancy. In the physical examination, maneuvers to accentuate the skin changes such as "hands on hips" or "arms raised over the head" assist in evaluating for these findings. Most clinicians excise any dominant 3D mass occurring in a woman older than 35 years or in those with an increased likelihood of mammary cancer (family history). Histologic analysis from the excisional biopsy will most likely confirm the diagnosis of cancer.

46.4 **A.** In females in the adolescent years or in their twenties, the most common cause of a dominant breast mass is a fibroadenoma. These tumors are firm, rubbery, mobile, and solid in consistency. The best way to image the breast of a woman less than age 30 is usually ultrasound due to the dense fibrocystic changes that interfere with mammographic interpretation. Ultrasound can differentiate a solid versus a cystic mass, and sometimes can suggest a fibroadenoma; nevertheless, tissue should be obtained to confirm the diagnosis.

46.5 **B.** In a woman who has a "red tender indurated breast" who is nonlactating, inflammatory breast cancer must be ruled out. Biopsy of the breast is critical. Inflammatory breast cancer is aggressive in nature, and the skin changes occur due to the cancer cells within the subdermal lymph channels. Immediate diagnosis and therapy are crucial, whereas delay with various antibiotics would be detrimental. Interestingly, inflammatory breast cancer occurs more in younger patients, although women of any age can be affected.

46.6 **B.** In a patient who develops bilateral or premenopausal breast cancer, BRCA testing should be offered to the patient. If BRCA testing is positive, then first degree relatives should be notified, so that these individuals can consider whether BRCA testing is desired. If BRCA testing is negative in this index patient, then no further testing is needed to other relatives. This is the most efficient approach. Chemoprophylaxis with tamoxifen or bilateral mastectomy is not needed unless BRCA mutation is present.

CLINICAL PEARLS

▶ A firm, nontender, smooth mobile breast mass in a young woman (less than age 25 years) is most likely a fibroadenoma.

▶ Ultrasound is the best initial imaging modality in a younger patient.

▶ Although the biggest risk factor for breast cancer in general is age, breast malignancy does occur in younger patients.

▶ A red inflamed breast in a nonlactating woman should be evaluated for possible inflammatory breast cancer.

▶ BRCA testing is indicated for conditions of high risk for genetic breast and/or ovarian cancer.

REFERENCES

American College of Obstetricians and Gynecologists. Breast cancer screening. *ACOG Practice Bulletin 122*. Washington, DC; 2011. (Reaffirmed 2014.)

American College of Obstetricians and Gynecologists. Breast concerns in children and adolescents with cancer. *ACOG Committee Opinion 607*. Washington, DC; 2014.

Hacker NF, Friedlander ML. Breast disease: a gynecologic perspective. In: Hacker NF, Gambone JC, Hobel CJ, eds. *Essentials of Obstetrics and Gynecology*. 5th ed. Philadelphia, PA: Saunders; 2009: 332-344.

Valea FA, Katz VL. Breast diseases. In: Lentz GM, Lobo RA, Gershenson DM, Katz VL, eds. *Comprehensive Gynecology*. 6th ed. St. Louis, MO: Mosby-Year Book; 2012:301-335.

CASE 47

A 50-year-old G4P4 woman comes in for a well-woman examination. She had used the contraceptive diaphragm for birth control until she went into menopause 1 year ago. Her family history is unremarkable for cancer. Her surgical history includes a myomectomy for symptomatic uterine fibroids 10 years ago. On examination, her blood pressure (BP) is 120/74 mm Hg, heart rate (HR) is 80 beats per minute (bpm), and she is afebrile. Her thyroid is normal on palpation. Her heart and lung examinations are normal. The breast examination reveals a 1.5-cm, mobile, nontender mass in the upper outer quadrant of the right breast. No adenopathy or skin changes are appreciated. Mammography and ultrasound examinations of the breasts are normal.

▶ What is your next step?

ANSWER TO CASE 47:
Dominant Breast Mass

Summary: A 50-year-old postmenopausal woman comes in for a well-woman examination. The breast examination reveals a 1.5-cm, mobile, nontender mass of the upper outer quadrant of the right breast. No adenopathy or skin changes are appreciated. Mammography and ultrasound examinations of the breasts are normal.

- **Next step:** Core needle biopsy.

ANALYSIS
Objectives

1. Understand that a dominant breast mass requires tissue for histologic analysis.
2. Understand that the age of the patient is usually the biggest risk factor for breast cancer.
3. Understand that normal imaging of a palpable breast mass does not rule out cancer.

Considerations

This 50-year-old woman came in for a well-woman examination. The physical examination is aimed at screening for common and/or serious conditions, such as hypertension, thyroid disease, cervical cancer (Pap smear), colon cancer (stool for occult blood), and breast cancer. A single 1.5-cm breast mass is palpated, without any associated skin changes, such as nipple retraction or dimpling of the skin. There is no associated adenopathy. Furthermore, the imaging tests (mammography and ultrasonography) are normal. Despite the normal imaging, there is a possibility that the breast mass is malignant. Therefore, biopsy of the mass is indicated.

The usual approach is a core needle biopsy based on palpation. Fine-needle aspiration is an acceptable diagnostic modality, but would not be able to discern ductal carcinoma in situ versus invasion. Needle biopsy is usually preferred rather than excision to better plan future surgeries. The combination of the clinical examination, the imaging, and the needle biopsy is called the triple test. When all three tests agree (benign or malignant), this concordant result is >99% accurate. If any one parameter suggests cancer, even in the face of the other two being negative, most experts will recommend excision of the mass to assess for malignancy.

APPROACH TO:
Breast Masses

DEFINITIONS

DOMINANT BREAST MASS: A mass that, on palpation, is felt to be separate from the remainder of the breast tissue.

EXCISIONAL BIOPSY: Surgical procedure removing the entire mass.

SENTINEL NODE BIOPSY: Removal and examination of the first lymph nodes that cancer cells are likely to spread from the primary tumor, determined by injecting radioactive or color dye near the tumor, and probing the lymph nodes which are affected.

SKIN DIMPLING: Retraction of the skin, which is suspicious for an underlying malignancy, due to the cancer being fixed or pulling on the skin.

BRCA GENE MUTATIONS: BRCA1 gene is located on chromosome 17 and BRCA2 gene is located on chromosome 13. These are tumor suppressor genes, such that a mutation in the gene confers a markedly increased risk of breast cancer and ovarian cancer.

INFLAMMATORY BREAST CANCER: A rare but aggressive type of breast cancer in which the cancer cells obstruct the lymphatic vessels of the skin and subdermal breast tissue. The presentation is warmth and redness and diagnosed by biopsy.

CLINICAL APPROACH

Breast cancer is the most common cancer in women, excluding skin cancer. It is the second leading cause of female cancer deaths in the United States, exceeded only by lung cancer. It is also the most frequently diagnosed cause of death from cancer in women worldwide. Established risk factors for breast cancer include age, personal or family history of breast cancer or precancerous lesions, reproductive factors (early menarche and late menopause), hormonal treatment, postmenopausal obesity, alcohol consumption, exposure to ionizing radiation, and genetic predisposition. The prevalence of breast cancer is age specific, and **age is the most important risk factor.** One in 2500 women will develop breast cancer at the age of 20 years; whereas 1 in 30 women will develop breast cancer at the age of 60 years, giving an overall lifetime risk of 1 in 8.

Early diagnosis improves survival. One common way breast cancer is first discovered is a mass palpated by the patient. Unfortunately, this frequently occurs at an advanced stage. Routine screening is preferable. Clinical breast examination every 3 years should be performed for women from ages 20 to 39 years. Routine self-breast examination is no longer recommended due to false positive rates; however, breast self awareness still has utility. In other words, the patient may be aware of the texture and consistency of her breasts and should report changes. **Women over the age of 40 years should have a yearly clinical breast examination and** mammography according to ACOG (The American College of Obstetricians and Gynecologists) and American Cancer Society guidelines. **In contrast, the United States Preventive Services Task Force recommend biennial mammography in women aged 50–74 years. However, mammography** may be performed sooner if risk factors warrant the need. In general, age is the most significant risk factor for breast cancer, but other parameters are important to consider.

Mammograms carry a false-negative rate of up to 10%. Thus, **any palpable dominant mass, regardless of mammographic findings, requires histologic diagnosis.**

Other imaging methods include breast ultrasound (handled or automated), tomosynthesis, magnetic resonance imaging (MRI) (with or without the administration of contrast material), positron-emission tomography, and positron-emission mammography. Those technologies are not alternatives to mammography for women with average risk of breast cancer.

Ultrasonography is an established adjunct to mammography, useful in evaluating young patients and other women with dense breast tissue and in differentiating a cyst from a solid mass. Magnetic resonance is the recommended imaging modality for screening women with 20% or greater lifetime risk of breast cancer including women with BRCA1 or BRCA2 gene mutation according to the American cancer society.

If a mammogram detects a suspicious lesion, a biopsy is usually performed. For nonpalpable lesions, the biopsy requires ultrasound-guided core needle biopsy or stereotactic core needle biopsy. In selected cases, excisional biopsy with needle localization may be required.

Nearly 30% of breast cancers have some familial component, but <10% are caused by inherited mutations in major breast cancer susceptibility genes. A patient who has two first-degree relatives with breast cancer is a candidate for genetic testing, such as BRCA1 and BRCA2 testing. Patients of Ashkenazi Jewish ancestry are particularly of increased risk (see Table 47–1). A mutation of the BRCA1 or

Table 47–1 • INDICATIONS FOR BRCA TESTING
Recommended due to 20% risk
Patient has had both breast and ovarian cancer
Patient with ovarian cancer and close relative with ovarian cancer or premenopausal breast cancer
Patient with ovarian cancer who are of Ashkenazi Jewish descent
Patient with breast cancer at an early age (<50) and a close relative with breast cancer
Patient diagnosed with breast cancer below age 40 of Ashkenazi Jewish descent
Patient with a close relative with a known BRCA1 or BRCA2 mutation
Counseled about possible testing due to 5%-10% risk
Patient with breast cancer diagnosed below age 40
Patient with cancer of ovary, peritoneum or fallopian tube of high grade, serous histology (regardless of age)
Patient with breast cancer at early age (<50) and close relative diagnosed with breast cancer at early age (<50)
Patient with breast cancer diagnosed at early age (<50) and of Ashkenazi Jewish descent

Close relative: first degree relative (mother, sister, daughter) or second degree relative (grandmother, granddaughter, aunt, niece).

TABLE 47–2 • SCREENING, MEDICAL AND SURGICAL PREVENTION OF BREAST AND OVARIAN CANCER IN HIGH RISK PATIENTS

Prevention of breast cancer

Lifestyle: early childbirth, breast feed; exercise, normal weight, minimize alcohol
Clinical examination every 6 months
Mammography annually beginning age 25-30
Consider MRI of breast beginning age 25-30 (not yet consensus)
Consider tamoxifen (raloxifene or aromatase inhibitor may also be used)
Consider bilateral mastectomy age 35-40

Prevention of ovarian cancer

Pelvic examination every 6-12 months
Consider CA125 and pelvic ultrasound every 6-12 months
Consider oral contraceptive agent for 6 years
Recommend bilateral salpingo-ophorectomy at age 40 (reduces breast cancer and ovarian cancer risk)

BRCA2 gene is associated with a 60% to 70% risk of breast cancer. BRCA1 mutation is associated with a 40% to 50% of ovarian cancer, and BRCA2 mutation is associated with 12% to 20% of ovarian cancer. Identification of these risks also allow for risk-reduction medications and possibly surgery such as bilateral mastectomy or prophylactic salpino-oophorectomy after childbearing (See Table 47–2).

CASE CORRELATION

- See also Case 46 (Fibroadenoma) and compare the diagnostic approach to a younger patient with features consistent with a fibroadenoma versus an older patient with a breast mass.

COMPREHENSION QUESTIONS

47.1 A 36-year-old woman is noted to have a 2-cm palpable breast mass noted on physical examination. A mammogram is performed suggestive of a cyst. Ultrasound confirms a cystic mass. A fine-needle aspiration is performed with 8 cc of blood-colored fluid obtained. The mass is no longer palpable. Which of the following is the next best step for this patient?

A. Expectant management as the prognosis is excellent

B. Send the fluid for cytology

C. Lumpectomy and lymph node dissection

D. Tamoxifen therapy

47.2 A 26-year-old woman is referred for genetic counseling because her mother died from breast cancer, and her sister has been diagnosed with breast cancer. The patient is noted to have a BRCA1 mutation. Which of the following best describes the genetic transmission of this disorder?
   A. Autosomal dominant
   B. Autosomal recessive
   C. X-linked dominant
   D. X-linked recessive

47.3 A 49-year-old woman is noted to have a 1.5-cm mass of the right breast. It is nontender, and there are no skin changes or adenopathy. The mammogram and ultrasound findings are normal. A core needle biopsy reveals an infiltrating intraductal carcinoma. Which of the following would most significantly impact on the patient's prognosis?
   A. Hormone receptor status
   B. Lymph node status
   C. Size of the primary cancer
   D. Presence of skin changes

47.4 A 35-year-old G0P0 woman complains of right breast redness and tenderness. The patient denies a family history of breast or ovarian cancer. Which of the following is the next best step in managing this patient?
   A. Antibiotic therapy to cover *Staphylococcus aureus*
   B. Biopsy of the breast
   C. Ultrasound of the breast
   D. Begin combination chemotherapy

ANSWERS

47.1 **B.** When the fluid obtained from a breast cyst is straw-colored and the mass disappears, then the fluid can be discarded and no further therapy is needed. However, when the fluid is a different color such as bloody, then the fluid should be sent for cytology. Lumpectomy and lymph node sentinel node biopsy is performed for proven breast cancer for staging. Tamoxifen therapy may be used for postmenopausal women with estrogen receptor positive breast cancer after surgery.

47.2 **A.** A mutation to BRCA1 gene is associated with an increased risk of breast and ovarian cancer. This is an autosomal dominant disorder. Half the offsprings would be affected, and both sexes would be equally affected.

47.3 **B.** The patient's lymph node status is the most significant impact on the patient's prognosis. Hormone receptor status does play some role but not as significantly as the lymph node condition. Infiltrating intraductal carcinoma is the most common histological subtype of breast cancer. The size of the primary tumor likewise does play a role. Optimally, the smaller the tumor, the better the survival.

47.4 **B.** This patient very well could have inflammatory breast cancer since she has redness and warmth of the breast and is not lactating. She is nulliparous. Chemotherapy should not be initiated until a diagnosis is made.

CLINICAL PEARLS

▶ A breast mass must be biopsied, regardless of the imaging results.
▶ Early detection of breast cancer leads to better survival.
▶ In general, the biggest risk factor for the development of breast cancer is age.
▶ Two first-degree family members with breast cancer suggest a familial syndrome, such as mediated by the BRCA1 or BRCA2 gene.
▶ For women who test positive for BRCA1 or BRCA2 mutations, enhanced screening is recommended (such as twice-yearly clinical breast examinations, annual mammography, annual breast MRI, and instruction in breast self-examination beginning at age 25 years or sooner based on earliest age onset in the family), and risk reduction methods should be discussed.
▶ Women at the age of 35 years or greater with a family history of breast cancer should have annual mammography.
▶ The most common cause of unilateral serosanguineous nipple discharge from a single duct is intraductal papilloma.
▶ Infiltrating ductal carcinoma is the most common histological type of breast cancer.
▶ A breast cyst in which the fluid is straw-colored or clear and the breast mass upon aspiration disappears may be observed.
▶ Upon aspiration of a breast cyst, fluid that is other than straw-colored should be sent for cytology, and a mass that persists after aspiration should be biopsied.

REFERENCES

American College of Obstetricians and Gynecologists. Breast cancer screening. *ACOG Practice Bulletin 42*. Washington, DC; August 2011. (Reaffirmed 2014.)

American College of Obstetricians and Gynecologists. Hereditary breast and ovarian cancer syndrome. *ACOG Practice Bulletin 103*. Washington, DC; April 2009. (Reaffirmed 2015.)

Béatrice L.-S., Chiara S, Dana L, et al. Breast-cancer screening—viewpoint of the IARC working group. *N Engl J Med.* 2015;372:2353-2358. DOI: 10.1056/NEJMsr150436.

Hoffman BL, Schorge JO, Schaffer JI, et al. Breast disease. *Williams Gynecology.* 2nd ed. McGraw-Hill Education; 2012:345-352.

Lentz GM, Lobo RA, Gershenson DM, et al. Breast diseases. *Comprehensive Gynecology.* 6th ed. Philadelphia, PA: Elsevier Mosby; 2012:309-332.

CASE 48

A 59-year-old woman comes into the doctor's office for a health maintenance examination. Her past medical history is remarkable for mild hypertension controlled with an oral thiazide diuretic agent. Her surgical history is unremarkable. On examination, her blood pressure is 140/84 mm Hg, heart rate is 70 beats per minute, and she is afebrile. The thyroid is normal to palpation. The breasts are nontender and without masses. The pelvic examination is unremarkable. Mammography revealed a small cluster of calcifications around a small mass.

▶ What is your next step?

ANSWER TO CASE 48:
Breast, Abnormal Mammogram

Summary: A 59-year-old woman comes into the doctor's office for a health maintenance examination. The breasts are nontender and without masses. Mammography revealed a small cluster of calcifications around a small mass.

- **Next step:** Stereotactic core needle biopsy.

ANALYSIS
Objectives

1. Understand the role of mammography in screening for breast cancer.
2. Know that mammography is not perfect in identifying breast cancer.
3. Know the typical mammographic findings that are suspicious for cancer.

Considerations

This 59-year-old woman is going to her doctor for routine health maintenance. She is taking a thiazide diuretic for mild hypertension. Her blood pressure is mildly elevated. The mammogram reveals a small cluster of calcifications around a small mass, which is one of the classic findings of breast cancer. With this mammographic finding, it is of paramount importance to obtain tissue for histologic diagnosis. Because of the high risk of malignancy, a stereotactic-directed core biopsy is indicated.

APPROACH TO:
The Abnormal Mammogram

DEFINITIONS

SUSPICIOUS MAMMOGRAPHIC FINDINGS: A small cluster of calcifications, or masses with ill-defined borders.

NEEDLE LOCALIZATION: Procedure in which a sterile wire is placed via mammographic guidance such that the end of the wire is placed in the center of the suspicious area. The surgeon uses this guide to assist in excising breast tissue.

STEREOTACTIC CORE BIOPSY: Procedure in which the patient is prone on the mammographic table and biopsies are taken as directed with computer-assisted techniques.

CLINICAL APPROACH

Although a clinical history and proper clinical breast examinations are important in detecting breast cancer, mammography remains the best method of detecting breast cancer at an early stage.

A mammogram is an x-ray of the breast tissue. Current radiation levels from mammography have been shown to be safe and cause no increased risk in developing breast cancer. The radiation exposure is <10 rad per lifetime if annual mammograms begin at age 40 years and continue up to age 90. Both false positives and false negatives of up to 10% have been noted. **Hence, a palpable breast mass in the face of a normal mammogram still requires a biopsy.** Breast implants can diminish the accuracy of a mammogram, particularly if the implants are in front of the chest muscles. Magnetic resonance imaging has recently been shown to be effective in screening for breast cancer, particularly in younger patients and those at risk for breast cancer such as due to BRCA mutation. Magnetic resonance imaging (MRI) may identify early breast cancers missed by mammography.

Mammographic findings strongly suggestive of breast cancer include a mass, often with spiculated and invasive borders, or an architectural distortion, or an asymmetric increased tissue density when compared with prior studies or a corresponding area in the opposite breast (Figure 48–1). An isolated cluster of irregular calcifications, especially if linear and wispy, is an important sign of breast cancer.

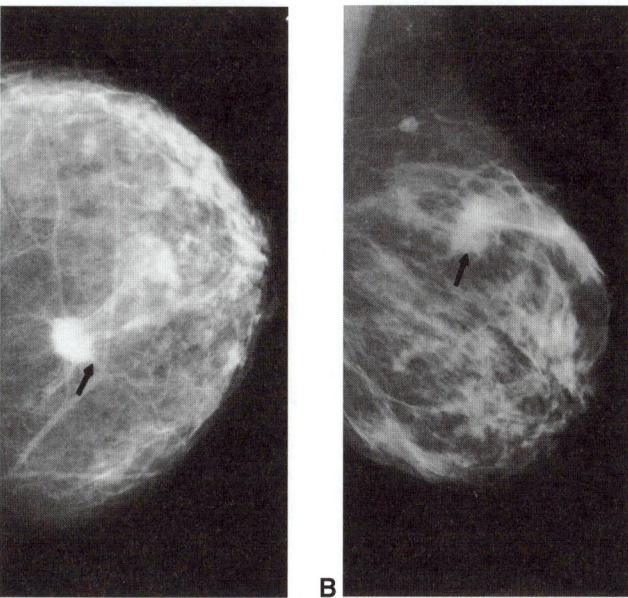

Figure 48–1. Mammogram showing spiculated mass. Early intraductal carcinoma of the right breast. Craniocaudal (**A**) and oblique mediolateral (**B**) views of the right breast show a spiculated mass in the upper outer quadrant. (*Reproduced with permission from Schwartz SI, Shires GT, Spencer FL, et al, eds. Principles of Surgery. 7th ed. New York, NY: McGraw-Hill; 1999:545.*)

If a breast cancer is suspected, biopsy is warranted. A stereotactic biopsy may be used to localize and sample the lesion. This method employs a computerized, digital, three-dimensional view of the breast and allows the physician to direct the needle to the biopsy site. The procedure carries a 2% to 4% "miss rate." Needle-localization biopsies employ multiple mammographic views of the breast and allow the surgeon to localize the lesion for evaluation. The latter procedure is more time-consuming, carries a comparable 3% to 5% miss rate, but excises more tissue, which is helpful in "borderline" histologic conditions, such as ductal carcinoma-in-situ.

As compared to conventional film mammography, digital mammography has a slightly higher sensitivity for women less than age 50, premenopausal women, and those with dense breasts. However, outside of those categories, film mammography and digital mammography have similar accuracy.

CASE CORRELATION

- See also Case 46 (Fibroadenoma) and Case 47 (Dominant Breast Mass). In these two cases, the mass is palpable and directed biopsy toward the palpable mass. In this current case, the imaging result is abnormal and no mass is palpable.

COMPREHENSION QUESTIONS

48.1 A 40-year-old woman undergoes a screening mammogram which reveals a lesion of the right breast, showing an ill-defined mass with a cluster of calcifications. She recalls bumping her right breast against a doorknob leading to a bruise approximately 1 year previously. Which of the following is the most likely diagnosis?

A. Ductal carcinoma-in-situ
B. Infiltrating intraductal carcinoma
C. Fat necrosis
D. Lobular carcinoma

48.2 A 39-year-old woman physicist is referred by her physician for a screening mammogram. She asks about the amount of radiation exposure, and the cumulative risk of cancers due to the radiation. Which of the following describes the radiation risk with modern mammography given once annually?

A. Increased risk for thyroid cancer
B. No increased risks
C. Increased risk for lung cancer
D. Increased risk of skin cancer in the chest area

48.3 A 55-year-old woman has several coarse calcifications found on mammographythat are suspicious for breast cancer. She has no family history of breast cancer and no mass is palpable. Which of the following is the most accurate statement?

A. The best diagnostic method for this patient is fine-needle aspiration.
B. The next best step is MRI of the lesion.
C. Since there is no palpable mass on physical examination, the patient may be observed for changes on mammography in 3 months.
D. One option for this patient is a core tissue biopsy by stereotactic means.

48.4 A 62-year-old woman is noted to have a 2-cm left breast mass detected on clinical examination. Stereotactic core needle biopsy reveals infiltrating ductal carcinoma. The patient is noted to have a triple negative tumor. Which of the following is more accurate about this condition?

A. The patient has a negative mammogram, MRI, and ultrasound.
B. The patient has a negative sentinel node biopsy, chest x-ray, and computed tomography scan.
C. The patient has a negative estrogen and progesterone receptor, and her2/neu expression status.
D. The patient has a negative surgical margin laterally, medially, and anteroposteriorly.

ANSWERS

48.1 **C.** Fat necrosis resulting from trauma to the breast often leads to mammographic findings that are identical to breast cancer. For instance, trauma to the breast due to a motor vehicle accident with the shoulder belt causing bruising of the breast is a common scenario. This patient recalls trauma to the breast in the location of the mammographic abnormality. To further evaluate the patient and confirm the diagnosis, a biopsy should be performed. Cancer is still a concern, and infiltrating ductal carcinoma is the most common histological subtype.

48.2 **B.** Modern mammography has very low radiation and no increased risk of cancer.

48.3 **D.** Mammographic findings that are suspicious for cancer must be addressed. Two viable methods include core biopsy via stereotactic guidance and needle-localization excision. Fine-needle aspiration is not sensitive enough, and no mass is palpable to be able to serve for localizing. MRI does not add to an already suspicious lesion.

48.4 **C.** The triple negative malignancy consists of estrogen receptor, progesterone receptor, and her2/neu expression negative. This finding is associated with a poor prognosis, and the malignancy is less treatable.

CLINICAL PEARLS

▶ Mammographic findings suggestive of cancer include a small cluster of calcifications or a mass with irregular borders.

▶ Stereotactic core biopsy or needle-localization excisional biopsy are two accepted methods of assessing suspicious mammographic nonpalpable masses. Core needle biopsy can decrease the number of surgical procedures for the patient.

▶ The amount of radiation from mammography is negligible and has no significant sequelae.

▶ Trauma to the breast may lead to fat necrosis and produce mammographic findings similar to that seen in breast cancer. These lesions should be excised to confirm the diagnosis.

REFERENCES

American College of Obstetrician and Gynecologists. Breast cancer screening. *ACOG Practice Bulletin 42*. Washington, DC; August 2011. (Reaffirmed 2014.)

American College of Obstetricians and Gynecologists. Management of gynecologic issues in women with breast cancer. *ACOG Practice Bulletin 126*; March 2012. (Reaffirmed 2014.)

Foulkes WD, et al. Triple-negative breast cancer. *N Engl J Med*. 2010:363;1938.

Hacker NF, Friedlander ML. Breast disease: a gynecologic perspective. In: Hacker NF, Gambone JC, Hobel CJ, eds. *Essentials of Obstetrics and Gynecology*. 6th ed. Philadelphia, PA: Saunders; 2015: 332-344.

Valea FA, Katz VL. Breast diseases. In: Katz VL, Lentz GM, Lobo RA, Gersenson DM, eds. *Comprehensive Gynecology*. 6th ed. St. Louis, MP: Mosby-Year Book; 2012:327-357.

CASE 49

A 33-year-old woman complains of 7 months of amenorrhea following a spontaneous abortion. She had a dilation and curettage (D&C) at that time. Her past medical and surgical histories are unremarkable. She experienced menarche at age 11 years and notes that her menses have been every 28 to 31 days until recently. Her general physical examination is unremarkable. The thyroid is normal to palpation, and breasts are without discharge. The abdomen is nontender. The pelvic examination shows a normal uterus, closed and normal-appearing cervix, and no adnexal masses. A pregnancy test is negative.

- What is the most likely diagnosis?
- What is the test to confirm the diagnosis?
- What would be the patient's response if a progestin challenge is administered?

ANSWERS TO CASE 49:
Amenorrhea (Intrauterine Adhesions)

Summary: A 33-year-old woman complains of 7 months of amenorrhea after she had a D&C for a spontaneous abortion. Her menstrual history was normal previously. The thyroid, pelvic, and breast examinations are normal. The pregnancy test is negative.

- **Most likely diagnosis:** Intrauterine adhesions (IUA; Asherman syndrome).
- **Test to confirm diagnosis:** Hysterosalpingogram or saline infusion sonohysterogram (or hysteroscopy).
- **Response to progestin challenge:** No bleeding due to unresponsive endometrium.

ANALYSIS
Objectives

1. Know the definition of secondary amenorrhea.
2. Understand how uterine curettage can cause endometrial adhesions and amenorrhea.
3. Know how to diagnose intrauterine adhesive disease (Asherman syndrome).

Considerations

This 33-year-old woman has had 7 months of amenorrhea since experiencing a miscarriage. She had undergone a uterine dilation and curettage at that time. Her menstrual history was unremarkable previously; hence, she meets the definition of secondary amenorrhea (6 months of no menses in a woman with previously normal menses). Pregnancy is the most common cause of secondary amenorrhea and thus, should be the first condition to be ruled out. The stepwise algorithm to assess for the etiology for amenorrhea is noted in Figure 49–1. Secondary amenorrhea may be caused by hypothalamic etiologies (such as hypothyroidism or hyperprolactinemia), pituitary conditions (such as Sheehan syndrome), or ovarian causes (such as premature ovarian failure). The patient does not have symptoms of hypothyroidism or galactorrhea, or hot flushes. Additionally, her history indicates that prior to an acute event, her miscarriage, she had regular menses. With no indication of a postpartum hemorrhage, the most probable source of her amenorrhea is an issue with the end organ, her uterus. Hence, the most likely diagnosis is intrauterine adhesions, arising from the curettage of the uterus. With this condition, the hypothalamus, pituitary, and ovary are working normally, but the endometrial tissue is not responsive to the hormonal changes. To confirm that the uterine cavity is obliterated with adhesions, a hysterosalpingogram, a radiologic study where radiopaque dye is injected into the uterine cavity via a transcervical catheter, or saline infusion ultrasound study can be used.

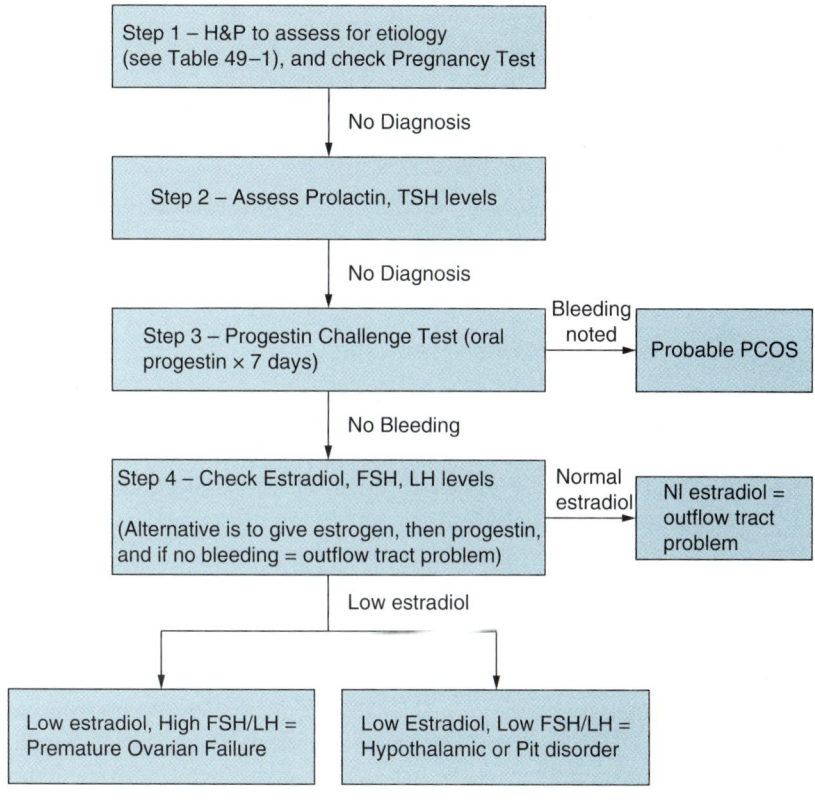

Figure 49–1. Algorithm to assess secondary amenorrhea.

APPROACH TO:
Suspected Intrauterine Adhesions

DEFINITIONS

PRIMARY AMENORRHEA: Not achieving menarche by age 16 while having normal breast development.

SECONDARY AMENORRHEA: Absence of menses in a previously menstruating women for a period of 6 months.

INTRAUTERINE ADHESIONS: Condition when scar tissue or synechiae form to obliterate the endometrial cavity, usually occurring because of uterine curettage following a pregnancy.

HYSTEROSALPINGOGRAM: A radiologic study in which radiopaque dye is injected into the endometrial cavity via a transcervical catheter, used to evaluate the endometrial cavity and/or the patency of the fallopian tubes.

HYSTEROSCOPY: Procedure of direct visualization of the endometrial cavity with an endoscope, a light source, and a distension media.

SALINE INFUSION SONOHYSTEROGRAPHY (SIS): A vaginal ultrasound procedure in which fluid is infused transcervically into the uterine cavity to provide enhanced visualization of the endometrial cavity.

UTERINE SOUNDING: Assessing the depth and direction of the cervical and uterine cavity with a thin blunt probe.

CLINICAL APPROACH

Intrauterine Adhesions (Asherman Syndrome)

Intrauterine scarring resulting in an unresponsive endometrium accounts for approximately 7% of cases of amenorrhea. It is most commonly due to injury to the pregnant or recently pregnant uterus secondary to curettage leading to damage of the endometrial basalis layer. However, any mechanical, infectious, or radiation factor can produce endometrial sclerosis and adhesion formation, including common uterine surgeries like cesarean sections and myomectomies. The adhesions are usually strands of avascular fibrous tissue, but they may also consist of inactive endometrium or myometrium. Myometrial adhesions are usually dense and vascular carrying a poor prognosis. Women with atrophic and sclerotic endometrium without adhesions carry the worst prognosis. This is usually found after radiation or tuberculous endometritis and is not amenable to any therapy. Postpartum curettage performed usually for concerns for retained products of conception, combined with hypoestrogenic states such as breast-feeding or hypogonadotropic hypogonadism, is associated with extensive intrauterine scar formation. Uterine curettage performed after a missed abortion is associated with a higher incidence of intrauterine synechiae than curettage performed after an incomplete abortion or a molar pregnancy. Adhesions may also form after a diagnostic D&C. In general, the routine use of uterine curettage at the time of a diagnostic laparoscopy is unwarranted and may damage the endometrium.

Intrauterine adhesions should be suspected if a woman presents with secondary amenorrhea, a negative pregnancy test, and does not have progestin-induced withdrawal bleeding (see Table 49–1 for etiologies). There is no consistent correlation between the menstrual bleeding patterns and the extent of intrauterine adhesions. The diagnosis of IUA should be suspected in every patient with infertility, recurrent abortions, uterine trauma, and menstrual abnormalities. **The most common methods of diagnosing IUA are by hysterosalpingogram or SIS.** Classic hysterosalpingogram findings include irregular, angulated filling defects within the uterine cavity. In cases of severe intrauterine adhesions, the cavity cannot be sounded, making the procedure very difficult to perform. Vaginal ultrasound without saline lacks specificity. Saline infusion sonohysterography is an excellent complement to the vaginal ultrasound and can allow for the evaluation of the uterine cavity. Magnetic resonance imaging (MRI) is expensive and does not offer a greater advantage over the other diagnostic modalities. Hysteroscopy allows for direct visualization of the uterine cavity and is considered the "gold standard" for the establishment of the diagnosis and extent of the IUA.

Table 49-1 • ETIOLOGIES OF SECONDARY AMENORRHEA
Hypothalamic causes
Excessive exercise, weight loss
Stress
Hypothyroidism, hyperprolactinemia
Pituitary causes
Sheehan syndrome (necrosis)
Irradiation or surgery on pituitary
Ovarian causes
Polycystic ovarian syndrome
Premature ovarian failure
Outflow tract causes
Intrauterine adhesions
Cervical stenosis

Operative hysteroscopy is the ideal treatment for IUA that allows direct transection of adhesions. The postoperative management may include the insertion of an IUD or preferentially a pediatric Foley catheter for 7 days postoperatively to prevent the recently lysed adhesions from reforming. In addition, the administration of conjugated estrogens and progesterone (medroxyprogesterone acetate) should be considered. Repetitive treatments may be necessary to regain reproductive potential. The uterine cavity should be re-evaluated prior to attempting conception. Although 70% to 80% of patients with IUA have been able to achieve pregnancies, these pregnancies are at an increased risk of being complicated by premature labor, placenta accreta, placenta previa, and/or postpartum hemorrhage.

CASE CORRELATION

- See also Case 12 (Placenta Accreta) which is more common when the placenta attaches to areas of uterine adhesions.

COMPREHENSION QUESTIONS

49.1 A 34-year-old woman states that she has had no menses since she had a uterine curettage and cone biopsy of the cervix 1 year previously. Since those surgeries, she complains of severe, crampy lower abdominal pain "similar to labor pain" for 5 days of each month. Her basal body temperature chart is biphasic, rising 1°F for 2 weeks of every month. Which of the following is the most likely etiology of secondary amenorrhea?

    A. Hypothalamic etiology

    B. Pituitary etiology

    C. Uterine etiology

    D. Cervical condition

49.2 A 29-year-old G2P0 woman underwent an evaluation for amenorrhea of 10 months duration. Her menses had been regular previously. A pregnancy test, thyroid stimulating hormone (TSH), prolactin level, follicle stimulating hormone (FSH), and luteinizing hormone (LH) levels were normal. The patient had sequential estrogen and progestin therapy without vaginal bleeding. Her presumptive diagnosis was intrauterine adhesions, which was confirmed with imaging. Which of the following statements is most accurate?

A. Her condition usually occurs after uterine curettage for a pregnancy-related process.

B. She would best be diagnosed by laparoscopy.

C. The patient likely has cramping pain every month.

D. Her treatment includes endometrial ablation.

49.3 A 32-year-old G1P1 woman presents with an 8-month history of amenorrhea. A pregnancy test is negative. TSH and prolactin levels are normal. The FSH level is elevated at 40 IU/L. Which of the following is the most likely complication for this patient?

A. She is at significant risk for endometrial cancer.

B. She is at increased risk for ovarian cancer.

C. She is at increased risk for osteoporosis.

D. She is at increased risk for multiple gestations.

49.4 If the patient in question 49.3 were to have a diagnostic work-up, which of the following is most likely to be noted?

A. Obliterated uterine cavity on saline infusion sono-HSG

B. No bleeding with a progestin challenge test

C. Normal level of estradiol

D. Abnormal MRI of the brain

49.5 A 41-year-old woman is suspected of having intrauterine adhesions because she has had irregular menses since a spontaneous abortion 18 months previously. Which of the following historical or laboratory pieces of information would support this diagnosis?

A. Presence of hot flushes

B. FSH level too low to be measurable

C. Normal estradiol levels for a reproductive-aged woman

D. Monophasic basal body temperature chart

ANSWERS

49.1 **D.** This patient has two potential causes for amenorrhea: IUA caused by the uterine curettage and cervical stenosis due to the cervical conization. The biphasic basal body temperature chart suggests normal functioning of the hypothalamus–pituitary–ovarian axis. The crampy abdominal pain most likely is due to retrograde menstruation; thus, this is most likely due to a cervical process, cervical stenosis. If untreated, this patient would likely develop severe endometriosis.

49.2 **A.** Uterine curettage for a pregnancy-related process predisposes to **IUA**. This is best diagnosed with **hysteroscopy** (direct visualization of endometrial cavity) and not laparoscopy (visualized intraperitoneal cavity). **Cervical stenosis**, and not IUA, is associated with cramping pain every month. Ideal treatment for Asherman is **operative hysteroscopy**. The patient has had a work-up for secondary amenorrhea, which is fairly standard consisting of pregnancy test, prolactin, and TSH levels, which would alter GnRH pulsations, and FSH and LH assessing ovarian failure. Sequential estrogen and progestin without bleeding indicates a uterine/cervical etiology.

49.3 **C.** This patient has secondary amenorrhea. Her pregnancy test is negative. The TSH and prolactin levels are normal. Her serum FSH level is elevated, indicating that she has premature ovarian failure. Due to the low estrogen levels, she is at risk for osteoporosis. She is not at risk for endometrial cancer. Patients with polycystic ovarian syndrome (PCOS) would be at risk for endometrial cancer due to unopposed estrogen.

49.4 **B.** This patient likely has premature ovarian failure since the gonadotropin levels are markedly elevated. The estradiol levels are most likely low, and the patient would not respond to the progestin challenge test since the endometrium is too thin to yield any endometrial shedding. The uterine cavity should be normal in shape. The MRI of the brain is normal.

49.5 **C.** With IUA, the hormonal status of the woman should be normal. This would exclude the possibility of ovarian failure (hot flushes), low FSH levels, and a monophasic basal body temperature chart since these are all indications of an *abnormal* hormonal status.

CLINICAL PEARLS

▶ After pregnancy is ruled out, the most common cause of secondary amenorrhea after uterine curettage is intrauterine adhesions.

▶ Secondary amenorrhea can be caused by abnormalities in one of four compartments: hypothalamus, pituitary, ovary, and uterus (outflow tract).

▶ Intrauterine adhesions are diagnosed by hysterosalpingogram or saline infusion sonohysterography and confirmed by hysteroscopy.

▶ Hysteroscopic resection is the best treatment of intrauterine adhesions.

▶ Uterine curettage, especially associated with pregnancy, is a risk factor for intrauterine adhesions.

▶ The evaluation of secondary amenorrhea includes a pregnancy test, prolactin level, TSH level, and assessment of gonadotropin levels.

REFERENCES

Alexander CJ, Mathur R, Laufer LR, Aziz R. Amenorrhea, oligomenorrhea, and hyperandrogenic disorders. In: Hacker NF, Gambone JC, Hobel CJ, eds. *Essentials of Obstetrics and Gynecology.* 6th ed. Philadelphia, PA: Saunders; 2015:355-367.

Hoffman BL, Schorge JO, Schaffer JI, Halvorson LM, Bradshaw KD, Cunningham FG. Amenorrhea. *Williams Gynecology.* 2nd ed. New York, NY: McGraw Hill Medical; 2012:440-459.

Lentz GM. Primary and secondary amenorrhea and precocious puberty. In: Katz VL, Lentz GM, Lobo RA, Gersenson DM, eds. *Comprehensive Gynecology.* 6th ed. St. Louis, MO: Mosby-Year Book; 2012:933-960.

Speroff L, Fritz MA. Amenorrhea. *Clinical Gynecologic Endocrinology and Infertility.* 7th ed. Philadelphia, PA: Lippincott Williams & Wilkins; 2005:401-463.

Tur-Kaspa I, Gal M, Hartman M, Hartman J, Hartman A. A prospective evaluation of uterine abnormalities by saline infusion sonohysterography in 1009 women with infertility or abnormal uterine bleeding. *Fertil Steril.* 2009;86(6):1731-1735.

CASE 50

A 30-year-old parous woman notes a watery breast discharge of 6 months' duration. Her menses have been somewhat irregular. She denies a family history of breast cancer. The patient had been treated previously with radioactive iodine for Graves disease. Currently, she is not taking any medications. On examination, she appears alert and in good health. The blood pressure is 120/80 mm Hg, and heart rate is 80 beats per minute. The breasts are symmetric and without masses. No skin retraction is noted. A white discharge can be expressed from both breasts. No adenopathy is appreciated. The pregnancy test is negative.

- What is the most likely diagnosis?
- What is your next step?
- What is the likely mechanism for this disorder?

ANSWERS TO CASE 50:
Galactorrhea Due to Hypothyroidism

Summary: A 30-year-old parous woman with irregular menses notes a watery breast discharge of 6 months' duration. She had been treated previously with radioactive iodine for Graves disease. The pregnancy test is negative.

- **Most likely diagnosis:** Galactorrhea due to hypothyroidism.
- **Next step:** Check serum prolactin and thyroid-stimulating hormone (TSH) levels.
- **Likely mechanism:** Hypothyroidism is associated with an elevated thyroid-releasing hormone (TRH) level, which acts as a prolactin-releasing hormone. The hyperprolactinemia then induces the galactorrhea.

ANALYSIS
Objectives

1. Know the clinical presentation of galactorrhea.
2. Know some of the major causes of hyperprolactinemia.
3. Understand that hyperprolactinemia can induce hypothalamic dysfunction leading to oligo-ovulation and irregular menses.

Considerations

This patient complains of oligomenorrhea and a white, watery breast discharge, which is likely to be milk (galactorrhea). The first investigation should be a pregnancy test. Causes of galactorrhea include a pituitary adenoma, pregnancy, breast stimulation, medications, chest wall trauma, or hypothyroidism. She does not have headaches or visual disturbances. This woman had been treated previously with radioactive iodine for Graves disease and is not taking thyroid replacement. Thus, she likely has hypothyroidism. With primary hypothyroidism, both the thyroid-releasing hormone and thyroid-stimulating hormone are elevated. TRH acts as a prolactin-releasing hormone. Hence, elevated TSH and prolactin levels will be noted in this patient. Hyperprolactinemia results in a reflex increase in dopamine in the brain. Dopamine stimulates receptors on cells of the hypothalamus that produce GnRH interrupting its pulsatile release. Thus, gonadotropin release is inhibited. In turn, follicle development is disrupted, estradiol decreases, and menstrual cycles become irregular or cease. This patient would have no bleeding in response to a progestin challenge test due to insufficient endometrium. (See Case 49, Intrauterine adhesions.)

APPROACH TO:
Galactorrhea

DEFINITIONS

GALACTORRHEA: Nonpuerperal watery or milky breast secretion that contains neither pus nor blood. The secretion can be manifested spontaneously or obtained only by breast examination.

PITUITARY SECRETING ADENOMA: A tumor in the pituitary gland that produces prolactin; symptoms include galactorrhea, headache, and peripheral vision defect (bitemporalhemianopsia).

CLINICAL APPROACH

Galactorrhea is a milky breast secretion that occurs in a nonlactating patient. It is usually bilateral. To determine if the breast discharge is truly galactorrhea, a smear under microscope will reveal multiple fat droplets. Patients with galactorrhea often have associated oligomenorrhea or amenorrhea. See Table 50–1 for the different etiologies for hyperprolactinemia.

Galactorrhea and hyperprolactinemia require a careful diagnostic approach. A thorough history and physical should be done. All medications that can stimulate prolactin production should be discontinued. A magnetic resonance scan is the most sensitive test to detect pituitary adenomas, providing 1-mm resolution; it can detect virtually all microadenomas. Prolactin should be evaluated in the morning when it is at its lowest physiological level. Nonpregnant prolactin is less than 20 ng/mL. **Microadenomas are <10 mm diameter; macroadenomas are >10 mm.** Macroadenomas of any cell type, not merely prolactinomas, should be imaged by magnetic resonance(MRI) because macroadenomas can damage the pituitary stalk and thereby decrease the normal dopamine inhibition of pituitary lactotropes. MRI is performed with and without gadolinium. Those with a markedly high prolactin level, or those with neurologic symptoms, should have an MRI of the pituitary. Hyperprolactinemia is a common cause of menstrual disturbances. Hence, a woman with galactorrhea, regular menses, and normal serum prolactin is at low risk for having a prolactinoma. These patients can be followed with annual serum prolactin tests.

Table 50–1 • CAUSES OF HYPERPROLACTINEMIA
Drugs (tranquilizers, tricyclic antidepressants, antihypertensives, narcotics, oral contraceptive pills)
Hypothyroidism
Hypothalamic causes (craniopharyngioma, sarcoidosis, histiocytosis, leukemia)
Pituitary causes (microadenoma [<1 cm], macroadenoma [>1 cm])
Hyperplasia of the lactotrophs
Empty sella syndrome
Acromegaly
Renal disease (acute or chronic)
Chest surgery or trauma (breast implants, herpes zoster at the T_2 dermatome of the chest)

However, even in the face of normal prolactin assays, women with oligomenorrhea and galactorrhea should undergo an anteroposterior and lateral coned-down view of the sellaturcica. If necessary, a skull MRI will confirm the diagnosis of empty sella. Patients with secondary amenorrhea and low levels of serum estrogen (<40 pg/mL) have a significantly greater risk of having a pituitary adenoma as well as early onset of osteoporosis.

Women with galactorrhea but normal menses and normal serum prolactin levels may be observed. Also, patients with microadenomas who do not wish to conceive and do not have estrogen deficiency may be expectantly managed. Other patients with pituitary adenomas should receive treatment, which is primarily medical management and rarely surgical.

If the hyperprolactinemia is found to be due to hypothyroidism, the patient should be treated with thyroxine. Symptomatic patients with hyperprolactinemia due to a pituitary microadenoma or asymptomatic patients with a macroadenoma should be treated with a dopamine agonist, such as bromocriptine, a nonselective dopamine receptor agonist. Its side effects (orthostatic hypotension, fainting, dizziness, and nausea and vomiting). Bromocriptine is particularly useful for patients desiring fertility. Cabergoline is a selective type 2 dopamine receptor agonist for patients and has less side effects and lowers prolactin levels more effectively; it is also available in depot form. Both bromocriptine and cabergoline can be given vaginally if the patient does not tolerate the oral form. Patients with hyperprolactinemia, with or without microadenoma, with adequate estrogen levels (>40 pg/mL) and who do not desire pregnancy should be treated with periodic progestin withdrawal.

Patients who fail medical therapy may require surgery, which involves transsphenoidal microsurgical exploration of the sellaturcica with removal of the pituitary adenoma while preserving the functional capacity of the remaining gland. Complications of the surgery include transient diabetes insipidus (occurs in about one-third), hemorrhage, meningitis, cerebrospinal fluid leak, and panhypopituitarism. Cure rate is directly related to the pretreatment prolactin levels (prolactin level of 100 ng/mL has an excellent prognosis, whereas 200 ng/mL has a poor prognosis). It may be preferable to reduce the size of the macroadenoma with bromocriptine before surgical removal of these tumors.

CASE CORRELATION

- See also Case 49 (Intrauterine Adhesions). With uterine adhesions, the hormonal axis (hypothalamus, pituitary, ovary) is normal. Many medical conditions can affect hypothalamic GnRH pulsatile release.

COMPREHENSION Questions

50.1 A 25-year-old woman presents with galactorrhea and irregular menses of 10 months' duration. Her pregnancy test is negative. Laboratory tests reveal normal TSH and serum-free T_4 and hyperprolactinemia. Which of the following is most likely to be a cause of her condition?
  A. Posterior pituitary adenoma
  B. Abdominal wall trauma
  C. Psychotropic medication
  D. Hyperthyroidism

50.2 A 38-year-old woman is seen by her physician because of headaches, amenorrhea, and galactorrhea. Her pregnancy test was negative. Her prolactin level was markedly elevated and TSH was normal. The physician makes a presumptive diagnosis of pituitary adenoma and orders an MRI of the brain. Which of the following clinical presentations is consistent with a prolactin-secreting pituitary adenoma?
  A. Diabetes insipidus
  B. Occipital cerebral defect
  C. Central field visual defect
  D. Amenorrhea at the hypothalamus level

50.3 A 47-year-old woman is being evaluated for a possible pituitary tumor. She complains of headaches and has some visual difficulties. The MRI shows a mass in the **posterior** pituitary gland, which the radiologist notes is unusual. Which of the following is a hormone contained in the posterior pituitary gland?
  A. Follicle-stimulating hormone (FSH)
  B. Prolactin
  C. Thyroid-stimulating hormone
  D. Oxytocin

50.4 A 33-year-old woman with a microadenoma of the pituitary gland becomes pregnant. When she reaches 28 weeks' gestation, she complains of headaches and visual disturbances. Which of the following is the best therapy?
  A. Craniotomy and pituitary resection
  B. Tamoxifen therapy
  C. Oral bromocriptine therapy
  D. Expectant management
  E. Lumbar puncture

ANSWERS

50.1 **C.** Medications are a common cause of hyperprolactinemia, especially psychotropic medications. Pregnancy is associated with elevated prolactin levels. The anterior, not posterior, pituitary secretes prolactin; an anterior pituitary adenoma is more likely to be a cause of hyperprolactinemia. Symptoms may include galactorrhea, headache, and peripheral vision defect (bitemporalhemianopsia). Hypothyroidism may lead to hyperprolactinemia. With primary hypothyroidism, both TRH (secreted by the hypothalamus) and TSH (secreted by anterior pituitary) levels are elevated. TRH acts as a prolactin-releasing hormone in addition to being a thyroid-releasing hormone. Chest wall trauma, and not abdominal wall trauma, can cause hyperprolactinemia.

50.2 **D.** Elevated prolactin levels inhibit GnRH pulsations from the hypothalamus. Without the signal from GnRH, gonadotropins (FSH/LH) are not released from the anterior pituitary and no estrogen (or progesterone) is released from the ovaries; this results in amenorrhea. Pituitary adenomas impinge on the optic chiasm, causing deficits of the peripheral vision (bitemporalhemianopsia) and not the central visual field. The pituitary is located in the anterior half of the cerebrum; therefore, an occipital cerebral defect is unlikely to be a clinical presentation relating to a pituitary adenoma. Diabetes insipidus results from a deficiency in antidiuretic hormone (ADH) from the posterior pituitary, and would not be a clinical presentation consistent with an anterior pituitary tumor.

50.3 **D.** Oxytocin and ADH are posterior pituitary hormones. The other answer choices are released by the anterior pituitary. Whereas prolactin acts on the breast to produce milk, oxytocin acts on the breast to stimulate ejection of the milk in a lactating woman. Oxytocin is also responsible for uterine contractions during labor. The main function of FSH is to stimulate follicular development and maturity in the ovaries. ADH acts on the kidney to conserve water and is released when the body is dehydrated. TSH causes release of thyroid hormones, T_3 and T_4, which are involved in essential metabolic processes throughout the body.

50.4 **C.** Bromocriptine therapy is indicated during pregnancy if symptoms (eg, headache or visual field abnormalities) arise. No studies have shown bromocriptine to be unsafe to the developing fetus. A craniotomy and pituitary resection is a very high-risk surgery. It is typically reserved for patients with a macroadenoma, who have failed medical treatment. Surgery would not be indicated for this patient who has a microadenoma and has not attempted medical therapy. Plus, any procedure that may induce hemorrhage in a patient would be considered risky in pregnancy. Tamoxifen is not indicated because it is a selective estrogen receptor modulator used in the treatment of breast cancer. It therefore binds to estrogen receptors to inhibit estrogen action, and does not affect the microadenoma or prolactin production and action. A lumbar puncture would not be an option for managing a prolactinoma, but might worsen the patient's headache. Expectant management would not be a good option because a microadenoma can continue to grow during pregnancy from hormonal influences. Therefore, the patient's symptoms would only worsen, and treatment should be initiated promptly.

CLINICAL PEARLS

▶ Galactorrhea in the face of normal menses and a normal prolactin level may be observed. The normal menses indicates normal hypothalamic function.

▶ The first evaluation in a woman with oligomenorrhea and galactorrhea should be a pregnancy test.

▶ Osteoporosis is a danger with hypoestrogenemia due to hyperprolactinemia.

▶ Hypothyroidism can lead to hyperprolactinemia and galactorrhea.

▶ Both hypothyroidism and hyperprolactinemia lead to hypothalamic (interfere with pulsatile GnRH) amenorrhea; this is a hypogonadotropic hypogonadism.

▶ MRI is the most sensitive imaging test to assess pituitary adenomas.

REFERENCES

Alexander CJ, Mathur R, Laufer LR, Aziz R. Amenorrhea, oligomenorrhea, and hyper-androgenic disorders. In: Hacker NF, Gambone JC, Hobel CJ, eds. *Essentials of Obstetrics and Gynecology*. 6th ed. Philadelphia, PA: Saunders; 2015:355-367.

Fritz M, Speroff L. Amenorrhea. In: Fritz M, Speroff L, eds. *Clinical Gynecologic Endocrinology and Infertility*. 8th ed. Philadelphia, PA: Lippincott Williams and Wilkins; 2010.

Halvorson LM. Hypothalamic amenorrhea. In: Schorge J, Schaffer J, Halvorson LM, et al., eds. *Williams Gynecology*. 2nd ed. New York, NY: McGraw-Hill; 2012:400-439.

Lobo RA. Hyperprolactinemia, galactorrhea, and pituitary adenomas. In: Katz VL, Lentz GM, Lobo RA, Gersenson DM, eds. *Comprehensive Gynecology*. 6th ed. St. Louis, MO: Mosby-Year Book; 2012:963-978.

CASE 51

A 24-year-old G2P2 woman delivered vaginally 8 months previously. Her pregnancy was unremarkable and she states that she had no medical problems. Her delivery was complicated by postpartum hemorrhage requiring curettage of the uterus and a blood transfusion of four units of erythrocytes. She complains of amenorrhea since her delivery. She denies taking medications or having headaches or visual abnormalities. Her pregnancy test is negative. She was not able to breastfeed her baby.

- ▶ What is the most likely diagnosis?
- ▶ What is the likely mechanism for the condition?
- ▶ What are other complications that are likely with this condition?

ANSWERS TO CASE 51:
Amenorrhea (Sheehan Syndrome)

Summary: A 24-year-old G2P2 woman has had amenorrhea since a vaginal delivery complicated by postpartum hemorrhage and uterine curettage. She was not able to lactate.

- **Most likely diagnosis:** Sheehan syndrome (anterior pituitary necrosis).
- **Mechanism:** Pregnancy-associated enlargement of the anterior pituitary gland and hypotension leading to hemorrhage into the anterior pituitary gland.
- **Other complications that are likely with this condition:** Anterior pituitary insufficiency, such as hypothyroidism or adrenocortical insufficiency.

ANALYSIS
Objectives

1. Be able to differentiate the clinical presentation of Sheehan syndrome from intrauterine adhesions (IUAs; Asherman syndrome).
2. Understand the mechanism of Sheehan syndrome.
3. Know the other tropic hormones that may be affected by anterior pituitary necrosis.

Considerations

This patient developed amenorrhea from the time of her vaginal delivery that was complicated by postpartum hemorrhage. This patient has **secondary amenorrhea** (see also Case 49). The initial evaluation should be a pregnancy test (which is negative). The patient also underwent a uterine curettage in the treatment of the postpartum bleeding. In this setting, there are two explanations: (1) Sheehan syndrome and (2) intrauterine adhesions (Asherman syndrome). Sheehan syndrome is caused by hypotension in the postpartum period, leading to hemorrhagic necrosis of the anterior pituitary gland. Asherman syndrome is caused by the uterine curettage, which damages the decidua basalis layer, rendering the endometrium unresponsive. The key to differentiating between Sheehan syndrome and intrauterine adhesions is to assess for whether or not the anterior pituitary is functioning, and whether the outflow tract (uterus) is responsive to hormonal therapy. For instance, since this patient's history was "unable to breastfeed after delivery," it would suggest that the anterior pituitary was not functioning (lack of prolactin). Had the patient been able to breastfeed, the most likely diagnosis would have been intrauterine synechiae. This patient was given a combination oral contraceptive agent, and if the endometrium were responsive to the hormonal therapy, then proliferation of the endometrium should occur followed by stabilization of the endometrium with the progestin component, and then finally bleeding when the placebo pills are taken (days 21–28). Other evidences of anterior pituitary dysfunction may include low thyroid hormones, gonadotropin (follicle-stimulating hormone [FSH] and luteinizing hormone [LH]), or cortisol levels. A definitive diagnosis of IUA can be made with saline infusion sonohysterogram or hysterosalpingogram.

APPROACH TO:
Postpartum Amenorrhea

DEFINITIONS

AMENORRHEA: No menses for 6 months.

SHEEHAN SYNDROME: Anterior pituitary hemorrhagic necrosis caused by hypertrophy of the prolactin-secreting cells in conjunction with a hypotensive episode, usually in the setting of postpartum hemorrhage. The bleeding in the anterior pituitary induces pressure necrosis.

INTRAUTERINE ADHESIONS (ASHERMAN SYNDROME): Scar tissue that forms in the endometrium, leading to amenorrhea caused by unresponsiveness of the endometrial tissue.

POSTPARTUM HEMORRHAGE: Classically defined as bleeding >500 mL for a vaginal delivery and >1000 mL for a cesarean delivery. From a more pathophysiologic standpoint, it is the amount of bleeding that results in, or threatens to result in, hemodynamic instability if left unabated.

CLINICAL APPROACH

Amenorrhea can ensue after a term delivery for 2 to 3 months; breast feeding may inhibit the hypothalamic function, and lead to a greater duration of amenorrhea. However, in a nonlactating woman, when no menses resumes by 12 weeks after delivery, then pathology must be suspected. Overall, **the most common cause of amenorrhea in the reproductive years is pregnancy.** Therefore, a pregnancy test is the appropriate initial test. If the patient does not have a history of postpartum hemorrhage, evaluation of hypothalamic causes, such as hypothyroidism or hyperprolactinemia, is often fruitful. If the patient is somewhat obese, or has a history of irregular cycles, then polycystic ovarian syndrome (PCOS) would be entertained. Findings consistent with PCOS include a positive progestin withdrawal bleed (vaginal bleeding after the ingestion of a progestin, such as medroxyprogesterone acetate or Provera). Polycystic ovarian syndrome is characterized by estrogen excess without progesterone, obesity, hirsutism, and glucose intolerance. Elevated luteinizing hormone to follicle-stimulating hormone ratios are often seen (eg, LH:FSH is of 2:1). Polycystic ovarian syndrome should be suspected in patients with obesity, hirsutism, and oligomenorrhea. When women are hypoestrogenic, then two broad categories of causes are common: hypothalamic/pituitary diseases or ovarian failure. The FSH level can distinguish between these two causes, with an elevated FSH indicative of ovarian failure.

Table 51–1 • DIFFERENCES BETWEEN SHEEHAN SYNDROME AND ASHERMAN SYNDROME

Hormone Function	Sheehan Syndrome	Intrauterine Adhesions
Thyroid hormone (T_4)	Low	Normal
TSH	Low	Normal
FSH	Low	Normal
Estradiol levels	Low	Normal
LH surge (biphasic basal body temperature chart)	Absent	Normal biphasic
Cortisol levels	Low	Normal
Prolactin levels (able to breastfeed)	Low (unable to lactate)	Normal
Bleeding in response to estrogen and progestin (oral contraceptive)	Yes	No

The patient in this case had amenorrhea after a vaginal delivery and postpartum hemorrhage, making Sheehan syndrome or intrauterine adhesions the two most likely causes. Distinguishing between these two entities involves assessing whether the patient has normal or abnormal anterior pituitary function, or some evidence of unresponsiveness of the outflow tract to hormonal treatment (Table 51–1). The treatment of Sheehan syndrome consists of replacement of hormones, such as thyroxine, cortisol, and mineralocorticoid, and estrogen and progestin therapy. Intrauterine adhesions are treated by hysteroscopic resection of the scar tissue.

CASE CORRELATION

- See also Case 49 (Intrauterine Adhesions) and Case 50 (Hypothalamic Dysfunction Due to Galactorrhea) as two other causes of secondary amenorrhea. Pituitary causes are the least common. See also Case 6 (Postpartum Hemorrhage).

COMPREHENSION QUESTIONS

51.1 A 19-year-old G1Ab1 woman underwent a uterine curettage after a miscarriage. She has had no menses since then and is not pregnant. The physician is suspecting intrauterine adhesions. Which of the following is a feature of intrauterine synechiae (Asherman syndrome)?

A. Usually occurs after uterine curettage
B. Associated with low gonadotropin levels
C. Associated with a monophasic basal body temperature chart
D. Associated with low cortisol levels

51.2 A 24-year-old G1P1 woman is seen in the office with secondary amenorrhea after her delivery. She is given a tentative diagnosis of pituitary necrosis (Sheehan syndrome). Which of the following is consistent with her presumed diagnosis?

A. Usually associated with hypertensive crisis at or soon after a delivery
B. Caused by an ischemic necrosis of the posterior pituitary gland
C. Associated with decreased prolactin levels
D. Often associated with elevated thyroid-stimulating hormone (TSH) levels

51.3 A 32-year-old G2P1Ab1 woman presents to the gynecologist with 6 months of amenorrhea. Which of the following is the best description of the mechanism of intrauterine synechiae (Asherman syndrome)?

A. Trophoblastic hyperplasia
B. Pituitary engorgement
C. Myometrial scarring
D. Decidual hypertrophy
E. Endometrial disruption

51.4 A 25-year-old woman presents with a 6-month history of amenorrhea. Her pregnancy test is negative. She is evaluated for other causes of secondary amenorrhea, and is given a diagnosis of PCOS. Which of the following is consistent with this disorder?

A. Estrogen deficiency and vaginal atrophy
B. Osteoporosis
C. Endometrial hyperplasia
D. Hypoglycemia
E. A history of regular menses each month prior to 6 months

ANSWERS

51.1 **A.** Intrauterine adhesions are associated with a biphasic basal temperature chart that reflects normal pituitary function and normal ovulation. This indicates the presence of progesterone, which elevates the temperature. Intrauterine adhesions usually occur after curettage of the uterus. It is with Sheehan syndrome, and not with Asherman syndrome, that due to anterior pituitary hemorrhagic necrosis, the patient is unable to breastfeed after delivery, has a monophasic basal body temperature chart, and has low cortisol levels. The necrotic anterior pituitary is unable to secrete prolactin, FSH/LH, ACTH, TSH, or growth hormone, and patients must take hormone replacements to restore function of the organs and systems these hormones acted upon.

51.2 **C.** Sheehan syndrome involves the anterior pituitary undergoing hemorrhagic necrosis after a hypotensive episode, usually in the setting of postpartum hemorrhage. The anterior pituitary is, therefore, unable to secrete prolactin among a few other hormones. The posterior pituitary is not involved because it has a direct arterial supply. Hypothyroidism is a result of Sheehan syndrome due to the low or absent TSH secretion from the anterior pituitary. A patient may have an associated hypotensive episode, and not a hypertensive one, in their peripartum period caused by the postpartum hemorrhage.

51.3 **E.** In Asherman syndrome, large patches of endometrium are defective because of intrauterine adhesions. The endometrium is unresponsive, so estrogen exposure will have no effect on the lining of the uterus, and therefore, cannot pose a risk for endometrial hyperplasia. Endometrial, and not myometrial, scarring is involved. Pituitary engorgement occurs during pregnancy due to the hypertrophy and hyperplasia of lactotrophs. There is no associated increase in vascular supply, so when postpartum hemorrhage occurs, the anterior pituitary is particularly vulnerable to ischemia. Trophoblastic hyperplasia originates from placental tissues. It does not directly induce intrauterine synechiae; however, if the patient undergoes a dilation and curettage for management of the trophoblastic disease, Asherman syndrome may develop.

51.4 **C.** PCOS is a condition characterized by chronic anovulation, hyperandrogenism where other causes have been eliminated, and possible evidence of small ovarian cysts on ultrasound. It is associated with unopposed estrogen and estrogen excess. This setting increases the patient's risk of endometrial hyperplasia or endometrial cancer. Osteoporosis is a risk in hypoestrogenic states, and this patient has estrogen excess, so osteoporosis is not a concern; in fact, bone mineral density is usually quite good. Vaginal atrophy is associated with estrogen deficiency, not excess. Glucose intolerance, diabetes mellitus, and a history of oligomenorrhea since menarche are consistent with the diagnosis of PCOS.

> **CLINICAL PEARLS**
>
> ▶ The two most common causes of secondary amenorrhea after postpartum hemorrhage are Sheehan syndrome and intrauterine adhesions.
>
> ▶ A pregnancy test should be the first test in evaluating a woman with secondary amenorrhea.
>
> ▶ Normal function of the anterior pituitary points toward intrauterine adhesions.
>
> ▶ Hypothyroidism or a monophasic basal body temperature chart suggests Sheehan syndrome.
>
> ▶ The treatment of Sheehan syndrome consists of replacement of the hormones governed by the anterior pituitary gland.
>
> ▶ The most common cause of ovulatory dysfunction in a reproductive-aged woman is PCOS, which is characterized by obesity, anovulation, hirsutism, glucose intolerance, and estrogen excess.

REFERENCES

Alexander CJ, Mathur R, Laufer LR, Azziz R. Amenorrhea, oligomenorrhea, and hyper-androgenic disorders. In: Hacker NF, Gambone JC, Hobel CJ, eds. *Essentials of Obstetrics and Gynecology.* 5th ed. Philadelphia, PA: Saunders; 2010:355-367.

Lobo RA. Primary and secondary amenorrhea and precocious puberty. In: Katz VL, Lentz GM, Lobo RA, Gershenson DM, eds. *Comprehensive Gynecology.* 6th ed. St. Louis, MO: Mosby-Year Book; 2012:933-961.

CASE 52

A 23-year-old G0P0 woman presents to the office with complaints of irregular cycles since menarche. Upon further questioning, she has also noticed an increase in facial hair and acne for many years. She denies any history of medical problems and has a strong family medical history of diabetes. On examination, she is noted to have a normal blood pressure (BP), pulse, respiratory rate, and temperature. She is obese with a body mass index (BMI) of 34 kg/m². She is noted to have some hirsutism and acanthosis nigricans (of neck and inner thighs). Her pelvic examination is limited by her obesity but normal. She does not desire pregnancy at this time. Her pregnancy test is negative.

- ▶ What is the most likely diagnosis?
- ▶ What complications is the patient at risk for?
- ▶ What is your next diagnostic step?
- ▶ What is your therapeutic plan for this patient?

ANSWERS TO CASE 52:
Polycystic Ovarian Syndrome

Summary: A 23-year-old woman with a long-standing history of irregular cycles, obesity, hirsutism, and acne.

- **Most likely diagnosis:** Polycystic ovarian syndrome.
- **Complications:** Diabetes mellitus (DM), endometrial cancer, hyperlipidemia, metabolic syndrome, cardiovascular disease.
- **Diagnostic steps:** Thyroid-stimulating hormone (TSH), prolactin, serum testosterone, dehydroepiandrosterone sulfate (DHEA-S), and 17-hydroxyprogesterone, pelvic ultrasound.
- **Therapeutic plan:** Regulate menstrual cycles with combination oral contraceptives and screen for metabolic abnormalities (diabetes, lipid panel, etc). Encourage diet and exercise.

ANALYSIS
Objectives

1. Know the clinical presentation and diagnostic criteria of polycystic ovarian syndrome (PCOS).
2. Understand the work-up needed for the diagnosis.
3. Become familiar with basic management strategies.

Considerations

The patient is a 23-year-old G0P0 woman with classic presentation of PCOS. The diagnostic criteria require two out of the three following signs and symptoms: oligomenorrhea/amenorrhea, hyperandrogenism (not otherwise explained), or evidence of small multiple ovarian cysts on transvaginal ultrasound. The ratio of luteinizing hormone (LH) to follicle-stimulating hormone (FSH) is often cited as a supporting diagnostic factor; however, this lab finding is inconsistent and unreliable. She has chronic menstrual cycle irregularities, obesity, and signs of hyperandrogenism (acne, hirsutism). The presence of acanthosis is a sign of insulin resistance. After exclusion of secondary causes of hyperandrogenism (late onset congenital adrenal hyperplasia, hyperprolactinemia, adrenal/ovarian tumors, Cushing syndrome, thyroid disorders), the diagnosis can be made. Management depends on fertility desires. When the patient does not desire a pregnancy, her menstrual cycles are best regulated with combined oral contraceptive pills. Diet and exercise are important in treating the patient. She should be assessed for metabolic abnormalities, as this patient is at high risk for chronic conditions such as type 2 diabetes and cardiovascular disease. Ovulation induction may be necessary if the patient desires a pregnancy.

SECTION II: CASES 491

> APPROACH TO:
> Polycystic Ovarian Syndrome

DEFINITIONS

POLYCYSTIC OVARIAN SYNDROME: A condition of unexplained hyperandrogenic chronic anovulation associated with excessive estrogen.

Criteria for diagnosis: (need two out of three): (1) Hyperandrogenism, (2) oligomenorrhea or amenorrhea, and (3) polycystic ovaries by ultrasound.

HIRSUTISM: Excessive terminal hair growth in male pattern of distribution.

BMI: Statistical measurement used to identify obesity taking into account a person's height and weight (weight in kg divided by height in m^2). The normal BMI range is considered to be 18.5 to 24.9.

ACANTHOSIS NIGRICANS: Velvety, mossy, verrucous, hyperpigmented skin usually noted on the back of the neck, in the axilla, and under the breasts, usually a sign of insulin resistance.

CLINICAL APPROACH

One would think by the name PCOS, the development of polycystic ovaries is a central feature for the hyperandrogenic chronic anovulation state. However, the polycystic ovary can occur with any state of anovulation and should be viewed as a sign but not a disease. Consequences of persistent anovulation include infertility, menstrual irregularities, androgen excess (hirsutism, acne, and alopecia), and increased risk of endometrial cancer, cardiovascular disease, and diabetes mellitus. **Hyperandrogenic anovulation is reported to occur in 4% to 6% of women.**

When evaluating patients with suspected PCOS, a thorough history and physical should be performed. Other causes of hyperandrogenic anovulation should be excluded. Important information to obtain from the patient includes her menstrual history, onset, and duration of androgen excess, medications, family history (especially of diabetes and cardiovascular disease), and lifestyle factors (exercise, smoking, alcohol). The physical examination, should carefully evaluate the body hair distribution and other signs of androgen excess (acne, temporal balding). The presence of acanthosis should be noted, and a pelvic examination should be performed to assess for ovarian enlargement.

Laboratory studies which need to be considered are **TSH, prolactin, lipid profile, glucose-intolerance screening, endometrial biopsy** (in patients with long-standing anovulation and unopposed estrogen exposure), and **17-hydroxyprogesterone** (congenital adrenal hyperplasia). **Testosterone and DHEA-S** levels can be assessed when clinical signs of excess androgen stimulation are present or if an androgen-secreting tumor is suspected. The majority of testosterone is produced by the ovary, whereas, DHEA-S is almost exclusively secreted by the adrenal gland.

Besides the clinical examination, pelvic sonography revealing multiple small follicles on the ovaries is often one of the diagnostic criteria. More specifically, usually the presence of 12 or more follicles in each ovary measuring 2 to 9 mm in diameter or increased ovarian volume >10 mL is considered to be polycystic. It is called the "string of pearls" sign since the small follicles line the periphery of the ovary.

Overall treatment goals are to:

1. Reduce circulating androgen levels
2. Protect the endometrium from unopposed estrogen and reduce risk of endometrial cancer
3. Encourage weight loss and healthy lifestyle changes
4. Induce ovulation when pregnancy is desired
5. Monitor for the development of diabetes and cardiovascular disease and modify risk factors if possible (smoking cessation, lipid-lowering agents, etc)

Combination oral contraceptives have been the primary management of long-standing PCOS. They are effective in regulating dysfunctional bleeding, limiting unopposed estrogen (thus reducing endometrial cancer risk), increasing the sex hormone-binding globulin (decreases free androgen levels), and suppressing ovarian androgen production. Weight loss can reduce both hyperinsulinemia and hyperandrogenism. These benefits can be seen with as little as 5% weight loss. Insulin-lowering agents, such as **metformin** can be helpful in reducing the hyperinsulinism and thus limiting the risk of developing cardiovascular disease and diabetes mellitus.

For patients desiring pregnancy with a BMI <30, clomiphene citrate is the agent of choice; however, for those patients with a BMI >30, letrozole (aromatase inhibitor) is the first-line. Metformin should only be used for glucose intolerance.

CASE CORRELATION

- Secondary amenorrhea can be due to **pregnancy** or abnormalities in one of the four areas:
- Hypothalamus (pulsatile GnRH)—Case 50 (Galactorrhea and Hypothyroidism)
- Pituitary (no FSH or LH)—Case 51 (Anterior Pituitary Necrosis)
- Ovarian (a) estrogen excess and anovulation: PCOS (current case) or (b) premature ovarian failure (hypoestrogenic)
- Uterine/Cervical—Case 49 (Intrauterine Adhesions)

COMPREHENSION QUESTIONS

52.1 A 32-year-old G0P0 woman is noted to have irregular menses and hirsutism. Which of the following is consistent with polycystic ovarian syndrome?

A. Elevated 17-hydroxyprogesterone level
B. Finding of a 9-cm right ovarian mass
C. Vaginal bleeding after a 5-day course of progesterone oral therapy
D. DEXA scan showing osteopenia

52.2 A 29-year-old G0P0 woman with a diagnosis of PCOS is being counseled about the dangers of her condition. In particular, she is cautioned about the possibility of developing metabolic syndrome. Which of the following is the most significant consequence of metabolic syndrome?

A. Hyperthyroidism
B. Cardiovascular disease
C. Breast cancer
D. Renal insufficiency

52.3 A 28-year-old G0P0 woman has a chronic history of oligomenorrhea and amenorrhea. She undergoes an endometrial biopsy in light of her long history of anovulation, which returns as Grade 1 adenocarcinoma of the endometrium. Magnetic resonance imaging seems to indicate that the endometrial cancer is isolated to the uterus. The patient desires to have children if possible. Which of the following is the best therapy for this patient?

A. Endometrial ablation
B. Radical hysterectomy
C. Cervical conization
D. High-dose progestin therapy
E. Oral contraceptive agent

ANSWERS

52.1 **C.** PCOS is characterized by obesity, anovulation, hyperandrogenism due to ovarian secretion of testosterone, after excluding other etiologies such as congenital adrenal hyperplasia (CAH), Sertoli–Leydig cell tumor, hypothyroidism and hyperprolactinemia. An elevated 17-hydroxyprogesterone level would indicate CAH. A 9-cm ovarian mass would suggest a Sertoli–Leydig cell tumor. With PCOS, the DEXA scan usually shows good bone density due to the excess estrogen environment. Women with PCOS usually will have a positive progestin challenge test; in other words, they have bleeding with a 5- to 10-day course of oral progestin.

52.2 **B.** Metabolic syndrome is characterized by hyperlipidemia, glucose intolerance, hypertension, and central obesity. Patients with metabolic syndrome are at greatly increased risk of cardiovascular disease, particularly when the glucose intolerance is present.

52.3 **D.** Young patients with chronic anovulation due to PCOS are at risk for endometrial cancer. The lesions are almost always Grade 1, and are usually treated with hysterectomy and surgical staging. In selected circumstances, high-dose progestin therapy and repeat of the endometrial sampling in 2 to 3 months is possible for those who desire a pregnancy. Hysterectomy is usually recommended after childbirth. The chronic estrogen exposure without progestin is the reason for development of endometrial cancer.

CLINICAL PEARLS

► Polycystic ovary syndrome is a common cause of chronic hyperandrogenic anovulation, and its diagnosis is made after other secondary causes have been ruled out.

► Testosterone is largely secreted by the ovary whereas DHEA-S is secreted by the adrenal gland.

► Patients with PCOS should be screened for glucose intolerance and lipid abnormalities.

► Combined oral contraceptive pills are the primary management for irregular cycles and also decrease androgen levels.

► An endometrial biopsy should be considered in patients with long-standing anovulation and unopposed estrogen.

REFERENCES

Alexander CJ, Mathur R, Laufer LR, Aziz R. Amenorrhea, oligomenorrhea, and hyperandrogenic disorders. In: Hacker NF, Gambone JC, Hobel CJ, eds. *Essentials of Obstetrics and Gynecology*. 6th ed. Philadelphia, PA: Saunders; 2015:355-367.

American College of Obstetricians and Gynecologist. Polycystic ovary syndrome. *ACOG Practice Bulletin 108*. Washington, DC; 2009. (Reaffirmed 2013.)

Fritz M, Speroff L. Anovulation and the polycystic ovary. In: *Clinical Gynecologic Endocrinology and Infertility*. 8th ed. New York, NY: Lippincott Williams and Wilkins; 2010:465-498.

Legro, RS, Brzyski RG, Diamond MP, et al. Letrozole versus Clomiphene for Infertility in the Polycystic Ovary Syndrome. *N Engl J Med*. 2014;371(2):119-129.

Lobo RA. Hyperandrogenism. In: Katz VL, Lentz GM, Lobo RA, Gersenson DM, eds. *Comprehensive Gynecology*. 6th ed. Philadelphia, PA: Mosby-Year Book; 2012:849-867.

CASE 53

A 42-year-old parous woman has noticed increasing hair growth on her face and abdomen over the past 6 months. She denies the use of steroid medications, weight changes, or a family history of hirsutism. Her menses previously had been monthly, and now occur every 35 to 70 days. Her past medical and surgical histories are unremarkable. On examination, her thyroid is normal to palpation. She has excess facial hair and male-pattern hair on her abdomen. Acne is also noted on the face. The cardiac and pulmonary examinations are normal. The abdominal examination reveals no masses or tenderness. Examination of the external genitalia reveals possible clitoromegaly. Pelvic examination shows a normal uterus and cervix and an 8-cm, right adnexal mass.

- ▶ What is the most likely diagnosis?
- ▶ What is the probable management?

ANSWERS TO CASE 53:
Hirsutism, Sertoli–Leydig Cell Tumor

Summary: A 42-year-old woman with a 6-month history of increasing hirsutism and irregular menses. She denies the use of steroid medications, weight changes, or a family history of hirsutism. Pelvic examination shows an 8-cm, right adnexal mass.

- **Most likely diagnosis:** An ovarian tumor, probable Sertoli–Leydig cell tumor.
- **Probable management:** Ovarian cancer (surgical) staging.

ANALYSIS
Objectives

1. Understand the differential diagnosis of hirsutism.
2. Know the work-up and approach to a woman with virilism and hirsutism.
3. Know the typical history and physical examination and treatment for the various causes of hirsutism.

Considerations

This 42-year-old woman has the onset of excess male-pattern hair over the past 6 months, as well as features of virilism (clitoromegaly). This is evidence of excess androgens. The rapid onset speaks of a tumor. Adrenal or ovarian tumors are possibilities. This woman has a large adnexal mass, and so the diagnosis is straightforward. She has irregular menses because of the androgen effect of inhibiting ovulation. The patient does not have the stigmata of Cushing disease, such as hypertension, buffalo hump, abdominal striae, and central obesity. Likewise, she does not take any medications containing anabolic steroids. Polycystic ovarian syndrome (PCOS) is the most common cause of hyperandrogenism; however, PCOS does not fit this clinical scenario. PCOS most commonly presents with an insidious onset of hirsutism and irregular menses since menarche. A Sertoli–Leydig cell tumor of the ovary is a solid stromal type of tumor, the androgen counterpart of granulosa-theca cell tumor (which secretes estrogens). These tumors are usually of low malignant potential and slow growing, but nevertheless may metastasize and often recur. As with all ovarian malignancies, surgical staging is the treatment of choice.

APPROACH TO:
Hirsutism

DEFINTIONS

HIRSUTISM: Excessive male-pattern hair in a woman.

VIRILISM: Androgen effect other than hair pattern, such as clitoromegaly, male balding, deepening of the voice, and acne.

CLINICAL APPROACH

Hirsutism should be viewed both as an endocrine and a cosmetic problem. It is most commonly associated with anovulation; however, other causes of increased androgen levels, such as adrenal and ovarian diseases, need to be ruled out. The most sensitive marker of excess androgen production is hirsutism, followed by acne, oily skin, increased libido, and virilization. **Virilization** consists of clitoromegaly, deepening of the voice, balding, increased muscle mass, and male body habitus. Adrenal hyperplasia or androgen-secreting tumors of the adrenal gland or ovary are causes of virilization. Of note, virilization is rarely associated with PCOS. The treatment depends on the underlying etiology.

The pattern of hair growth is genetically predetermined. Differences in hair growth between ethnic groups are secondary to variations in hair follicle concentration and 5-alpha-reductase activity. Hair growth can be divided into three phases: anagen (growing phase), catagen (involution phase), and telogen (quiescent phase). The hair length is determined by the length of the anagen phase. The stability of hair is determined by the length of the telogen phase. Hairs found on the face, axilla, chest, breast, pubic area, and anterior thighs are termed "sex hair" because they respond to sex hormones. Androgens (especially testosterone) initiate the growth of pubic hair and increase the diameter and pigmentation of pubic hair. Androgens may be produced by the ovary, adrenal gland, or by peripheral conversion. Dehydroepiandrosterone sulfate (DHEA-S) is derived almost exclusively from the adrenal gland. Dihydrotestosterone (DHT) is metabolized from testosterone by 5-alpha-reductase; increased activity of 5-alpha-reductase leads to an increase in DHT and stimulation of hair growth. The majority of testosterone is bound to sex hormone-binding globulin (SHBG), and it is the unbound portion that is primarily responsible for androgenicity. Hyperandrogenism decreases SHBG, and thus, exacerbates hirsutism.

The appearance and cosmetic changes associated with hirsutism depend on the number of follicles present, ratio of growth to resting phases, asynchrony of growth cycles, and thickness and degree of pigmentation of individual hairs. **The history should focus on the onset and duration of symptoms (faster growth is associated with tumors of the adrenal gland and ovary, whereas slow onset since menarche is more likely polycystic ovarian syndrome).** The severity of symptoms should also be characterized (eg, virilization is rare and is usually associated with androgen-secreting tumors). The regularity of the menses and symptoms of thyroid disease should also

Table 53–1 • DIFFERENTIAL DIAGNOSIS OF HIRSUTISM

Disease	History	Physical Examination	Laboratory Test	Treatment
Cushing syndrome	Glucose intolerance	Hypertension, buffalo hump, central obesity	Dexamethasone suppression test	Surgical
Adrenal tumor	Rapid-onset virilism	Abdominal mass	DHEA-S	Surgical
Congenital adrenal hyperplasia	Ambiguous genitalia, family history	Hypotension	Elevated 17-hydroxyprogesterone	Replace cortisol and mineralocorticoid
Polycystic ovarian syndrome	Onset since menarche	Hirsutism, rarely virilization	Elevated LH-FSH ratio	Oral contraceptive pills
Sertoli–Leydig cell tumor	Rapid onset	Hirsutism, virilism, adnexal mass	Elevated testosterone level	Surgical

be sought. The physical examination should focus on the location of hair growth and its severity, thyromegaly, body shape and habitus, the presence of breast discharge, skin changes (acanthosis or abdominal striae), adnexal or abdominal masses, and the external genitalia. Helpful laboratory tests include assays for serum testosterone, DHEA-S, 17-hydroxyprogesterone (which is elevated with congenital adrenal hyperplasia), prolactin, and thyroid-stimulating hormone (TSH). A markedly elevated testosterone level suggests an androgen-secreting ovarian tumor, such as a Sertoli–Leydig cell tumor. With a high DHEA-S level, the examiner should be suspicious of an adrenal process, such as adrenal hyperplasia or a tumor.

The differential diagnosis for hirsutism (Table 53–1) includes anovulation, late-onset adrenal hyperplasia, androgen-secreting tumors (adrenal or ovarian in origin), Cushing disease, medications, thyroid disease, and hyperprolactinemia.

A genetic defect in the enzyme 21-hydroxylase causes most of the cases of congenital adrenal hyperplasia (CAH). While **classic CAH is the most common cause of ambiguous genitalia in the newborn**, late onset of nonclassical CAH can present in adult women with symptoms of hirsutism and anovulation. An elevated morning fasting 17-hydroxyprogesterone level is highly suggestive of CAH. Treatment depends on the etiology; however, in general, the goal is to decrease the amount of DHT available. This can be accomplished by inhibiting adrenal or ovarian androgen secretion, changing SHBG binding, impairing peripheral conversion of androgen to active androgen, and inhibiting activity at target tissues. Treatment options include weight loss, combined oral contraception pills, spironolactone (a diuretic that is an androgen antagonist), progesterone-containing medications, electrolysis, laser vaporization, waxing, and shaving. The patient must be warned that there is a slow response to treatment with medications (an average of 6 months). To help with more immediate results, nonmedical therapies (waxing and shaving) may be used initially until the new medication begins to work effectively.

COMPREHENSION QUESTIONS

53.1 A 6-year-old girl is noted to have breast development and vaginal spotting. No abnormal hair growth is noted. A 10-cm ovarian mass is palpated on rectal examination. Which of the following is the most likely diagnosis?

A. Benign cystic tumor (dermoid)
B. Idiopathic precocious puberty
C. Sertoli–Leydig cell tumor
D. Congenital adrenal hyperplasia
E. Granulosa-theca cell tumor

53.2 A 15-year-old G0P0 girl complains of increasing hair over her face and chest. She also has a deepening voice and clitoromegaly. There have been two neonatal deaths in the family. Which of the following is the best diagnostic test for the likely diagnosis?

A. Testosterone level
B. Dexamethasone suppression test
C. 17-Hydroxyprogesterone level
D. Luteinizing hormone (LH) and follicle-stimulating hormone (FSH) levels
E. Karyotype

53.3 A 22-year-old nulliparous woman with irregular menses of 7 years' duration complains of primary infertility. She has a family history of diabetes. She has mild hirsutism on examination. Which of the following is the most likely therapy?

A. Cortisol and mineralocorticoid replacement
B. Excision of an adrenal tumor
C. Surgical excision of an ovarian tumor
D. Oral clomiphene citrate
E. Intrauterine insemination

53.4 A 24-year-old woman complains of bothersome hirsutism and skipping periods. She does not have evidence of voice changes, hair loss, or clitoromegaly. The pelvic examination does not reveal adnexal masses. The serum DHEA-S, testosterone, and 17-hydroxyprogesterone levels are normal. The LH-to-FSH ratio is 1:1. Which of the following is the most likely diagnosis?

A. Polycystic ovarian syndrome
B. Familial hirsutism
C. Ovarian tumor
D. Adrenal tumor
E. Cushing syndrome

ANSWERS

53.1 **E.** Isosexual (no virilization) **precocious puberty** with an **adnexal mass** usually is a **granulosa cell tumor** of the ovary. **Dermoid cysts** are also found in the ovary. They present as a pelvic mass that causes pain due to its rapidly enlarging size, however, they do not cause isosexual precocious puberty. A **Sertoli–Leydig cell tumor** is the androgen counterpart to the granulose-theca cell tumor. With a Sertoli–Leydig cell tumor, testosterone levels are markedly elevated, and patients typically present with hirsutism, virilism, and an adnexal mass. **Congenital adrenal hyperplasia** is the most common cause of ambiguous genitalia in the newborn; however, late onset can present in adult women with symptoms of hirsutism and anovulation.

53.2 **C.** The most common neonatal endocrine cause of death (salt wasting) is **congenital adrenal hyperplasia (21-hydroxylase deficiency)**. An elevated testosterone level would be found with a **Sertoli–Leydig cell tumor**. A dexamethasone suppression test is used in the diagnosis of **Cushing syndrome**. An elevated LH-to-FSH ratio is found with **PCOS**. A **karyotype** may be used in finding the etiology behind a young girl's presentation of primary amenorrhea or pubertal delay.

53.3 **D.** This patient most likely has **PCOS**; the initial treatment for **infertility** is **clomiphene citrate**. Since the symptoms were not of rapid onset, the etiology is not likely to involve a tumor. Intrauterine insemination is usually indicated for the rare cervical factor infertility, and not **ovulatory dysfunction**.

53.4 **A.** Polycystic ovarian syndrome is the **most common cause of hirsutism and irregular menses**. Treatment may be **spironolactone** (androgen antagonist) and **oral contraceptives**. Familial hirsutism usually is not associated with oligomenorrhea. Symptoms do not correlate with an ovarian tumor (since the patient has abnormal hair growth, hirsutism); also, laboratory values indicate normal adrenal function, thus ruling out adrenal tumor and Cushing syndrome. Notably, a normal LH:FSH ratio does not rule out PCOS, although often there is an increased LH:FSH ratio.

CLINICAL PEARLS

▶ The rapid onset of hirsutism or virilization usually indicates the presence of an androgen-secreting tumor.

▶ The two most common locations of androgen production and secretion are the ovary and the adrenal gland.

▶ The most common cause of hirsutism and irregular menses is polycystic ovarian syndrome.

▶ The most common cause of ambiguous genitalia in the newborn is congenital adrenal hyperplasia, usually due to 21-hydroxylase enzyme deficiency.

▶ Hyperandrogenism in the face of an adnexal mass usually indicates a Sertoli–Leydig cell tumor of the ovary, and is treated surgically.

REFERENCES

Alexander CJ, Mathur R, Laufer LR, Aziz R. Amenorrhea, oligomenorrhea, and hyperandrogenic disorders. In: Hacker NF, Gambone JC, Hobel CJ, eds. *Essentials of Obstetrics and Gynecology.* 6th ed. Philadelphia, PA: Saunders; 2012:355-367.

Schorge W, Schaffer J, Horson L, et al. Ovarian germ cell and sex cord stromal tumors. In: Schorge W, Schaffer J, Horson L, eds. *Williams Gynecology.* 2nd ed. New York, NY: McGraw-Hill; 2012: 738-754.

Speroff L. Hirsutism. In: Fritz MA, Speroff L. eds. *Clinical Gynecologic Endocrinology and Infertility.* 8th ed. Philadelphia, PA: Lippincott Williams and Wilkins; 2010:499-530.

CASE 54

A 16-year-old adolescent female is referred for never having menstruated. She is otherwise in good health. She has an older sister who experienced menarche at the age of 12 years. She denies excessive exercise or having an eating aversion. There is no family history of depression. On examination, she is 50 in tall and weighs 100 lb. The neck is supple and without masses. Her breasts appear to be Tanner stage I, and her pubic hair pattern is also consistent with Tanner stage I. Abdominal examination reveals no masses. The external genitalia are normal for a prepubescent female. A normal-appearing small cervix is seen on speculum examination. On bimanual examination, a small uterus and no adnexal masses are palpated.

▶ What is the most likely diagnosis?
▶ What is the next step in diagnosis?

ANSWERS TO CASE 54:
Pubertal Delay, Gonadal Dysgenesis

Summary: A healthy 16-year-old adolescent woman is referred for never having menstruated. She denies excessive exercise or an eating aversion. On examination, she is 50 in tall and weighs 100 lb. The neck is supple and without masses. Her breasts and pubic hair are both Tanner stage I. The abdominal examination reveals no masses. The pelvic examination is consistent with a prepubescent woman.

- **Most likely diagnosis:** Gonadal dysgenesis (Turner syndrome).
- **Next step in diagnosis:** Serum follicle-stimulating hormone (FSH).

ANALYSIS
Objectives

1. Know that the absence of secondary sexual characteristics by the age of 14 years constitutes delayed puberty.

2. Know that the most common cause of sexually infantile delayed puberty, gonadal dysgenesis, is usually associated with a chromosomal abnormality.

3. Understand that the FSH level can help determine whether the delayed puberty is due to a central nervous system (CNS) problem or an ovarian problem.

4. Know that the definition of precocious puberty is the onset of secondary sexual characteristics >2 standard deviations from the mean (age 7 years in Caucasian women and 6 years in African-American women).

5. Know that the most common cause of precocious puberty in women is idiopathic and treated with gonadotropin-releasing hormone agonist.

Considerations

This 16-year-old adolescent woman has never menstruated and, therefore, has primary amenorrhea. Furthermore, she has not yet experienced breast development (which should occur by an age of 14 years) and thus has delayed puberty. The lack of breast development means a lack of estrogen, which may be caused by either a central nervous system problem (low gonadotropin levels) or an ovarian problem (elevated gonadotropins). She is also of short stature, confirming the lack of estrogen. The absent pubic and axillary hair are consistent with delayed puberty. The most likely diagnosis without further information would be gonadal dysgenesis, such as Turner syndrome. An elevated FSH level would be confirmatory.

APPROACH TO:
Pubertal Delay

See also Case 55 (Primary Amenorrhea).

DEFINITIONS

DELAYED PUBERTY: Lack of secondary sexual characteristics by the age of 14 years.

GONADAL DYSGENESIS: Failure of development of gonads (ovaries or testes), usually associated with a karyotypic abnormality (such as 45,X) and often associated with streaked gonads. Less commonly, the karyotype may be 46,XX or 46,XY.

CLINICAL APPROACH

Delayed Puberty

Maturation of the hypothalamic–pituitary–ovarian axis leads to the onset of puberty. There are four stages of pubertal development: (1) thelarche, (2) pubarche/adrenarche, (3) growth spurt, and (4) menarche. The first sign of puberty is the appearance of breast budding (thelarche), which occurs at a mean age of 10.8 years. This is followed by the appearance of pubic and axillary hair (pubarche/adrenarche), usually at 11 years. The growth spurt typically occurs 1 year after thelarche. The onset of menses (menarche) is the final event of puberty, occurring approximately 2.3 years after thelarche, at a mean age of 12.9 years. Normal puberty takes place between the ages of 8 and 14 years, with an average duration of 4.5 years. Delayed puberty is the absence of secondary sexual characteristics by the age of 14 years.

Thelarche → Adrenarche → Growth spurt → Menarche
Breast bud → Axillary and pubic hair → Menses

Delayed puberty can be subdivided on the basis of two factors: the gonadotropic and the gonadal state. The FSH level defines the gonadotropic state. The ovarian production of estrogen refers to the gonadal state. The FSH level differentiates between brain and ovarian causes of delayed puberty. Central nervous system defects result in low FSH levels secondary to disruption of the hypothalamic–pituitary axis. With ovarian failure, the negative feedback of estrogen on the properly functioning hypothalamic–pituitary axis is not present, resulting in high FSH levels.

Hypergonadotropic hypogonadism (high FSH, low estrogen) is due to gonadal deficiency. The most common cause of this type of delayed puberty is Turner syndrome. These individuals have an abnormality in, or the absence of one of the X chromosomes leading to gonadal dysgenesis and a 45,X karyotype. They do not have true ovaries, but rather a fibrous band of tissue referred to as gonadal streaks. Thus, they lack ovarian estrogen production and, as a result, secondary sexual characteristics. The internal and external genitalia are that of a normal woman, but remain infantile even into adult life. Other characteristic physical findings are short stature, webbed neck, low set ears and posterior hairline, widely spaced nipples or "shield chest," and increased carrying angle at the elbow. Turner syndrome should be suspected in an individual who presents with primary amenorrhea, prepubescent secondary sexual characteristics, and sexually infantile external genitalia. The definitive diagnosis can be made with an elevated FSH level and a karyotypic evaluation. Occasionally, the karyotype with gonadal dysgenesis may be 46,XX or 46,XY. When affected with 46,XY, the gonads should be removed surgically to avoid neoplastic changes. Other causes of hypergonadotropic hypogonadism are ovarian damage due to exposure to ionizing radiation, chemotherapy, inflammation, or torsion.

Hypogonadotropic hypogonadism (low FSH and low estrogen) is usually secondary to a central defect. Hypothalamic dysfunction may occur due to poor nutrition or eating disorders (anorexia nervosa and bulimia), extremes in exercise, and chronic illness or stress. Other causes are primary hypothyroidism, Cushing syndrome, pituitary adenomas, and craniopharyngiomas (the most commonly associated neoplasm). Kallmann syndrome (absence of gonadotropin releasing hormone [GnRH]-releasing neurons in the hypothalamus) is another rare cause of hypogonadotropic hypogonadism.

The diagnostic approach to delayed puberty begins with a meticulous history and physical examination. The history should query chronic illnesses, exercise and eating habits, and age of menarche of the patient's sisters and mother. The physical examination should search for signs of chronic illness, such as a goiter, or neurologic deficits, such as visual field defects indicative of cranial neoplasms. Skull imaging should be obtained to look for intracranial lesions. The laboratory evaluation should include serum measurements of FSH, estradiol, prolactin, TSH, free T_4, and appropriate adrenal steroids. A karyotype evaluation should be performed when the FSH level is elevated.

The management goals for those with delayed puberty are to initiate and sustain sexual maturation, prevent osteoporosis from hypoestrogenemia, and promote the full height potential. Hormonal therapy and human growth hormone can be used to achieve these objectives. Patients with hypergonadotropic hypogonadism presenting with delayed puberty should be started on unopposed estrogen for 2 to 3 years before a progestin is added. They are started on low-dose estrogen and then gradually increased every 3 months. Estrogen will promote growth of the long bones and development of the breasts. Exposure to progestins during the first 2 to 3 years of estrogen therapy would lead to abnormal development of the breasts (tubular breast formation). Once the breasts are formed and are at Tanner stage 3 or 4, a progestin is added. Combination of oral contraceptives provides the adequate amount of estrogen needed to prevent osteoporosis, and the progestin protects against endometrial cancer.

Patients with hypogonadotropic hypogonadism with no apparent cause need imaging of the brain to rule out a brain tumor. If a cause is identified (hyperprolactinemia, hypothyroidism, behavioral), therapy is tailored to correct the underlying cause. In non-treatable conditions such as gonadal dysgenesis, estrogen replacement is started then followed with combination estrogen/progestin therapy.

Precocious Puberty

On the other end of the spectrum, girls who develop secondary sexual characteristics too early are said to have precocious puberty. In general, the definition is breast development prior to age 7, and in African-American women, prior to age 6. **The most common cause of female precocious puberty is idiopathic**, with the GnRH pulse generator initiating early without anatomical pathology. This is a diagnosis of exclusion. Serum FSH, luteinizing hormone (LH), and estradiol levels help to distinguish central (brain causes) versus peripheral causes. FSH and LH levels that are barely detectable are consistent with a peripheral cause, whereas FSH and LH levels in the reproductive range would suggest a central cause. Central causes can include brain tumors, meningitis, hydrocephalus, or head trauma. Peripheral causes can include granulosa cell tumors of the ovary, McCune-Albright syndrome, or adrenal tumors. Peripheral precocious puberty usually presents at an early age (<4 years). If precocious puberty is untreated, the girl will be taller than her peers initially, but due to early long bone epiphyseal closure, the eventual height will be shorter. Central precocious puberty is treated with GnRH agonists.

COMPREHENSION QUESTIONS

54.1 A 15-year-old adolescent female is diagnosed with gonadal dysgenesis on the basis of delayed puberty, short stature, and elevated gonadotropin levels. Which of the following is generally present?

A. Secondary amenorrhea

B. 69,XXY karyotype

C. Tanner stage IV breast development

D. Osteoporosis

E. Polycystic ovaries

54.2 A 16-year-old adolescent female is brought into the pediatrician's office due to no breast development. The patient's mother notes that both of patient's sisters had onset of breast development at age 10, and also all of her friends have already begun menstruating. Examination reveals Tanner stage I breast and pubic/axillary hair, and is otherwise unremarkable. Which of the following is the most likely diagnosis?

A. Delayed puberty

B. Development is within normal limits and should be observed

C. Primary amenorrhea

D. Likely craniopharyngioma

54.3 A 16-year-old adolescent female is evaluated for lack of pubertal development. She is diagnosed with gonadal dysgenesis. Which of the following laboratory findings is likely to be elevated in this patient?
   A. Follicle-stimulating hormone levels
   B. Estrogen levels
   C. Progesterone levels
   D. Prolactin levels
   E. Thyroxine levels

54.4 A 20-year-old individual with a 46,XY karyotype is noted to be a sexually infantile phenotypic woman and is diagnosed as having gonadal dysgenesis. Which of the following is the most important treatment for this patient?
   A. Progestin therapy to reduce osteoporosis
   B. Estrogen and androgen therapy to enhance height
   C. Progesterone therapy to prevent endometrial cancer
   D. Gonadectomy
   E. Estrogen therapy to initiate breast development

54.5 A 6-year-old Caucasian girl is noted to have Tanner 3 breast development and menses. Which of the following is the probable treatment for this patient?
   A. Adrenal tumor excision
   B. Brain tumor excision
   C. GnRH agonist therapy
   D. Replacement of thyroid hormone

ANSWERS

54.1 **D.** Breast tissue usually is infantile (**Tanner stage I**) with gonadal dysgenesis because no estrogen is produced; these patients are at risk for **osteoporosis**. Breast tissue is a reflection of endogenous estrogen. They have **primary amenorrhea**, and usually a **45,X karyotype**. They have **streak ovaries**, and not polycystic ovaries (PCOS). PCOS is a condition in which there is unopposed estrogen, high levels of circulating androgens, and normal timing of puberty onset.

54.2 **A. Delayed puberty** is defined as no secondary sexual characteristics by the age of 14 years. **Primary amenorrhea** is defined as no menarche by the age of 16 years in the presence of secondary sexual characteristics, or age 14 in the absence of secondary sexual characteristics . This patient has primary amenorrhea. Her work-up would include TSH, prolactin, FSH and estradiol levels. If estradiol is low and FSH is high, karyotype is needed. If Estradiol and FSH are both low, then a hypothalamic or pituitary cause must be considered (MRI will be needed).

54.3 **A.** With gonadal dysgenesis, the **FSH level is elevated**. This distinguishes ovarian failure from a central nervous system dysfunction (central defect). The FSH level determines the gonadotropic state, and the ovarian estradiol level dictates the gonadal state. **Estrogen and progesterone levels are low**; the prolactin, and thyroxin levels remain unchanged.

54.4 **D.** The **Y chromosome predisposes intra-abdominal gonads to malignancy.** Even a mosaic karyotype, such as 46,XX/46,XY, would predispose to gonadal malignancy. Had the patient had a karyotype similar to that in Turner syndrome (45,X), another gonadal dysgenesis disorder, a gonadectomy on the streak ovaries, would not be indicated.

54.5 **C.** The most common cause of female precocious puberty is idiopathic. The treatment is GnRH-agonist therapy. The patient should have an evaluation such as FSH and LH levels to determine central versus peripheral causes. If the FSH and LH are consistent with a central (brain) etiology, then the brain is imaged to assess for central nervous system etiologies. Bone age and assessment of thyroid function tests are also important. Interestingly, only hypothyroidism causes precocious puberty with **delayed** bone age. All other etiologies of precocious puberty are associated with **accelerated** bone age (bone age "older" than chronological age).

CLINICAL PEARLS

- The most common cause of sexually infantile primary amenorrhea is gonadal dysgenesis.
- The most common karyotype associated with gonadal dysgenesis is 45,X, although 46,XX or 46,XY may be seen.
- Delayed puberty is defined as no development of secondary sexual characteristics by the age of 14 years.
- The FSH level distinguishes ovarian failure from central nervous system dysfunction.
- The FSH level determines the gonadotropic state, and the ovarian estradiol level dictates the gonadal state.
- The most important initial test for primary amenorrhea with normal breast development is a pregnancy test.
- The most common cause of precocious puberty in women is idiopathic, which is a central cause, and a diagnosis of exclusion.
- The treatment of central precocious puberty is GnRH-agonist therapy.

REFERENCES

De Ugarte CM, Buyalos RP, Laufer LR. Puberty and disorders of pubertal development. In: Hacker NF, Moore JG, Gambone JC, eds. *Essentials of Obstetrics and Gynecology*. 6th ed. Philadelphia, PA: Saunders; 2015:386-397.

Fritz MA, Speroff L. Normal and abnormal growth and puberty. In: Fritz MA, Speroof L. *Clinical Gynecology and Infertility*. 8th ed. Philadelphia, PA: Lippincott Williams and Wilkins; 2012:391-410.

Pisarska MD, Alexander CJ, Azziz R, Buyalos RP. Puberty and disorders of pubertal development. In: Hacker NF, Gambone JC, Hobel CJ, eds. *Essentials of Obstetrics and Gynecology*. 6th ed. Philadelphia, PA: Saunders; 2015:345-354.

CASE 55

An 18-year-old nulliparous adolescent woman complains that she has not yet started menstruating. She denies weight loss or excessive exercise. Each of her sisters achieved menarche by 13 years of age. The patient's mother recalls a doctor mentioning that her daughter had a missing right kidney on an abdominal x-ray film. On examination, she is 5 ft 6 in tall and weighs 140 lb. Her blood pressure is 110/60 mm Hg. Her thyroid gland is normal on palpation. She has Tanner stage IV breast development and female external genitalia. She has Tanner stage IV axillary and pubic hair. There are no skin lesions.

▶ What is the most likely diagnosis?
▶ What is the next step in diagnosis?
▶ What is the most likely finding on pelvic examination?

ANSWERS TO CASE 55:
Amenorrhea (Primary), Müllerian Agenesis

Summary: An 18-year-old nulliparous adolescent woman, who may have only one kidney, presents with primary amenorrhea. She denies weight loss or excessive exercise. On examination, she is 5 ft 6 in tall and weighs 140 lb. Her blood pressure is 110/60 mm Hg. Her thyroid gland is normal. She has appropriate Tanner stage IV breast development, axillary and pubic hair, and female external genitalia.

- **Most likely diagnosis:** Müllerian (or vaginal) agenesis.
- **Next step in diagnosis:** Serum testosterone or karyotype.
- **Most likely finding on pelvic examination:** Blind vaginal pouch or vaginal dimple.

ANALYSIS
Objectives

1. Know the definition of primary amenorrhea, that is, no menses by the age of 16 years.
2. Know that the two most common causes of primary amenorrhea when there is normal breast development are müllerian agenesis and androgen insensitivity.
3. Understand that a serum testosterone level or karyotype would differentiate the two conditions.

Considerations

This 18-year-old adolescent woman has never had a menstrual period; therefore, she has primary amenorrhea. She has **normal Tanner stage IV breast development** as well as **normal axillary and pubic hair.** Breast development connotes the presence of estrogen, and axillary and pubic hair suggests the presence of androgens. She also has a history of only one kidney. The most likely diagnosis is müllerian agenesis because a significant fraction of such patients will have a urinary tract abnormality. Also, with androgen insensitivity, there is typically scant axillary and pubic hair since there is a defective androgen receptor. The diagnosis can be confirmed with a serum testosterone, which would be normal in müllerian agenesis, and elevated (in the normal male range) in androgen insensitivity. **In both conditions, there is no uterus, tubes, or cervix, and a blind vaginal pouch or vaginal dimple.** A karyotype would also help to distinguish the two conditions. Notably, **absence of breast development** would point to a hypoestrogenic state such as **gonadal dysgenesis (Turner syndrome).**

APPROACH TO:
Primary Amenorrhea

DEFINITIONS

PRIMARY AMENORRHEA: No menarche by the age of 16 years.

ANDROGEN INSENSITIVITY: An androgen receptor defect in which 46,XY individuals are phenotypically female with normal breast development.

MÜLLERIAN AGENESIS: Congenital absence of development of the uterus, cervix, and fallopian tubes in a 46,XX female, leading to primary amenorrhea.

CLINICAL APPROACH

When a young woman presents with primary amenorrhea, the differential diagnosis can be narrowed on the basis of whether or not normal breast tissue is present, and whether a uterus is present or absent. After pregnancy is excluded, the two most common etiologies that cause primary amenorrhea associated with normal breast development and an absent uterus are androgen insensitivity syndrome and müllerian agenesis (Table 55–1).

An individual with androgen insensitivity syndrome, also known as testicular feminization, has a 46,XY karyotype with normally functioning male gonads that produce normal male levels of testosterone. However, due to a defect in the androgen receptor synthesis or action, there is no formation of male internal or external genitalia. The external genitalia remain female, as it occurs in the absence of sex steroids. There are no internal female reproductive organs, and the vagina is short or absent. Without androgenic opposition to the small circulating levels of estrogen secreted by the gonads and adrenals, and produced by peripheral conversion of androstenedione, breast development is normal or enhanced. **Pubic and axillary hair is absent or scant due to defective androgen receptors.** Therefore, these individuals are genotypically male (46,XY karyotype) but phenotypically female (look like a woman). The abnormal intra-abdominal gonads are at increased risk for malignancy, but this rarely occurs before puberty. Thus, gonadectomy is not performed until after puberty is completed to allow full breast development and linear growth

Table 55–1 • MÜLLERIAN AGENESIS VERSUS ANDROGEN INSENSITIVITY

	Müllerian Agenesis	Androgen Insensitivity
Breast tissue	Normal breast development	Normal breast development
Axillary and pubic hair	Normal	Scant or absent
Uterus and vagina	Absent uterus and blind vagina	Absent uterus and blind vagina
Testosterone level	Normal testosterone	High testosterone (male range)
Karyotype	46,XX	46,XY
Complications	Renal anomalies	Need gonadectomy

to occur. After these events take place, usually around the age of 16 to 18 years, the gonads should be removed. The diagnosis of **androgen insensitivity syndrome** should be suspected when a patient has **primary amenorrhea**, an **absent uterus, normal breast development**, and **scant or absent pubic and axillary hair**. The diagnosis can be confirmed with a karyotype evaluation and/or elevated testosterone levels (male normal range).

Women with müllerian agenesis have a 46,XX karyotype, no uterus or fallopian tubes, and a short or absent vagina. Externally, they resemble individuals with androgen insensitivity. They do, however, have normal functioning ovaries since the ovaries are not müllerian structures, and have normal breast development. They also have **normal pubic and axillary hair** growth because there is no defect in their androgen receptors. Congenital renal abnormalities occur in about one-third of these individuals. These women are genotypically and phenotypically female (46,XX). The diagnosis of müllerian agenesis should be suspected when a patient has primary amenorrhea, an absent uterus, normal breast development, and normal pubic and axillary hair. The presence of normal pubic and axillary hair is what differentiates them from individuals with androgen insensitivity syndrome, and laboratory confirmation can be accomplished with a karyotype examination and/or testosterone level.

Another type of müllerian defect is a uterine septum. In these cases, there is a midline septum that is of varying lengths due to incomplete dissolution of the fused midline portion of the müllerian ducts. Patients often have recurrent miscarriage due to the avascular nature of the septum and inability to sustain a pregnancy. Diagnosis is performed by hysterosalpingogram, saline infusion sonohysterography, or magnetic resonance imaging. Hysteroscopic resection of the septum is the treatment, and outcomes are very good.

CASE CORRELATION

- See also Case 54 (Delayed Puberty) to distinguish between that condition (no breast development by age 14) and müllerian agenesis (primary amenorrhea) where affected women have normal breast development but no menses by age 16.

COMPREHENSION QUESTIONS

55.1 An 18-year-old nulliparous adolescent woman complains of not having started her menses. Her breast development is Tanner stage V. She has a blind vaginal pouch and no cervix. Which of the following describes the most likely diagnosis?

A. Müllerian agenesis
B. Kallmann syndrome
C. Gonadal dysgenesis
D. Polycystic ovarian syndrome

55.2 A 20-year-old G0P0 woman is told by her doctor that there is a strong probability that her gonads will turn malignant. She has not had her menses yet. She has Tanner stage I breast development. Which of the following describes the most likely diagnosis?

A. Müllerian agenesis
B. Androgen insensitivity
C. Gonadal dysgenesis
D. Polycystic ovarian syndrome

55.3 A 19-year-old woman has primary amenorrhea, Tanner stage IV breast development, and a pelvic kidney. Which of the following describes the most likely diagnosis?

A. Müllerian agenesis
B. Androgen insensitivity
C. Gonadal dysgenesis
D. Polycystic ovarian syndrome

55.4 Which of the following is the best explanation for breast development in a patient with androgen insensitivity?

A. Gonadal production of estrogens
B. Adrenal production of estrogen
C. Breast tissue sensitivity to progesterone
D. Peripheral conversion of androgens
E. Autonomous production of breast-specific estrogen

55.5 A 15-year-old adolescent female is brought into the pediatrician due to the absence of breast development and short stature. A karyotype is performed which reveals 46,XY. Which of the following is the most likely diagnosis?

A. Androgen insensitivity
B. Gonadal dysgensis
C. Kallman syndrome
D. Testicular atrophy syndrome

ANSWERS

55.1 **A.** Normal breast development, no cervix, and a blind vaginal pouch may be caused by either müllerian agenesis or androgen insensitivity. The serum testosterone level will help to distinguish the two conditions. Kallmann syndrome is associated with delayed puberty (Tanner stage I breasts).

55.2 **C**. The Y-chromosome gonad may become malignant. This patient likely has gonadal dysgenesis since she has Tanner stage I breast development. Although usually 45,X is associated with gonadal dysgenesis, the karyotype can also be 46,XX or 46,XY. In other words, this patient has delayed puberty. This is XY gonadal dysgenesis.

55.3 **A**. A **pelvic kidney** most likely is associated with a **müllerian abnormality**. These women have no uterus or fallopian tubes, and have a short or absent vagina. They do, however, have **normally functioning ovaries** because the ovaries are not müllerian structures, and as a result, they have normal breast development.

55.4 **D**. Individuals with androgen insensitivity usually have full breast development due to the **peripheral conversion of androgens to estrogens**. Also, because of the defective androgen receptor, the high endogenous androgens do not inhibit breast development as in a normal male, but **pubic and axillary hair is scant or absent**. The gonads and adrenals also produce a small circulating amount of estrogen, but do not contribute as much as the peripheral androgen conversion. Progesterone sensitivity does not influence breast development, nor does a breast-specific estrogen.

55.5 **B**. The most common cause of delayed puberty (**absent breast tissue** after the age of 14 years) is **gonadal dysgenesis**, which can also occur with a 46,XY karyotype (along with androgen insensitivity). The most common karyotype of gonadal dysgenesis, however, is **45,XO** in **Turner syndrome**. In androgen insensitivity, normal breast development occurs. **Kallmann syndrome** is an example of a hypogonadotropic hypogonadism, or hypothalamic hypogonadism, disorder caused by a deficiency in the gonadotropin-releasing hormone (GnRH) secreted by the hypothalamus (and, therefore, decreased LH and FSH production). Gonadal dysgenesis, on the other hand, is a state of hypergonadotropic hypogonadism. Patients with Kallmann syndrome also typically have a **deficiency or inability to smell**. Women present with delayed puberty and lack of breast development, but have a normal karyotype (46,XX). Treatment is hormone replacement.

CLINICAL PEARLS

▶ A pregnancy test should be the first test for any woman with primary or secondary amenorrhea.

▶ The two most common causes of primary amenorrhea in a woman with normal breast development are androgen insensitivity and müllerian agenesis.

▶ Scant axillary and pubic hair suggest androgen insensitivity.

▶ A karyotype and testosterone level help to differentiate between müllerian agenesis and androgen insensitivity.

▶ Renal anomalies are common with müllerian abnormalities.

REFERENCES

Lobo RA. Primary and secondary amenorrhea and precocious puberty. In: Katz VL, Lentz GM, Lobo RA, Gersenson DM, eds. *Comprehensive Gynecology*. 6th ed. St. Louis, MO: Mosby-Year Book; 2012:933-960.

Pisarska MD, Alexander CJ, Azziz R, Buyalos RP. Puberty and disorders of pubertal development. In: Hacker NF, Gambone JC, Hobel CJ, eds. *Essentials of Obstetrics and Gynecology*. 6th ed. Philadelphia, PA: Saunders; 2015:345-354.

CASE 56

A 31-year-old G1P1 woman presents with a history of infertility of 2-year duration. She states that her menses began at age 12 years, and they occur at regular 28-day intervals. A biphasic basal body temperature (BBT) chart is recorded. She denies sexually transmitted diseases, and a hysterosalpingogram (HSG) shows patent tubes and a normal uterine cavity. Her husband is 34 years old and his semen analysis is normal.

▶ What is the most likely etiology of the infertility?

ANSWER TO CASE 56:
Infertility, Peritoneal Factor

Summary: An infertile couple is evaluated. Her menses are regular, and a biphasic basal body temperature chart is recorded. She denies sexually transmitted diseases, and a hysterosalpingogram shows patent tubes and a normal uterine cavity. The semen analysis is normal.

- **Most likely etiology:** Endometriosis (peritoneal factor).

ANALYSIS
Objectives

1. Know the five basic etiologies of infertility.
2. Understand the history and laboratory tests for these five factors.
3. Understand that endometriosis is more common than cervical factor infertility.

Considerations

This 31-year-old woman has secondary infertility, meaning she has had a pregnancy in the past. In approaching infertility, there are five basic factors to examine: (1) ovulatory, (2) uterine, (3) tubal, (4) male factor, and (5) peritoneal factor (endometriosis). Her history is consistent with regular ovulation; this is further supported by the biphasic basal body temperature chart. The uterine and tubal factors are normal based on the normal hysterosalpingogram (a radiologic study in which dye is placed into the uterine cavity via a transcervical catheter). The male factor is essentially ruled out based on the normal semen analysis. Therefore, the remaining factor not addressed is the peritoneal factor. If the patient had prior cryotherapy to the cervix, the examiner might be directed to consider cervical factor (rare); similarly, if the patient complained of the three Ds of endometriosis (dysmenorrhea, dyspareunia, and dyschezia), then the clinician would be pointed toward the peritoneal factor. Since there are no hints favoring one factor over another, the clinician must pick the most common condition, which is endometriosis.

APPROACH TO:
Infertility

DEFINITIONS

ASSISTED REPRODUCTIVE TECHNOLOGY: Procedures in which the oocytes and/or sperm are handled in the laboratory in an effort to enhance fertilization. These include in vitro fertilization (IVF), intracytoplasmic spermatic injection, preimplantation genetic diagnosis, and other procedures.

IN VITRO FERTILIZATION: The handling of a woman's oocyte and sperm in the laboratory environment, fertilization of the oocyte, and then injection of the blastocyst into the endometrium.

INFERTILITY: Inability to conceive after 1 year of unprotected intercourse.

PRIMARY INFERTILITY: A woman has never been able to get pregnant.

SECONDARY INFERTILITY: A woman has been pregnant in the past, but has 1 year of inability to conceive.

CLINICAL APPROACH

Infertility affects approximately 10% to 15% of couples in the reproductive age group. **Fecundability,** defined as the probability of achieving a pregnancy within one menstrual cycle, has been estimated at **20% to 25%** for a normal couple. On the basis of this estimate, approximately 90% of couples should conceive after 12 months. The physician's initial encounter with the couple is very important and sets the tone for further evaluation and treatment. It is extremely important that after the initial evaluation, a realistic plan be established and followed (Table 56–1).

The five main causes of infertility are as follows:

1. **Ovulatory disorders (ovulatory factor).** Ovulatory disorders account for approximately 30% to 40% of all cases of female infertility. A history of regularity or irregularity of the menses is fairly predictive of the regularity of ovulation. The basal body temperature chart is the easiest and least expensive method of detecting ovulation (Figure 56–1).

    The temperature should be determined orally, preferably with a basal body thermometer, before the patient arises out of bed, eats, or drinks. The chart documents the rise of temperature of about 0.5°F that occurs after ovulation due to the release of progesterone (a thermogenic hormone) by the ovary. The rise of temperature accounts for the biphasic pattern indicative of ovulation.

Table 56–1 • APPROACH TO INFERTILITY			
Factor	History	Test	Therapy
Ovulatory dysfunction	Irregular menses, obesity	Basal body temperature chart, LH surge, or progesterone level	Clomiphene citrate
Uterine disorder	Uterine fibroids	Hysterosalpingogram showing abnormal uterine cavity	Hysteroscopic procedure
Male factor	Hernia, varicocele, mumps	Semen analysis	Repair of hernia or varicocele, in vitro fertilization
Tubal disorder	Chlamydial or gonococcal infection	Hysterosalpingogram	Laparoscopy; in vitro fertilization
Peritoneal factor (endometriosis)	3 Ds: dysmenorrhea, dyspareunia, dyschezia	Laparoscopy (some advocate CA-125)	Ablation/excision of endometriosis, medical therapy

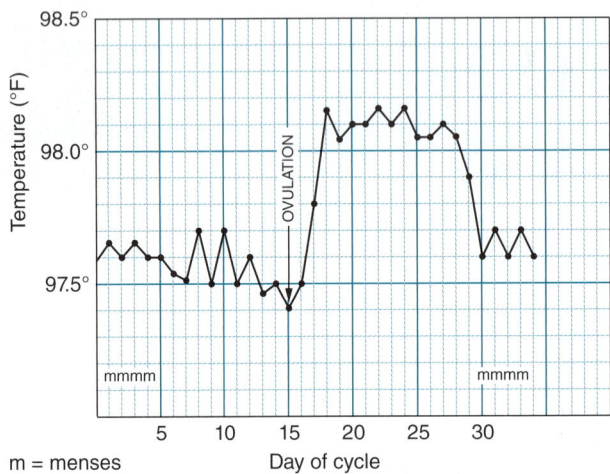

Figure 56–1. Basal body temperature chart. After ovulation, the temperature rises by 0.5°F for 10 to 12 days.

Midluteal (day 21) serum progesterone level is an indirect method of documenting ovulation. Luteinizing hormone (LH) and, particularly the LH surge, can be detected with self-administered urine test kits. Ovulation occurs predictably about 36 hours after the onset of the LH surge. Other tests include the endometrial biopsy showing secretory tissue, or an ultrasound documenting a decrease in follicular size and presence of fluid in the cul-de-sac, suggesting ovulation. For women older than age 30, assessment of ovarian reserve such as day 3 follicle-stimulating hormone (FSH), or anti-müllerian hormone level testing may be helpful (see Case 30).

2. **Uterine problems.** The hysterosalpingogram is the initial test for intrauterine shape and tubal patency. It should be performed between days 6 and 10 of the cycle. Hysteroscopy likewise provides direct visualization of the uterine cavity when the HSG suggests an intrauterine defect. Saline infusion sonohysterography can also be performed to image the endometrial cavity. Uterine abnormalities have been associated with recurrent pregnancy losses. Uterine myomata and, in particular, submucosal myomata may interfere with implantation and fertility.

3. **Tubal factor.** A history of chlamydial or gonococcal cervicitis or salpingitis may point toward tubal disease. Yet, the majority of women with tubal factor infertility have no history of sexually transmitted infections (STIs), owing to the asymptomatic nature of the infections. The hysterosalpingogram is fairly accurate but not perfect. A normal test shows a thin line of dye through the tubes and spillage into the peritoneal cavity outlining the bowel. Abnormal findings should be confirmed with laparoscopy, which is considered the "gold standard" for diagnosing tubal and peritoneal disease. In addition, operative laparoscopy can provide for the treatment of tubal and peritoneal disease through a minimally invasive technique.

4. **Abnormalities in the semen (male factor).** The semen analysis is a very basic and noninvasive test and should be one of the initial examinations. Even men who have fathered other children should have a semen analysis. The semen should be evaluated in terms of: volume (nl > 2.0 mL), sperm concentration (nl > 20 million/mL), motility (nl > 50%), and morphology (nl > 30% normal forms). An abstinence period of 2 to 3 days prior to semen collection is recommended. One abnormal test is not sufficient to establish the diagnosis of a male factor abnormality, and the test should be repeated after 2 to 3 months (the process of transforming spermatogonia into mature sperm cells requires 74 days).

5. **Peritoneal factor (endometriosis).** Endometriosis, a common condition associated with infertility, should be suspected in any infertile woman. The prevalence of endometriosis ranges from 0.5% to 5% in fertile and 25% to 40% in infertile women. Fecundity, defined as the probability of a woman achieving a livebirth in a given month, ranges from 0.15 to 0.20 in normal couples and 0.02 to 0.10 in untreated women with endometriosis. The suspicion should increase if she complains of dysmenorrhea and dyspareunia, but often is present even in asymptomatic women. Although not completely understood, endometriosis may cause infertility by inhibiting ovulation, inducing adhesions, and, perhaps, interfering with fertilization. Laparoscopy is the gold standard for the diagnosis of endometriosis, and can allow for surgical ablation/excision of the lesions. Lesions can be of various appearances, from clear to red to the classic "powder burn" color.

Current evidence indicates that medical therapy is not as beneficial for endometriosis-associated infertility. Surgical treatment in the form of laparoscopy or laparotomy is the efficacious choice with the former providing shorter hospitalization, shorter recovery, potentially less adhesions, and less discomfort to the patient. Restoration of the anatomy with excision of endometrial nodules, removal of endometriomas, and adhesiolysis is the mainstay in the treatment of advanced stages of endometriosis associated with infertility. However, despite surgical excision, conception rates seem to be less in women with extensive disease. Regardless, it seems intuitive that a structural normalization of severely distorted pelvic anatomy can improve conception outcomes, quality of life for the patient, and facilitate egg retrieval in cases of in vitro fertilization. Surgical options remain controversial in early stages of endometriosis without anatomical distortion. However, excision of early lesions can retard the progression of the disease. There is an absence of qualified evidence to indicate that fertility is enhanced with preoperative or postoperative medical therapy. The theoretical benefits do not seem to outweigh the increased costs and rates of morbidity. Medical therapy alone or in combination with surgery may only serve to delay fertility.

Assisted Reproductive Technologies

Assisted reproductive technologies now account for 1% to 2% of pregnancies in the United States. The indications include severe tubal factor, male factor, endometriosis, or unexplained or other infertility not responsive to medical therapy. IVF involves transvaginal extraction of oocytes using ultrasound guidance, typically

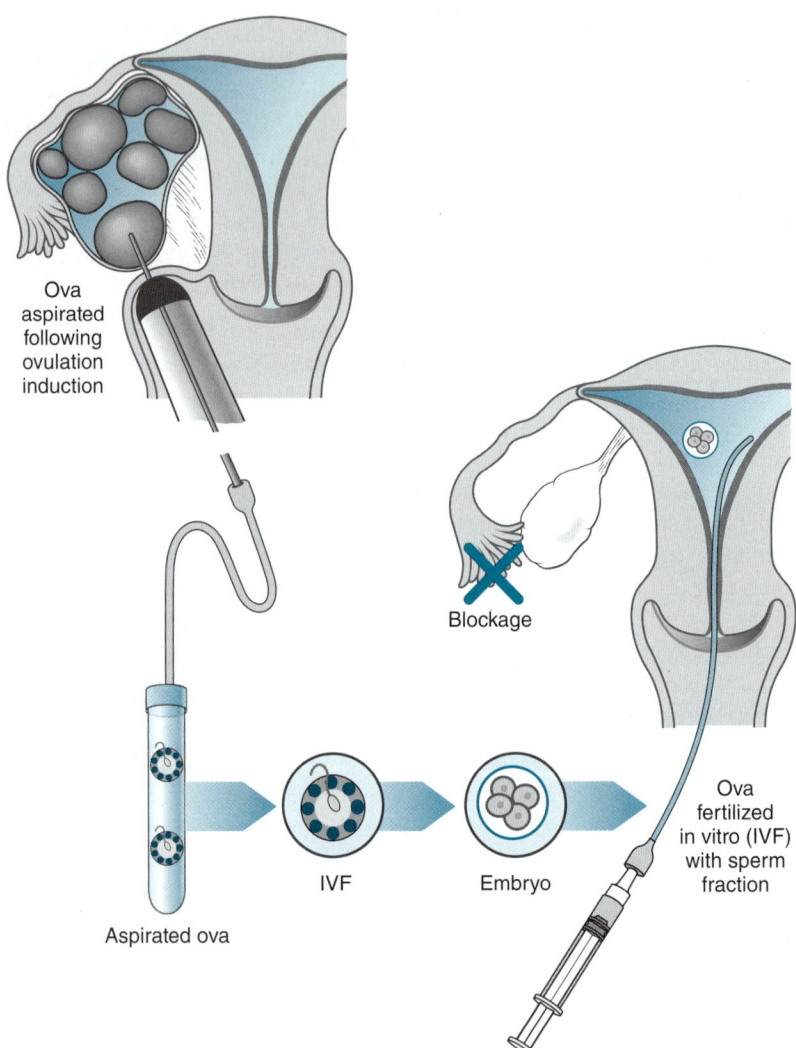

Figure 56–2. IVF sequence: ova aspirated, fertilized in laboratory, and then embryo transfer performed in this patient with tubal factor infertility.

after follicle stimulation, fertilization with sperm, and then replacement of fertilized blastocyst(s) into the endometrial cavity through a transcervical catheter (see Figure 56–2). Careful monitoring of the patient with serial ultrasounds and estradiol levels is important to avoid the dangerous ovarian hyperstimulation syndrome. Other complications include multiple gestation, preterm labor, and miscarriage.

In general, **the "quality" of the oocyte is the single most important factor dictating successful pregnancy.** Donor eggs can be used if the patient's oocytes are of questionable quality. With male factor infertility, intracytoplasmic spermatic injection (ICSI) can be used, by directly injecting a single sperm through the zonapellucida and oocyte cell membrane using micromanipulation techniques. Preimplantation genetic diagnosis can be performed by removing 1 or 2 cells at the 6 to 8 cell blastocyst stage, to test for single gene disorders or translocations. Cryopreservation is often used for those fertilized oocytes that are not implanted, and can be thawed and used at a later time. Surrogates have been used for gestation. There are numerous other issues that are controversial and ethical dilemmas.

Note: **Cervical factor** is considered an **infrequent etiology** and may be suspected with thick viscid cervical mucus before ovulation. Intrauterine insemination, using a catheter to inject washed sperm through the cervix, bypasses the cervix.

COMPREHENSION QUESTIONS

56.1 A 22-year-old G0P0 woman complains of irregular menses every 30 to 65 days. The semen analysis is normal. The hysterosalpingogram is normal. Which of the following is the most likely treatment for this patient?

A. Laparoscopy
B. Intrauterine insemination
C. In vitro fertilization
D. Clomiphene citrate

56.2 A 26-year-old G0P0 woman has regular menses every 28 days. The semen analysis is normal. The patient had a postcoital test revealing motile sperm and stretchy watery cervical mucus. She has been treated for chlamydial infection in the past. Which of the following is the most likely etiology of her infertility?

A. Peritoneal factor
B. Male factor
C. Cervical factor
D. Tubal factor
E. Ovulatory factor
F. Uterine factor

56.3 A 28-year-old G1P1 woman complains of painful menses and pain with intercourse. She has menses every month and denies a history of sexually transmitted diseases. Which of the following tests would most likely identify the etiology of the infertility?

A. Semen analysis
B. Laparoscopy
C. Basal body temperature chart
D. Hysterosalpingogram
E. Progesterone assay

56.4 A 34-year-old infertile woman is noted to have evidence of blocked fallopian tubes by hysterosalpingogram. Which of the following is the best next step for this patient?

A. FSH therapy
B. Clomiphene citrate therapy
C. Laparoscopy
D. Intrauterine insemination

ANSWERS

56.1 **D.** Irregular menses usually means irregular ovulation, and therefore, infertility could most likely be attributed to an ovarian factor. The three conditions to consider are polycystic ovarian syndrome (PCOS), which is most common, hypothalamic disturbances, and premature ovarian failure (POF). Causes of hypothalamic disturbances affect pulsatile gonadotropin-releasing hormone, such as hypothyroidism and hyperprolactinemia. Thus, the evaluation of a woman with irregular ovulation usually includes checking TSH and prolactin levels. Elevated FSH levels would suggest POF. Clomiphene citrate is a treatment for anovulation, particularly polycystic ovarian syndrome. The diagnosis of PCOS is a clinical one, with characteristics of obesity, anovulation, hirsutism, and possibly glucose intolerance. A laparoscopy would be indicated if there was suspicion of a tubal factor causing infertility (such as a prior history [PMH] of chlamydia or gonorrhea) or peritoneal factor (three Ds of endometriosis). Intrauterine insemination is indicated when a cervical factor is thought to be the cause of infertility, such as thick viscid cervical mucus before ovulation. This procedure bypasses the unfavorable cervix using a catheter to inject washed sperm. The patient in this scenario does not present with symptoms consistent with cervical factor infertility. In vitro fertilization can be considered if the problem was a tubal factor or male factor.

56.2 **D.** The history of chlamydial infection strongly suggests tubal factor infertility. Laparoscopy would be the next step in management and is considered the "gold standard" for diagnosing **tubal and peritoneal** disease. The patient does not present with any of the "three Ds" of peritoneal factor, and the semen analysis is normal which excludes male factor as the cause for infertility. There is no mention of a history of fibroids, and she reports regular menses; this eliminates uterine and ovulatory factors as the etiology of her infertility.

56.3 **B.** This patient's history of dysmenorrhea and dyspareunia (two out of the three Ds of peritoneal factor symptoms) suggests endometriosis, which is best diagnosed by laparoscopy. A hysterosalpingogram visualizes the inside of the uterus and would not be helpful in the diagnosis of endometriosis, since it manifests outside the uterus, tubes, and ovaries. She has menses every month; therefore, her basal body temperature chart should be normal. A progesterone assay may be used to assess whether ovulation occurs, or the adequacy of the corpus luteum (a so-called luteal phase defect).

56.4 **C.** This patient presents with findings suggestive of tubal factor infertility. The hysterosalpingogram (radiologic study in which dye is injected into the uterus) is not specific and should be followed up with laparoscopy; sometimes tubal spasm can prevent dye from flowing into the tubes. Laparoscopy can provide the treatment of tubal and peritoneal disease through a minimally invasive technique. Clomiphene is not effective in patients with tubal factor, and is indicated with anovulation. FSH therapy and intrauterine insemination would be ineffective for the same reasons.

CLINICAL PEARLS

▶ The five basic factors causing infertility are: ovulatory, uterine, tubal, male, and peritoneal.

▶ Irregular menses usually means irregular ovulation; regular menses usually indicates regular ovulation. In general, ovulatory disorders are fairly amenable to therapy.

▶ A history of salpingitis or chlamydial cervicitis suggests tubal factor infertility.

▶ Laparoscopy is the "gold standard" in diagnosing endometriosis, and lesions may have a variety of appearances.

▶ Surgery is the main therapy for endometrial or tubal abnormalities associated with infertility.

▶ Assisted reproductive technologies involve isolation and handling of the oocyte and procedures include IVF and ICSI.

REFERENCES

Barnhart K, Dunsmoor-Su R, Coutifaris C. Effect of endometriosis on in vitro fertilization. *Fertil Steril.* 2002;77:1148-1155.

Brown J, Farquhar C. Endometriosis: an overview of Cochrane reviews. *Cochrane Database Syst.* Rev, 2014.

ESHRE Endometriosis Guideline Development Group. ESHRE guideline for the diagnosis and treatment of endometriosis; 2013.

Houston DE, Noller KL, Melton LJ, et al. Incidence of pelvic endometriosis in Rochester, Minnesota, 1970-1979. *Am J Epidemiol.* 1987;125(6):959-969.

Lobo RA. Infertility. In: Katz VL, Lentz GM, Lobo RA, Gersenson DM, eds. *Comprehensive Gynecology.* 6th ed. St. Louis, MO: Mosby-Year Book; 2012:1001-1038.

Meldrum DR. Infertility and assisted reproductive technologies. In: Hacker NF, Gambone JC, Hobel CJ, eds. *Essentials of Obstetrics and Gynecology.* 6th ed. Philadelphia, PA: Saunders; 2015:371-378.

CASE 57

A 60-year-old nulliparous woman who underwent menopause at age 55 years complains of a 4-week history of vaginal bleeding. Prior to menopause, she had irregular menses for about 20 years. She denies the use of estrogen-replacement therapy. Her medical history is significant for diabetes mellitus controlled with an oral hypoglycemic agent. On examination, she weighs 190 lb, her height is 5 ft 3 in, blood pressure is 150/90 mm Hg, and temperature is 99°F (37.2°C). The heart and lung examinations are normal. The abdomen is obese, and no masses are palpated. The external genitalia appear normal, and the uterus seems to be of normal size without adnexal masses.

- ▶ What is the next step?
- ▶ What is your concern?

ANSWERS TO CASE 57:
Postmenopausal Bleeding

Summary: A 66-year-old diabetic, nulliparous woman complains of postmenopausal vaginal bleeding. Prior to menopause, which occurred at age 55, she had irregular menses. She denies the use of estrogen-replacement therapy. Her examination is significant for obesity and hypertension.

- **Next step:** Perform an endometrial biopsy.
- **Concern:** Endometrial cancer.

ANALYSIS
Objectives

1. Understand that postmenopausal bleeding requires endometrial sampling or vaginal ultrasound assessment of the endometrial stripe to assess for endometrial cancer.
2. Know the risk factors for endometrial cancer.
3. Know that endometrial cancer is staged surgically.

Considerations

This patient has postmenopausal vaginal bleeding, which should always be investigated, because it can indicate malignant or premalignant conditions. The biggest concern should be endometrial cancer. She also has numerous risk factors for endometrial cancer including obesity, diabetes, hypertension, prior anovulation (irregular menses), late menopause, and nulliparity. The endometrial sampling or biopsy can be performed in the office by placing a thin, flexible catheter through the cervix. Either endometrial biopsy or transvaginal ultrasound is acceptable initial tests to assess for endometrial cancer. This patient is not taking unopposed estrogen-replacement therapy, which would be another risk factor. If endometrial cancer were diagnosed, the patient would need surgical staging. If the endometrial sampling is negative for cancer, another cause for postmenopausal bleeding, such as atrophic endometrium or endometrial polyp, is possible. A blind sampling of the endometrium, such as with the endometrial biopsy device, has 90% to 95% sensitivity for detecting cancer. If this patient, who has so many risk factors for endometrial cancer, were to have a negative endometrial sampling, many practitioners would go to a direct visualization of the endometrial cavity such as hysteroscopy. If the clinician were to elect to observe this patient after the endometrial biopsy, any further bleeding episodes would necessitate further investigation.

APPROACH TO:
Postmenopausal Bleeding and Endometrial Cancer

DEFINITIONS

ENDOMETRIAL SAMPLING (BIOPSY): A thin catheter is introduced through the cervix into the uterine cavity to aspirate endometrial cells (see Figure 57–1).

ENDOMETRIAL POLYPS: A growth of endometrial glands and stroma, which projects into the uterine cavity, usually on a stalk; it can cause postmenopausal bleeding.

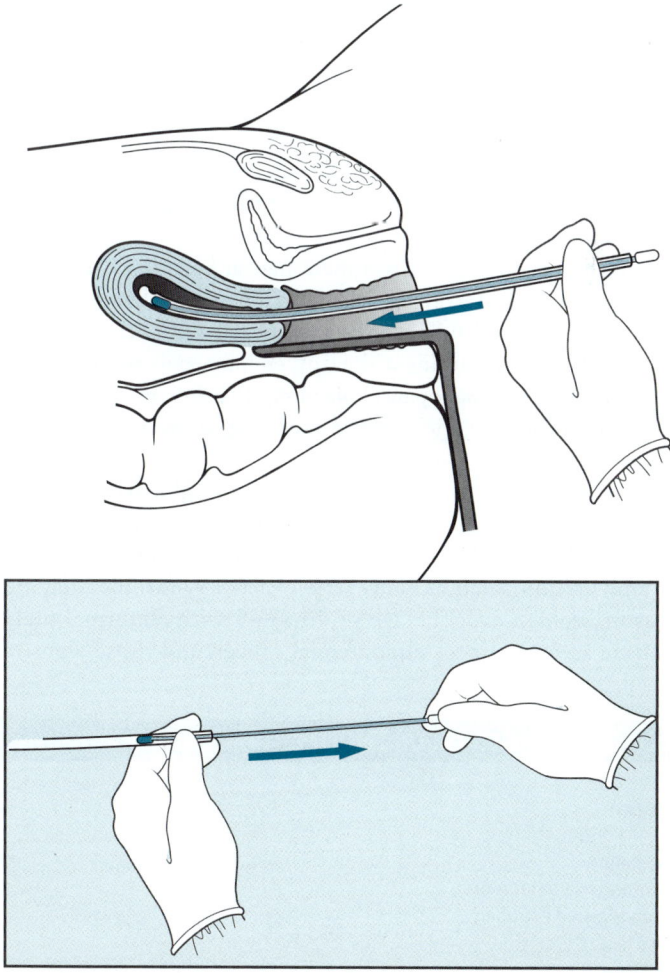

Figure 57–1. Endometrial biopsy. Pipelle is a thin flexible catheter and placed through the cervix into the uterus via speculum. The stylet is withdrawn creating a suction, and then the apparatus is gently withdrawn while rotating to get a sampling of the entire endometrium.

ATROPHIC ENDOMETRIUM: The most common cause of postmenopausal bleeding is friable tissue of the endometrium or vagina due to low estrogen levels.

ENDOMETRIAL STRIPE: Transvaginal sonographic assessment of the endometrial thickness; a thickness greater than 4 mm is abnormal in a postmenopausal woman.

TYPE I ENDOMETRIAL CANCER: This is the typical endometrioid cell type which is estrogen dependent, occurring in the perimenopausal or early menopause patient with the classic risk factors of unopposed estrogen. This type of cancer is typically lower grade and not as aggressive.

TYPE II ENDOMETRIAL CANCER: This is usually an aggressive disease with cell types of papillary serous or clear cell, and is estrogen independent (ER negative). These cancers involve late menopausal women, thin patients, or those with regular menses.

CLINICAL APPROACH

Postmenopausal bleeding always needs to be investigated because it can indicate malignant disorders or premalignant conditions, such as endometrial hyperplasia. Notably, complex hyperplasia with atypia is associated with endometrial carcinoma in 30% to 50% of cases.

The most common etiology of postmenopausal bleeding is **atrophic** endometritis or vaginitis. Vaginal spotting can occur in a patient taking hormonal therapy. However, since endometrial malignancy can coexist with atrophic changes or in women taking hormone-replacement therapy, **endometrial carcinoma must be ruled out in any patient with postmenopausal bleeding.** Possible methods for assessment of the endometrium include endometrial sampling, hysteroscopy, or transvaginal sonography.

Risk factors for endometrial cancer are listed in Table 57–1. They primarily include conditions of estrogen exposure without progesterone. Although endometrial cancer typically affects older women, a woman in her 30s with a history of chronic anovulation, such as polycystic ovarian syndrome, may be affected. For this reason, women over the age of 40 to 45 with abnormal uterine bleeding should have assessment for endometrial cancer, and those women less than

Table 57–1 • RISK FACTORS FOR ENDOMETRIAL CANCER
Early menarche
Late menopause
Obesity
Chronic anovulation
Estrogen-secreting ovarian tumors
Ingestion of unopposed estrogen
Hypertension
Diabetes mellitus
Personal or family history of breast or ovarian cancer or genetic cancer syndrome (Lynch syndrome)
Older age
History of infertility

age 40 to 45 with risk factors should also be considered for a diagnostic procedure. Endometrial hyperplasia especially with cellular atypia is strongly associated with the development of endometrial cancer.

When the endometrial sampling is unrevealing, the patient with persistent postmenopausal bleeding, or with numerous risk factors for endometrial cancer, should undergo further evaluation, such as by hysteroscopy. Direct visualization of the intrauterine cavity can identify small lesions that may be missed by the office endometrial sampling device. Additionally, endometrial polyps can be identified by hysteroscopy. More recently, saline infusion sonohysterography has been used to identify endometrial pathology such as polyps. These polyps still need surgical management since they could be malignant.

Endometrial Cancer

Endometrial carcinoma is the most common female genital tract malignancy. Although endometrial cancer is not the most common cause of postmenopausal bleeding, it is the one that is most concerning. Fortunately, because endometrial cancer is associated with an early symptom, abnormal uterine bleeding, it is usually detected at an early stage. Once diagnosed, endometrial cancer is staged surgically (Table 57–2). The subset of women who have grade 1 (well differentiated), endometriod carcinoma that is minimally invasive may not necessarily need lymph node sampling. Minimally invasive surgery has advantages particularly in obese patients, but power morcellation should not be used (see also Case 41 for FDA warning).

Sometimes endometrial cancer may occur in the atypical patient such as a **thin** patient; these cancers tend to be of the **Type II variety (clear cell and papillary serous type)** and more **aggressive and associated with extrauterine metastases**. In fact, clear cell carcinoma only accounts for 10% of uterine cancer but is associated with 40% of deaths. African-American women are more likely to have Type II disease. Also, those patients with uterine cancer with a thin endometrial stripe (<4 mm) postmenopausal bleeding are likely to have Type II cancer.

Women with Lynch syndrome are at increased risk of developing colon cancer, ovarian cancer, and Type I endometrial cancer. This is an autosomal dominant disorder and associated with mutations of one of the mismatch repair genes. The lifetime risk of developing endometrial cancer varies from 16% to 61% depending on the exact mutation.

Emerging Concepts

Young women with endometrial carcinoma may strongly desire to have a child. Although extensive data are lacking, patients are sometimes given high-dose progestins or less commonly the levonorgestrel intrauterine device (IUD) with

Table 57–2 • STAGING PROCEDURE FOR ENDOMETRIAL CANCER
Total hysterectomy, bilateral salpingo-oophorectomy
Omentectomy if papillary serous or clear cell pathology[a]
Lymph node sampling
Peritoneal washings

[a]Papillary serous or clear cell histology is associated with a worse prognosis and more aggressive spread.

frequent periodic endometrial sampling. Strict criteria are used in these settings: grade 1, no myometrial invasion, no extrauterine involvement, and strong desire for fertility sparing procedure. Most experts recommend definitive surgical management immediately after childbearing.

> **CASE CORRELATION**
> - See also Case 52 (Polycystic Ovarian Syndrome) which is a risk factor for endometrial cancer.

COMPREHENSION QUESTIONS

57.1 A 60-year-old woman presents to her physician's office with postmenopausal bleeding. She undergoes endometrial sampling, and is diagnosed with endometrial cancer. Which of the following is a risk factor for endometrial cancer?

A. Multiparity
B. Herpes simplex infection
C. Diabetes mellitus
D. Oral contraceptive use
E. Smoking

57.2 A 48-year-old healthy postmenopausal woman has a Pap smear performed, which reveals atypical glandular cells. She does not have a history of abnormal Pap smears. Which of the following is the best next step?

A. Repeat Pap smear in 3 months
B. Colposcopy, endocervical curettage, endometrial sampling
C. Hormone-replacement therapy
D. Vaginal sampling

57.3 A 57-year-old postmenopausal woman with hypertension, diabetes, and a history of polycystic ovarian syndrome complains of vaginal bleeding for 2 weeks. The endometrial sampling shows a few fragments of atrophic endometrium. Estrogen-replacement therapy is begun. The patient continues to have several episodes of vaginal bleeding 3 months later. Which of the following is the best next step?

A. Continued observation and reassurance
B. Unopposed estrogen-replacement therapy
C. Hysteroscopic examination
D. Endometrial ablation
E. Serum CA-125 testing

57.4 A 52-year-old woman, who has hypertension and diabetes, is diagnosed with endometrial cancer. Her diseases are well controlled. Her physician has diagnosed the condition as tentatively stage I disease (confined to the uterus). Which of the following is the most important therapeutic measure in the treatment of this patient?

A. Radiation therapy
B. Chemotherapy
C. Immunostimulation therapy
D. Progestin therapy
E. Surgical therapy

57.5 A 35-year-old woman is diagnosed with endometrial cancer. Which of the following is most likely to be present?

A. Ascites
B. BRCA-1 mutation
C. Galactorrhea
D. Pelvic irradiation
E. Polycystic ovarian syndrome

ANSWERS

57.1 **C.** Diabetes mellitus is associated with endometrial cancer. Other risk factors include advanced age, early menarche, late menopause, obesity, chronic anovulation, estrogen-secreting ovarian tumors, hypertension, family history, and, the biggest risk factor, ingestion of unopposed estrogen. Taking a combination oral contraceptive decreases the risk of endometrial cancer due to the progestin component in the pill that prevents the endometrium from becoming hyperprolific. Smoking is associated with a lower estrogenic state, which would, therefore, also decrease a patient's risk for endometrial cancer. But this poses a major public health risk, since smoking itself is associated with an overall increase in morbidity and mortality. Multiparity decreases the risk of endometrial cancer as well, and herpes simplex infection does not influence a patient's chance of acquiring endometrial cancer.

57.2 **B.** Atypical glandular cells on the Pap smear may indicate cervical, endometrial, or ovarian cancer. Therefore, a colposcopic examination of the cervix, curettage of the endocervix, and endometrial sampling are indicated. Because endometrial carcinoma is the most common female genital tract malignancy and is very treatable when detected at an early stage, the benefit of using multiple techniques to further examine the cervix and endometrium at a microscopic level should not be delayed. Delaying further investigation by repeating a Pap smear in 3 months may allow progression of any sort of malignancy the patient might have. An abnormal Pap smear is not very specific, so waiting to repeat the test and again obtaining abnormal results would still not specify whether or not the patient has cancer or another pathologic process. Vaginal sampling would not give us information as to the patient's likelihood of having an endometrial or cervical malignancy. In addition, vaginal cancer is not nearly as common as endometrial or cervical cancer and vaginal sampling would not be cost-effective if there are no symptoms associated with vaginal carcinoma. Hormone-replacement therapy (estrogen) would either worsen the situation if it were endometrial cancer. Unopposed estrogens increase the proliferation of endometrial cells and the likelihood of developing endometrial hyperplasia and eventually, endometrial carcinoma.

57.3 **C.** Persistent postmenopausal bleeding, especially in a woman with risk factors for endometrial cancer, must be evaluated. Hysteroscopy would be very cost-effective in this patient, who presents with persistent postmenopausal bleeding with many risk factors. Hysteroscopy is one of the best methods for assessing the uterine cavity since it allows for direct visualization and guided biopsy of the uterine cavity. Continued observation and reassurance would not be indicated since there is a high suspicion that this patient may be presenting with endometrial cancer. Any delay in treatment may allow progression of the cancer, making it more difficult to treat, and reassurance would be misleading. Unopposed estrogen-replacement therapy would not be indicated for this patient who already has so many risk factors and symptoms for endometrial cancer. Endometrial ablation may be beneficial in stopping bleeding in patients with menorrhagia who no longer wish to bear children, but it is not a method for diagnosing or treating endometrial carcinoma. Endometrial ablation in this patient would delay the diagnosis and treatment of endometrial cancer. The serum antigen CA-125 is not a specific cancer marker, and is mostly associated with epithelial tumors of the ovary.

57.4 **E. Surgery is a fundamental aspect of the treatment and staging of endometrial carcinoma.** Radiotherapy is used as an adjunctive treatment when the surgery performed for staging shows high suspicion of spread. Chemotherapy would be indicated if the surgery revealed metastasis. Progestin therapy is effective in shedding the endometrial lining, but not at inhibiting cellular proliferation or treating endometrial cancer.

57.5 **E.** Endometrial cancer usually affects postmenopausal women. Less commonly, women who are below 40 are affected, and almost always with a long history of anovulation (unopposed estrogen). Ascites typically is present with ovarian cancer and not as often with endometrial cancer. A BRCA-1 mutation usually presents with breast and ovarian cancer, and not endometrial cancer. Galactorrhea causes hypothalamic dysfunction and a hypoestrogenic state. Pelvic irradiation is associated with uterine sarcomas and not endometrial cancer.

CLINICAL PEARLS

▶ An endometrial assessment (sampling vs ultrasound) should be performed in a woman with postmenopausal bleeding to assess for endometrial carcinoma.

▶ Unopposed estrogen is generally the biggest risk factor for the development of endometrial cancer.

▶ Endometrial cancer is staged surgically, and surgery is a fundamental part of its treatment.

▶ Persistent postmenopausal bleeding warrants further investigation (such as hysteroscopy) even after a normal endometrial sampling.

▶ Endometrial cancer is usually discovered at an early stage due to an early symptom: abnormal uterine bleeding.

▶ Type II endometrial cancer, involving clear cell or papillary serous subtypes, occurs in an atypical patient without a history of anovulation; it tends to be more aggressive.

▶ Women with Lynch syndrome have a high risk of developing endometrial cancer.

REFERENCES

American College of Obstetricians and Gynecologists. Management of abnormal cervical cancer screening test results and cervical cancer precursors. *ACOG Practice Bulletin 140*. Washington, DC; 2013.

American College of Obstetricians and Gynecologists. Management of endometrial cancer. *ACOG Practice Bulletin 149*. Washington, DC; 2015.

American College of Obstetricians and Gynecologists. The role of transvaginal ultrasonography in the evaluation of postmenopausal bleeding. *ACOG Committee Opinion 440*. Washington, DC; 2009. (Reaffirmed 2013.)

Hacker NF. Uterine corpus cancer. In: Hacker NF, Moore JG, Gambone JC, eds. *Essentials of Obstetrics and Gynecology*. 6th ed. Philadelphia, PA: Saunders; 2015:428-434.

Lu K, Slomovitz BM. Neoplastic diseases of the uterus. In: Katz VL, Lentz GM, Lobo RA, Gersenson DM, eds. *Comprehensive Gynecology*. 6th ed. St. Louis, MO: Mosby-Year Book; 2012:813-839.

CASE 58

A 50-year-old G5P5 woman complains of postcoital spotting over the past 6 months. Most recently, she complains of a malodorous vaginal discharge. She states that she has had syphilis in the past. Her deliveries were all vaginal and uncomplicated. She has smoked 1 pack per day for 20 years. On examination, her blood pressure is 100/80 mm Hg, temperature is 99°F (37.2°C), and heart rate is 80 beats per minute. Her heart and lung examinations are within normal limits. The abdomen reveals no masses, ascites, or tenderness. Her back examination shows right costovertebral angle tenderness (CVAT). The pelvic examination reveals normal external female genitalia. The speculum examination reveals a 3-cm exophytic lesion on the anterior lip of the cervix. No other masses are palpated. Her right leg is more swollen than her left leg.

- What is your next step?
- What is the most likely diagnosis?
- What is the best treatment for this condition?

ANSWERS TO CASE 58:
Cervical Cancer

Summary: A 50-year-old G5P5 woman complains of a 6-month history of postcoital spotting and malodorous vaginal discharge. She has had a prior infection with syphilis, and is a smoker. The speculum examination reveals a 3-cm exophytic lesion on the anterior lip of the cervix. There is right CVAT and right leg swelling.

- **Next step:** Biopsy of the cervical lesion.
- **Most likely diagnosis:** Cervical cancer with metastases to the right pelvic sidewall.
- **Best treatment:** Radiotherapy with a chemosensitizer (such as a platinum agent).

ANALYSIS
Objectives

1. Understand that a cervical biopsy and not a Pap smear (which is a screening test) is the best diagnostic procedure when a cervical lesion is seen.
2. Know that postcoital spotting is a symptom of cervical cancer.
3. Know the risk factors for cervical cancer.
4. Know that radiotherapy is the best treatment for advanced cervical cancer.

Considerations

This 50-year-old woman presents with postcoital spotting. Abnormal vaginal bleeding is the most common presenting symptom of invasive cervical cancer, and in sexually active women, postcoital spotting is common. This patient's age is close to the mean age of presentation of cervical cancer, 51 years. She also complains of a malodorous vaginal discharge that is because of the large, necrotic tumor. Notably, the woman has right flank tenderness, which is very suspicious for metastatic obstruction of the ureter, leading to hydronephrosis; her leg swelling is also consistent with involvement with the pelvic sidewall. A cervical biopsy and not Pap smear is the best diagnostic test to evaluate a cervical mass. A Pap smear is a screening test and appropriate for a woman with a normal-appearing cervix. Risk factors for cervical cancer in this woman include multiparity, cigarette smoking, and history of a sexually transmitted disease (syphilis). Other risk factors not mentioned would be early age of coitus, multiple sexual partners, and human immunodeficiency virus (HIV) infection (Table 58–1).

Table 58-1 • RISK FACTORS FOR CERVICAL CANCER

Early age of coitus
Sexually transmitted diseases
Early childbearing
Low socioeconomic status
Human papillomavirus
HIV infection
Cigarette smoking
Multiple sexual partners

APPROACH TO:
Cervical Cancer

DEFINITIONS

CERVICAL INTRAEPITHELIAL NEOPLASIA (CIN): Preinvasive lesions of the cervix with abnormal cellular maturation, nuclear enlargement, and atypia.

HUMAN PAPILLOMAVIRUS (HPV): Circular, double-stranded DNA virus that can become incorporated into cervical squamous epithelium, predisposing the cells for dysplasia and/or cancer.

RADICAL HYSTERECTOMY: Removal of the uterus, cervix, and supportive ligaments such as the cardinal ligament, uterosacral ligament, and proximal vagina.

RADIATION BRACHYTHERAPY: Radioactive implants placed near the tumor bed.

RADIATION TELETHERAPY: External beam radiation where the target is at some distance from the radiation source.

HUMAN PAPILLOMAVIRUS VACCINE: Killed virus vaccine, FDA approved, for females and males aged 9 to 26. The quadrivalent vaccine contains antigens of HPV types 16 and 18 (which are associated with about 50% of cervical cancer and dysplasia in females) and 6 and 11 (which cause venereal warts in males and females).

CLINICAL APPROACH

Cervical Cancer

When a woman presents with postcoital spotting or has an abnormal Pap smear, cervical dysplasia or cancer should be suspected. An abnormal Pap smear is usually evaluated by colposcopy with biopsies, in which the cervix is soaked with 3% or 5% acetic acid solution. The colposcope is a binocular magnifying device that allows visual examination of the cervix. **The majority of cervical dysplasia and cancers arise near the squamocolumnar junction of the cervix.** Typically, cervical intraepithelial lesions will turn white with the addition of acetic acid, the so-called "acetowhite change." Along with the change in color, dysplastic lesions will often have vascular

Table 58–2 • STAGING PROCEDURE FOR CERVICAL CANCER
Examination under anesthesia
Intravenous pyelogram
Chest radiograph
Barium enema or proctoscopy
Cystoscopy

changes, reflecting the more rapidly growing process; in fact, the vascular pattern usually characterizes the severity of the disease. An example of mild vascular pattern is punctuations (vessels seen end-on) versus atypical vessels (such as corkscrew and hairpin vessels). A biopsy of the worst-appearing area should be taken during colposcopy for histologic diagnosis. Hence, the next step to evaluate an abnormal Pap smear is colposcopic examinations with directed biopsies.

When a woman presents with a cervical mass, biopsy of the mass, not a Pap smear, is appropriate. Because the Pap smear is a screening test, used for asymptomatic women, it is not the best test for a visible lesion. The Papanicolaou smear test has a false-negative rate and may give false reassurance.

When cervical cancer is diagnosed, the next step is staging the severity. Cervical cancer is staged clinically, meaning using physical examination, imaging tests, or nonsurgical procedures (Table 58–2). Early cervical cancer (generally less than 4 cm in diameter and contained within the cervix) may be treated equally well with surgery (radical hysterectomy) or radiation therapy. However, **advanced cervical cancer is best treated with radiotherapy, consisting of brachytherapy (implants) with teletherapy (whole pelvis radiation) along with chemotherapy, usually platinum-based (*cis*-platinum), to sensitize the tissue to the radiotherapy.**

Since HPV is the etiologic agent in the vast majority of cervical cancer, the advent of the HPV vaccine promises to prevent much of cervical dysplasia and cancer. At the time of this publication, the FDA has approved three HPV vaccines. The original quadrivalent vaccine Gardasil® (Merck) prevents infection of four strains of HPV (6, 11, 16, and 18) gained FDA approval in 2006 for use in males and females ages 9 to 26. In December 2014, the FDA approved Gardasil 9, which protects against the four strains in the previous Gardasil vaccine and also 31, 33, 45, 52, and 58. In 2009, GlaxoSmithKline's bivalent vaccine, Cervarix® protects against HPV strains 16 and 18, was approved for females aged 10 to 25.

HPV subtypes 6 and 11 cause the majority of condyloma acuminata (venereal warts), and more importantly **subtypes 16 and 18,** which cause 50% to 70% of cervical cancer. Clinical research seems to indicate a protection against the acquisition of HPV infection from these subtypes; however, because other subtypes can still cause cervical dysplasia or cancer, regular Pap smears are still required even after vaccination. Ideally, the vaccine should be administered at an age prior to sexual activity. Cervical cancer often spreads through the cardinal ligaments toward the pelvic sidewalls. It can obstruct one or both ureters leading to hydronephrosis. In fact, **bilateral ureteral obstruction leading to uremia is the most common cause of death due to this disease.**

Pap Smear and Cervical Cancer Prevention

The purpose of cervical cytology is to detect premalignant conditions, and intervene before it becomes invasive cancer. In general, abnormal Pap smears as a screening test require colposcopy and biopsy to determine the full extent of the dysplasia. Recently, the strategy of cervical cytology has undergone substantial changes due to the availability of HPV testing, and recognition that adolescents often clear the HPV and dysplasia spontaneously.

Cervical cytology is generally begun at age 21 years regardless of the age of onset of sexual intercourse (see Table 58-3). Pap smear every 2 years is then recommended up to age 30 years. For patients with three consecutive cervical cytology tests that are negative for intraepithelial lesions and malignancy at age 30, the interval of screening can be extended to every 3 years. Cotesting of HPV plus Pap smear is appropriate after age 30. If cervical cytology and HPV subtype testing are both negative, Pap smears do not need to be performed any sooner than every 3 years. Women with CIN risk factors, including HIV, immunosuppression, exposure to diethylstilbestrol (DES), and previous treatment for CIN 2, 3 or cancer may require more frequent screening. Screening can be stopped at age 65 to 70 after three negative cytology screening tests and no abnormal tests in the past 10 years. Finally, routine cervical cytology is not recommended in women who have had a total hysterectomy for benign indications, and no history of cervical dysplasia. However, **if hysterectomy is performed for cervical dysplasia (ie, CIN III), then Pap smear of the vaginal cuff is still needed.**

HPV typing is helpful in triaging cytology showing atypical squamous cells of undetermined significance (ASCUS), but is generally not helpful with any higher dysplasia. Thus, cytology showing low-grade squamous intraepithelial lesion or high-grade squamous intraepithelial lesion (HSIL) generally requires colposcopic examination. Adolescents and pregnant women with ASCUS may be observed instead of immediate colposcopy or even HPV testing. Women younger than age 25 with biopsy proven CIN 1 or 2 may be observed with serial Pap smears since the resolution rate is high, and excisional procedures on the cervix may lead to cervical insufficiency and preterm delivery.

Once colposcopic-directed biopsies have delineated the extent of the dysplasia, appropriate therapy may be used. This may include observation in younger patients and/or mild disease, cryotherapy (freezing of the cervix), or excisional procedures such as loop electrosurgical excision procedure for more significant dysplasia.

Atypical glandular cells (AGCs) are more rarely found on Pap smears, and can indicate squamous pathology, or also endometrial or endocervical disease. For this

Table 58-3 • SUMMARY OF CERVICAL CYTOLOGY SCREENING

- <21 years: No screening recommended
- 21-29 years: Cytology (Pap smear) alone every 3 years
- 30-65 years: Two options: Cytology with human papillomavirus (HPV) cotesting every 5 years (preferred) or cytology alone every 3 years (acceptable)
- 65+ years: No screening recommended if adequate prior screening has been negative and high risk is not present

reason, women with AGC Pap smears usually undergo colposcopy, endocervical curettage, and endometrial biopsy.

Emerging Concepts

Cervical cancer is typically treated with either radical hysterectomy if early (small tumor) invasive cancer is found or radiation therapy if advanced disease is found. However, in younger women who desire children, radical trachelectomy (removal of the cervix and upper vagina while leaving the uterus) can be performed. The surgeon places a purse-string suture at the uterine neck. This treatment attempts to remove the cervical cancer while allowing the patient to be able to achieve a pregnancy. Long-term results are pending for this rare procedure.

CASE CORRELATION

- See also Case 29 (Health Maintenance) for more details regarding cancer screening.

COMPREHENSION QUESTIONS

58.1 A 48-year-old woman who presents with postcoital vaginal bleeding is noted to have a cervical exophytic mass. A biopsy of the mass confirms squamous cell carcinoma. If molecular analysis of the cancer is performed, which of the following HPV subtypes is most likely to be found in the specimen?

A. 6 and 11
B. 16 and 18
C. 55 and 57
D. 89 and 92

58.2 A 39-year-old woman is diagnosed with advanced cervical cancer that appears to have spread to her right pelvic sidewall. She has right hydronephrosis as evidenced by the intravenous pyelogram (IVP). The biopsy specimen confirms that it is a poorly differentiated carcinoma. Which of the following statements regarding this patient's condition is most accurate?

A. The best therapy for her is surgical excision.
B. Both brachytherapy and teletherapy are important in the treatment of this patient.
C. Radical hysterectomy is an option in the therapy of this patient.
D. The majority of cervical cancers are of adenomatous cell type.

58.3 A 45-year-old woman is diagnosed with an early cervical cancer, noted to be confined to the cervix and about 3 cm in diameter. Which of the following is a risk factor for cervical cancer?

A. Early age of coitus
B. Nulliparity
C. Obesity
D. Late menopause
E. Family history of cervical cancer

58.4 A 33-year-old woman has a Pap smear showing moderately severe cervical dysplasia (high-grade squamous intraepithelial neoplasia). She denies a smoking history and does not recall having any sexually transmitted infections. Which of the following is the best next step?

A. Repeat Pap smear in 3 months
B. Conization of the cervix
C. Colposcopy-directed biopsies
D. Radical hysterectomy
E. Computed tomography scan of the abdomen and pelvis

58.5 A 40-year-old woman is referred for a Pap smear showing high-grade squamous intraepithelial lesions. Which of the following statements is most accurate?

A. If HPV subtyping reveals no high-risk virus present, then routine cytology is recommended.
B. If colposcopy demonstrates the entire transformation zone, then no further analysis is needed.
C. If an endocervical curetting shows cervical dysplasia, then an excisional procedure of the cervix is appropriate.
D. Cervical cancer is highly unlikely due to the Pap smear revealing only HSIL.

58.6 A 47-year-old woman G4P4 has a Pap smear which shows HSIL. Colposcopy is performed which is adequate, and reveals CIN III. An endocervical curettage is negative. The patient also has menorrhagia caused by uterine fibroids. Thus, the patient undergoes a total abdominal hysterectomy, including removal of the cervix. The patient asks whether Pap smears need to be performed now that her cervix has been surgically removed. Which of the following is the most accurate statement?

A. The patient should continue to have annual Pap smears of the vaginal cuff.
B. The patient should have Pap smears every 2 to 3 years, which may be discontinued if negative after 10 years.
C. The patient does not need Pap smears any longer.
D. The patient should have the HPV vaccine.

ANSWERS

58.1 **B.** HPV subtypes 6 and 11 are associated with condylomata acuminata (venereal warts), whereas subtypes 16 and 18 are associated with cervical dysplasia and cancer. The other answer choices are uncommon subtypes and not associated with cervical cancer. Cervical dysplasia or cancer should be suspected when a woman presents with postcoital spotting or an abnormal Pap smear.

58.2 **B.** For patients with advanced cervical cancer (such as this patient with extension to the pelvic side walls), radiotherapy is superior to surgical therapy. Major advantages of radical hysterectomy over radiotherapy are preservation of sexual function (owing to vaginal agglutination caused by the radioactive implants—essentially closes the vagina) and preservation of ovarian function. Radiotherapy can be performed on women who are poor operative candidates and is the best therapy for advanced disease, consisting of **brachytherapy and teletherapy**. Advanced disease involves spread to the pelvic sidewalls or hydronephrosis. Early-stage cervical cancer can be treated equally well with surgery or radiation therapy. The majority of cervical dysplasia and cancers arise near the squamocolumnar junction of the cervix and are of the squamous, not adenomatous, type.

58.3 **A.** Early age of coitus, a history of STDs, early childbearing, low socioeconomic status, HPV, HIV, cigarette smoking, and multiple sex partners are all risk factors for developing cervical cancer. HPV is the main risk factor, and is usually acquired from sexual exposure. Late menopause, obesity, and nulliparity are risk factors for endometrial cancer, not cervical cancer. Family history is not shown to be a risk factor for cervical cancer.

58.4 **C.** Colposcopic examination with directed biopsies is the next step to evaluate abnormal cytology on Pap smear.

58.5 **C.** When high-grade SIL is present, colposcopic examination is important. HPV typing has a role in triaging atypical cells of undetermined significance, but not HSIL. Demonstration of the entire transformation zone during colposcopy allows biopsy of the worst area. A cervical excisional procedure (loop electrosurgical excisional procedure) or cone biopsy is indicated when there is the possibility of endocervical disease.

58.6 **A.** When the patient has a history of cervical dysplasia, even after total hysterectomy (removal of uterine corpus and cervix), annual Pap smears should be performed of the vaginal cuff. This is because vaginal cancer may arise. In contrast, when total hysterectomy is performed for benign reasons, and no history of cervical dysplasia, then no further Pap smears need to be performed.

CLINICAL PEARLS

▶ The main risk factors for cervical cancer are sexually related, especially exposure to human papillomavirus.

▶ Human papillomavirus 16 and 18 are the most commonly isolated subtypes in cervical dysplasia and cancer.

▶ Flank tenderness or leg swelling indicate advanced cervical cancer, which is best treated by radiotherapy with a chemotherapeutic radiosensitizer.

▶ A visible lesion of the cervix should be evaluated by biopsy and not Pap smear.

▶ An abnormal Pap smear is usually evaluated with colposcopy-directed biopsies.

▶ The HPV vaccine is approved for females and males aged 9 to 26 to reduce the likelihood of cervical dysplasia or cancer in females, and venereal warts in males and females.

▶ Cervical cytology no longer needs to be performed after age 65 to 70 years, and after total hysterectomy for benign reasons and when there is no history of cervical dysplasia.

REFERENCES

American College of Obstetricians and Gynecologists. Cervical Cancer Screening and Prevention. *ACOG Practice Bulletin 157*. Washington, DC; 2016.

American College of Obstetricians and Gynecologists. Evaluation and management of abnormal cervical cytology and histology in the adolescent. *ACOG Committee Opinion 330*. Washington, DC; 2006.

American College of Obstetricians and Gynecologists. Human papillomavirus vaccination. *ACOG Committee Opinion 641*. Washington, DC; 2015.

American College of Obstetricians and Gynecologists. Management of abnormal cervical cancer screening test results and cervical cancer precursors. *ACOG Practice Bulletin 140*. Washington, DC; 2013.

Hacker NF. Cervical cancer. In: Berek JS, Hacker NF, eds. *Practical Gynecologic Oncology*. 6th ed. Philadelphia, PA: Lippincott Williams and Wilkins; 2014:345-406.

Hacker NF. Cervical dysplasia and cancer. In: Hacker NF, Gambone JC, Hobel CJ, eds. *Essentials of Obstetrics and Gynecology*. 6th ed. Philadelphia, PA: Saunders; 2015:402-411.

Jhingran A, Levenback C. Malignant diseases of the cervix. In: Katz VL, Lentz GM, Lobo RA, Gersenson DM, eds. *Comprehensive Gynecology*. 6th ed. St. Louis, MO: Mosby-Year Book; 2012:759-780.

Massad SL, Einstein MH, Huh WK et al for the 2012 ASCCP Consensus Guidelines Conference. 2012 Updated consensus guidelines for the management of abnormal cervical cancer screening tests and cancer precursors. *Obset Gynecol* 2013;121(4):829-46.

Noller KL. Intraepithelial neoplasia of the lower genital tract (cervix, vulva). In: Katz VL, Lentz GM, Lobo RA, Gersenson DM, eds. *Comprehensive Gynecology*. 6th ed. St. Louis, MO: Mosby-Year Book; 2012:743-754.

CASE 59

A 62-year-old parous woman complains of a 3-month history of weight loss, abdominal bloating, unable to eat much without "indigestion." She has no prior medical problems. On examination, her blood pressure is 110/60 mm Hg, heart rate is 80 beats per minute, and she is afebrile. She is alert and in no distress. Her heart and lung exams are normal. Her abdomen is moderately protuberant, and nontender and with normal bowel sounds. There is a fluid wave present. Based on the clinical findings, the physician suspects a gynecologic malignancy.

▶ What is the most likely diagnosis?
▶ What is likely to be best management of this patient?

ANSWERS TO CASE 59:
Ovarian Cancer (Epithelial)

Summary: A 62-year-old parous woman with no medical history has a 3-month history of weight loss, abdominal bloating, and early satiety. She has a protuberant abdomen and a fluid wave. A gynecologic malignancy is suspected.

- **Most likely diagnosis:** Epithelial ovarian cancer.
- **Management of this patient:** Surgical staging and ovarian cancer debulking, followed by combination chemotherapy.

ANALYSIS
Objectives

1. Know that epithelial ovarian cancer presents abdominal bloating and indigestion, and is associated with ascites.
2. Know that benign cystic teratomas (dermoid cysts) are the most common ovarian tumors in women younger than 30 years.
3. Know that surgical therapy and cancer debulking followed by combination chemotherapy is the treatment of choice for epithelial ovarian cancer.
4. Understand how to evaluate and manage adnexal masses in the various age groups.

Considerations

This 62-year-old woman has a 3-month history of weight loss, abdominal bloating, and indigestion. She is noted to have a protuberant abdomen which shows a fluid wave, which is most likely ascites. Based on the clinical presentation, the physician suspects a gynecologic malignancy. The presence of ascites would be consistent with epithelial ovarian cancer. The treatment of choice for epithelial ovarian cancer is surgical staging and debulking. Staging includes a total hysterectomy, bilateral salpingo-oophorectomy, omentectomy, lymph-node sampling, pelvic washings, and peritoneal biopsies. After maximal surgical debulking, the patient is usually treated with combination chemotherapy, such as with a paclitaxel and platinum combination. Endometrial cancer is the most common gynecologic malignancy, and usually presents with postmenopausal vaginal bleeding. Cervical cancer is the second most common gynecologic malignancy and classically presents with abnormal vaginal bleeding and/or a cervical mass. Ovarian cancer is the third most common malignancy but the leading cause of gynecologic cancer death, principally due to discovery at a late stage. Vulvar cancer presents with itching, and/or a labial ulcer or mass.

SECTION II: CASES   551

APPROACH TO:
Adnexal Masses and Ovarian Cancer

DEFINITIONS

CYSTIC TERATOMA (DERMOID CYST): A germ cell tumor that may contain all three germ cell layers. These are almost always benign (mature), although rarely they can be malignant (immature).

STRUMA OVARII: Benign cystic teratoma containing thyroid tissue, which can cause symptoms of hyperthyroidism.

OVARIAN NEOPLASM: An abnormal growth (either benign or malignant) of the ovary; most will not regress.

EPITHELIAL OVARIAN TUMOR: Neoplasm arising from the outer layer of the ovary, which can imitate the other epithelium of the gynecologic or urologic system. This is the most common type of ovarian malignancy, usually occurring in older women.

GERM CELL OVARIAN TUMOR: Neoplasm of the ovary derived from germ cells. This is the second most common type of ovarian neoplasm, occurring in young women.

SEX CORD-STROMAL TUMORS: Neoplasm of the ovary derived from the sex cords and supporting stroma of the ovary.

FUNCTIONAL OVARIAN CYST: Physiologic cysts of the ovary, which occur in reproductive-aged women, of follicular, corpus luteal, or theca lutein in origin.

CLINICAL APPROACH

Germ Cell Tumors

Germ cell tumors (Table 59–1) represent about one-quarter of all ovarian tumors, and are the second most frequent type of ovarian neoplasms. They are found mainly in young women, usually in the second and third decades of life. The most common germ cell tumor is the benign cystic teratoma (dermoid). A germ cell malignancy usually presents as a pelvic mass and causes pain due to its rapidly enlarging size. Because of these symptoms, 60% to 70% of patients present as stage I, limited to one or both ovaries.

Table 59–1 • GERM CELL CLASSIFICATION
Dysgerminoma
Endodermal sinus tumor
Embryonal carcinoma
Polyembryoma
Choriocarcinoma
Teratoma

Teratomas

Mature (benign) cystic teratomas constitute over 95% of all ovarian teratomas. They make up 15% to 25% of all ovarian tumors, especially in the second and third decades of life. Teratomas contain tissues of all three embryonic layers, including endoderm, mesoderm, and ectoderm. The most common elements are ectodermal derivatives such as skin, hair follicles, and sebaceous or sweat glands. Although most are unilateral, they can appear bilaterally 10% to 15% of the time. Ultrasound features of dermoid cysts include a hypoechoic area or echoic band-like strand in a hypoechoic medium or the appearance of a cystic structure with a fat fluid level. Ultrasound is generally very accurate in the diagnosis of dermoid cysts. Torsion is the most frequent complication, with severe acute abdominal pain as the typical presenting symptom. This is more commonly seen during pregnancy, the puerperium, and in children or younger patients. Rupture is an uncommon complication and may present as shock or hemorrhage. A chemical peritonitis can be caused by the spill of the contents of the tumor into the peritoneal cavity. The treatment is usually a cystectomy or unilateral oophorectomy with inspection of the contralateral ovary.

Immature (malignant) teratomas contain all three germ layers, as well as immature or embryonal structures. They are uncommon and comprise less than 1% of ovarian cancers. They occur primarily in the first and second decades of life and are rare after menopause. Malignant teratomas contain immature neural elements and that quantity alone determines the grade. They are almost always unilateral. The prognosis is directly related to the stage and the grade or degrees of cellular immaturity. The treatment is a unilateral salpingo-oophorectomy with excision or extensive sampling of peritoneal implants. If the primary tumor is grade 1, no further treatment is warranted. However, if the primary tumor is grade 2 or 3 and if there are implants or recurrences, combination chemotherapy is usually indicated.

Struma Ovarii

Struma ovarii is a teratoma in which thyroid tissue is a major or exclusive element. They are usually unilateral, occurring more frequently in the right adnexa, and generally measure less than 10 cm in diameter. Preoperative clinical or radiologic diagnosis is very difficult. On magnetic resonance imaging, these tumors appear as complex multilobulated masses with thick septa, thought to represent multiple large thyroid follicles. Most of these tumors are benign, but about 10% can have malignant changes. They will rarely produce sufficient thyroid hormone to induce hyperthyroidism, with less than 5% leading to thyrotoxicosis. The treatment is usually cystectomy or salpingo-oophorectomy.

Epithelial Tumors

Epithelial tumors (Table 59–2) represent about two-thirds of all ovarian tumors, and are the most frequent type of ovarian neoplasms, typically occurring in women over 30 years.

The **serous subtype** is **most common** and more often **bilateral**. **Mucinous** tumors are characterized by their large size, and if ruptured, may lead to pseudomyxomaperitonei, a condition in which the mucinous material spills out into the

Table 59–2 • EPITHELIAL OVARIAN TUMORS
Serous
Mucinous
Endometrioid
Brenner
Clear cell

intra-abdominal cavity. This can lead to repeat bouts of bowel obstruction. Endometrioid tumors of the ovary may coexist with a primary endometrial carcinoma of the uterus.

Epithelial Ovarian Cancer

Epithelial ovarian cancer is the most common cause of gynecologic cancer death and fifth most frequent cause of cancer death in women. Approximately 5% to 10% of cases are familial with first-degree relatives having ovarian cancer or ovarian–breast cancer; some of these involve the BRCA 1 or 2 mutation. Most patients have widespread metastasis at the time of diagnosis because of the early spread of the malignant cells to peritoneal and bowel surfaces. Gastrointestinal symptoms such as bloating, early satiety, increased abdominal girth, or abdominal pain are frequently ignored, but noted in retrospect.

The physical examination may show an abdominal or pelvic mass, ascites, or omental nodules. The tumor marker cancer antigen (CA)-125 is elevated in most epithelial ovarian tumors. CA-125 is more specific in postmenopausal women, since a variety of diseases during the reproductive years can elevate the CA-125 level. Imaging is important to characterize the pelvic mass. Malignant ascites is common with cancer, as it is spread to the small bowel, omentum, and lymphatics.

The treatment of epithelial tumors is surgical, and if malignancy is confirmed, cancer staging is indicated. Treatment of epithelial ovarian cancer involves a combination of surgical staging with maximum removal of the tumor (debulking) and combination chemotherapy especially with a platinum agent (cisplatinum or carboplatinum) and a taxane.

Sex Cord-Stromal Tumors

Sex cord-stromal (Table 59–3) represents approximately 6% of ovarian neoplasms and the majority of hormonally active neoplasms. Granulosa cell tumors contain functional granulosa cells which produce estrogen and supporting theca cells. Approximately 5% of these tumors occur before puberty and can lead to precocious puberty. Sertoli–Leydig tumors secrete androgens which can lead to

Table 59–3 • SEX CORD-STROMAL TUMORS
Granulosa cell
Sertoli–Leydig
Gynandroblastoma
Thecoma
Fibroma

masculinization and hirsutism. Sex cord-stromal tumors appear solid on ultrasound, with fibromas being the most common benign solid neoplasm of the ovary.

Adnexal Masses

The evaluation of adnexal masses is guided by the suspicion of neoplasm (benign or malignant). At the extremes of ages, there are few functional ovarian cysts and the management is straightforward (Table 59-4).

During the reproductive years, functional ovarian cysts, such as follicular and corpus luteal cysts, sometimes make the evaluation difficult. In general, any adnexal mass greater than 10 cm in size is likely to be a tumor and should be excised. Any adnexal mass less than 5 cm in size suggests a functional cyst. Between 5 and 10 cm, the sonographic features may help to distinguish functional versus neoplasm. Septations, solid components, or excrescences (growth on surface or inner lining) are consistent with a neoplastic process, whereas a simple cyst is more suggestive of a functional cyst. Sometimes, a practitioner will choose to observe and repeat imaging in an adnexal mass that is between 5 and 10 cm in size and operate if it is persistent.

Emerging Concepts

Over the past several years, the proposed etiology of several types of epithelial ovarian cancer (serous, endometrioid, clear cell) is speculated to arise from the fallopian tube, particularly the fimbriated end. These seem to be associated with high grade and undifferentiated malignancies. Many experts recommend salpingectomy at the time of hysterectomy as a means of reducing ovarian cancer risk. Regarding therapy, several randomized trials have shown increased survival with the combination of intraperitoneal and intravenous (IV) chemotherapy versus only IV chemotherapy for epithelial ovarian cancer. There seems to be more adverse complications with intraperitoneal chemotherapy.

Table 59-4 • EVALUATION OF ADNEXAL MASSES BASED ON AGE		
Age Group	Ovarian Size (cm)	Plan
Prepubertal	>2	Operate
Reproductive age	<5	Observe
	5-10	Sonogram; if septations, solid components or excrescences, then operate; otherwise observe for 1 month
	>10	Operate
Menopausal	>5	Operate

CASE CORRELATION

- See also Case 36 (Pelvic Inflammatory Disease), Case 40 (Uterine Fibroids), Case 53 (Sertoli–Leydig Cell Tumor of the Ovary), and Case 56 (Endometriosis) for a differential diagnosis of pelvic masses:
- Uterine fibroids—typically midline and irregular.
- Tubo-ovarian abscess—typically with some adnexal tenderness.
- Sertoli–Leydig cell tumor—usually androgen effects.
- Endometrioma—usually less than 8 cm, associated with dysmenorrhea and dyspareunia.

COMPREHENSION QUESTIONS

59.1 A 5-year-old girl is noted to have breast enlargement, vaginal bleeding, and an 8-cm pelvic mass. Which of the following is the most likely etiology?
   A. Benign cystic teratoma (dermoid)
   B. Endodermal sinus tumor
   C. Brenner tumor
   D. Choriocarcinoma
   E. Granulosa-theca cell tumor

59.2 A 25-year-old woman is noted to have a 4-cm simple cyst of the right ovary. She denies any abdominal pain, nausea, or vomiting. Which of the following is the next best step?
   A. Expectant management
   B. Laparoscopy
   C. Exploratory laparotomy
   D. Chemotherapy

59.3 Which of the following is the best treatment for a suspected dermoid cyst found in an 18-year-old nulliparous woman?
   A. Total abdominal hysterectomy
   B. Unilateral salpingo-oophorectomy
   C. Ovarian cystectomy
   D. Observation

Match the following sonographic findings (A-D) with the ovarian tumor type (59.4-59.6)?
   A. Completely solid
   B. Simple cyst
   C. Complex
   D. Ascites is commonly seen

59.4 Granulosa cell tumor

59.5 Benign cystic teratoma (dermoid cyst)

59.6 Follicular cyst

59.7 A 44-year-old woman is noted to have a 30-cm tumor of the ovary. Which of the following is the most likely cell type?
   A. Dermoid cyst
   B. Granulosa cell tumor
   C. Serous tumor
   D. Mucinous tumor

ANSWERS

59.1 **E.** This is a young child with precocious puberty, which suggests an estrogen-secreting tumor. This is most likely a granulosa-theca cell tumor, best treated by surgery. These are sex cord-stromal tumors.

59.2 **A.** When the ovarian cyst in the reproductive-aged female is less than 5 cm in diameter, the most likely cause is a physiologic cyst such as a follicular cyst or corpus luteum. Expectant management and reassessment in 1 to 3 months is the best next step.

59.3 **C.** Ovarian cystectomy is the best treatment for benign cystic teratomas in a younger patient especially when future childbearing is desired. Because of the 15% to 20% risk of bilaterality, the contralateral ovary should be inspected for a possible dermoid.

59.4 **A.** Granulosa cell tumors and Sertoli–Leydig cell tumors are usually solid on ultrasound, and may secrete sex hormones. Typically, granulosa-theca cell tumors produce estrogens, whereas Sertoli–Leydig cell tumors make androgens.

59.5 **C.** Benign cystic teratomas (dermoid cysts) are complex cysts since they usually have both solid and cystic components. The best treatment of a dermoid in a young woman is ovarian cystectomy. Ovarian torsion is the most frequent complication. Immature teratomas contain all three germ layers, as well as immature or embryonal structures. Malignant teratomas contain immature neural elements, and the grade of the tumor is determined by the amount of neural tissue involved.

59.6 **B.** Follicular cysts are generally simple cysts without septations or solid parts. They are among the physiologic cysts of the ovary, which occur in reproductive-aged women. Other physiologic, or functional, cysts include corpus luteal or theca lutein cysts.

59.7 **D.** Mucinous tumors of the ovary can grow to be very large. If they rupture intra-abdominally, they may cause pseudomyxomaperitonei, which leads to repeated bouts of bowel obstruction. They are of epithelial origin. The most common type of epithelial ovarian tumor is the serous type, which unlike the mucinous tumors, usually occurs bilaterally. The tumor marker CA-125 is elevated in most epithelial ovarian tumors and is more specific in postmenopausal women because a variety of diseases that occur during the reproductive years can show an elevated CA-125 level.

CLINICAL PEARLS

- The most common ovarian tumor in a woman younger than 30 years is a benign cystic teratoma (dermoid cyst). The best treatment of a dermoid in a young woman is ovarian cystectomy.
- The most common ovarian tumor in a woman older than 30 years is epithelial in origin, most commonly serous cystadenoma.
- An ovarian mass larger than 5 cm in a postmenopausal woman most likely represents an ovarian tumor and should generally be removed. An ovarian mass that is larger than 2 cm in a prepubertal girl likewise should be investigated and usually requires removal.
- During the reproductive years, functional ovarian cysts are common and are usually smaller than 5 cm in diameter. Any ovarian cyst larger than 10 cm in a reproductive-aged woman is probably a neoplasm and should be excised.
- The tumor marker CA-125 is elevated in most epithelial ovarian cancers. It is more specific in postmenopausal women.
- Mucinous tumors of the ovary can grow to be very large. If they rupture intra-abdominally, they may cause pseudomyxomaperitonei, which can lead to repeated bouts of bowel obstruction.
- Ascites is a common sign of ovarian malignancy.
- Ovarian cancer staging consists of total hysterectomy, bilateral salpingo-oophorectomy, omentectomy, peritoneal biopsies, peritoneal washings or sampling of ascitic fluid, and lymphadenectomy.
- After maximum debulking of the epithelial cancer, combination chemotherapy with a platinum agent and a taxane is used.

REFERENCES

American College of Obstetricians and Gynecologists. Management of adnexal masses. *ACOG Practice Bulletin 83*. Washington, DC; July 2007 (Reaffirmed 2015).

American College of Obstetricians and Gynecologists. Salpingectomy for Ovarian Cancer Prevention. *ACOG Committee Opinion 620*; Jan 2015.

Coleman RL, Gershenson DM. Neoplastic diseases of the ovary. In: Katz VL, Lentz GM, Lobo RA, Gersenson DM, eds. *Comprehensive Gynecology*. 6th ed. St. Louis, MO: Mosby-Year Book; 2012: 839-882.

Katz VL. Benign gynecologic lesions. In: Katz VL, Lentz GM, Lobo RA, Gersenson DM, eds. *Comprehensive Gynecology*. 6th ed. St. Louis, MO: Mosby-Year Book; 2012:419-471.

National Cancer Institute. Ovarian epithelial cancer treatment. http://www.cancer.gov/cancertopics/pdq/treatment/ovarianepithelial/HealthProfessional/page1; Accessed 1.10.2015.

Nelson AL, Gambone JC. Congenital anomalies and benign conditions of the ovaries and fallopian tubes. In: Hacker NF, Gambone JC, Hobel CJ, eds. *Essentials of Obstetrics and Gynecology*. 6th ed. Philadelphia, PA: Saunders; 2015:248-255.

Stany MP, Hamilton CA. Benign disorders of the ovary. *Obstet Gynecol Clin North Am*. 2008;35(2): 271-284.

CASE 60

A 51-year-old parous woman complains of a 4-year history of vaginal and vulvar itching. She scratches the area nearly every day and reports that the itching is worse at nighttime. She has diabetes, well controlled, is postmenopausal of 3 years, denies any sexually transmitted diseases or abnormal Pap smear history, and has four children delivered vaginally. Her blood pressure is 130/70 mm Hg and heart rate is 80 bpm. On inspection and examination of the external female genitalia, the following is revealed: atrophic-appearing external female genitalia, tissue over the labia minora is white and thin, the clitoris is hard to appreciate, excoriations are noted on bilateral labia majora, and some small bruising noted at the vaginal introitus. She is very tender on examination and speculum insertion is difficult, because the introitus is constricted. The cervix is visualized and no discharge is noted. Bimanual examination reveals a small uterus and no adnexal masses are appreciated.

- What is the most likely diagnosis?
- What is the next step in making the diagnosis?
- What is the most likely therapy?

ANSWERS TO CASE 60:
Lichen Sclerosis of Vulva

Summary: A 51-year-old woman is noted to have vaginal and vulvar itching for 4 years. Inspection of the external female genitalia reveals atrophic, white, thin excoriated tissue and retraction of the clitoris and constriction of the vaginal introitus with some bruising.

- **Most likely diagnosis:** Lichen sclerosis (LS).
- **Next step:** Biopsy of the affected areas.
- **Most likely therapy:** Corticosteroid ointment each evening.

ANALYSIS
Objectives

1. Describe the characteristics of patients that present with lichen sclerosis, and the natural history of the disease.
2. Recognize the anatomical boundaries of the vulva and aspects of good vulvar hygiene.
3. Identify current treatment regimes for lichen sclerosis and the follow-up that is requisite.
4. Describe some of the other common vulvar diseases and their treatment.

Considerations

This postmenopausal woman is suffering from lichen sclerosis given her history and physical finding. The diagnosis is confirmed with biopsy of the affected vulvar tissue, revealing a thinned epidermis, hyperkeratosis, and elongation of the rete pegs. Lichen planus can also present similarly, but usually involves the vagina which LS does not. An experienced dermatopathologist should be able to differentiate the two on biopsy specimen. Long-standing candidal infection of the vulva may lead to similar symptoms. Since our patient is postmenopausal, therefore lacking estrogen, the pH of the area is raised and not amenable to candidal infection unless she has poorly controlled diabetes or is immunosuppressed. Sometimes vaginal atrophy in the postmenopausal patient can lead to pruritus, but usually not to this extent. Psoriasis may present with pruritus but not usually, and the lesions are classically described as silver scales, and are also present on the extensor surfaces of the extremities. Cancer of the vulva or vulvar intraepithelial neoplasia commonly presents with pruritus and is often associated with LS, which is why biopsy of the affected area and frequent surveillance of the vulva is warranted.

APPROACH TO:
Vulvar Disorders

DEFINITIONS

LICHEN SCLEROSIS: Chronic, inflammatory dermatologic disease characterized by pruritus and pain, which mainly affects the anogenital region.

VULVA: The external genitalia of the female comprised of the mons pubis, the labia majora and minora, the clitoris, the vestibule of the vagina and its glands, and the opening of the urethra and of the vagina.

CLINICAL APPROACH

The anatomic boundaries of the vulva extend from the mons pubis superiorly to the anus inferiorly and the genitocrural folds laterally. It is made up of the labia majora and minora, mons pubis, clitoris, vestibule of the vagina, urethral meatus, Skene glands, vaginal orifice, hymen, and Bartholin glands.

Lichen Sclerosis

Lichen sclerosis is a chronic progressive inflammatory medical condition of which there is no definitive cure. LS is more common in women than men, and the onset can occur at any age, peaking in the prepubertal and postmenopausal period. LS usually presents in the anogenital region, with extragenital disease only 15% to 20% of the time. Women with the disease usually present with the complaint of itching which can be worse at night, and is described by the patient as vaginal itching. Appreciate that the itching is localized to the tissue of the vulva. **Differential diagnosis** of LS is **lichen planus, psoriasis, vulvar intraepithelial neoplasia, and vitiligo.** On examination of the external genitalia, a figure-eight pattern is seen around the vulva and anus. The skin is classically described as **"cigarette paper" as it appears crinkled and is fragile, thinned, and atrophic.** Abrasions may develop from scratching or attempted intercourse, and ultimately scarring may cause narrowing or a complete closure of the vaginal introitus, even in the parous woman. The labia minora may fuse burying the clitoris behind the fused clitoral hood. The scratching of the areas worsens the disease and can also lead to dyschezia, from constriction of the anus.

Counseling of the patient is important including discussing components of vulvar hygiene, avoiding irritants to the skin such as soaps and bubble baths, cessation of scratching the lesions, and wearing all cotton, white underwear. The patient should be made aware of the chronicity of the disease and the need for yearly surveillance. Treatment of the disease is aimed at preventing relapses of intense pruritus and the mainstay is corticosteroids. Initially, a potent steroid ointment, Clobetasol, may be necessary to provide relief, and should be used daily until symptoms abate and then tapered to intermittent use.

Bartholin Gland Abscess

The Bartholin or greater vestibular glands are located at the 5- and 7-o'clock locations of the labia majora. Usually, they are too small to palpate but with inflammation, they can be enlarged and painful. The treatment options include incision and placement of a small balloon catheter into the gland or marsupialization which is surgical fixation of the cyst wall everted against the mucosa of the vulva. The purpose of both of these techniques is to allow drainage of the infection for several weeks. **A simple incision and drainage is prone to recurrence.** Bartholin gland infections are usually **polymicrobial** and not usually sexually transmitted. Involvement in women over the age of 40 years can be associated with cancer and should have a biopsy.

Vulvar Cancer

Because vulvar cancer can present with no symptoms or with itching, any suspicious lesion of the vulva especially in a postmenopausal woman should undergo biopsy. Unfortunately, delay in diagnosis is usually the rule due to lack of clinical suspicion and prescription of various topical agents. Younger women such as those in their 30s may develop vulvar cancer due to human papillomavirus; smoking is also a risk factor. Again, biopsy is the rule. Regardless of the age, if vulvar cancer is diagnosed, then the patient should have surgical staging, with the primary lesion removed and the adjacent (ipsilateral) inguinal lymph nodes. Most vulvar cancers are squamous cell, but **melanoma**, basal cell carcinoma, and other subtypes can occur. Thus, pigmented lesions of the vulva should be carefully considered for biopsy.

> ### CASE CORRELATION
>
> - See also Case 39 (Syphilitic Chancre) as a differential diagnosis of vulvar lesions, and also Case 57 (Endometrial Cancer), Case 58 (Cervical Cancer), and Case 59 (Ovarian Cancer) to see the differences in risk factors, presentation, and treatment.

COMPREHENSION QUESTIONS

Match the vulvar lesion (A-E) to the clinical presentation (60.1-60.5).

A. Lichen sclerosis
B. Psoriasis
C. Vulvar cancer
D. Vulvar candidiasis
E. Postmenopausal vulvar atrophy

60.1 A 60-year-old postmenopausal woman is recently remarried and has pain with intercourse.

60.2 A 52-year-old postmenopausal woman complains of intense itching around her vagina and anus which makes intercourse and defecating painful.

60.3 A 45-year-old woman with poorly controlled diabetes reports that she has tears on her vagina causing pain with intercourse and defecation.

60.4 A 59-year-old postmenopausal woman presents with a 10-year history of vaginal itching, which she scratches frequently, and a bump near her clitoris.

60.5 A 54-year-old postmenopausal woman complains of itching in her vagina and, the physician notices scaly lesions on both of her elbows.

60.6 A 34-year-old G2P2 woman is noted to have a painful mass of the vulvar area at the 5:00 location. An incision and drainage procedure is performed. If culture is done, which of the following organisms is most likely to be found?
   A. *Treponema pallidum*
   B. *Neisseria gonorrhea*
   C. *Chlamydia trachomatis*
   D. *Haemophilus ducreyi*
   E. Peptostreptococci

60.7 A 56-year-old woman is seen for a 2-cm ulcerating lesion of the right labia majora that has been present for 5 months. You perform a punch biopsy of the lesion which reveals moderately differentiated squamous cell carcinoma. Which of the following is the most likely location of the metastasis?
   A. Left labia majora
   B. Uterosacral ligament
   C. Inguinal lymph nodes
   D. Pelvic lymph nodes
   E. Hypogastric arterial plexus

ANSWERS

60.1 **E.** Complaints of dyspareunia, or painful intercourse, are not uncommon in the postmenopausal state. In the first 5 years after menopause, atropic changes are not as common. This patient is 60 years old, and likely 10+ years postmenopausal. Without estrogen, the vaginal and vulvar tissue can atrophy leading to bruising, tearing, and even bleeding of the vulva vagina with intercourse. Topical estrogen can alleviate these symptoms. The vaginal and vulvar area should be inspected for lesions.

60.2 **A.** Pruritus of the vulva is not unique to lichen sclerosis, although the predilection for the vulva and anus is. Examination of the vulva and anus with indicated biopsies and topical steroid ointment is the treatment of choice.

60.3 **D.** Diabetes can lead to candidal infection of the vulva which can cause fissures in the labial folds, and the scratching of the disease can sometimes spread the infection. Women who present with vulvar candidiasis should be evaluated for diabetes.

60.4 **C.** Lichen sclerosis (LS) left untreated and with repeated scratching can predispose to carcinoma of the vulva. Nevertheless, this is fairly rare, since only about 5% of women with LS will ultimately develop vulvar cancer.

60.5 **B.** Psoriasis can affect the genital area, and the silver plaques on the elbow are a dead giveaway to the disease. Treatment of this disease may prove difficult, and consultation with an experienced dermatologist is requisite.

60.6 **E.** The most common bacteria found in a Bartholin gland abscess are polymicrobial such as skin organisms, Gram-negative rods, and anaerobes. It is rare to have STI-related organisms in these abscesses.

60.7 **C.** The most common location for spread of a squamous cell carcinoma of the labia majora is the ipsilateral inguinal lymph nodes. After spread to these nodes, the cancer may progress to the pelvic lymph nodes. A midline lesion may travel to bilateral inguinal nodes, but a lateral lesion will almost always be isolated to the ipsilateral nodes.

CLINICAL PEARLS

▶ Itching of the vulva, especially in a postmenopausal woman, should prompt a thorough history and examination with indicated biopsies of the affected areas.

▶ Lichen sclerosis is a chronic condition characterized by thin, cigarette paper-like, crinkly epithelium. Frequent surveillance of the vulva is necessary as to prevent squamous cell carcinoma of the vulva.

▶ Vulva cancer is staged surgically including dissecting the ipsilateral inguinal lymph nodes.

▶ Bartholin gland cysts are treated by Word catheter or marsupialization so that drainage for several weeks can occur. Simple incision and drainage is associated with a high rate of recurrence.

REFERENCES

American College of Obstetricians and Gynecologists. Diagnosis and management of vulvar skin disorders. *ACOG Practice Bulletin 93*. Washington, DC; 2008. (Reaffirmed 2013.)

Brown D. Non-neoplastic epithelial disorders of the skin and mucosa (vulvar dystrophies). In: Kaufman R, Faro S, Brown D, eds. *Benign Diseases of the Vulva and Vagina*. 5th ed. Philadelphia, PA: Elsevier; 2005:274-290.

FIGO Committee on Gynecologic Oncology. Revised FIGO staging for carcinoma of the vulva, cervix, and endometrium. *Int J Gynecol Obst*. 2012;119S2:S90-96.

Frumovitz M, Bodurka DC. Neoplastic diseases of the vulva. In: Katz VL, Lentz GM, Lobo RA, Gershenson DM, eds. *Comprehensive Gynecology*. 6th ed. St. Louis, MO: Mosby-Year Book; 2012:781-800.

SECTION III

Review Questions

SECTION III: REVIEW QUESTIONS   567

The following are strategically designed review questions to assess whether the student is able to integrate the information presented in the cases. The explanations to the answer choices describe the rationale, including which cases are relevant.

REVIEW QUESTIONS

R-1. A 5-year-old female child is brought into the physician's office for breast development and menses. On examination, the child is found to have Tanner IV breast development and Tanner IV pubic and axillary hair. Which of the following is the most likely therapy for this patient?
   A. Aromatase inhibitor
   B. Gonadotropin-releasing hormone (GnRH) agonist
   C. Oral contraceptive use
   D. Reassurance and expectant management
   E. Surgical therapy and removal of an ovarian tumor

R-2. A 32-year-old woman is noted to have 1200 cc of blood loss following a spontaneous vaginal delivery and delivery of the placenta. The uterine fundus is palpated and noted to be firm. Which of the following is the most likely treatment for this patient?
   A. Intramuscular prostaglandin
   B. Replacement of coagulation factors
   C. Replacement of inverted uterus
   D. Surgical repair via vaginal route

R-3. A 32-year-old woman comes into the office not having menstruated for 3 months. Her menarche occurred at age 11, and she had regular menses each month until 3 months ago. The patient's breasts are Tanner V, and she has normal Tanner V axillary and pubic hair. Her pregnancy test is negative. Which of the following mechanisms is most likely responsible for this patient's amenorrhea?
   A. False negative pregnancy test
   B. Gonadotropin-releasing hormone insufficiency
   C. Pituitary dysfunction
   D. Ovarian dysfunction
   E. Uterine anomaly

R-4. If the patient in R3 is prescribed and takes a 28-day package of combination oral contraceptive pills, which of the following is most likely to occur?
   A. The patient will have bleeding during the drug-free (placebo) phase (days 21-28).
   B. The patient will have no bleeding during any of the days of the pills.
   C. The patient will have bleeding during the first half the pills (days 1-14).
   D. The patient will have light bleeding throughout the pills.

R-5. A 23-year-old woman is noted to have 4 months of amenorrhea. Her pregnancy test is negative. Oral progestin is given for 7 days leading to vaginal bleeding after the progestin therapy. Which of the following is most likely to be found in this patient's examination prior to the progestin therapy?
   A. Gonadotropin levels elevated in the menopausal range
   B. Vaginal pH <4.5 range
   C. Ultrasound shows the endometrial stripe to be thin (<5 mm)
   D. Atrophy noted of the vulvar and vaginal epithelium

R-6. A 55-year-old woman is noted to have an abdominal mass and increased abdominal girth. On examination, there is shifting dullness and a fluid wave. Which of the following malignancies is most likely to be found in this patient?
   A. Colon cancer
   B. Endometrial cancer
   C. Cervical cancer
   D. Ovarian cancer
   E. Vulvar cancer

R-7. A 29-year-old G1P0 woman is noted to be at 39 weeks' gestation, and comes into the hospital complaining of significant shortness of breath. On examination, her heart rate (HR) is 120 bpm and respiratory rate is 32 and labored. Her O_2 saturation is 85% (normal 95%). The chest radiograph reveals bilateral pulmonary infiltrates and also an enlarged cardiac silhouette. Which of the following is the mechanism for this patient's symptoms?
   A. Decreased cardiac contractility
   B. Bronchospasm and reactive airway disease
   C. Capillary leakage and pulmonary injury, acute respiratory distress syndrome
   D. Inflammation, interstitial pneumonitis
   E. Hypercoagulable state

R-8. A 33-year-old G2P1 woman at 29 weeks' gestation is seen in the office for a prenatal visit. The fundal height is 35 cm and fetal parts are difficult to palpate. On ultrasound, there are two cystic structures noted in the fetal abdomen—one on the left side, and another cystic structure on the right side. Which of the following is most accurate regarding this pregnancy?

A. The fetus likely has a fetal kidney abnormality.
B. The fetus is at increased risk for leukemia.
C. The fetus likely has an elevated middle cerebral artery Doppler velocity.
D. The fetus likely has been infected with parvovirus.

R-9. A 19-year-old G1P0 woman at 7 weeks' gestation is seen in the emergency center for vaginal spotting. The patient is noted to have an ultrasound that reveals no gestational sac and no adnexal masses. Which of the following statements is most accurate regarding the management for this patient?

A. This patient should have a laparoscopy for probable ectopic pregnancy.
B. This patient should have a repeat human chorionic gonadotropin (hCG) level in 48 hours.
C. This patient should be offered methotrexate for ectopic pregnancy provided her vital signs are normal.
D. There is insufficient information to manage this patient at this time.

R-10. A 38-year-old woman is seen in the office desiring contraception. She has a 7-year history of chronic hypertension, which is controlled with sustained release nifedipine (Procardia). She smokes about a pack of cigarettes each day. She complains of dysmenorrhea and heavy menses with clots. Which of the following is the best contraceptive agent for this patient?

A. Copper intrauterine device (IUD)
B. Levonorgestrel IUD
C. Combination oral contraceptive agent
D. Condom (barrier method)

R-11. A 48-year-old woman has a 1-cm right breast mass noted on physical examination. Stereotactic biopsy reveals intraductal carcinoma. Which of the following would indicate a poor prognostic finding for this patient?

A. Her2/neu positive
B. Outer breast involvement
C. The patient is postmenopausal
D. Estrogen receptor positive

R-12. A 22-year-old nulliparous woman is seen by her gynecologist and given a routine Pap smear. The Pap smear revealed LSIL, and a colposcopy is performed. A biopsy at 3:00 shows CIN2. Which of the following is the best therapy for this patient?

A. Conization of the cervix with top hat to address any endocervical involvement
B. LEEP excision of the cervix
C. Offer hysterectomy
D. Repeat Pap smear in 6 months

R-13. A 28-year-old G2P1 woman at 34 weeks' gestation is noted to have chronic hypertension. Her weekly fetal assessment includes a nonstress test (NST), which shows a fetal heart rate of 140 bpm, and no accelerations, and no decelerations. What is the best next step for this patient?

A. Schedule for cesarean delivery immediately
B. Schedule for induction of labor in the next 24 hours
C. Repeat the NST in 1 week
D. Perform a biophysical profile

R-14. A 27-year-old G3P2 woman at 12 weeks' gestational age comes in for her first prenatal visit. On exam, her BP is 110/60 and urine dips 2+ glucose. The fetal heart tones are 150 bpm. Which of the following is the most likely explanation for the glucosuria?

A. The patient likely has gestational diabetes.
B. The patient likely has pregestational diabetes.
C. The patient likely has a degree of renal insufficiency.
D. The patient's increased glomerular filtration rate (GFR) is responsible for the finding.

R-15. A 34-year-old woman is hospitalized for presumed PID. On ultrasound, she is noted to have a 7-cm left adnexal mass. The patient is treated with intravenous antibiotics and on hospital day 2, the nurses call you due to the patient being confused and having tachycardia. On exam, the BP is 84/44 and HR is 130 bpm. Which of the following is the best therapy for this patient?

A. Interventional radiology to drain the ovarian cyst
B. Immediate surgery
C. Change the antibiotics due to probable medication adverse effect
D. Administer digoxin for probable atrial fibrillation

R-16. A 28-year-old patient sees you in the office and states that although born as a male, she identifies more as a woman. She has been using "street hormones" to have the appearance of a female. She says she has always thought of herself as a female even at a young age. Which of the following is the most likely diagnosis?

   A. Androgen insensitivity syndrome
   B. Cross-dressing
   C. Gender dysphoria
   D. Gender mutilation syndrome
   E. Intersex disorder

R-17. A 17-year-old G0P0 female complains of severe pain with her menses, and misses school for 4 days per month. Oral contraceptives and nonsteroidal anti-inflammatory drugs (NSAIDs) are prescribed and after 6 months, the pain is unchanged. Which of the following is the best next step?

   A. Continued expectant management
   B. GnRH agonist therapy
   C. Laparoscopy
   D. Opiate medication during menses
   E. Psychiatric referral

R-18. A 35-year-old G0P0 presents to her doctor for infertility. She also has heavy vaginal bleeding that persisted for 3 weeks. She has a long history of oligomenorrhea. An endometrial biopsy shows Grade 1 endometrial carcinoma. Which of the following is the best treatment for this patient?

   A. Clomiphene citrate
   B. Combination chemotherapy
   C. Progestin therapy
   D. Radiation therapy
   E. Surgical staging

ANSWERS

R-1. **B.** This child presents with precocious puberty, which is defined as secondary sexual characteristics prior to age 8. The most common cause is idiopathic, which means the hypothalamic GnRH pulse generator initiates too early. The diagnosis is of exclusion, and other causes must be ruled out including central nervous system (CNS) tumors, head trauma or CNS infections, ovarian or adrenal tumors. Idiopathic precocious puberty is treated with a GnRH agonist, which downregulates the hypothalamus and pituitary hormone secretion. With precocious puberty, it is important to assess whether it is purely female characteristics (estrogen) versus hirsutism (androgens).

It is important to remember that *the most common cause of precocious puberty is idiopathic*, but the most common cause of *delayed puberty* is a pathological cause such as gonadal dysgenesis.

Please also see Cases 54 (Delayed Puberty—Note Tanner I Breasts) and 55 (Primary Amenorrhea—Tanner IV Breasts).

R-2. D. The most common cause of postpartum hemorrhage overall is uterine atony, which is treated by uterotonic agents, and if unresponsive, then intrauterine balloon or surgical therapy. The most common cause of postpartum hemorrhage with a well-contracted uterus is a genital tract laceration, usually involving the cervix. Surgical therapy, usually involving suturing the defect, is the most appropriate treatment for lacerations. See Case 6 (Postpartum Hemorrhage) for more discussion on postpartum hemorrhage. The other common causes of PP hemorrhage include retained products of conception, placenta accreta (Case 12), and inverted uterus (Case 3).

R-3. B. When a patient has **regular** menses and has an isolated amenorrhea, the most common cause is hypothalamic dysfunction, causing GnRH inhibition. Causes include hypothyroidism, hyperprolactinemia, excessive exercise, malnutrition from an eating disorder, stress, and some drugs. The evaluation of secondary amenorrhea (no menses for 3 months in a woman who has previously had menses) includes: (a) pregnancy test, (b) thyroid-stimulating hormone, and (c) prolactin level. If these are normal, then the next step is typically to assess luteinizing hormone and follicle-stimulating hormone and administer progestin to see if the outflow tract (uterus) responds normally and has sufficient estrogen to have caused proliferation of the endometrium (see Cases 49-51; Case 49 contains a diagnostic algorithm). Bleeding after progestin alone indicates anovulation, typically caused by polycystic ovary syndrome (PCOS) (see Case 52).

R-4. A. Because the patient in R-3 most likely has a hypothalamic dysfunction as discussed, she is in a hypoestrogenic state. Hence, progestin alone will not lead to bleeding because there is no endometrium to shed. However, because she has a normal outflow tract (uterus), she should respond normally to the oral contraceptive agent and bleed normally during the drug-free days (days 21-28). In other words, because the combination OC contains both estrogen and progestin, this regimen will stimulate growth of the endometrium, and the progestin withdrawal during the drug-free pills will lead to bleeding. A patient with intrauterine adhesions (see Case 49) will not have bleeding after the combination OCP.

R-5. B. This patient has bleeding following progestin therapy indicative of anovulation, and indicative of the presence of sufficient estrogen to have caused endometrial growth. The presence of estrogen causes a normal endometrial stripe (6-12 mm), normal rugae, and growth of the vulvar and vaginal epithelium. The normal estrogen environment also promotes *Lactobacilli* growth, which lowers the vaginal pH to <4.5. This patient likely has PCOS with anovulation and estrogen excess. In contrast, the postmenopausal hypoestrogenic state is associated with an elevated vaginal pH > 4.5 and a thin and atropic vulvar and vaginal epithelium (see Cases 49-51).

R-6. **D.** Ovarian cancer is associated with a pelvic mass and ascites. The majority occurs in older (postmenopausal) women, and the majority are epithelial in nature. Symptoms of epithelial carcinoma are subtle including early satiety, bloating, and increased abdominal girth. The cancer cells spread early to the peritoneal cavity, the bowel, and the omentum. The peritoneal seeding incites ascites. The most common way that ovarian cancer kills women is by cachexia (starvation) as a result of widespread small bowel metastasis. The most common way that cervical cancer kills is by bilateral ureteral metastases, leading to uremia (see Case 59, Ovarian Cancer (Epithelial)).

R-7. **A.** A dilated cardiac silhouette is highly suggestive of a cardiomyopathy, and when it occurs in pregnancy, it is commonly due to peripartum cardiomyopathy. The etiology of peripartum cardiomyopathy is unknown, but it is a four-chamber dilated cardiomyopathy and thus has a negative effect on cardiac contractility. Treatment is diuretics, digoxin, and afterload reduction. The majority of patients will improve and the cardiac output normalizes, but there is a significant recurrence of the cardiomyopathy with future pregnancies.

R-8. **B.** This patient has hydramnios (also known as polyhydramnios). The combination of size greater than dates, and fetal parts being difficult to palpate indicates hydramnios. Hydramnios may be caused by fetal intestinal abnormalities because the baby eliminates amniotic fluid by swallowing. The ultrasound showing cystic areas in both the right and the left abdomen is consistent with duodenal atresia, which is a sonographic finding oftentimes referred to as the "double bubble sign." Duodenal atresia is associated with Down syndrome, and children with Down syndrome are at risk for leukemia. Fetal kidney anomalies are associated with oligohydramnios because fetal urine is the main component of amniotic fluid. Increased middle cerebral artery flow is associated with fetal anemia, which should not occur with this situation (see Case 19, Parvovirus Infection in Pregnancy).

R-9. **D.** This is an important question to assess whether the student has a clear understanding of the role of the hCG and vaginal ultrasound in assessing early pregnancy bleeding. A patient with a threatened abortion in the first trimester will have one of three possible causes: (a) a normal intrauterine pregnancy and the bleeding will stop (about 50% of cases), (b) an abnormal intrauterine pregnancy or miscarriage (about 40% of cases), or (c) an ectopic pregnancy (about 10% of cases). The scenario notes the transvaginal ultrasound results, but does not give the hCG level to be able to interpret the ultrasound findings. For instance, if the hCG level is below the "discriminatory zone" of 1200 to 1500 mIU/mL (see Cases 42-43), then in a stable patient, a follow-up hCG in 48 hours is the appropriate next step. If instead the hCG level is above the threshold (Case 43), then the next step is laparoscopy because the risk of ectopic pregnancy is high.

R-10.   B. This patient is over the age of 35 and a heavy smoker (>15 cigarettes/d), and thus the oral contraceptive and any estrogen containing contraceptive agent is contraindicated. The presence of dysmenorrhea and menorrhagia would be made worse with the copper IUD, which causes inflammation. Condoms (barrier method) is acceptable but has a higher failure rate. The levonorgestrel IUD would be ideal in this patient because there would not be an increased risk of thrombosis, and the progestin would thin the endometrium and decrease the menstrual blood flow (see Case 44, Contraception).

R-11.   A. Breast cancer that is her2/neu positive tends to be more aggressive. Estrogen receptor (ER) and progesterone (PR) receptor positive tumors tend to be less aggressive and respond to hormonal therapy. Breast cancers that are ER, PR, and her2/neu negative (so-called triple negative) have a poor prognosis (see Cases 46-48). A majority of breast cancers are located in the upper/outer quadrant of the breast; however, this does not affect prognosis.

R-12.   D. The trend recently is to be less aggressive with cervical dysplasia in younger patients less than age 25. Women less than age 25 with CIN2 have been observed to clear the cervical intraepithelial neoplasia 70% to 80% of the time, and thus observation with surveillance Pap smears is a reasonable management approach. Also for younger women, the treatment such as LEEP excisions of the cervix can lead to preterm labor or cervical insufficiency (see Case 58, Cervical Cancer).

R-13.   D. The nonstress test is a good test for assurance of fetal well-being when it is reactive with accelerations present. However, the NST is not reliable when there is an absence of accelerations and decelerations, so-called nonreactive. More than half of the time, the fetal status is normal with a nonreactive NST. Thus, another fetal test such as biophysical profile should be used to further assess fetal well-being. NST and BPP are both tests of fetal well-being and used in settings when there is an increased risk of stillbirth (see also Cases 14 and 22 for fetal testing).

R-14.   D. Glucose in the urine is a common finding due to the 50% increase in GFR and increased glucose to the renal tubules, which is greater than the resorption capability. Whereas glycosuria may be a finding of diabetes mellitus in a nonpregnant individual, it is not indicative of diabetes in pregnancy. The next step in this patient is either fingerstick glucose to assess glucose level, or screening test for diabetes (see Case 28, Prenatal Care).

R-15.   B. This patient likely has a tubo-ovarian abscess, a complication of PID. The patient is treated with intravenous (IV) antibiotics which is the appropriate therapy. There is no description of the type of antibiotics, but anaerobic coverage is important. This patient develops a shock-like picture with confusion, hypotension, and tachycardia which is likely due to rupture of the TOA. Immediate surgical management is important in this setting, due to high mortality without prompt treatment. IV antibiotic therapy successfully treats the majority of patients with a TOA (see Case 36, Salpingitis, Acute).

Table R–1 • GENDER DISORDERS	
Term	Description
Gender dysphoria	Internal conflict between a personal's physical gender and the gender he or she identifies with; usually originates as a child. The term "Gender Identity Disorder" is now considered outdated.
Transgender	An umbrella term for people whose gender identity and/or gender expression differs from what is typically associated with the sex they were assigned at birth.
Cross-dresser	Wearing the clothes of the opposite gender, as a form of gender expression. Cross-dressers do not wish to permanently change their sex or live full time as the opposite gender.
Transition	The process of changing from one physical gender to the preferred gender, and includes changing one's preferred name/nickname, dressing differently, hormonal therapy, and sometimes surgery. (Previously referred as undesirable term "sex change.")
Intersex condition	A variation of sex characteristics including chromosomes, gonads, or genitalia that do not allow an individual to be distinctly identified as male or female. This can include genital ambiguity or discordant genotype/phenotype (example: other than XY male or XX female).

R16. **C.** This patient describes findings consistent with gender dysphoria, in which an individual identifies with the opposite gender from their chromosomal (anatomical) gender, and does not have intersex disorder, such as ambiguous genitalia due to 21 hydroxylase deficiency or true hermaphroditism. Typically, the gender identification occurs at a young age, and DSM V criteria indicate that this occurs prior to puberty. Cross-dressing is not the same as gender dysphoria in that these individuals are aware of their chromosomal gender and do not necessarily desire to be the opposite gender. This topic is not currently covered in case files, but has emerged as an important area within our specialty (see Table R-1).

R-17. **C.** In an adolescent with dysmenorrhea, the most likely etiology is primary dysmenorrhea with the etiology is elevated prostaglandin F2-alpha in the endometrium and myometrium leading to intense uterine contractions. The best treatment is NSAIDs, which is typically very helpful. Oral contraceptive agents, particularly used continuously, also offer relief. When an adequate trial of NSAID and oral contraceptive therapy is unhelpful, a large fraction of these adolescents will have endometriosis. Laparoscopy is the appropriate procedure for diagnosis. GnRH agonist therapy should not be used "blindly" due to the side effects and also the importance of establishing a diagnosis (see Case 37, Chronic Pelvic Pain).

R-18. **C.** In a patient who strongly desires child-bearing and has a low grade (Grade 1), minimally invasive cancer, high-dose progestin therapy followed by frequent endometrial sampling is possible. After child-bearing is complete, definitive surgical staging should be undertaken (see Case 57, Postmenopausal Bleeding).

INDEX

Page numbers followed by *f* or *t* represent figures or tables, respectively.

A

Abdominal examination, 6
Abdominal pain
  ectopic pregnancy, 139
  in pregnancy
    analysis, 136
    appendicitis, 138
    cholecystitis, 138
    clinical approach, 137–139
    differential diagnosis, 137t
    ovarian torsion, 136, 138
    placental abruption, 138–139
    ruptured corpus luteum, 139
Abnormally retained placenta, 53
Abnormal mammogram
  analysis, 460
  breast implants and, 461
  clinical approach, 461–462
  clinical pearls, 464
  definitions, 460
Abortion. *See also* Spontaneous abortion; Threatened abortion
  completed, 406
  history of, 3
  incomplete, 406, 407
  inevitable, 406
  missed, 406, 407
  septic. *See* Septic abortion
Abruptio placentae
  abdominal pain, 138–139
  analysis, 120
  clinical approach, 121–122
  clinical pearls, 125
  clinical presentation, 119–120
  definitions, 121
  differential diagnosis, 137t
  risk factors for, 121t
Abscesses
  Bartholin gland, 109
  tubo-ovarian, 16
Absent end-diastolic flow, 228
Acanthosis, 498
Acanthosis nigricans, 491
Accelerations, heart rate, 23
Acetowhite change, 541
Acquaintance rape, 307
Active phase, labor
  arrest of, 23, 24
  defined, 23
  stages of, 23
Acute chest syndrome, 48, 49
Acute fatty liver of pregnancy (AFLP), 148
Acute management of severe hypertension, 170
Acute pelvic pain, 363
Acute respiratory distress syndrome, 237
  pathophysiology, 236
  treatment, 236–237
Acyclovir, for herpes simplex virus, 106–107, 109
Adnexal mass, 500
  evaluation of, 554, 554t
Advanced maternal age, 280
AFP (α-Fetoprotein), 87–88
Age, in patient history, 3
Allergies, in patient history, 5
α-Fetoprotein (AFP), 87–88

Altered mental status, 220
Amenorrhea (intrauterine adhesions)
　analysis, 466–467
　clinical approach, 468–469
　clinical pearls, 472
　definitions, 467–468
Amenorrhea (Sheehan syndrome), 484t
　analysis, 482–483
　clinical pearls, 487
　definitions, 483
　distinguishing between Asherman syndrome, 484t
　treatment, 484
Amniocentesis, 92, 230
Amnioinfusion, 38
Amnionicity, 97, 98t
Amniotic fluid embolism (AFE), 158
Androgen insensitivity, 513–514, 513t
Androgen-secreting tumors, 498
Anemia
　defined, 43
　hemolytic, 43
　iron deficiency, 43, 48
　macrocytic, 44, 47
　megaloblastic, 48
　microcytic, 47
　in pregnancy, 42–49
　　analysis, 42
　　clinical approach, 43–45
　　clinical pearls, 48–49
　　hemoglobinopathies, 43–44
　　physiology of pregnancy, 43
Anion gap, 265
Anovulation, 498
Antenatal steroids, 181, 182
Antenatal testing, 280
Antepartum hemorrhage, 114
Antepartum vaginal bleeding. *See also* Abruptio placentae; Placenta previa
　analysis, 112
　clinical approach, 114–115
　clinical pearls, 117
　clinical presentation, 111–112
　definitions, 113–114
Anthropoid pelvis, 37
Anticoagulation therapy, 139
Appendicitis, 137t, 138
Arrest, active phase of labor, 23, 24
Artificial rupture of membranes, 69
ASB. *See* Asymptomatic bacteriuria (ASB)
Ascending infection, 351
Asherman syndrome, 468–469, 483, 484t
Aspirin, 173
Assisted reproductive technology, 520, 523–525
Asymmetric IUGR, 227–228
Asymptomatic bacteriuria (ASB), 238, 280
Atrophic endometrium, 532
Atropine, 73
Atypical squamous cells of undetermined significance (ASCUS), 543
Autosomal recessive disorders, 47

B

Back and spine examination, 6
Bacterial vaginosis (BV). *See also* Vaginal infections
　Amsel's criteria, 371
　analysis, 370
　causes of infectious vaginal discharge, 370
　clinical approach, 371
　clinical pearls, 375
　definitions, 370
　substaging, 12
　treatment, 371
Bacteriuria, 389
Barker hypothesis, 228

Barrier contraceptives, 425–426
Bartholin gland abscess, 109, 561–562
Basal body temperature chart, 522f
Basic obstetrical ultrasound, 280
Behcet disease, 379
β-Agonist, 69
β-Thalassemia, 43–44
Biliary colic, 138
Bilobed placenta, 97
Bimanual pelvic examination, 6–7, 7f
Biophysical profile (BPP), 149t
Bladder neck sling, 340–341
Bleeding
    antepartum vaginal. See also Abruptio placentae; Placenta previa
        analysis, 112
        clinical approach, 114–115
        clinical pearls, 117
        clinical presentation, 111–112
        definitions, 113–114
        placenta previa, 111–112
    postmenopausal vaginal
        analysis, 530
        clinical approach, 532–534
        clinical pearls, 537
        definitions, 531–532
    postpartum hemorrhage. See Postpartum hemorrhage (PPH)
        analysis, 76
        clinical approach, 77–79
        clinical pearls, 82
        clinical presentation, 76
        definitions, 77
        treatment for, 78t
Bloody show, 37
Body mass index (BMI), 491
Bone mineral density (BMD) testing, 300
BRCA gene mutations, 453–455, 461, 537, 553
BRCA testing, 446, 454, 454t

Breast
    abscess, 256
    examination, 6
    infections
        clinical approach, 257
        clinical pearls, 260
        definitions, 256–257
        galactocele, 257
        postpartum mastitis, 256–257
    mammogram, abnormal
        analysis, 460
        clinical approach, 461–462
        clinical pearls, 464
        definitions, 460
    masses
        BRCA testing, 446, 454, 454t
        clinical approach, 445–446, 453–455
        clinical pearls, 448
        definitions, 445, 453
        dominant, 445, 452–453
        fibroadenoma, 445–446
Breast cancer
    biopsy of, 454, 462
    diagnosis, 453
        screening tests, 453–454, 455t
    inflammatory, 453
    mammogram, 452, 454, 461f. See also abnormal mammogram
    risk factor, 453
Breast-feeding, benefits of, 258, 271
BV. See Bacterial vaginosis (BV)

C
Cancer
    breast
        biopsy of, 454, 462
        diagnosis, 453–454, 455t
        inflammatory, 453
        mammogram, 452, 454, 461f
        risk factor, 453

Cancer (*Cont.*):
  cervical
    analysis, 540
    cervical cytology screening, 543, 543t
    clinical approach, 541–544
    definitions, 541
    prevention, 543–544
    risk factors, 540–541t
    staging procedure, 542t
    treatment, 542, 544
  endometrial, 533
    clinical pearls, 537
    diagnosis and sampling, 536
    risk factors for, 532, 532t
    staging procedure for, 533t
    treatment, 536
    type I and II, 532–533
  inflammatory breast, 453
  ovarian cancer (epithelial), 553
    analysis, 550
    clinical approach, 551–555
    clinical pearls, 557
    definitions, 551
  vulvar, 562
Cancer antigen (CA)-119, 553
Candida vulvovaginitis, 371. *See also* vaginal infections
Candidiasis, 373
Cardiac arrhythmia, 220
Cardiac examination, 6
Cardinal ligament, 319
Carneous degeneration, 395
CBC (complete blood count), 8
Cell-free fetal DNA (cfDNA), 89–90
Cephalopelvic disproportion, 24
Cervical cancer
  analysis, 540
  cervical cytology screening, 543, 543t
  clinical approach, 541–544
  definitions, 541
  prevention, 543–544
  risk factors, 540–541t
  staging procedure, 542t
  treatment, 542, 544
Cervical cap, 426
Cervical cytology screening, 543, 543t
Cervical dysplasia, 541
Cervical factor, 525
Cervical intraepithelial lesions, 541
Cervical intraepithelial neoplasia (CIN), 541
Cervical length assessment, 181
Cervical motion tenderness, 351
Cervicitis
  chlamydial. *See* Chlamydia trachomatis
  gonococcal. *See* Gonorrhea
  mucopurulent, 351
Cesarean delivery
  herpes simplex virus, 108
  placenta previa, 116
  primary, safe prevention of, 30
cfDNA (cell-free fetal DNA), 89–90
Chancre, syphilitic. *See* Syphilis
Chancroid, 109, 381–382
Chief complaint, 4
Child sexual abuse, 307
Chlamydial conjunctivitis, 209
Chlamydial neonate infection, 209
Chlamydia trachomatis
  analysis, 208
  antiviral therapy, 211
  clinical approach, 209
  clinical pearls, 214
Cholecystitis, 137t, 138
Chorioamnionitis. *See* Intra-amniotic infection
Chorionicity, 97, 98t
Chronic hypertension, 167, 169
Chronic pelvic pain
  analysis, 362–363

appropriate consultation for, 365
character of the pain in, 363–364
clinical approach, 363–366
clinical pearls, 367
definitions, 363
gynecologic causes of, 364t
laboratories and imaging studies, 365
nongynecologic causes of, 365t
pain persisting without identifiable cause, 365–366
patient examination in, 364–365
psychological or psychosocial reasons for, 364
Chronic pelvic pain syndrome, 363
Cigarette paper, 561
Cleft palate/lip, 92
Clinical problem solving
approach to, 11–13
reading, 13–18
Clomiphene, 98
Clomiphene citrate, 500
Coagulopathy, 78, 121
consumptive, 124
Cocaine, 125
Complete blood count (CBC), 8
Complete placenta previa, 113f
Complications, of disease, 16–17
Comprehensive (targeted) ultrasound, 280
Computed tomography (CT), 10
Concealed abruption, 121. See also Abruptio placentae
Condoms, 426
Congenital adrenal hyperplasia (CAH), 498, 500
Congenital infections, 201
Consumptive coagulopathy, 124
Contraception. See also Oral contraceptive (OCP)
agents, 427t–429t
analysis, 424–425
barrier contraceptives, 426
clinical approach, 425–433
clinical pearls, 435
condoms, 426
contraceptive patch, 430
contraceptive ring, 430
contraindications to, 424
definitions, 425
emergency, 431, 432t
failure rates, 426t
injectable contraceptive, 430
levonorgestrel-releasing intrauterine device (LNG-IUD), 424–425, 431
main risks of combined hormonal, 430
oral, 430, 492, 500
spermicides, 430
subdermal implant, 430
usage, history of, 4
Contraction, uterine, 22, 24. See also Labor
Contraction stress test, 149t
Copper IUD, 433
Copper T380A, 431
Cord prolapse, 68–70, 70f
Core needle biopsy, 445
Corticosteroids, 101
Cost-effectiveness, 291
Couvelaire uterus, 121
Cryopreservation, 525
CT (computed tomography), 10
Cultures, herpes, 105
Cushing disease, 498
Cushing syndrome, 500, 506
Cystectomy, 552
Cystic teratoma (dermoid cyst), 551
Cystitis, 12, 389. See also Urinary tract infection
Cystocele, 327, 328f, 340

Cystometric evaluation
  (urodynamics), 342
Cystoscopy, 319
Cytomegalovirus (CMV), 201

D
Date rape, 307
Dating error, 228
Decelerations, heart rate, 23, 27–29f
  prolonged, interventions for, 31t
Deep incision, 335
Deep venous thrombosis, 155
Dehydroepiandrosterone sulfate
  (DHEA-S), 490, 491
Delayed puberty. *See* Pubertal delay
Depot medroxyprogesterone acetate
  (DMPA), 424
Dermoid cysts, 136, 500
Diabetes in pregnancy, 264. *See also*
  gestational diabetes;
  pregestational diabetes
  analysis, 264–265
  clinical pearls, 274
  definitions, 265–266
Diabetes mellitus, 535
Diabetic ketoacidosis (DKA), 264,
  265
  diagnostic difficulties, 264
  FHR pattern, 265
  management of, 265
  in pregnancy, 265
    diagnostic criteria, 266t, 268
    electrolyte replacement in, 269
    fetal heart rate pattern, 270
    insulin therapy, 269
    management, 269
    maternal and neonatal
      complications of, 266t
    physiological factors, 269
    precipitating factors, 269
    prevalence rate, 268–269
    signs and symptoms, 269, 269t

Diabetic retinopathy, 267
Diarrhea, 220
DIC (disseminated intravascular
  coagulation), 124
Digital examination, 117
Dilantin, 92
Disseminated intravascular coagula-
  tion (DIC), 124
Dizygotic twins, 97–98, 101
Dominant breast mass, 445, 452–453
Down syndrome, 87, 88–89
Duodenal atresia, 92
Duplex ultrasound flow study, 155
Dysmenorrhea, 363
Dyspareunia, 363
Dyspnea in pregnancy, 156f

E
Eclampsia, 167, 169, 173. *See also*
  Preeclampsia
Ectopic pregnancy, 405
  analysis, 416
  clinical approach, 417
  clinical pearls, 422
  definitions, 417
  differential diagnosis of, 418t
  rare types of, 420
  risk factors for, 417t
  treatment, 418–419
Ectopic pregnancy
  abdominal pain, 139
  differential diagnosis, 137t
EDD (estimated date of delivery), 4
Efavirenz, 211
EGA (estimated gestational age), 4
Elderly abuse, 308, 311–312
Endometrial cancer, 533. *See also*
  polycystic ovarian syndrome
  (PCOS)
  clinical pearls, 537
  diagnosis and sampling, 536
  risk factors for, 532, 532t

staging procedure for, 533t
treatment, 536
type I and II, 532–533
Endometrial polyps, 531, 533
Endometrial sampling (biopsy), 531, 531f
Endometrial stripe, 532
Endometriosis (peritoneal factor), 520, 523
Endomyometritis, postpartum. *See* postpartum endomyometritis
Endotoxin, 236
Engagement, 69
Enterocele, 327
Ephedrine, 38, 69
Epidural anesthesia, 73
Epithelial ovarian tumor, 551–553, 553t
Epstein Barr virus (EBV) infection, 379
Erb palsy, 62, 63
Ergot alkaloids, 77, 82
Estimated date of delivery (EDD), 4
Estimated gestational age (EGA), 4
Evisceration, 335
Excisional biopsy, 445, 453

F

Famciclovir, 107
Fascial disruption
analysis, 334
clinical approach, 335–336
clinical pearls, 338
definitions, 335
Febrile morbidity, 251
Fecundability, 521
Fecundity, 523
Fetal bradycardia
analysis, 68
clinical approach, 69
clinical pearls, 74
clinical presentation, 68

cord prolapse and, 68–70
definitions, 69
fetal heart rate assessment, 70
steps to take with, 69t
Fetal fibronectin assay, 181
Fetal heart rate (FHR)
accelerations, 23
assessment, 70
baseline, 23
decelerations, 23, 27–29f, 31t
monitoring, 24
patterns, 24
tracings, 30, 34–36f
Fetal hydrops, 199
Fetal macrosomia, 62, 63
Fetal scalp electrode, 73
Fetal testing, 147
test for fetal health, 148, 149t
Fetal-to-maternal hemorrhage, 122
Fetomaternal hemorrhage, 121
FHR. *See* Fetal heart rate (FHR)
Fibroadenoma of the breast
analysis, 444
clinical approach, 445–446
clinical pearls, 448
definitions, 445
Fifth disease, 199, 200f
Fine-needle aspiration, 445
Firm contracted uterus, 78
First-trimester screening, 87
Fitz-Hugh–Curtis, 351
Folate deficiency, 47
Follicle-stimulating hormone (FSH), 490, 505–509, 522, 527
Footling breech presentation, 70f
Forceps-assisted deliveries, 63
Forendometriosis-associated infertility, 523
Free thyroxine (T_4), 219
Functional ovarian cyst, 551
Fundally implanted placenta, 56
Fundal pressure, 63

G

Galactocele, 257
Galactorrhea
  analysis, 474
  clinical approach, 475–476
  clinical pearls, 479
  definitions, 475
  diagnostic approach, 475
  due to hypothyroidism, 474–476
Gardasil vaccine, 542
Genetic counseling, 92, 280
Genital herpes. *See* Herpes simplex virus (HSV)
Genital tract lacerations, 78, 81
Genuine stress incontinence, 342
Germ cell ovarian tumor, 551, 551*t*
Gestational diabetes, 264, 265
  clinical approach, 266
  controversies, 271
  diagnosis, 270–271, 270*t*
    IADPSG diagnostic strategy, 270–271
    traditional diagnostic strategy, 270
  postpartum management, 271
  risk factors, 271
  treatment, 271
Gestational diabetes, 60, 62, 64, 92, 124
Gestational hypertension, 167, 168
Glucose-6-phosphate dehydrogenase deficiency (G6PD), 43, 44
GnRH-agonist therapy, 507, 509
Gonadal dysgenesis, 516. *See also* Turner syndrome
  analysis, 504
  clinical approach, 505–507
  definitions, 505
Gonadectomy, 513–514
Gonorrhea
  Chlamydia and, 209
  clinical approach, 209

G6PD (glucose-6-phosphate dehydrogenase deficiency), 43, 44
G3P0020 type 1 insulin-requiring diabetes, 264
Granuloma inguinale (GI), 382
Granulosa cell tumor, 500
Graves disease, 219, 474
Gravidity, in patient history, 3
Group A streptococcal toxic shock syndrome, 245
Gynecologic history, 4

H

Haemophilus ducreyi, 109
Hair growth, 497
Hair length, 497
Halothane, 54
HBsAg (hepatitis B surface antigen), 8
HCG. *See* Human chorionic gonadotropin (hCG)
HCG threshold, 405
Head and neck examination, 5
Health maintenance
  analysis, 290
  in older women, 291
    annual pelvic examinations, 292
    bimanual examination, 292
    clinical approach, 291–292
    clinical pearls, 295
Heart rate. *See* Fetal heart rate (FHR)
Helical computed tomography pulmonary angiogram, 155
HELLP syndrome (hemolysis elevated liver enzymes low platelets), 45, 48, 167
Hemoglobin electrophoresis, 43
Hemoglobinopathies, 43–44
Hemolysis, 48, 49
Hemolysis elevated liver enzymes low platelets (HELLP syndrome), 45, 48, 167

Hemolytic anemia, 43.
    See also Anemia
Hemorrhage. See Postpartum
    hemorrhage (PPH)
Hepatitis B surface antigen (HBsAg),
    8
Hepatitis testing, 211
Herpes gestationis, 147–148
Herpes simplex virus (HSV),
    379–380
  categories of, 106t
  gold standard diagnostic test, 380
  in pregnancy
    analysis, 104
    clinical approach, 105–107
    clinical presentation, 103–104
    controversies, 107
    definitions, 104–105
    depiction of, 105f
  prodromal symptoms, 104
  subtypes of, 106–107
  treatment, 380
Herpes zoster infection, 108
High-grade squamous intraepithelial
    lesion (HSIL), 543
Hirsutism, 491, 500
  analysis, 496
  appearance and cosmetic changes
    associated with, 497
  clinical approach, 497
  clinical pearls, 501
  definitions, 497
  differential diagnosis, 498t
  physical examination and laboratory
    tests, 498
  severity of symptoms, 497
History, patient, 3–5
HIV infections, 210–211
Hot flushes (flashes), 299
  treatment, 298–299
Human chorionic gonadotropin
    (hCG), 88, 405

Human immunodeficiency virus
    (HIV)
  screening test for obstetric patients,
    8
Human papillomavirus (HPV), 541
  vaccine, 541
Hydramnios, 199, 200, 200t
Hydronephrosis, 319
Hydrops fetalis, 200
21-hydroxylase deficiency, 498, 500.
    See also congenital adrenal
    hyperplasia (CAH)
17-hydroxyprogesterone, 491, 498
Hyperandrogenic anovulation,
    491
Hyperglycemia and adverse pregnancy
    outcome (HAPO) trial, 271
Hypergonadotropic hypogonadism,
    505–506
Hyperparathyroidism, 220–221
Hyperprolactinemia, 476, 498
  causes of, 475t
  diagnostic approach, 475
Hypertension, 220. See also
    Preeclampsia
  acute management of severe, 170
Hypertensive disorders, 267
Hyperthermia, 220
Hypogonadotropic hypogonadism,
    506
Hypothyroidism, 220, 222
Hysterectomy, 396, 543, 554
  postpartum hemorrhage, 81
Hysterosalpingogram, 10, 467, 514,
    522
Hysteroscopy, 18, 467, 469, 533,
    536

I
Immature (malignant) teratomas, 552
Incest, 308
Incontinence. See urinary incontinence

Infectious vulvar ulcers. *See also* Syphilis; Syphilitic chancre
  clinical approach, 379–382
  clinical pearls, 384
  definitions, 379
Infertility, 500
  abnormalities in the semen (male factor), 523
  analysis, 520
  approach to, 521*t*
  clinical approach, 521–525
  clinical pearls, 527
  definitions, 520–521
  ovulatory disorders (ovulatory factor), 521–522
  peritoneal factor (endometriosis), 523
  primary, 521
  secondary, 521
  tubal factor, 522
  uterine problems, 522
Inflammatory breast cancer, 453
Infrequent etiology, 525
Injectable contraceptive, 430
Intimate partner violence, 307, 313
Intra-amniotic infection, 190
  during postpartum, 251
Intracytoplasmic spermatic injection (ICSI), 524
Intrahepatic cholestasis of pregnancy (ICP), 146, 147
  diagnosis, 147
  risk of fetal demise and adverse fetal outcomes, 147
  treatment, 147
Intramural fibroid, 395
Intramuscular (IM) antenatal steroids, 180
Intrauterine adhesions (IUA), 467, 483. *See also* amenorrhea (intrauterine adhesions)
Intrauterine contraceptive device, 425, 430–431
  levonorgestrel-releasing intrauterine device (LNG-IUD), 424–425, 431
Intrauterine growth restriction (IUGR), 201–202
  analysis, 226–227
  antenatal corticosteroid therapy, 230
  asymmetric, 227–228
  clinical approach, 228–230
  clinical pearls, 233
  definitions, 227–228
  diagnosis, 229–230
  Doppler flow measurements, 227–228, 230
  etiology, 229
  evaluation, 229*t*
  fetal factors, 229
  guidelines for timing of delivery, 231*t*
  management, 230
  maternal factors, 229
  morbidity and mortality in, 228
  neonatal morbidities associated with, 228
  risk factors, 227*t*, 229
  symmetric, 227–228
  treatment, 230
  uterine/placental factors, 229
Intrauterine infections, 202*t*
Intravenous pyelogram, 10, 319, 320*f*–321*f*
Intravenous zidovudine (ZDV), 211, 214
Inverted uterus. *See* Uterine inversion
In vitro fertilization (IVF), 521, 523–524*f*
Iron deficiency anemia, 43, 48
Isoimmunization, 92, 280
Isosexual (no virilization) precocious puberty, 500

K

Kallmann syndrome, 506, 516
Karyotype, 500
   45,XO, 508, 516
   46,XX, 514, 516
Kegel exercises, 340
Kleihauer–Betke test, 122

L

Labor
   abnormal, 23–24
   active phase, 23
   defined, 23
   latent phase, 22–24
   management, algorithm for, 25f
   normal, 23–24, 23t, 37
Laboratory assessment, 8–9
Laparoscopy, robotics vs., 18
Laser ablation, 99, 101
Last menstrual period (LMP), 4, 86
Latency period, 191
Latent phase, labor, 22–24. See also Labor
   defined, 23
Late-onset adrenal hyperplasia, 498
Late postpartum endometritis, 213
Late postpartum hemorrhage, 82
Late preterm gestation, 181
Leak point pressure, 342
Leiomyomata, 395
Leiomyosarcoma, 395
Leukemia, 48
Levator ani, 327
Levonorgestrel-releasing intrauterine device (LNG-IUD), 424–425, 431
Lichen sclerosis (LS)
   analysis, 560
   clinical approach, 561–562
   clinical pearls, 564
   definitions, 561
   differential diagnosis, 561
   treatment, 561

LMP (last menstrual period), 4, 86
Long chain 3-hydroxyacyl-coenzyme A dehydrogenase (LCHAD) deficiency, 148
Lower genital tract, 351
   infections, 351–353, 352f
Low-lying placenta, 113f, 114
Luteinizing hormone (LH), 507, 522
Lymphogranuloma venereum (LGV), 382
Lynch syndrome, 533

M

Macrocytic anemia, 44, 47
Magnesium sulfate, 54, 57
Magnetic resonance angiography, 155
Magnetic resonance imaging (MRI), 10, 454
Mammography, 454
Marginal placenta previa, 113f, 114
Marital rape, 308
Maternal mortality, 158–159
   etiology, 159
Maternal oxygenation, 69
Maternal serum α-fetoprotein (msAFP)
   defined, 87
   elevated/low, causes of, 88t
   serum screening, 86
   twin gestation, 99
McBurney point, 138
McCune-Albright syndrome, 507
McRoberts maneuver, 60, 61f, 62, 64, 65
   defined, 61
Mean arterial pressure (MAP), 245
Medications, in patient history, 5
Megaloblastic anemia, 48
Menopause
   clinical pearls, 304
   definitions, 299
Menstrual history, 4
Meperidine, 73

Metformin, 492
Methergine (methylergonovine maleate), 77
Methylergonovine maleate (Methergine), 77
Microcephaly, 202
Microcytic anemia, 47
Middle cerebral artery (MCA) Doppler examination, 201
Midurethral sling procedures, 341
Milk-retention cyst. *See* galactocele
Misoprostol, 72, 77, 82
Missed or incomplete abortion, 407
Modified biophysical profile, 149*t*
Molar pregnancy, 408–409
Monozygotic twins, 97–98, 98*t*, 101
Montevideo units, 24, 26*f*
Mucinous tumors, 552
Mucopurulent cervicitis, 351
Müllerian abnormality, 516
Müllerian (or vaginal) agenesis
  analysis, 512
  vs. androgen insensitivity, 513*t*
  clinical approach, 513–514
  clinical pearls, 516
  definitions, 513
  diagnosis, 514
Myocardial infarction, 430
Myomectomy, 132, 396

N

Necrotizing fasciitis
  analysis, 244
  antibiotic therapy, 245
  clinical approach, 245
  clinical pearls, 247
  definitions, 245
Neonatal herpes infection, 104–105, 106
Nephrolithiasis, 389
Neural tube defect, 87
Neurologic examination, 8

Nexplanon, 424
Nitrofurantoin, 44, 47
Nonstress test (NST), 149*t*
Nontreponemal tests, 379
Nuchal translucency, 87, 89
Nucleic acid amplification testing (NAAT), 390

O

Obstetric history, 5
OCP. *See* Oral contraceptive (OCP)
Oligohydramnios, 92, 204
Open neural tube defect, 87
Operative hysteroscopy, 469
Operative vaginal delivery, 63
Oral contraceptive (OCP), 430, 492, 500
  and twinning, 97
Osteoporosis, 508
Ovarian cancer (epithelial), 553
  analysis, 550
  clinical approach, 551–555
  clinical pearls, 557
  definitions, 551
Ovarian cystectomy, 136
Ovarian neoplasm, 551
Ovarian teratomas, 552
Ovarian torsion, 136, 137*t*, 138
Overflow incontinence, 342–344
Ovulatory disorders (ovulatory factor), 521–522
Ovulatory dysfunction, 500
Oxytocin, 24, 37, 54, 57, 73, 79

P

Pancytopenia, 48
Papanicolaou smear test, 542
Pap smears, 8, 9*f*, 536, 540, 543
  abnormal, 541
Paravaginal defect, 327
Parity, in patient history, 3
Parvovirus infection in pregnancy
  clinical approach, 199–202

clinical pearls, 205
definitions, 199
diagnosis, 199–200
pregnant patient exposed to parvovirus B13, 199, 199t
Past medical history, 5
Past surgical history, 5
Patient, approach to
history, 3–5
physical examination, 5–10
PCR (polymerase chain reaction), 105
Pedunculated fibroid, 395
Pelvic diaphragm, 327
Pelvic examination, 6
Pelvic inflammatory disease (PID), 351
criteria for hospitalization, 354t
Pelvic kidney, 516
Pelvic organ prolapse (POP)
analysis, 326–327
clinical approach, 327–329
clinical pearls, 331
definitions, 327
Percreta, 131
Percutaneous nephrostomy, 319
Perfect use effectiveness, 425
Perimenopause. *See also* health maintenance
analysis, 298–299
clinical approach, 299–300
clinical pearls, 304
definitions, 299
short-term hormone-replacement therapy, 300
Peritoneal factor (endometriosis), 520, 523
Pessaries, 340, 342
Pessary devices, 329f
Physical examination, 5–10
Pituitary secreting adenoma, 475
Placenta
abnormally retained, 53
bilobed, 97

low-lying, 113f, 114
polyps, 132
separation, 52, 53
succenturiate-lobed, 97
Placenta accreta
analysis, 128
bleeding, 114
clinical approach, 129–130
clinical pearls, 132
clinical presentation, 127–128
definitions, 128
PPH in, 78
risk factors for, 129t
uterine inversion, 54
Placenta increta, 128
Placental abruption. *See* Abruptio placentae
Placenta percreta, 128
Placenta previa
analysis, 112
clinical approach, 114–115
clinical pearls, 117
clinical presentation, 111–112
complete, 113f
definitions, 113–114
management, 116
marginal, 113f, 114
risk factors for, 114t
Plan B one-step, 425, 431
Plan B (progestin only), 425, 431
POC (products of conception), 79, 81
Point of maximal impulse, 6
Polycystic ovarian syndrome (PCOS), 483, 496, 500, 532
analysis, 490
clinical approach, 491–492
clinical pearls, 494
definitions, 491
diagnostic criteria, 491–492
treatment, 492
Polyhydramnios, 116, 199, 204
Polymerase chain reaction (PCR), 105
Polyps, placental, 132

Postcoital spotting, 116
Posterior reversible encephalopathy syndrome (PRES), 167
Postmenopausal vaginal bleeding
  analysis, 530
  clinical approach, 532–534
  clinical pearls, 537
  definitions, 531–532
Postoperative fever, 321, 322t
Postpartum, with breast pain and fever, 256
Postpartum amenorrhea
  cinical approach, 483–484
  definitions, 483
Postpartum endomyometritis
  analysis, 250
  antibiotic therapy, 251
  clinical approach, 251–252
  definitions, 251
  risk factors for, 250
Postpartum fever, approach to, 252t
Postpartum hemorrhage (PPH), 121, 483
  analysis, 76
  causes of, 14
  clinical approach, 77–79
  clinical pearls, 82
  clinical presentation, 76
  definitions, 77
  secondary, 78
  treatment for, 78t
Postpartum mastitis, 256–257
Postpartum thyroiditis, 220
Posttraumatic stress disorder, 308
PPH. See Postpartum hemorrhage (PPH)
PPROM. See Preterm premature rupture of membranes (PPROM)
Precocious puberty, 507
Preeclampsia
  analysis, 166–167
  clinical approach, 168–173
  clinical evaluation, 169–170
  clinical pearls, 178
  definitions, 167–168
  diagnosis, 168t, 170
  management, 170–173
  pathophysiology, 169
  risk factors, 169
  severe features, 168, 169t
  superimposed, 168
  symptoms, 5
Preeclampsia-pulmonary edema, 238
Pregestational diabetes, 264, 265
  clinical approach, 266
  fetal risks, 267
  glycemic control for, 268
  management, 268–270
  maternal risks, 267
  monitoring, 268
  preconception counseling, 268
Pregnancy
  abdominal pain in. See Abdominal pain, in pregnancy
  algorithm for management of hypertension in, 172f
  anemia in. See Anemia, in pregnancy
  dyspnea in, 156f
  herpes simplex virus in. See Herpes simplex virus (HSV), in pregnancy
  management of hypertension in, 171t
  normal arterial blood gas changes in, 157t
  parvovirus infection in, 198–202, 205
  physiological changes in, 279t, 281
  physiology of, 43
  pruritus in. See Pruritus, in pregnancy
  pulmonary embolus in, 154–159, 162

serum screening. *See* Serum
   screening, in pregnancy
thyroid storm, 218–221, 223
thyrotoxicosis in, 218–221, 223
Premature ovarian failure, 299
Premature rupture of membranes, 191
Prenatal care, 278–284
   analysis, 279–280
   clinical approach, 281
   clinical pearls, 288
   definitions, 280
   screening for conditions of risk, 281
   summary of prenatal laboratories,
      ramifications, and evaluation,
      282*t*–283*t*
Prenatal genetic tests, 88*t*
Preterm labor
   analysis, 180–181
   clinical approach, 182–184
   clinical pearls, 186
   common tocolytic agents, 183*t*
   definitions, 181
   risk factors for, 182*t*
   symptoms, 182
   treatment, 182
   work-up for, 183*t*
Preterm labor with tocolytic agent,
   238
Preterm premature rupture of
      membranes (PPROM), 190
   algorithm for the management of,
      193*f*
   analysis, 190
   clinical approach, 191–192
   clinical evaluation, 191
   clinical pearls, 196
   controversies in, 192
   definitions, 191
   etiologies, 191
   outcome, 192
   placental abruption, 125
   risk factors, 191*t*
   treatment, 192

Primary amenorrhea, 467, 508
   analysis, 512
   clinical approach, 513–514
   definitions, 513
Primary infertility, 521
Primary prevention, 291
Primary syphilis, 378
Procidentia, 328
Products of conception (POC), 79,
   81, 438
Profuse hemorrhage, 54
Progesterone, during gestation,
   139
Prolactin, 491
Prostaglandin F_2-alpha, 77
Pruritic urticarial papules and plaques
      of pregnancy (PUPPP),
      147
   lesions of, 148
Pruritus, in pregnancy
   analysis, 146
   clinical approach, 147–148
   clinical pearls, 152
   definitions, 147
Pseudogestational sac, 418
Pubertal delay
   analysis, 504
   clinical approach, 505–507
   clinical pearls, 509
   definitions, 505
   diagnostic approach to,
      506
Pubococcygeus, 327
Puborectalis, 327
Pulmonary edema, 101, 182
Pulmonary embolism, 238
Pulmonary embolus in pregnancy
   analysis, 154–155
   clinical approach, 155–158
   clinical pearls, 162
   definitions, 155
Pulmonary examination, 6
Pulse oximetry, 155–156

Pyelonephritis, 236, 238, 390
  in pregnancy
    analysis, 236
    antibiotic therapy, 237
    clinical approach, 237–238
    clinical pearls, 241
    definitions, 236–237
    prevention, 237–238
    treatment, 237
  urinary tract infection, 12

R
Radical brachytherapy, 541
Radical hysterectomy, 541
Radical teletherapy, 541
Rape-trauma syndrome, 311
Reading, clinical problem-oriented approach to, 13–18
Rectal examination, 7
Rectocele, 327, 328f
Renal damage, 267
Reproductive aging, 301t
Retropubic colposuspension (Burch procedure), 341
Reverse end-diastolic flow, 228
Review of systems, 5
Risk factors, 16
Robotics, laparoscopy $vs.$, 18
Rubella titer, 8
Ruptured corpus luteum, 137t, 139

S
Sacrospinous ligament fixation procedure, 329
Saline infusion sonohysterography (SIS), 468, 533
Salpingitis, 16
  analysis, 350
  clinical approach, 351–354
  definitions, 351
  placenta previa, 116
  signs and symptoms, 353t
Salpingo-oophorectomy, 552

Salpingostomy, 419, 419f
Screening tests, 291
  breast cancer, 453–454, 455t
  cervical cytology screening, 291t
  in HIV-positive women, 292
Secondary amenorrhea, 467
  etiologies, 469t
Secondary infertility, 521
Secondary postpartum hemorrhage, 78–79
Secondary prevention, 291
Secondary syphilis, 380
Sentinel node biopsy, 453
Septic abortion
  analysis, 438
  antibiotic therapy, 439
  clinical approach, 439–440
  clinical pearls, 442
  definitions, 439
  signs and symptoms, 439
  treatment, 438, 439–440
Septic pelvic thrombophlebitis (SPT), 251, 252
Septic shock, 245, 439
Serologic tests, 379
Serosanguineous, 335
Sertoli-Leydig cell tumor, 496, 498, 500, 553
  analysis, 496
Serum screening, in pregnancy
  analysis, 86
  clinical approach, 87–90
  clinical pearls, 93
  clinical presentation, 86
  definitions, 87
Sex cord-stromal tumors, 551, 553–554, 553t
Sex hair, 497
Sex hormone-binding globulin (SHBG), 497–498
Sexual assault
  analysis, 306–307

antibiotic therapy for sexually transmitted infections, 310
clinical approach, 308–313
clinical pearls, 315
definition, 307
examination of a sexual assault victim, 309f
life-threatening injuries, 308–310
post-exposure prophylaxis, 310–311, 311t
risk for, 308
risk of pregnancy after, 310
Sexual coercion, 308
Sexually transmitted diseases, 4
Shock, 245
Shoulder dystocia
analysis, 60
clinical approach, 62–63
clinical pearls, 65
clinical presentation, 60
definitions, 61–62
treatment of, maneuvers for, 62t
Sickle cell disease, 44, 47, 49
Simple cystitis, 389
Sinusoidal heart rate pattern, 199, 201
Skin dimpling, 453
Sonography, 124
Sonohysterography, 10
Speculum examination, 6, 117
Spermicides, 430
Spironolactone, 500
Spontaneous abortion, 407
classification of, 409t
symptoms, 407
treatment, 407
Spotting, postcoital, 116
Station, defined, 37
Statutory rape, 307
Stereotactic core needle biopsy, 454, 462
Steroid hormone contraception, 425
Streak ovaries, 508
Strokes, 430

Struma ovarii, 551–552
Subacute pelvic pain, 363
Subdermal implant, 430
Submucosal fibroid, 395
Subserosal fibroid, 395
Suburethral slings, 340
Succenturiate-lobed placenta, 97
Superimposed preeclampsia, 169
Suppressive antiviral therapy, 107
Suprapubic pressure, 61, 61f, 62, 65
Surgery, approach to, 18
Surgical history, 5
Surgical site infection (SSI), 335
Symmetric IUGR, 227–228
Syphilis
analysis, 378
chancres, 380
clinical presentation, 109
genital condylomalata of secondary, 381f
latency of varying duration, 380
primary, 380
secondary, 380
test, 8
treatment, 378, 381t

T

Tachysystole, 37
Tension-free vaginal tape (TVT), 341–342
Teratogens, 87, 90
select listing of, 90t
Teratomas, 552
Terbutaline, 37, 54, 57, 69, 73
Testicular feminization, 513
Testosterone, 491
Tetracycline effect, 209
Thalassemia, 43–45
classification of, 43–44
defined, 43
Thionamide antithyroid medications, 219

Third stage of labor
  active management, 52, 55t
  controversy on, 54–55, 55t
  defined, 53
  physiologic management, 52, 55t
Threatened abortion
  algorithm for management of, 408f
  analysis, 404–405
  in asymptomatic women, 406
  clinical approach, 406–409
  clinical pearls, 412
  definitions, 405–406
  differential diagnosis, 408
Three Ps (powers, passenger, and pelvis), 23
Thrombocytopenia, 48
Thrombocytopenic purpura, 202
Thyroid-stimulating hormone (TSH), 219, 222, 490–491
Thyroid storm
  clinical approach, 219–221
  clinical pearls, 223
  complications, 220
Timed prenatal tests, 9
TOA (tubo-ovarian abscesses), 16
Tobacco cessation, 291–292
Tocolysis, 101, 181–182
Toxoplasmosis, 201
Transobturator tape (TOT) procedure, 342
Transvaginal tape procedure, 341
Trendelenburg position, 68
Trichomonas vaginalis, 371–372. *See also* Vaginal infections
Triple assessment, 446
Triple test, 452
Trisomy (triple) screen, 87
Trophotropism, 130
TTT (twin-twin transfusion) syndrome, 97, 99, 101
Tubo-ovarian abscesses (TOA), 16, 351
Turner syndrome, 504–506, 509, 516. *See also* Gonadal dysgenesis
Turtle sign, 60

Twin gestation
  analysis, 96
  clinical approach, 97–100, 98f, 99f
  clinical pearls, 102
  definitions, 97
  with vasa previa, 96
Twin–twin transfusion (TTT) syndrome, 97, 99, 101
Type 1 diabetes, 265
Type 2 diabetes, 266
Type I endometrial cancer, 532
Type II endometrial cancer, 532
Typical use effectiveness, 425

U
Ulipristal (ella), 425
Ultrasonography, 454
  overview, 9–10
  placenta previa, 117
Ultrasound-guided core needle biopsy, 454, 462
Umbilical cord prolapse. *See* Cord prolapse
Umbilical Doppler velocity, 149t
Unconjugated estriol, 88
Upper genital tract, 351
  infections, 353–354
Ureteral injuries after hysterectomy
  analysis, 318
  clinical approach, 319–322
    at cardinal ligament, 319
    prevention of complications, 321
    types, 319–320
  clinical pearls, 324
  definitions, 319
Urethral syndrome, 389
Urethritis, 389, 390
Urge incontinence, 342–343
Urinalysis, 8
Urinary incontinence
  analysis, 340–341
  clinical pearls, 348
  definitions, 341–342
  differential diagnosis of, 345t

evaluation of, 344
mechanisms of incontinence, 342–343
Urinary tract infection
  analysis, 388
  clinical approach, 389–390
  clinical pearls, 392
  common form of, 389
  definitions, 389
  treatment, 389
Uterine artery embolization, 397
Uterine atony, 14, 77, 79, 81, 121
  risk factors for, 77t
Uterine contraction, 22, 24
Uterine hyperstimulation, 72
Uterine inversion, 53f, 78
  analysis, 52
  clinical approach, 54
  clinical pearls, 58
  clinical presentation, 52
  definitions, 52–53
  treatment, 54
Uterine leiomyomata, 395f
  analysis, 394
  clinical approach, 396–397
  clinical pearls, 400
  definitions, 395
  physical examination of, 396
  treatment, 396
Uterine relaxing agent, 57
Uterine rupture, 72
Uterine septum, 514
Uterine sounding, 468
Uterine suction curettage, 406–407, 409, 439

V

Vacuum deliveries, 63
Vaginal diaphragm, 426
Vaginal epithelial "clue cells," 372f
Vaginal epithelium, 370
Vaginal infections. See also bacterial vaginosis
  characteristics of various, 371t
  clinical approach, 371–373
  clinical pearls, 375
  definitions, 370–371
Vaginitis, 532
Valacyclovir, 107
Vasa previa, 96, 97, 100
  defined, 114
Velamentous cord insertion, 97
Venous thromboembolism, 430
Ventilation-perfusion scan imaging procedure, 155
Vertical transmission, 280
Virilism, 497
Virilization, 497
Vital signs, 5
Vomiting, 220
VTE prophylaxis, 322t
Vulva, 561
Vulvar cancer, 562
Vulvar disorders
  Bartholin gland abscess, 109
  carcinoma, 109
  definitions, 561

W

White classification, 266–267
Wood's corkscrew, 62
Wound complications
  antibiotic prophylaxis for, 335–336
  clinical approach, 335–336
  clinical pearls, 338
  definition, 335
  prevention of, 335–336
Wound dehiscence, 335

Y

Yuzpe regimen, 425

Z

Zavanelli maneuver, 62
"0" station, 37